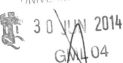
The loan period may be shortened if the item is requested.

Functional Brain Imaging

Functional Brain Imaging

William W. Orrison, Jr., M.D.
Chief, Division of Neuroradiology
Veterans Affairs Medical Center
Professor of Radiology
Associate Professor of Neurology
The University of New Mexico School of Medicine
Albuquerque, New Mexico

Jeffrey David Lewine, Ph.D.
Scientific Director, MSI
Veterans Affairs Medical Center
Research Assistant Professor of Radiology and Psychology
The University of New Mexico School of Medicine
Albuquerque, New Mexico

John A. Sanders, Ph.D.
Scientific Director, MRI
Veterans Affairs Medical Center
Research Assistant Professor of Radiology
The University of New Mexico School of Medicine
Albuquerque, New Mexico

Michael F. Hartshorne, M.D.
Chief, Joint Imaging Service
Veterans Affairs Medical Center
Professor of Radiology
The University of New Mexico School of Medicine
Albuquerque, New Mexico

with 874 illustrations

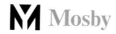

St. Louis Baltimore Boston Carlsbad Chicago Naples New York Philadelphia Portland
London Madrid Mexico City Singapore Sydney Tokyo Toronto Wiesbaden

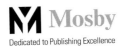
Mosby

Dedicated to Publishing Excellence

A Times Mirror
Company

Executive Editor: Susan M. Gay
Developmental Editor: Sandra Clark Brown
Project Managers: Peggy Fagen, Carol Weis
Manufacturing Supervisor: Kathy Grone
Book Designer: Staff Design

Printed in the United States of America
Composition by Graphic World, Inc.
Printing/Binding by Maple Vail, York

Mosby–Year Book, Inc.
11830 Westline Industrial Drive
St. Louis, MO 63146

International Standard Book Number 0-8151-6509-9

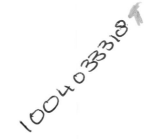

95 96 97 98 99 / 9 8 7 6 5 4 3 2 1

TO

Mary Espinosa, R.N.

With gentle, guiding touch from one hand and a firm push
from the other, Mary got us to finish this book.
It is as much a product of her skill, expertise, and finesse as it is ours.
We will be forever in her debt.

Preface

At the end of the eighteenth century, Franz Joseph Gall postulated that the various sensory, motor, and cognitive faculties of man arose from different organs and centers of the brain. These centers, although independent, were believed to interact in the expression of complex human behaviors. Unfortunately, Gall also argued that, because the skull is modified by the shape and size of the brain, measurement of the bumps of the skull allowed one to deduce the moral and intellectual characteristics of individuals. Few today believe that palpation of the skull can allow one to distinguish between the criminal and the average citizen, but the basic concept of Gall's phrenology of the mind—the view that different mental abilities arise from the interactions between functionally distinct brain processing modules—remains prevalent in modern neuroscientific thought.

Indeed, it is almost embarrassing how closely most modern-day attempts to image the neuronal correlates of language and memory, and even such conditions as anxiety and depression, resemble the phrenology of the nineteenth century. We have traded in our $5 calipers for measuring skull size for million dollar high-tech machines (such as CAT, MRI, and PET scanners) that measure the anatomy, biochemistry, and physiology of brain regions. Yet, through these non-invasive neuroimaging tools that measure the brain directly, we have entered into an unprecedented time of discovery of the workings of the human mind.

Previous books of this type have focused on only a subset of available neuroimaging methods (e.g., electrophysiologic techniques or metabolic techniques), whereas this text explores all of the dominant clinical neuroimaging methods, with the goal of providing an integrated view of brain structure, chemistry, and physiology. More so than any other set of methodologies, neuroimaging techniques have brought the neurosciences to the clinical forefront and the public mind. Indeed, the new possibilities afforded by non-invasive neuroimaging methods provided the driving force for the Congressional declaration of the 1990s as the decade of the brain. Progress in the field is very rapid, and new exciting developments not cited here will have undoubtedly occurred after the publication of this text. Despite this unavoidable limitation, it is hoped that when readers finish this text, they will be inspired by the potential of brain imaging techniques for unraveling the mysteries of the human psyche and brain.

This text is intended as an introductory overview to this exciting and emerging field. Readers will no doubt be from various backgrounds and fields of endeavor, both within and outside the neurosciences, so we have attempted to integrate basic biophysical, neuroscientific, and clinical information into our discussion of each imaging technique. As a consequence, there is some minor repetition of concepts between chapters, but each is intended to provide new insights into neuroimaging. We have attempted to provide an even balance of technical and clinical information in each chapter, although some are more heavily biased one way or the other. It should be noted that cognitive neuroscience has benefitted tremendously from the development of brain imaging techniques, but our discussions of these developments have been truncated in favor of clinical information. Neuroimaging techniques have opened a new doorway into both the normal and the diseased brain, and the curious reader need merely step through via this text.

We wish to acknowledge the many individuals who

have contributed to the completion of this text, most notably Mary Espinosa, R.N., and Donna Skinner, R.N., whose dedicated efforts have actually resulted in a finished product, and Carol Garner, whose tireless efforts produced the exquisite drawings that accompany the written text. We also wish to thank Jonathan Briggs, our department editor, Sheila Mulligan-Webb, our division editor, and staff for their help and support. Special thanks also go to Jim Janis and Sheila Lieuwen for their work on the photography, much of which was completed, because of us, on a rush basis. We also wish to acknowledge the many collaborators who have made this work possible, particularly our colleagues at the Los Alamos National Laboratories, Sandia National Laboratories, and multiple clinical centers throughout the world. Dr. Larry Davis, our Chief of Neurology, has been an integral part of our functional imaging program and the source of not only a great number of our patient referrals but also a wealth of clinical neurologic correlations.

We extend our sincerest appreciation to our dedicated clinical and support staff: Robyn Adams, Robert Astur, Randall Barker, Dorothy Baros, Stacy Conviser, Marc Cottrell, Jerri Cruz, John Davis, Mike Davis, Brian Dorotik, Todd Ellis, Nancy Gotti, Geneva Ham, Brad Jones, Adria Lawson, Kim McGonigle, Herman Mettling, Jeff Meyer, Terry Mills, Joe Monasterio, Kim Paulson, Sherri Provencal, Julie Ptacek, Pedro Quiroga, Sheila Rhodus, Lori Russo, Donna Skinner, Jonathan Stearley, Joanna Stein, Linda Vera, Cipriano Wildenstein, Dan Williamson, Vardaman Wash, and Bill Zoeckler. It is through your hard work and dedication to the well-being of our patients that we are able to provide the information in this book.

William W. Orrison, Jr.
Jeffrey David Lewine
John A. Sanders
Michael F. Hartshorne

Contents

Functional Brain Imaging

1

Introduction to Brain Imaging

William W. Orrison, Jr.

In a sense, it might be said that experimentalists have left clinicians and psychologists stranded upon the vast shores of the cerebral cortex with no chart and no compass to guide them.
WILDER PENFIELD
HERBERT JASPER

Historical Perspectives on Neuroimaging
Clinical Applications
Future Directions

The human adult brain is a gelatinous organ weighing approximately 1400 grams and containing more than 100 billion nerve cells. Nerve cells are more varied than cells in other organ systems, with as many as 10,000 different cell types interconnected by miles of complex fiber tracts.[1] It is most remarkable that this highly developed and integrated system of circuitry can adapt to virtually any situation on the planet and can process information in a broad range of forms with lightening speed. It is not so surprising, then, that our understanding of the human brain remains severely limited. This same organ that we struggle so hard to comprehend can only, in the final analysis, be approached in understanding by that exact same organ itself, the human brain.

Our analysis of the human brain is lacking, but our actual knowledge of the human mind remains virtually beyond comprehension. What is commonly referred to as the "mind" is generally considered to consist of certain functional aspects of the brain. It is not an insignificant advance to go from defining the locations of motor, speech, or memory activities of the brain to the intricacies of the human mind. Imagination, creativity, and fantasy are valued components of the human mind that defy modern technology in its various forms. No matter how well we begin to understand the basic functions that allow us to walk and talk, it is the highest order activities that fascinate us. It is our own "mind power" that drives this desire to know ourselves and in this sense creates a self-propagating process.

It is through elucidating the brain-code that modern neuroscience hopes to be able to unravel the mysteries of the human mind. The brain-code is that mechanism by which the brain so adeptly responds to symphony or sonnet, geometry or astronomy, love or hate, war or peace. Through understanding the

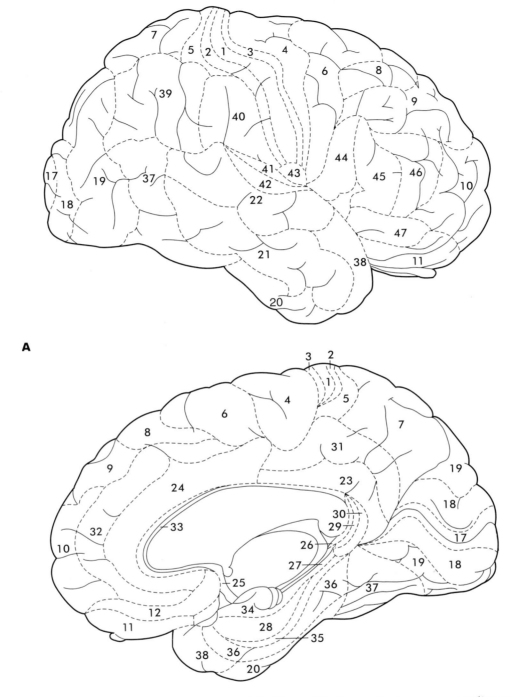

Fig. 1-1. A, Chart of the architectonic subdivisions of the human brain cortex according to Brodmann (1909[2]).

brain-code comes not only advanced knowledge of why we are the way we are but also the hope of a cure for the many dreaded afflictions that attack the human mind.

Disorders of the brain manifest in a variety of manners. From feeling (affect) or thought (cognition) abnormalities to total paralysis, each type of disorder can be seen as a specific form of brain dysfunction that may involve minute areas or massive regions of the brain. Regardless of the etiology of brain pathology, the final common pathway of each of the disorders is disruption of neuronal signals along myriad pathways. Indeed, the central theme in the broad range of normal and abnormal human behaviors is that this activity is a reflection of function or dysfunction of the brain.

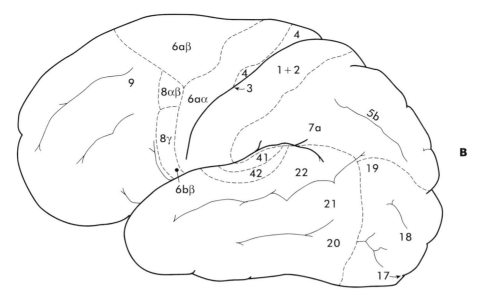

Fig. 1-1, cont'd.   B, Chart of the architectonic subdivisions of the human brain cortex according to Vogt (1926[2]).

The disruption of basic brain physiology can be detected or inferred by a number of methods, including computerized axial tomography (CT), magnetic resonance imaging (MR), positron emission tomography (PET), single photon emission computed tomography (SPECT), electroencephalography (EEG), magnetoencephalography (MEG), and magnetic resonance spectroscopy (MRS). In the past, most imaging methods of the brain have been limited to anatomic references, with little information about the actual function of the brain except that deduced from the clinical examination. The recent advent of a number of methods for actually evaluating the functional activity of the brain has resulted in new clinical applications for some previous methods of brain imaging as well as the arrival of entirely new clinical imaging modalities. However, this newly focused attention on the field of functional analysis of the human brain is not actually "new"; it began well over a century ago.

As early as 1861, Broca suggested that the human brain contained a specialized region for speech. This revolutionary concept of localized regions within the brain for specified functions was soon confirmed by experimentation. Along with physiologic confirmation of the principle of localization of cerebral function came numerous anatomic studies subdividing the cerebral gray matter. Cytologic organization of the brain was one readily available method; it has been referred to as cytoarchitectonics or myeloarchitectonics. The cerebral cortex has been divided into multiple areas using this method of architectonics, and as a result, there is much confusion regarding specific areas of the brain. These methods date from as early as 1903 and were modified or changed for the next quarter of a century. During this time period, over 200 cortical

areas were described, with the most commonly employed method being that of Brodmann. However, many of the described areas contradicted Brodmann, and no specialized function has been assigned to many of these architectonic fields[2] (Fig. 1-1).

Nonetheless, some areas of the brain—the calcarine fissure of the occipital lobe, for example—do subscribe to the architectonic method of analysis. This has led to further confusion regarding the use of such methods. The fact that architectonics has been available for nearly a century and that modern imaging, with its phenomenal detail, has not been significantly affected by these methods leads rapidly to the conclusion that such a detailed analysis of the anatomic variations in the brain are probably unnecessary. At best these methods appear overstated, and they may have resulted in a delay in our understanding of the more readily accessible regions of functional cortex. The suggestion that an understanding of brain function requires a detailed foundation in complex controversial brain maps (created almost a century ago) can be enough to discourage the most avid students in the area of functional analysis of the brain.

Even the well-established, more general terms for brain anatomy (such as frontal, parietal, occipital, or temporal) may be difficult to entirely define with the most modern imaging methods. Determination of the location of an important landmark, such as the central sulcus, may not be accurate even using sophisticated techniques like high-resolution MR.[3] Direct visualization of the cerebral cortex at surgery is also known to be inaccurate regarding brain function; before the advent of functional imaging techniques, the most widely accepted standard for functional localization on the cerebral cortex was direct intraoperative monitoring. This involves either direct electrical stimulation of the brain substance or placement of electrodes directly on the brain during surgery (electrocorticographic monitoring) for detection of the responses to peripheral stimulation.[4,5] Once such a determination is made, function remains variable between subjects and across subjects. For example, when direct human cortical measurements are obtained, 80% of motor responses will be accounted for by precentral gyral stimulation, with the remaining 20% from postcentral gyral stimulation. The reverse has been found for sensory responses, with 25% from the precentral gyrus and 75% from the postcentral gyrus.[2] Therefore, it becomes necessary to view the brain as a more dynamic and redundant system than traditional anatomic delineations would seem to indicate. Concepts such as individual variability in localizations of brain function as well as significant cerebral plasticity must now be considered an integral part of the studies on the functional capabilities of the human brain. Through the availability of modern imaging technologies, we can, for the first time in human history, examine the inner workings of the brain noninvasively.

HISTORICAL PERSPECTIVES ON NEUROIMAGING

Modern neuroimaging may be one of the greatest success stories in medicine. In less than one century remarkable progress and fantastic accomplishments have been achieved in central nervous system diagnosis and evaluation. Advances in neuroradiology, however, derive from extraordinarily humble beginnings.

In February of 1886, Thomas A. Edison accepted a challenge from William Randolph Hearst, publisher of the *New York Journal*, to make a "cathodograph of the human brain." Indeed, Edison did try to demonstrate the penetrating powers of the newly discovered x-ray by attempting to photograph a man's brain. However, within a month, Edison gave up on the project and declared that the experiment was a failure, partly because of the skull was an obstacle.[6] Harvey Cushing, commonly recognized as the father of modern neurosurgery, was the first diagnostician in the United States to use x-rays to evaluate a patient with neurologic disability.[6,7] This examination consisted of an x-ray of the cervical spine containing a bullet fragment. Unfortunately, an average exposure time of 35 minutes and several attempts were required to produce an image.[6,8] The first 25 years of neuroradiology were primarily confined to creating x-rays of the skull. These early radiographic studies of the skull included many important findings, such as "mass effect," which are used routinely in today's sophisticated neurodiagnostic modalities. The value of observing a shift in the calci-

fied pineal gland, as well as many other findings, were described in the early 1900s[6,9,10] (Fig. 1-2).

In 1918, Walter Dandy introduced a dramatic technical breakthrough in neuroradiology in the form of ventriculography and encephalography. Because of the toxic nature of most substances well visualized on x-rays, Dandy used air as a contrast medium for these procedures. Pneumoencephalography was performed by injecting air into the lumbar subarachnoid space, and ventriculography was performed by directly injecting air into the ventricles.[6,11,12] Although this technique revolutionized the practice of neurosurgery and resulted in much more accurate diagnoses of many types of intracranial abnormalities, particularly neoplasms, the technique was not without significant risk and caused severe patient discomfort. The post- pneumoencephalographic headache would frequently require hospitalization and the extensive use of pain relievers for protracted periods. In later years, the technique was frequently employed in conjunction with general anesthesia, required an elaborate "somersaulting" technique on a specialized chair, and continued to have a significant risk of herniation from altered intracranial pressures (Fig. 1-3).

In spite of the enthusiasm for the new diagnostic technique of pneumoencephalography, some radiologists realized that both the danger associated with air injections and the lack of precise diagnoses meant other diagnostic techniques were still needed. Egas Moniz pioneered the early work in cerebral arteriography during the late 1920s, and his technique rapidly became an adjunct to pneumoencephalography for the evaluation of intracranial pathology.[6,13,14] The earliest arteriograms performed required surgical access to the internal carotid artery; subsequently, the feasibility of direct percutaneous carotid artery puncture for cerebral angiography was demonstrated.[14] As early as 1949 the first neuroradiologic functional evaluations of the brain (using arteriography as an imaging guide) were described by Wada. He utilized sodium amytal injections directly into the carotid artery for the lateralization of speech dominance.[15] Then in 1953, Sven Ivar Seldinger reported success with the use of a flexible guide wire and catheter system allowing access to virtually any blood vessel in the body from a femoral artery.[16] By the early 1960s this technique had been combined with the Wada test, and functional evaluations of the brain using this method continue today. Subselective catheterization of distal branches of the middle cerebral artery allow for the evaluation of restricted brain regions using the Wada technique, and this method may also be beneficial in the localization of memory functions.[17] The combination of improved safety of contrast agents and the development of smaller catheters has resulted in cerebral angiography becoming an extremely safe

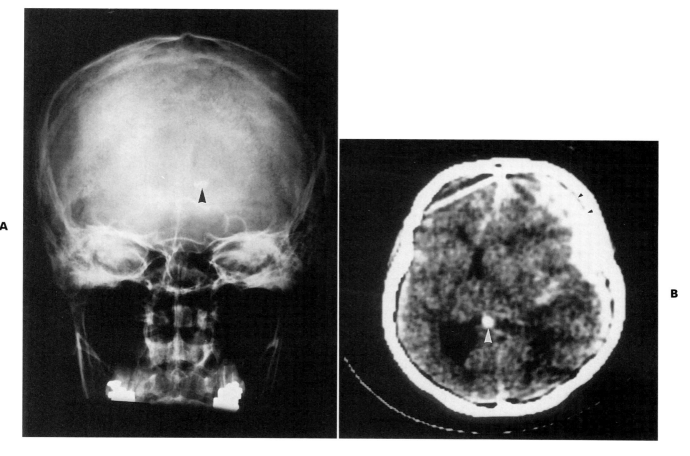

Fig. 1-2. A, AP view of the skull demonstrating shift of the calcified pineal gland *(arrow)* from its normal midline position. This patient had a subdural hematoma, which is shown on the CT scan in **B. B**, Axial CT scan through the level of the calcified pineal gland *(arrow)*, which is shifted away from the subdural hematoma *(double arrows)*. Note the "mass effect" on the underlying brain substance caused by the subdural hematoma.

and effective procedure. Until the availability of CT and magnetic resonance imaging (MR or MRI), angiography was the primary neuroradiologic imaging modality (Fig. 1-4).

In 1974, Charles A. Mistretta described a technique to improve arteriographic image quality and dramatically decrease procedure time.[18] This method of image analysis was the beginning of digital subtraction arteriography and has resulted in the immediate availability of arteriographic images in virtual real time. Immediate access to high-quality arteriographic images heralded the onset of an entirely new era of interventional neuroradiology. Now, catheters and guide wires hardly larger than a human hair can be placed in virtually any part of the brain for direct investigation or therapeutic intervention (Fig. 1-5).

As the developments in x-ray technology and interventional techniques were being made, other neuroimaging methods were also being developed. In 1948, George Moore reported the successful use of an intravenously injected radioactive substance for the detection of brain neoplasms.[6,19] Radionuclide brain scanning rapidly became an important part of neurodiagnostics since this is a minimally invasive procedure with virtually no morbidity (Fig. 1-6). The combination of pneumoencephalography, radionuclide brain scanning, and cerebral arteriography became the primary imaging tools of neurodiagnosticians during the 1950s, 1960s, and early 1970s.

The commercial availability of computerized axial tomography (CT) in the early 1970s heralded remarkable advances in the area of radionuclide brain scanning. The application of the computer reconstruction methods used in CT to nuclear medicine studies resulted in the clinical availability of techniques such as single photon emission computed tomography (SPECT) and positron emission tomography (PET). Although positron imaging was suggested as early as 1951 by Wrenn and colleagues, the first positron scanner was described by Brownell and Sweet in 1953.[20,21] The basic tenets of modern PET scanning were described by Phelps and coworkers in 1975, with

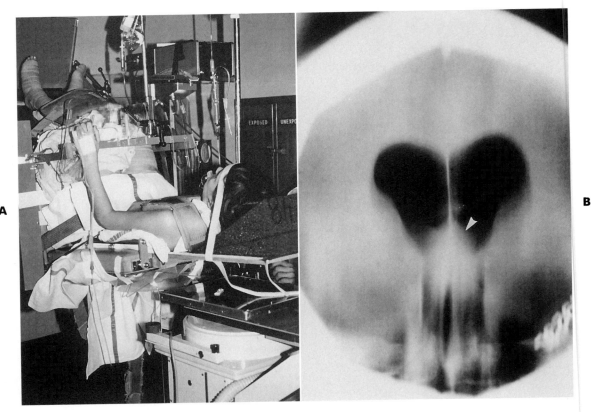

Fig. 1-3. A, Patient undergoing a pneumoencephalogram, circa 1976. The patient is positioned in a specialized chair that can be completely rotated (somersaulted), and the patient is under general anesthesia. **B,** Pneumoencephalogram from the patient examination in **A** demonstrating a mass in the region of the third ventricle *(arrow)*. Note the air-filled lateral ventricles on this AP projection.

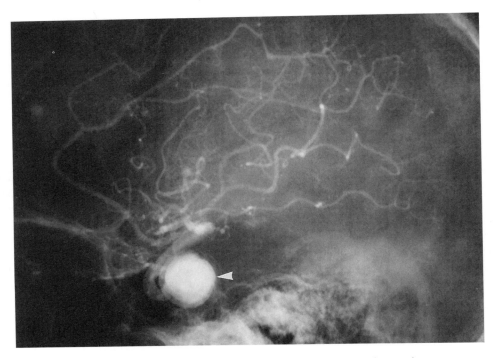

Fig. 1-4. Lateral view from an arteriogram (angiogram) demonstrating a giant aneurysm of the internal carotid artery *(arrow)*.

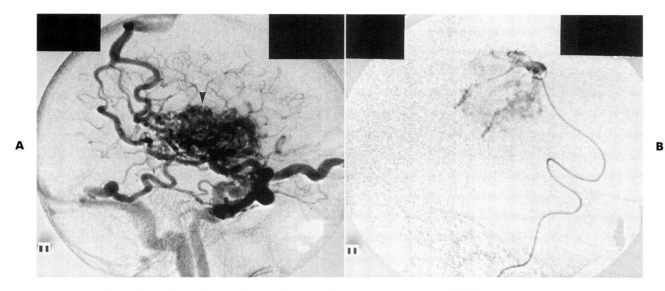

Fig. 1-5. A, Lateral view from a digital subtraction angiogram (DSA) demonstrating an arteriovenous malformation (AVM) *(arrow).* **B,** Digital subtraction angiogram from the same patient evaluation as **A** demonstrating subselective catheterization into the vasculature supplying the arteriovenous malformation for Wada testing. Note that this tiny catheter is positioned in the distal middle cerebral artery territory.

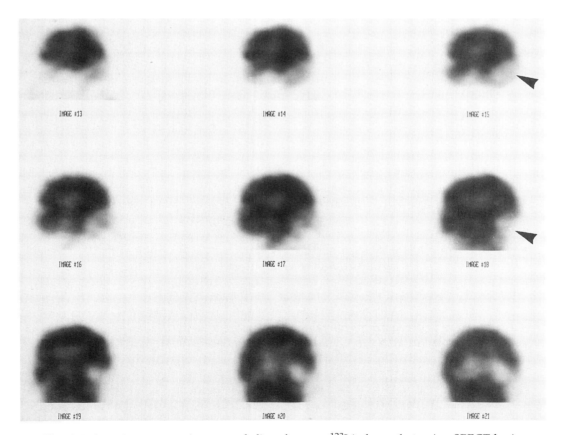

Fig. 1-6. Anterior to posterior coronal slices from an ^{123}I iodoamphetamine SPECT brain scan showing a marked decrease in the perfusion of the left temporal and inferior parietal regions from a low-grade glioma *(arrow).*

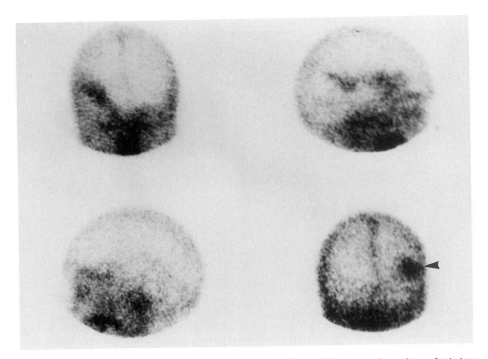

Fig. 1-7. Static images from a planar brain scan done 2 hours after the administration of ^{99m}Tc-DTPA showing a marked area of uptake in the center of the right middle cerebral artery territory. The patient had a cerebral infarct 3 weeks before the scan, which documents damage to the blood-brain barrier allowing ingress of the radiopharmaceutical.

continued impressive improvements in the technology since that time.[22,23] Cerebral SPECT imaging techniques have been utilized for more than 20 years; however, many of the most clinically significant advances have occurred in only the last 5 years or so. Improvements in image resolution and shorter imaging times have enabled this technology to be more widely applied in a variety of brain disorders. In addition, SPECT imaging has benefitted dramatically from a wide variety of single photon radiopharmaceuticals that are now available for the evaluation of cerebral disorders[24] (Fig. 1-7).

The development of CT in the late 1960s and early 1970s substantially transformed the field of neuroradiology. The first clinical prototype CT scanner was introduced in 1972 by Godfrey Hounsfield of EMI Limited in London.[6,25] Hounsfield's first experiments utilized a gamma-ray source and required 9 days for data acquisition. Computer technology was far less advanced at that time, and processing of the data required over 2 hours on a large mainframe computer. The scanning time was later reduced to 9 hours by replacing the gamma-ray source with an x-ray tube.[6] By the time that the first clinical scanner was introduced in 1972, the imaging and processing times had been reduced to minutes. Remarkable technologic advances have occurred since the introduction of the first clinical CT scanners, and these advances have

resulted in tremendous improvements in both image resolution and imaging times (Fig. 1-8).

The introduction of clinical MRI in the 1980s completed the modern transformation of neuroradiology and moved this radiologic specialty to the forefront of noninvasive medical imaging (see Fig. 1-8). Meanwhile, pneumoencephalography has become obsolete and cerebral angiography is primarily reserved for patients in whom magnetic resonance angiography (MRA) is nondiagnostic or when therapeutic intervention is required (Fig. 1-9). The first published MR image was by Paul Lauterbur in 1973.[6,26] However, it was not until 1977 that Damadian and cohorts published the first human images using MR.[6,27] As this new method of imaging gained popularity, three different magnet types were developed. These included permanent magnets made of ferromagnetic materials, resistive magnets that generate a magnetic field by current flow within multiple wire turns, and superconducting magnets that also generate a magnetic field from wire current flow. However, superconducting magnets use wire made of superconducting materials that give little or no resistance and thus produce a virtually perpetual current flow. The main drawback of these "super" systems is the expense of manufacturing and maintaining the superconducting state. By the mid-1980s MR technology became a standard part of many neuroradiologic

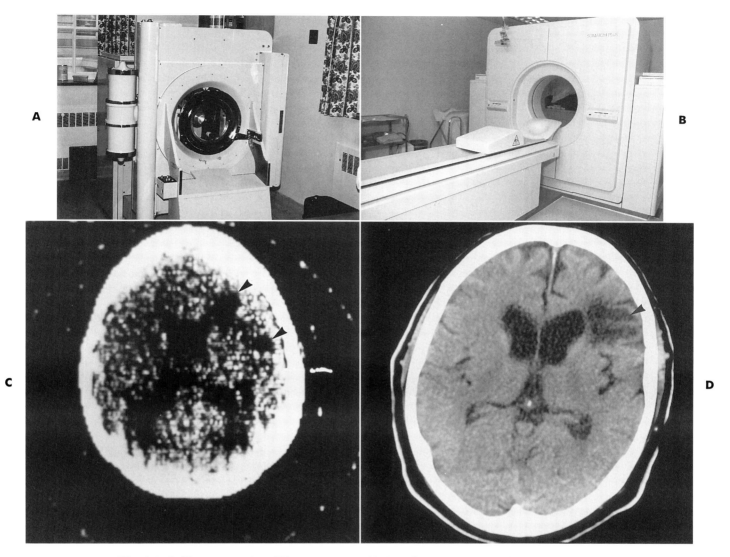

Fig. 1-8. A, First-generation CT scanner, circa 1976. **B**, Later-generation CT scanner, circa 1994. **C**, CT image from first-generation scanner, circa 1976. Note the focal areas of cortical and subcortical loss, probably representing ischemic disease *(arrows)*. **D**, CT image from later-generation scanner, circa 1994. Note the focal areas of cortical and subcortical loss, probably representing ischemic disease *(arrow)*. Compare to **C**.

practices and a name change occurred. In order to eliminate a perceived negative connotation in the original term "nuclear magnetic resonance (NMR)," the word "nuclear" was dropped. This left the terms magnetic resonance (MR) or magnetic resonance imaging (MRI), which continue to be used today. MR is now widely recognized as the imaging modality of choice for most central nervous system disorders.

Surprisingly, in the 1960s and early 1970s when CT and MR were beginning to be evaluated clinically, EEG reached a high point and functional evaluation techniques such as magnetoencephalography (MEG) first began. EEG, of course, had its origin in animal experiments dated as early as 1875 with the work of Richard Caton in Liverpool, England. The first re-

ported use of EEG in humans was by Hans Berger in 1929. By the 1950s, EEG had become commonplace in universities and teaching centers, and by the 1960s EEG could be found in virtually all moderate to large hospitals and in many private offices. During the 1970s and 1980s EEG and MEG efforts were largely overshadowed by the remarkable advances in imaging provided by CT and MR. However, with interest in the 1990s shifting toward the analysis of brain function or dysfunction, there has been a tremendous resurgence in the focus on the brain's electrical activity. This has included functional mapping of the brain by EEG that may prove particularly effective in the evaluation of epilepsy.[28]

MEG, which when combined with MRI forms a

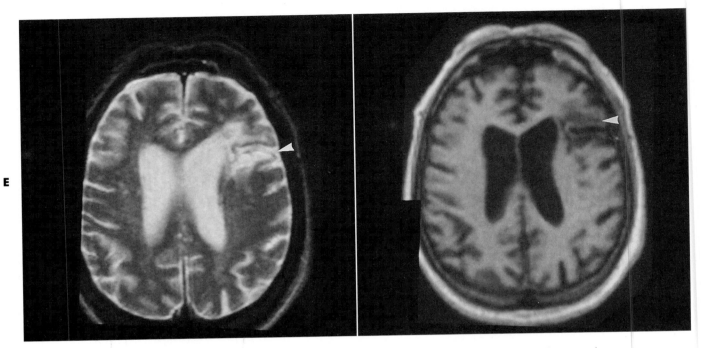

E

F

Fig. 1-8, cont'd. **E,** T2-weighted MR (TR 2500, TE 90) demonstrating focal area of subcortical and periventricular abnormal increased signal intensity resulting from cerebral ischemic disease *(arrow).* **F,** T1-weighted MR (TR 10, TE 4, FA 10) demonstrating focal area of abnormal decreased signal intensity resulting from cerebral ischemic disease *(arrow).*

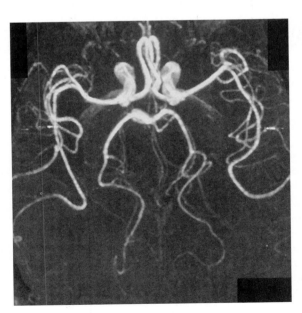

Fig. 1-9. Magnetic resonance angiogram with MIP (maximum intensity projection) reconstruction demonstrating exquisite detail of the intracerebral vasculature. (Compare to Figs. 1-4 and 1-5.)

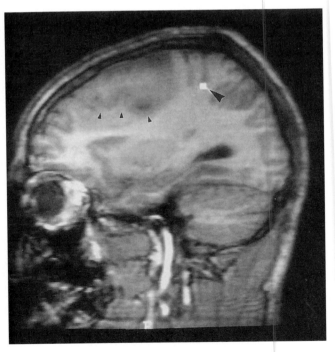

Fig. 1-10. MSI examination from a sagittal MR demonstrating abnormal decreased signal intensity from a brain tumor *(arrows)* and the localization of right-hand digit function represented by the white box *(arrow).*

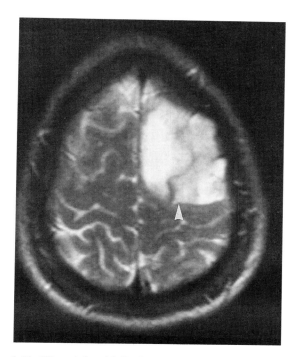

Fig. 1-11. T2-weighted MR (TR 2500, TE 90) demonstrating focal area of abnormal increased signal intensity from a low-grade astrocytoma detected after this patient had minor head trauma *(arrow)*. The neoplasm is unrelated to the head trauma and is an incidental finding at the time of the head trauma evaluation.

functional image of the brain or magnetic source imaging (MSI), was first used to measure brain activity by David Cohen in 1968.[29] However, unlike the remarkably rapid development in CT and MR, it was over two decades before clinical reports of the successful utilization of MEG and MSI began to emerge.[30] This long delay in clinical utility was due predominantly to the limitations of the equipment requiring extraordinarily long acquisition times and even longer processing times. While the early CT and MR examinations could require 60 to 90 minutes of patient evaluation time and an additional 30 to 60 minutes of analysis, early MEG examinations could easily require 8 to 12 hours of acquisition time and days or weeks for analysis. However, as larger array systems (37 channels or more) have become available and with more sophisticated computer analysis programs, these examinations can be conducted in 30 to 90 minutes with complete analysis in less than an hour for many procedures[31] (Fig. 1-10).

CLINICAL APPLICATIONS

The clinical applications of neuroradiologic procedures involve patients from virtually every discipline of medicine. In particular, patients with specific neurologic syndromes are frequently referred for neuroradiologic evaluation. Many times, the strength of these modalities is demonstrated in spite of the fact

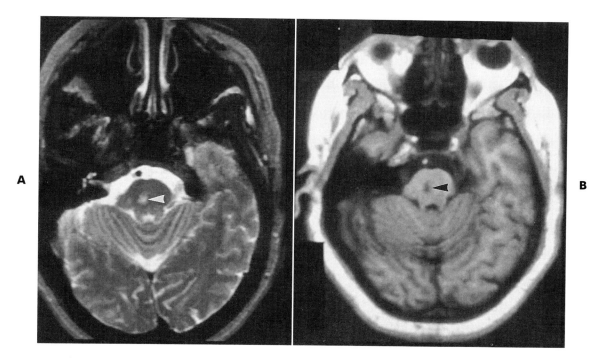

Fig. 1-12. A, T2-weighted MR examination demonstrating a small pontine infarct (TR 2500, TE 90) *(arrow)*. **B,** T1-weighted MR (TR 10, TE 4, FA 10) demonstrating a small pontine infarct *(arrow)*.

that the patient's clinical history, examination, and suspected diagnosis appear unrelated to the final diagnosis. For example, a patient may present with relatively minor head trauma, no other neurologic symptoms, and no abnormality on clinical examination, but CT and/or MRI may demonstrate a remarkable amount of brain pathology (Fig. 1-11). These cases have resulted in the increased use of CT and MRI, particularly in patients with minimal central nervous system complaints and normal clinical examinations. The remarkable sensitivity of these modalities to even the smallest regions of brain pathology is amazing, especially when the results are compared to those from the central nervous system evaluations performed less than 25 years ago (Fig. 1-12).

FUTURE DIRECTIONS

It is clear that the future of brain imaging includes functional brain imaging. The increasing number of modalities available for functional brain imaging and the exquisite anatomic detail available from MRI and CT make this future appear promising. The ability to identify a region of suspected pathology in individual brains with great precision and to superimpose detailed function (on a scale of millimeters of resolution and milliseconds of temporal activity) tests the limits of current technology. However, both millimeter spatial resolution and millisecond temporal resolution have been successfully demonstrated using current functional brain imaging techniques.[31] Currently, the primary limitation is in the ability to process the extraordinarily large amounts of data available from these techniques. Massive parallel supercomputers are becoming increasingly available to the medical community, and this technology may result in not only a new level of diagnostic image quality but also a new view of the real-time activities of the brain.

REFERENCES

1. Kandel ER, Schwartz JH, Jessell TM: Principles of neural science, New York, 1991, Elsevier.
2. Penfield W, Jasper H: Epilepsy and the functional anatomy of the human brain, Boston, 1954, Little Brown.
3. Sobel DF, Gallen CC, Schwartz BJ et al: Central sulcus localization in humans: comparison of MRI-anatomic and magnetoencephalographic functional methods, AJNR 14:915-925, 1993.
4. Penfield W, Boldrey E: Somatic motor and sensory representation in the cerebral cortex of man as studied by electrical stimulation, Brain 60:389-443, 1937.
5. Black PM, Ronner S: Cortical mapping for defining the limits of tumor resection, Neurosurgery 20(6):914-919, 1986.
6. Eisenberg RL. Radiology: an illustrated history, St Louis, 1992, Mosby.
7. Gutierrez C: The birth and growth of neuroradiology in the USA, Neuroradiology 21:227-237, 1981.
8. Cushing H: Hematomyelia from gunshot wound of the cervical spine, Bull Johns Hopkins Hosp 8:195-197, 1897.
9. Schüller A: Roentgen diagnosis of disease of head (translation F.F. Stocking), St Louis, 1918, Mosby.
10. Naffziger HC: A method for the localization of brain tumors — the pineal shift, Surg Gynecol Obstet 40:481-484, 1925.
11. Dandy WE: Ventriculography following the injection of air into the cerebral ventricles, Ann Surg 68:5-11, 1918.
12. Dandy WE: Roentgenography of the brain after the injection of air into the spinal canal, Ann Surg 70:397-403, 1919.
13. Moniz E: Arterial encephalography: importance in the localization of cerebral tumors, Rev Neurol (Paris) 34:72-90, 1927.
14. Loman J, Myerson A: Visualization of the cerebral vessels by direct intracarotid injection of thorium dioxide (Thorotrast). AJR 35:188-193, 1936.
15. Wada JA: A new method for the determination of the side of cerebral speech dominance: a preliminary report on the intracarotid injection of sodium amytal in man, Igaku Siebutsugaku 14:221-222, 1949.
16. Wada JA, Rasmussen T: Intracarotid injection of sodium amytal for the lateralization of cerebral speech dominance, J Neurosurg 17:266-282, 1960.
17. Seldinger SI: Catheter replacement of the needle in percutaneous arteriography: a new technique, Acta Radiol 39:368-376, 1953.
18. Mistretta CA: The use of a general description of the radiological transmission image for categorizing image enhancement procedures, Opt Eng 13:134-137, 1974.
19. Moore GE: Use of radioactive diiodofluorescein in the diagnosis and localization of brain tumors, Science 27:476-483, 1948.
20. Wrenn ER, Good ML, Handler P: The use of positron emitting radioisotopes for the localization of brain tumors, Science 113:525-527, 1951.
21. Brownell GL, Sweet WH: Localization of brain tumors with positron emitters, Nucleonics 11:40-45, 1953.
22. Phleps ME, Hoffman EJ, Mullani NA et al: Application of annihilation coincidence detection to transaxial reconstruction tomography, J Nucl Med 16:210-223, 1975.
23. Hoffman JM, Hanson MW, Coleman RE: Clinical positron emission tomography imaging, Radiol Clin North Am 31(4):935-959, 1993.
24. Van Heertum RL, Miller SH, Mosesson RE: SPECT brain imaging in neurologic disease, Radiol Clin North Am 31(4):881-907, 1993.
25. Hounsfield GN: Computerized transverse axial scanning (tomography): Part I. Description of a system, Br J Radiol 46:1016-1022, 1973.
26. Lauterbur PC: Image formation by induced local interactions: examples employing nuclear magnetic resonance, Nature 242:190-191, 1973.
27. Damadian R, Goldsmith M, Minkhoff L: NMR in cancer. XVI. FONAR image of the live human body, Physiol Chem Phys 9:97-108, 1977.
28. Niedermeyer E, Da Silva FL: Electroencephalography, Baltimore, 1993, Williams & Wilkins.
29. Cohen D: Magnetoencephalography: evidence of magnetic fields produced by alpha rhythm currents, Science 161:784-786, 1968.
30. Quencer RM: Magnetic source imaging: a future in CNS evaluation, AJNR 11:717-718, 1990.
31. Orrison WW, Davis LE, Sullivan GW et al: Anatomic localization of cerebral cortical function by magnetoencephalography combined with MR imaging and CT, AJNR 11:713-716, 1990.

Introduction to Functional Neuroimaging: Functional Neuroanatomy

Jeffrey David Lewine

Not only our pleasure, our joy and our laughter, but also our sorrow, pain, grief and tears arise from the brain, and the brain alone. With it we think and understand, see and hear, and we discriminate between the ugly and the beautiful, between what is pleasant and what is unpleasant and between good and evil.

HIPPOCRATES

The "mind-body" problem stands paramount in defining the intersection of scientific and philosophic endeavors.[1,2] In its simplest formulation, the issue is to elucidate the relationship between mental and physical events. Long before the birth of modern neuroscience, 400 years before the birth of Christ, members of the Hippocratic School of Physicians already suspected the intimate relationship between the nervous system and behavior.

Technologic advances in electronics, engineering, and other fields are allowing physiologists to begin deciphering the quantal elements of the neural-code that transmits information from one nerve cell to another. But the nature of the "brain-code," the cipher used by the brain to transmit cognitive data from one brain region to the next, remains elusive.[3] The neural-code is certainly the building block of the brain-code, but the emergent properties of the brain-code are likely to be as different from those of the constituent neural-code as the emergent properties of water are different from those of hydrogen and oxygen.

Elucidation of the brain-code requires an approach that is different from that used in cellular neuroscience. What is needed are techniques that provide data on the spatial and temporal pattern of neural activity within and across populations of cells. An understanding of the connectivity and interactions between brain regions is paramount, and techniques concerned with gross measures of brain function are certain to prove more useful than those that focus on individual neurons.

It is almost embarrassing that modern attempts to decipher the brain-code via neuroimaging so closely resemble nineteenth century phrenology, but phrenologic concepts on the localization of functional abilities remain prevalent. While we are amused by Franz Joseph Gall's early notions[4] that protruding eyes are a sign of a good memory, we are entranced by modern efforts to correlate mnemonic abilities with hippocampal size, anatomy, and physiology. Whereas the notion that specific bumps on the skull correlate with specific mental capacities is now dismissed as nonsense, observations that schizophrenics fail to show increases in blood flow to the frontal lobes during certain tasks are taken as indicative of the role of the frontal lobes in suppressing psychotic behaviors.

To understand how and why we are willing to accept neuroimaging observations as meaningful, it is necessary to understand the basic organization of the nervous system and the relationships between neurophysiology and the activities measured by noninvasive neuroimaging methods. Beginning with basic neuronal structure, this chapter will provide a brief overview of relationships between brain structure, function, and behavior.

CELLULAR COMPOSITION OF THE BRAIN

The brain is composed of two principal types of cells: neurons and glia. Neurons are the most differentiated cells of the body, and they are the dominant information processing units within the nervous system. The human brain contains more than 10^{12} neurons. Glial cells are 10 to 50 times more numerous than neurons. Glia play an important role in guiding neuronal migration during development, and they serve a variety of metabolic and structural support roles in maturity.

Neurons[5-7]

The functioning of the nervous system is intimately dependent on the precise anatomic arrangement and interconnectivity of its constituent elements. Whereas the individual cells making up most body tissues show relatively little between-cell variability in morphology, the structural diversity of nerve cells is one of the most

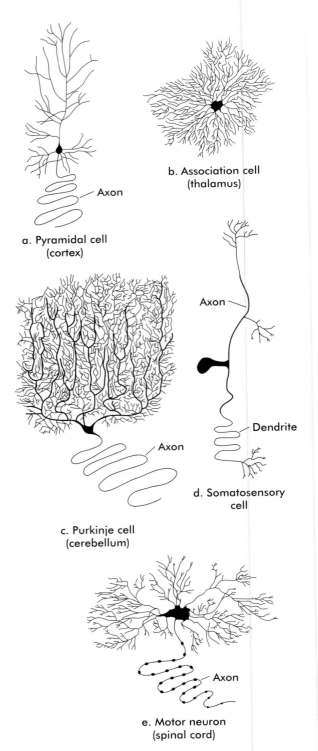

Fig. 2-1. The nervous system is composed of neurons with widely different morphologies. (Adapted from Kolb B, Whishaw IQ: Fundamentals of human neuropsychology, San Francisco, 1980, Freeman.)

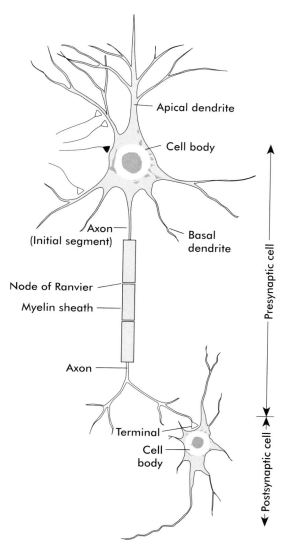

Fig. 2-2. Nerve cells have four major morphologic and functional regions: (1) the dendrites, (2) the cell body (soma), (3) the axon, and (4) the axonal terminal region and associated synaptic terminal contacts with other cells.

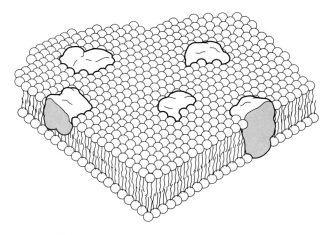

Fig. 2-3. Biologic membranes are formed by a bilayer of lipids (small spheres with wavy lines representing the phosphate head and fatty acid chains, respectively) with embedded proteins (large globular structures). (From Singer SJ, Nicholson GL: Science 175:720, 1972.)

striking features of the nervous system (Fig. 2-1). Nerve cells typically have four morphologically and functionally distinct regions: (1) the dendritic tree, (2) the cell body (soma), (3) the axon, and (4) the axon terminal region and associated synaptic specialization (Fig. 2-2).

Nerve cells, like all cells, are bounded by a plasma membrane 75 to 100 angstroms (Å) thick. The membrane is composed of water, lipids, and proteins.[8] The lipids are arranged into a bilayer. Some proteins are attached to the bilayer, while others span the bilayer or are embedded within (Fig. 2-3). The plasma membrane is a semipermeable membrane that allows certain substances to diffuse across it easily while restricting the transmembrane diffusion of others. Differences in the proteins found in the membrane of the dendrites,

soma, and axon convey different functional properties to each of these regions. For neurons, various chemical and electrical events can rapidly alter membrane permeability characteristics. As discussed later in this chapter, it is this property that gives neurons the ability to encode and transmit information by means of an electrochemical signal.

Contained within the boundaries of the plasma membrane are two distinct regions, the cytoplasm and the nucleus. The nucleus of a typical neuron is large and centrally located within the cell body. The nucleus contains the cell's genetic information in the form of DNA-rich chromatin. The chromatin of neurons is invariably pale, a common characteristic of cells that are very actively synthesizing new proteins.

The nucleus also contains one or more nucleoli made of densely packed RNA. The nucleus is bounded by a double-layered nuclear envelope, which may be highly convoluted (Fig. 2-4). Nuclear pores spanning portions of the nuclear membrane allow the nucleus to interact biochemically with the surrounding cytoplasm.

The cell bodies of neurons of the human brain range in size from 5 (for granule cells of the cerebellum) to 150 μm (for pyramidal Betz cells in the motor cortex). The soma cytoplasm is rich in cellular organelles (Fig. 2-5). The most prominent feature of the somatoplasm is the Nissl substance. Initially it was thought that Nissl bodies were a subcellular organelle unique to neurons, but electron microscopy (EM) has demonstrated that Nissl bodies are composed of rough endoplasmic reticulum (RER), a subcellular structure that is common to all cells. The endoplasmic reticulum (ER) is an extensive internal membrane system that is continuous with the nuclear membrane. It extends through-

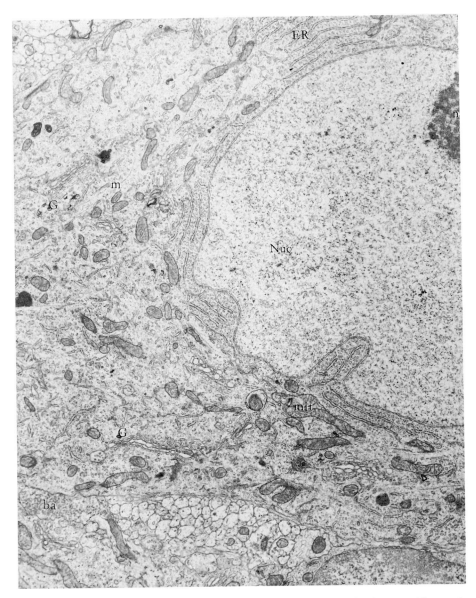

Fig. 2-4. This electron micrograph is of a Purkinje cell from the cerebral cortex. The nucleus (*NUC*) is bounded by a double-layered membrane with gaps known as nuclear pores. The nucleus contains an electron dense nucleolus (*ncl*). The cell cytoplasm is rich in subcellular organelles including mitochondria (*MIT*), endoplasmic reticulum (*ER*), Golgi apparatus (*G*), and microtubules (*m*). (From Peters A, Palay SL, Webster HdeF: The fine structure of the nervous system, Philadelphia, 1976, Saunders.)

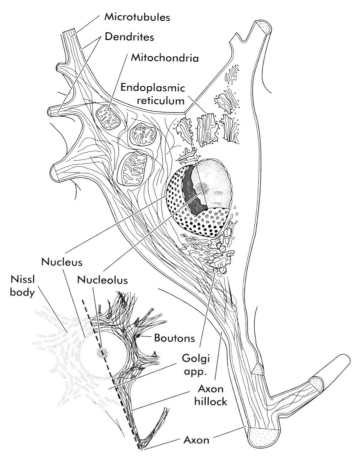

Fig. 2-5. Schematic of neuron showing subcellular organelles. (From Bullock TH, Orkand R, Grinnell A: Introduction to nervous systems, San Francisco, 1977, Freeman.)

out the cytoplasm as a system of membrane-bound channels. The RER of Nissl bodies is studded with ribosomes made mostly of ribonucleic acid. Ribosomes, and hence RER, play key roles in protein synthesis. It is the acidic nature of the ribosomes that causes Nissl bodies to stain darkly with basophilic dyes.

Smooth (agranular) ER is also common in the cell body, as are Golgi apparati. The Golgi apparatus is a particularly prominent organelle in neurons and other secretory cells. It plays an important role in the storage, modification, concentration, and packaging of proteins in secretory membrane vesicles.

Mitochondria play the dominant role in energy production, and they are found scattered throughout neurons. Mitochondria are typically spherical or rod shaped, and EM shows them to have a double-membrane structure, with the inner membrane drawn into folds known as cristae. Associated with the surface of the cristae are enzymes involved in the tricarboxylic acid cycle and cytochrome oxidase chain of oxidative respiration.

In addition to several other cytoplasmic organelles, neurons contain a variety of cytoskeletal elements.

The most prominent of these is the neurofibril. EM reveals that neurofibrils are composed of microtubules and neurofilaments. Microtubules consist of long, unbranched tubes with a hollow core and outer diameter of about 200 Å. Neurofilaments, which are unique to neurons, have a diameter of 100 Å. Neurons also contain microfilaments. Microfilaments have a diameter of 50 Å, and they are often associated with a variety of contractile proteins that allow for modification of neuronal shape.

Dendrites are true extensions of the cell body, and they show similar cytology (Fig. 2-6). At the gross morphologic level they arise smoothly from the cell body, with their diameter tapering with distance. A feature of many dendrites are spiny protuberances that increase the surface area available for synaptic contact with other cells. Many neurons are classified by characteristic branching patterns of their dendrites.

In marked contrast to dendrites, the cytology of axons is considerably different from that of the cell soma (Fig. 2-7). Axons arise abruptly from the soma at a region known as the axon hillock. While neurons may have many dendrites, they have at most one

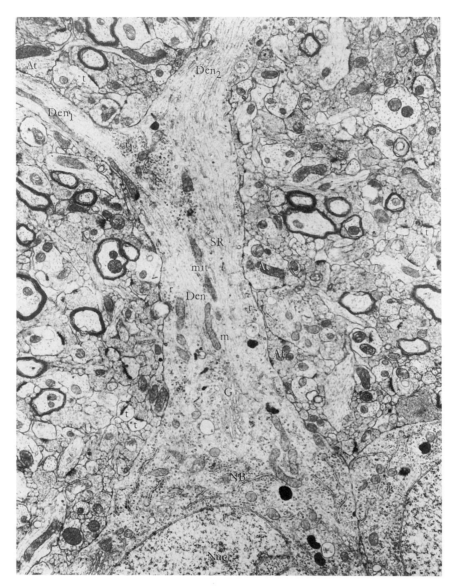

Fig. 2-6. Electron micrograph of the apical dendrite (*DEN*) of a pyramidal neuron. As the dendrite moves away from the nucleus (*Nuc*), it tapers and bifurcates (*Den1* and *Den2*). The dendrite arises smoothly from the cell body. It contains many of the same subcellular organelles as the cell body, including smooth endoplasmic reticulum (*SR*), mitochondria (*mit*), ribosomes (*r*), Golgi apparatus (*G*), and very prominent microtubules (*m*). (From Peters A, Palay SL, Webster HdeF: The fine structure of the nervous system, Philadelphia, 1976, Saunders.)

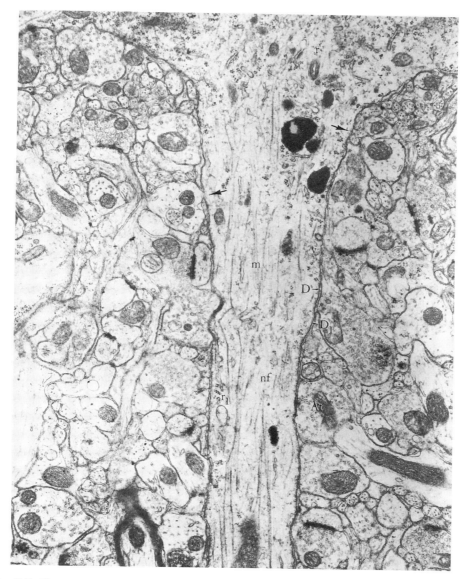

Fig. 2-7. Electron micrograph of axon hillock and axonal initial segment. The axon arises abruptly from the cell body. The axonal initial segment begins at the level defined by the arrows. In the region of the initial segment there is an electron dense undercoating (*D*) beneath the axolemma. The region of the hillock and the axon proper are mostly devoid of ribosomes, although occasional clusters are seen (*r, r1*). The hillock and initial segment are dense in microtubules (*m*) and neurofilaments (*nf*). (From Peters A, Palay SL, Webster HdeF: The fine structure of the nervous system, Philadelphia, 1976, Saunders.)

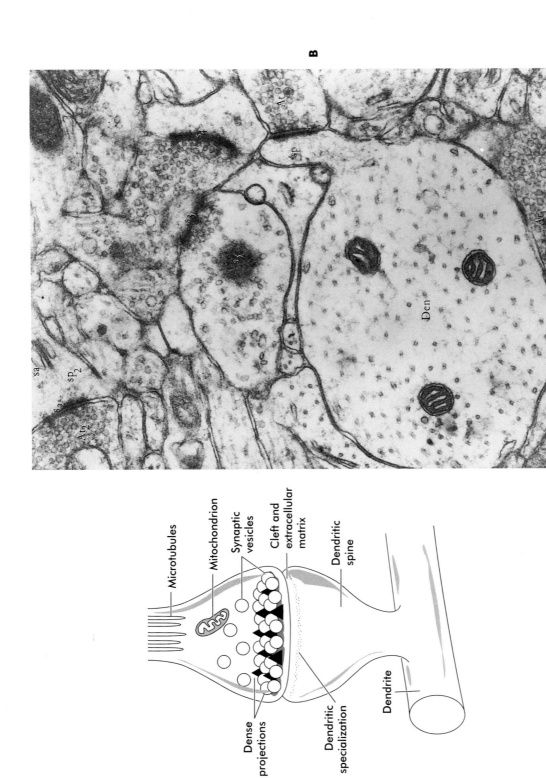

Fig. 2-8. A, Schematic of a spine synapse between an axon terminal and dendritic spine. **B,** Electron micrograph showing several synapses (*S*) between axon terminals (*At*), dendrites (*D*), and dendritic spines (*sp*). (From Peters A, Palay SL, Webster HdeF: The fine structure of the nervous system, Philadelphia, 1976, Saunders.)

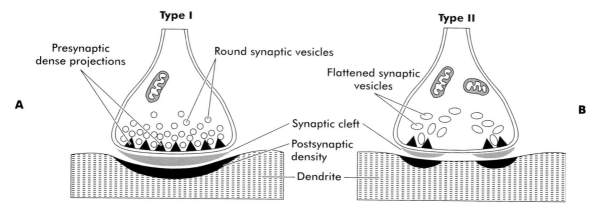

Fig. 2-9. A, Schematic of Gray's Type I synapse. **B**, Schematic of Gray's Type II synapse.

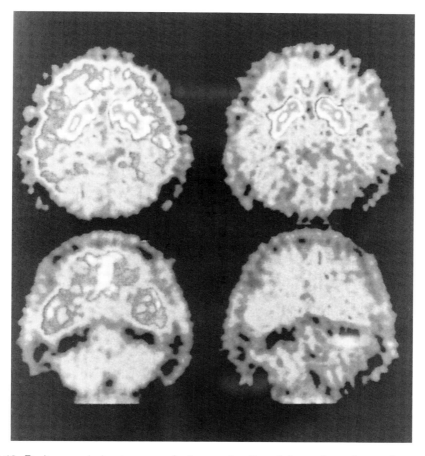

Fig. 2-10. Positron emission tomography images (sectioned through caudate and putamen) of dopamine receptors in the human brain. Leftmost images show D1 receptors, rightmost images show D2 receptors. (Reproduced in color in insert section.) (From Roland PE: Brain activation, New York, 1993, Wiley-Liss.)

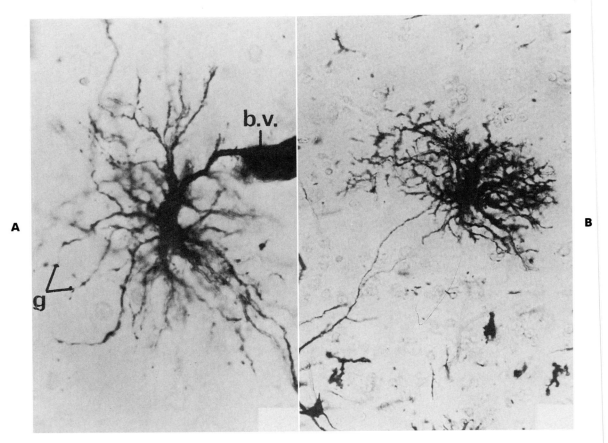

Fig. 2-11. **A**, Fibrous and **B**, protoplasmic astrocytes identified using a Golgi stain. Note the termination of some processes of the fibrous astrocyte on the nearby blood vessel (*b.v.*). (From Carpenter MB: Human neuroanatomy, ed 7, Baltimore, 1976, Williams & Wilkins.)

axonal process. The axon hillock is conspicuously devoid of Nissl substance. The general paucity of RER and free ribosomes in the axon is one of the prime features for distinguishing axons from dendrites in electron micrographs. Unlike dendrites, which taper gradually, axons maintain a relatively constant diameter near their point of termination. Axons may have an extensive terminal arborization, but they seldom branch near their cell body of origin.

The lack of ribosomes and RER in the axons of neurons places unique demands on nerve cells because this means that the synthesis of structural and secretory proteins all takes place at the cell body. It is therefore necessary to transport proteins to axonal sites that can be as much as 2 feet distant. Straightforward diffusion of proteins along a chemical gradient is too slow a process to meet the metabolic demands of neurons, so more rapid, energy-requiring processes have been developed. The processes by which proteins synthesized in the cell body are distributed to distant axonal sites are known as axoplasmic transport.[9]

There are two basic rates at which proteins move away from the cell body in the anterograde direction down the axon. Structural proteins generally move by means of slow axonal transport, at a rate of about 1 to 4 mm/day. In contrast, membrane-bound substances destined for secretion from axon terminals, and organelles such as mitochondria, typically move via fast axonal transport at a rate of 100 to 400 mm/day.

The cell body is the metabolic control center of the neuron, and it is important that information about the integrity and activity of distant axonal sites be relayed back to it. This is accomplished by retrograde axonal transport of a variety of trophic substances. In the retrograde direction, only the fast axonal transport mechanisms are believed to be active.

The exact structural basis for axoplasmic transport has yet to be elucidated. At the light microscopic level, substances move in a saltatory/jumping fashion. Materials appear to move along discrete pathways, and they may even slow and temporarily reverse direction in the course of transport. Microtubules almost certainly play a critical role in axoplasmic transport, since colchicine, a chemical that disrupts the organization of microtubules, also disrupts fast transport.

Nerve cells intercommunicate by means of specialized junctions known as synapses. For all synapses

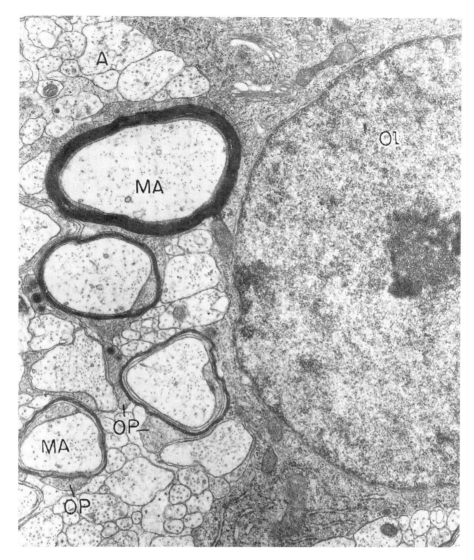

Fig. 2-12. Electron micrograph of an oligodendrocyte (*O*). Note the dense cytoplasm. Oligodendrocyte processes (*OP*) give rise to the myelin of myelinated axons (*MA*). (Courtesy Dr. J. Vaughn, City of Hope Medical Center, Duarte, CA; from Carpenter MB: Human neuroanatomy, ed 7, Baltimore, 1976, Williams & Wilkins.)

there are pre- and postsynaptic elements, with information transmitted from the pre- to postsynaptic sides. There is a small gap, the synaptic cleft, between pre- and postsynaptic membranes (Fig. 2-8). At the EM level, the most prominent characteristic of the chemical synapse is the existence of a neurotransmitter containing synaptic vesicles in the presynaptic element. The pre- and postsynaptic elements can be further identified by the presence of electron-dense materials that typically form a grid of spokelike projections presynaptically and a dense thickening postsynaptically. The presynaptic grid is believed to be related to subcellular structures that act to guide synaptic vesicles toward the terminal membrane. The postsynaptic density is believed to reflect the high

concentration of receptor proteins. Electron-dense materials may also be present within the synaptic cleft.

Synapses are commonly named for their pre- and postsynaptic elements. The most common type of synapse is between a presynaptic axon terminal and a postsynaptic dendrite. Such synapses are called axodendritic. Synapses where dendritic spines serve as the postsynaptic element are called spine synapses. Axosomatic synapses are also common. Axoaxonic and dendrodendritic synapses have been observed, but they are not very common.

Chemical synapses are often divided into Gray's Type I and Type II synapses. Type I synapses have a relatively large synaptic cleft (300 Å) and junctional area (1 to 2 μm), large spherical and clear synaptic

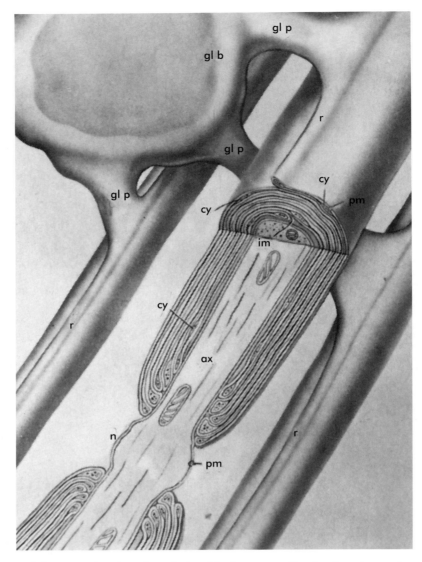

Fig. 2-13. Schematic showing the relationship between oligodendrocytes and a central myelin sheath. Each oligodendrocyte process forms the internode for one axon. *ax*, Axon; *glp*, glial cell process; *glb*, glial cell body; *cy*, cytoplasm of glial cell; *im*, inner mesaxon; *n*, node; *pm*, plasma membrane; *r*, ridge of cytoplasm. (From Bunge RP: Physiol Rev 48:197-251, 1968.)

vesicles, and a highly asymmetric junctional interface with an electron-dense, postsynaptic thickening (Fig. 2-9, *A*). Type II synapses have narrow clefts (100 to 200 Å), small junctional areas (<1 μm), dense oval or elliptical synaptic vesicles, and a relatively symmetric junctional interface (Fig. 2-9, *B*).

Type I synapses have been observed on cell bodies, dendrites, and dendritic spines. Type II synapses are found mostly on the cell soma and have not been observed on spines. There is a tendency for Type I synapses to be excitatory in nature while Type II synapses are inhibitory, but the exact excitatory or inhibitory nature of a particular synapse is determined by the membrane permeability changes induced by

transmitter binding to postsynaptic receptors, not the synaptic morphology per se.

Many different substances serve as transmitters in the nervous system. Some of the most prominent are acetylcholine; the catecholamines dopamine, adrenaline, and noradrenaline; and the indolamine serotonin. Several amino acids and more complex molecules also act as transmitters. Neurotransmitters and their biochemical analogues demonstrate very specific binding to postsynaptic receptor molecules. Some of these analogues can be "tagged" with positron-emitting atoms. This allows an important neuroimaging technique known as PET (positron emission tomography) to determine the distribution of particular types of

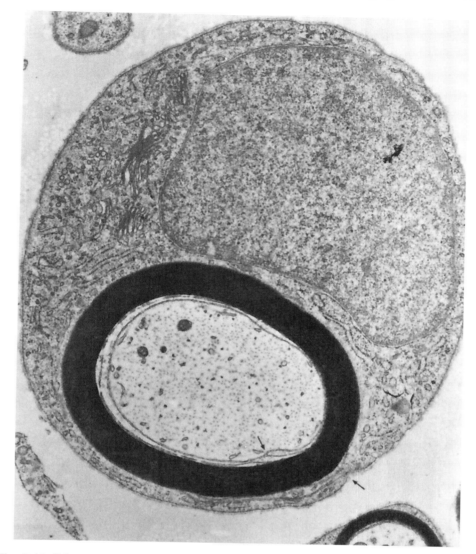

Fig. 2-14. Schwann cells give rise to myelin in the peripheral nervous system. Each Schwann cells gives rise to only a single internodal myelin segment. (From Raine CS: Neurocellular anatomy. In Siegel GJ, Albers RW, Katzman R, Arganoff BW, editors: Basic neurochemistry, ed 2, Boston, 1976, Little, Brown.)

receptors in the nervous system (Fig. 2-10). More details of this procedure are provided in subsequent chapters.

Glia[5-7,10]

The nervous system is subdivided into the central and peripheral nervous systems. The central nervous system (CNS) consists of the brain and spinal cord, and it contains two major classes of glial cells, macroglia and microglia. Macroglia are more numerous and come in two varieties: astrocytes and oligodendroglia. The dominant glial cell in the peripheral nervous system (PNS) is the Schwann cell.

Astrocytes (Fig. 2-11) are small star-shaped cells that generally contain little cytoplasm. They can be easily distinguished from other glia by their numerous microfilaments. Typically, they have a light EM appearance and are classified as either fibrous or protoplasmic. Protoplasmic astrocytes range in size from 10 to 40 μm. They have many thick, highly branched cytoplasmic processes, and they are found mostly in the gray matter, in association with capillaries. Fibrous astrocytes have many thin, mostly unbranched processes. They occur in the white matter and at the surface of the central nervous system where, with the pia mater, they form the pial-glial membrane.

One of the major roles of astrocytes is to provide structural and metabolic support for the nervous system. Astrocytes often ensheathe and isolate neural elements, and protoplasmic astrocytic processes

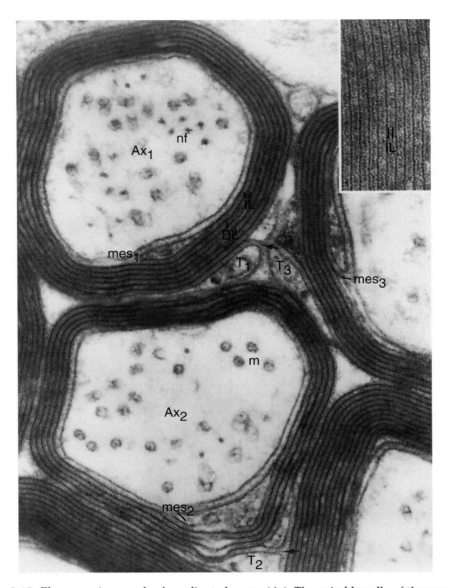

Fig. 2-15. Electron micrograph of myelinated axons (*Ax*). The spiral lamella of the myelin sheath starts at the internal mesaxon (*mes*). The intraperiod line (*IL*) is produced as the outer leaflets of two portions of the plasma membrane belonging to the myelinating oligodendrocyte come into apposition. The major dense line (*DL*) alternates with the intraperiod line. It is formed by apposition of inner leaflets of the plasma membrane, from which the normally intervening cytoplasm has been squeezed out. The major dense line terminates as the inner leaflets of the plasma membrane separate to surround the cytoplasm of the external tongue process (*T*). (From Peters A, Palay SL, Webster HdeF: The fine structure of the nervous system, Philadelphia, 1976, Saunders.)

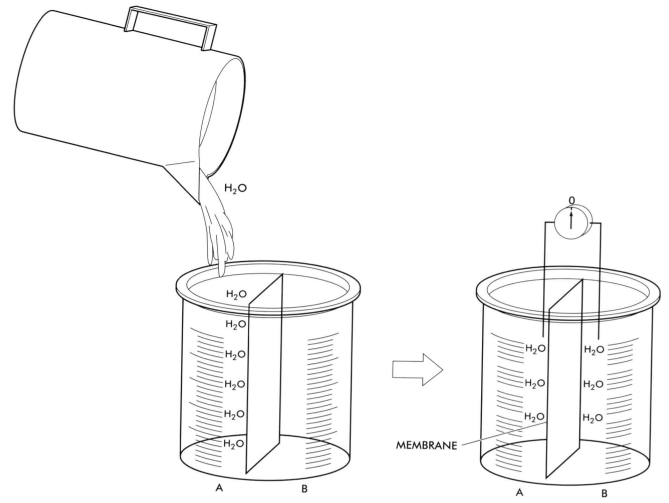

Fig. 2-16. Water distributes evenly across a permeable membrane. There is no voltage potential across the membrane.

known as endfeet are often found in close affiliation with blood vessels. Astrocytes play an important role during development: they provide structural support for migrating neurons. In response to trauma and injury to the nervous system, astrocytes proliferate and become highly phagocytotic, helping to clear neural debris.

Oligodendrocytes have small, dense nuclei with the chromatin clumping near the nuclear periphery (Fig. 2-12). The cytoplasm of oligodendroglia is typically dark, although immature oligodendrocytes may have a light EM appearance. One of the major functional roles of oligodendroglia is the formation of myelin segments that encase portions of some axons (Fig. 2-13). Schwann cells give rise to myelin in the peripheral nervous system (Fig. 2-14).

Myelin consists of spirally wrapped glial membrane where most of the cytoplasm has been squeezed out. Myelin serves as an electrical insulator that increases the speed and efficiency of neural transmission. At the

EM level, myelin has a very characteristic appearance (Fig. 2-15). The dark, major dense lines arise from fusion of the inner surfaces of glial membranes. The somewhat lighter interperiod lines come from approximation of the membrane outer surfaces. Regions of axon between adjacent myelin sheaths are referred to as nodes of Ranvier.

Microglia are of mesodermal origin, whereas neurons and macroglia are derived from the ectoderm. Microglia in the resting state have spindle-shaped cell bodies with a large nucleus and a thin rim of densely stained cytoplasm. In response to nearby injury, microglia become highly mobile and phagocytic.

BASIC NEUROPHYSIOLOGY[11-14]

The neural-code provides the foundation for the brain-code, and attempts to neuroimage brain function invariably take advantage of the electrophysiologic, biochemical, and metabolic characteristics of the neural-code. In order to understand the mecha-

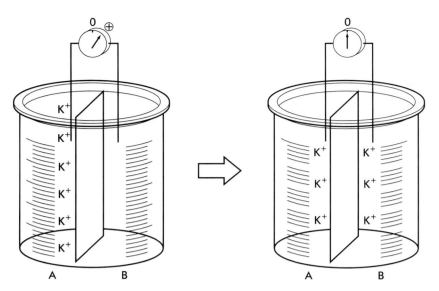

Fig. 2-17. When potassium ions are first added to compartment *A*, compartment *A* shows a positive charge relative to *B*. If the membrane is permeable to potassium, it distributes itself evenly across the membrane so that the potential difference is reduced to zero.

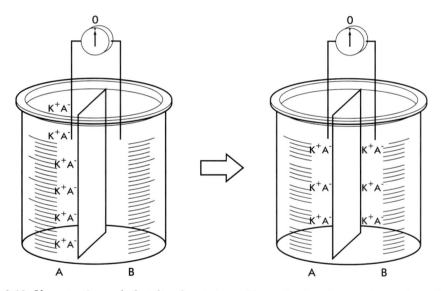

Fig. 2-18. If a potassium salt that dissolves into positive potassium ions and negative anions is added to *A*, initially there is no potential difference, because the salt, as a whole, is electrically neutral. If the membrane is permeable to both potassium and the anion, they diffuse across the membrane and distribute evenly. The electrical potential across the membrane remains zero.

nisms by which neurons encode information in the form of electrochemical signals, it is necessary to review some basic principles related to semipermeable membranes and ionic mechanisms.

Let us first consider a container of water divided into two compartments by a membrane that allows for free movement of all substances across it (Fig. 2-16). The water is electrically neutral and it will distribute evenly across the two sides of the membrane. If one

were to measure the electrical potential difference across the membrane, none would be found. Now consider the situation where positively charged potassium ions are added to compartment A (Fig. 2-17). Initially, there is a potential difference, with A more positive than B. With time, potassium ions diffuse along a chemical and electrical gradient to become distributed equally across the membrane. At that time, there is no longer a potential difference.

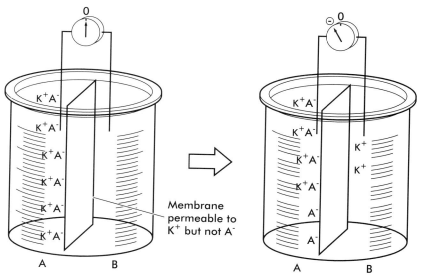

Fig. 2-19. If a potassium salt that dissolves into positive potassium ions and negative anions is added to *A*, initially there is no potential difference, because the salt, as a whole, is electrically neutral. If the membrane is permeable to potassium but not the anion, an electrical potential develops. Potassium ions move down their chemical gradient from compartment *A* to *B*. As electrical charges build up in *B*, an electrical gradient begins to work against the chemical gradient. Eventually, an electrochemical equilibrium is achieved. For the case shown, the potassium equilibrium potential will be negative.

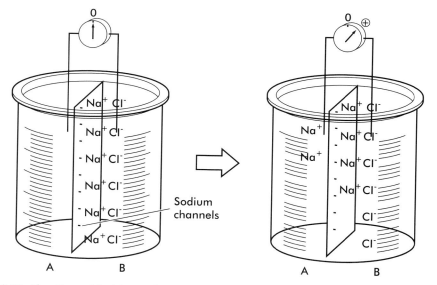

Fig. 2-20. If sodium chloride is added to compartment *B* and the membrane is permeable to sodium only, when electrochemical equilibrium is achieved, the transmembrane potential is positive.

Now imagine adding to compartment A a solution of a potassium salt that breaks down into positively charged potassium ions and negatively charged anions. If the membrane is completely permeable there is no transmembrane potential either initially or after the diffusion process (Fig. 2-18). However, if the membrane is fully permeable to potassium, but completely impermeable to the anions, an interesting situation develops. Initially there is no potential difference, but as potassium ions move across the membrane, a transmembrane potential develops (Fig. 2-19). Two factors influence the movement of potassium across the membrane: a chemical gradient and an electric gradient. The chemical gradient drives potassium from A to B in an effort to obtain an equal distribution of the ion. However, like charges repel and opposites attract, so, as a few positive charges move from A to B, an electrical gradient develops that tries to keep positively charged ions in compartment A. At some point in time, an equilibrium is achieved between the oppositely directed electrical and chemical gradients whereby there is no net flow of ions across the membrane. The membrane potential at this equilibrium is called the potassium equilibrium potential. For the described situation, compartment A will be negatively charged relative to compartment B, even though the overall number of positive potassium ions is greater in compartment A. The absolute magnitude of the potassium equilibrium potential depends on the concentration of ions across the membrane.

Now consider the situation if sodium chloride were added to compartment B (Fig. 2-20, *A*). If the membrane were completely impermeable, the salt would remain in compartment B and there would be no electrical potential. However, if the membrane were selectively permeable to sodium, sodium ions would distribute according to sodium's electrochemical equilibrium conditions. This leaves compartment A positive relative to compartment B (Fig. 2-20, *B*). That is, while the potassium equilibrium potential is negative, the sodium equilibrium potential is positive. Now consider the case where potassium salt is added to A and sodium salt to B. If the membrane is permeable only to potassium, then the potential difference across the membrane is determined by the potassium equilibrium potential. If the membrane is permeable only to sodium, then the sodium equilibrium potential applies.

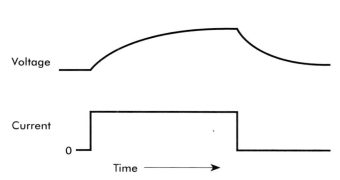

Fig. 2-21. When current is injected into a cell, it causes a change in the transmembrane potential. The time-course of change in the potential lags behind the time-course of injected current because the membrane acts partly like a leaky capacitor.

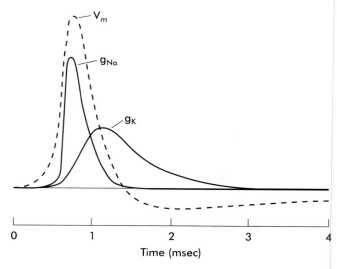

Fig. 2-23. Time-course of the change in membrane conductances and transmembrane voltage associated with an action potential.

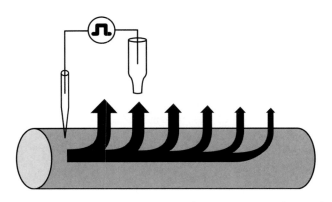

Fig. 2-22. Current pathways must be continuous. The total extracellular return current is equal to the current initially injected intracellularly. The transmembrane return current density (and hence the induced change in membrane potential) is highest near the site of injection, and it decreases exponentially with distance.

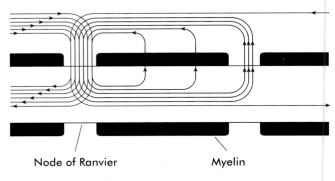

Fig. 2-24. Myelin decreases transmembrane capacitance and increases transmembrane resistance. This allows an action potential at one node to cause a threshold depolarization at the next node. The action potential thereby moves down the axon rapidly, by "jumping" from one node to the next.

At any point in time, the transmembrane potential is given by the Goldman-Hodgkin-Katz equation where the potential reflects the concentration of various ion species on the two sides of the membrane and the relative permeability of the membrane to these ions. For real neurons, the concentration of potassium is high intracellularly, whereas the concentration of sodium is high extracellularly. At rest, the membrane is far more permeable to potassium than sodium, so the membrane potential is mostly defined by the relevant potassium equilibrium potential.

If the transmembrane movement of sodium and

potassium ions along their gradients were allowed to continue unchecked, intracellular potassium levels would fall, while intracellular sodium levels would rise. The chemical gradient would dissipate, and the membrane potential would be reduced. This is prevented by the action of an energy-dependent sodium-potassium (Na-K) pump that moves sodium and potassium against their electrochemical gradients. That is, it moves sodium out of the cell and potassium into the cell.

Given this understanding of the resting membrane potential, it is possible to understand the action potential. Consider a resting axon with a typical resting membrane potential of -75 millivolts (mv). If a microelectrode is placed into the cell and a positive current is injected, there is a reduction of the membrane potential. The time course of the change in membrane potential does not follow the shape of the current pulse exactly because the membrane has both resistive and capacitive properties that are characterized by the membrane time constant (Fig. 2-21).

Current injected into a neuronal process by a microelectrode flows back to the return electrode in the extracellular fluid, with the net return current being equal to the injected current. Neurons have electrotonic properties that cause the amount of current flowing back across any point along the membrane to reflect the ratio of the transmembrane and intracellular resistances. Near the site of current injection there is a larger return current (and greater change in the transmembrane potential than that observed distant to the site [Fig. 2-22]). The change in membrane potential caused by focal current injection decreases exponentially with distance along the length of the process. The length constant of the membrane is defined by the distance along the membrane where the induced change in membrane

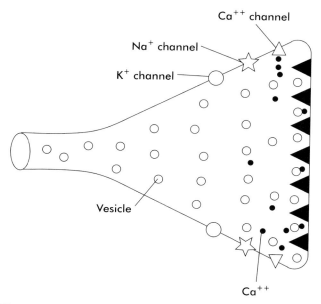

Fig. 2-25. When an action potential invades a presynaptic terminal, it causes opening of voltage-dependent calcium channels. Calcium moves down its electrochemical gradient into the cell, where it causes synaptic vesicles to bind with the presynaptic membrane and release their neurotransmitters into the cleft.

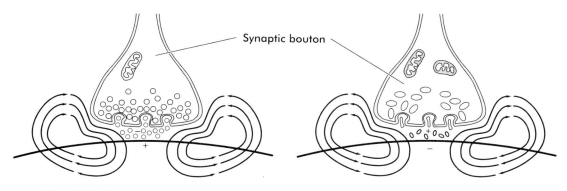

Fig. 2-26. Postsynaptic potentials are generated by chemically induced changes in membrane permeability. Postsynaptic potentials may be either excitatory (*left*) or inhibitory (*right*), depending on the involved ionic species. The electrotonic properties of dendritic membranes allow short-duration postsynaptic currents to produce long-duration postsynaptic potentials.

potential is 37% of that found at the site of current injection.

If the injected current is small, it causes a transient depolarization, with the resting membrane potential quickly reestablished once the current is turned off. The permeability characteristics of axonal membranes are dramatically influenced by the voltage difference across the membrane. The membrane contains both potassium and sodium ion channels. In the resting state, most potassium channels are open, so the membrane is highly permeable to potassium. In

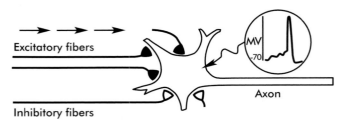

Fig. 2-27. Neurons demonstrate spatial and temporal summation. The membrane potential at any particular region of a neuron reflects electrotonic spread from all regions of the neuron.

contrast, most sodium ion channels are closed, so the membrane permeability to sodium is low. If a large amount of current is injected into the cell, so that the local membrane potential is brought from -75 mv to a threshold level of around -50 mv, voltage-gated sodium channels begin to open. As the membrane becomes more permeable to sodium, sodium ions move down their electrochemical gradient into the cell. This depolarizes the cell further so more sodium channels open, and the membrane potential is driven toward the sodium equilibrium potential of $+55$ mv. Some potassium channels are also voltage dependent, and these too open as the membrane potential is driven toward positive. Nevertheless, sodium is the dominant ionic force during generation of the action potential. After a millisecond or so, a poorly understood inactivation process occurs whereby individual sodium channels close. Hence, after the rapid rush of the membrane potential toward the sodium equilibrium potential, the membrane returns to being mostly permeable to potassium, and the membrane potential is driven back down toward the potassium equilibrium potential. In summary, the action potential is generated by a transient, local increase in the membrane's

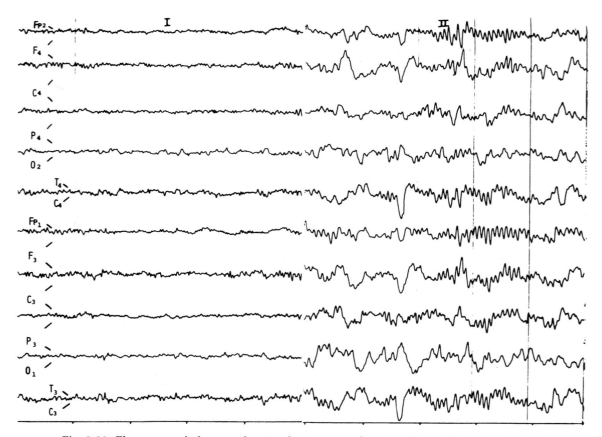

Fig. 2-28. Electroencephalogram showing brain waves during early stages of sleep (I and II). Stage I shows low-amplitude activity, whereas stage II is characterized by large-amplitude spindles and vertex and sharp transients. (From Hughes JR: EEG in clinical practice, Boston, 1982, Butterworth.)

permeability to sodium (Fig. 2-23). After resting permeability is restored, the Na-K pump works to reestablish the original concentration gradients.

When one small patch of membrane undergoes the described changes in ion permeability, the associated change in the local membrane potential is electrotonically propagated to adjacent membrane segments. At the peak of the action potential for one segment, electrotonic properties of the membrane ensure that adjacent membrane is depolarized to its threshold level. The adjacent membrane therefore undergoes a change in its permeability characteristics and a new action potential is generated. In this fashion, the action potential "moves" along the axon, with sodium inactivation preventing reverberant action potentials at previously active patches of membrane.

Myelin increases the efficiency of axonal transmission by increasing transmembrane resistance and decreasing membrane capacitance. This allows an action potential at one node of Ranvier to efficiently depolarize the membrane at the next node, so that an action potential is generated in rapid succession at each node (Fig. 2-24).

For a typical neuron, an action potential invading the region of the presynaptic membrane causes an opening of voltage-gated calcium channels (Fig. 2-25). Calcium then flows along its electrochemical gradient into the presynaptic region, where it interacts with calmodulin. This triggers the binding of synaptic vesicles to the presynaptic membrane and the release of neurotransmitters into the cleft. The neurotransmitters diffuse across the cleft and bind with specific receptor proteins at the postsynaptic membrane. Either through a conformational change or activation of an enzymatic cascade, transmitter-receptor binding causes a change in the local permeability of the postsynaptic membrane. Depending on the exact ionic changes in permeability, a local depolarization or hyperpolarization is produced. These postsynaptic potentials are generally small (on the order of 2 to 5 mv each) but of long duration (10 to 20 msec) (Fig. 2-26).

The surface area of the dendritic tree is quite large, and in general many hundreds of synapses are active in synchrony. This means that the Na-K pump must be especially active throughout the dendritic tree, especially in postsynaptic regions. The activity of the pump is partly governed by local intracellular ionic concentrations, so there is a coupling of the pump to the postsynaptic activity of cells. As shown by Mata and colleagues,[15] the energy demand of the pump has been shown to be the dominant factor in defining the local cerebral metabolic rate (CMR). This means the CMR is a reflection of pump activity and, hence, synaptic activity. Several neuroimaging techniques take advantage of this observation to infer levels of neuronal activity. For example, a common strategy in

positron emission tomography (PET) experiments is to measure regional cerebral glucose metabolism by using a metabolically inert, positron-emitting analogue of glucose, ^{18}F-labeled 2-deoxy-2-fluoro-D-glucose (FDG). Glucose is the main energy source for neurons, and active cells take up FDG as though it were normal glucose. FDG, however, cannot be fully metabolized, so it accumulates in active neurons. The amount of accumulated radioactivity in a particular region thereby provides an index of the extent of synaptic activity.

The electrotonic properties of neurons allow for both spatial and temporal summation of postsynaptic potentials. A rapid series of presynaptic action potentials results in several bursts of transmitter release, which in turn cause a large, local postsynaptic potential. Recall that a potential change at one point along the membrane is associated with smaller changes at a distance, as characterized by the membrane length constant. The membrane potential at any particular

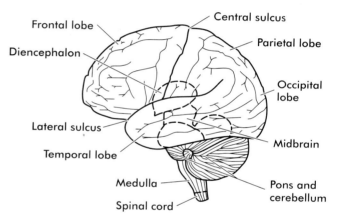

Fig. 2-29. Lateral surface view of the brain showing the major brain divisions. Note that several important brain regions are located internally (*dashed structures*).

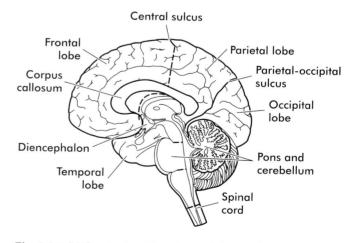

Fig. 2-30. Midsagittal section through brain showing major subdivisions.

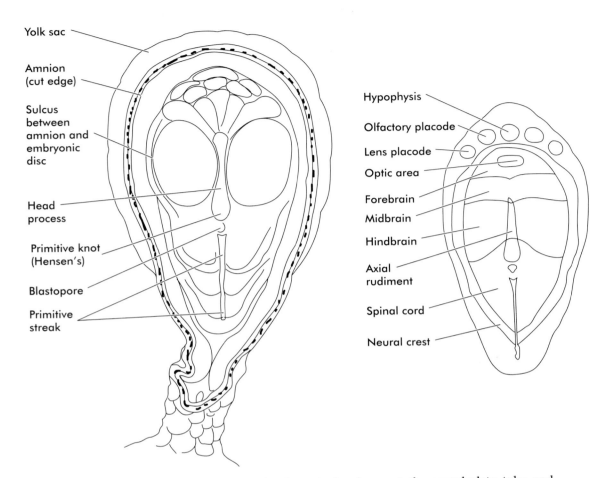

Fig. 2-31. At the eighteenth day of embryonic development, the neural plate, tube, and crest form. A biochemical interaction known as neural induction occurs between notochordal tissue located along the midline and anterior to the blastopore and the overlying head process. Neural induction establishes the fate of cell groups. The head process thickens to form the neural plate, which gives rise to the nervous system.

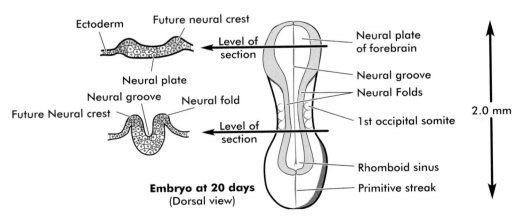

Fig. 2-32. The neural groove and neural folds are observable by embryonic day 20.

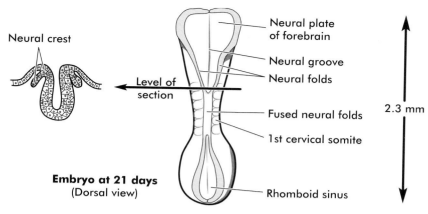

Fig. 2-33. Beginning on day 21, the neural folds fuse to form the neural tube.

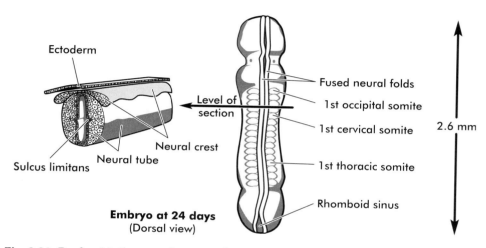

Fig. 2-34. By day 24, the neural crest and neural tube are distinct. The neural crest gives rise to elements of the peripheral nervous system, while the neural tube gives rise to the brain and spinal cord, the divisions of the central nervous system.

point in space therefore reflects summation of the electrotonic effects from potentials at all points along the membrane (Fig. 2-27).

Interestingly, with respect to the generation of action potentials in the postsynaptic cell, the only site of integration that really matters is that of the axonal initial segment, located just distal to the axon hillock. The region of the axonal initial segment is particularly dense in voltage-gated sodium channels, and it has the lowest depolarization threshold. Action potentials are generated if, and only if, the initial segment is depolarized to threshold through the electrotonic spread of postsynaptic potentials. The region of the axon hillock is therefore the final critical integration point for spatial and temporal summation of postsynaptic activity. A noteworthy consequence of this situation is that synapses on distal dendritic branches are not as effective as equivalent synapses located near the hillock region. The anatomic arrangement of synapses on a cell is therefore an important factor in determining the input-output characteristics of that cell.

Measurement of the brain's electrical activity is one of the most important means by which the functional integrity of the nervous system is evaluated.[16-20] The simplest noninvasive method for accomplishing this was developed by Hans Berger in the 1930s. Briefly, small metal disk electrodes are attached to the scalp surface, and differential amplifiers are used to record the time-varying changes in the magnitude of the electrical potential between two electrodes. The recorded brain waves, the electroencephalogram (EEG), are valuable for assessing conscious state and for diagnosing epilepsy and other forms of brain dysfunc-

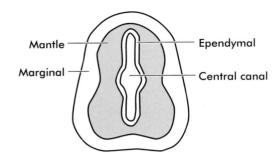

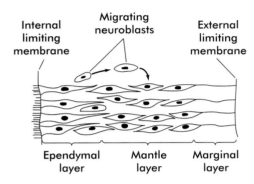

Fig. 2-35. The cells of the primitive neural tube are stratified into three pseudolayers: (1) the ependymal layer, which contains cells undergoing active mitosis; (2) the mantle layer, which contains cells that have migrated out of the ependymal zone; and (3) the marginal layer, which contains the outer processes of cells.

tion. The recorded electrical activity is a weighted sum of all electrophysiologic activity in the brain, although because of biophysical considerations (discussed in later chapters), it mostly reflects postsynaptic graded potentials in the apical dendrites of pyramidal cells (Fig. 2-28).

Magnetoencephalography (MEG) is another useful noninvasive tool for direct assessment of brain electrophysiology.[21-25] MEG measures the minute magnetic fields generated by intracellular currents flowing in the apical dendrites of pyramidal neurons oriented parallel to the skull surface. For both EEG and MEG, the recorded signals reflect synchronous activity in many thousands of neurons. Using signal-averaging techniques it is possible to extract, from the ongoing EEG or MEG, brain signals that are time-locked to specific sensory, motor, and cognitive events. EEG and MEG measure the spatiotemporal pattern of activation across cortical regions, and in some cases it is possible to link EEG and MEG signals to specific mental activities. In this fashion, encephalographers are beginning to use EEG and MEG to decipher the brain-code. Subsequent chapters discuss these techniques in detail.

While neuroimaging techniques have as their fundamental basis the neural-code and its associated biochemistry and physiology, the techniques yield fairly gross spatial measures of activation. An understanding of the large-scale functional organization of the nervous system is thus essential for the interpretation of neuroimaging data within the context of the brain-code.

GROSS NEUROANATOMIC ORGANIZATION OF THE NERVOUS SYSTEM

As previously mentioned, the nervous system can be subdivided into the anatomically distinct but functionally interrelated central and peripheral nervous systems. The central nervous system is composed of the brain and spinal cord. The peripheral nervous system has somatic and autonomic components. The somatic division includes motor neurons that innervate skeletal musculature and those neurons that provide sensory innervation of the skin, muscles, and joints. The autonomic nervous system has sympathetic and parasympathetic components that innervate the internal body viscera and provide for regulation of several body functions. Clinical neuroimaging techniques focus on CNS mechanisms, so the organization of the peripheral nervous system will be discussed in detail only when it pertains directly to understanding CNS activity.

As shown in Figs. 2-29 and 2-30, the CNS is divisible into six major parts: (1) the spinal cord, (2) the medulla, (3) the pons and cerebellum, (4) the midbrain, (5) the diencephalon, and (6) the cerebral hemispheres.

Each part of the CNS is characterized by distinct regions of gray matter that contain predominantly neuronal cell bodies and dendrites and regions of white matter that contain predominantly axonal fibers. Cell bodies in the gray matter are often aggregated to form structures known as nuclei. Alternatively, the cells may be arranged into sheets, as is the case for the cerebral cortex. The white appearance of the white matter is mostly a consequence of the high fat content of myelin sheaths that encase many of the white matter axons. Axons arising from and projecting to common regions tend to aggregate to form fiber tracts.

Development[26,27]

A developmental perspective is useful in understanding the organization of the central nervous system and its relationship to the peripheral nervous system. Immediately after mammalian egg cells are fertilized, a rapid series of cell divisions takes place. By the second embryonic week, three distinct cell layers can be observed. The inner layer is the endoderm, the middle layer the mesoderm, and the outer layer the ectoderm. The ectoderm gives rise to almost all of the nervous system. This layer also generates the epithelial cells of the skin and other organs.

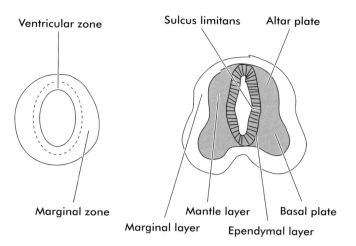

A

Ventricular zone

Marginal zone

B

Sulcus limitans   Altar plate

Mantle layer   Basal plate

Marginal layer   Ependymal layer

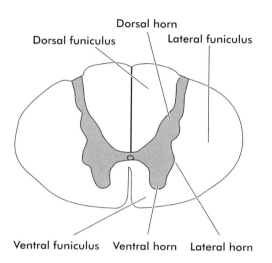

C

Dorsal horn

Dorsal funiculus   Lateral funiculus

Ventral funiculus   Ventral horn   Lateral horn

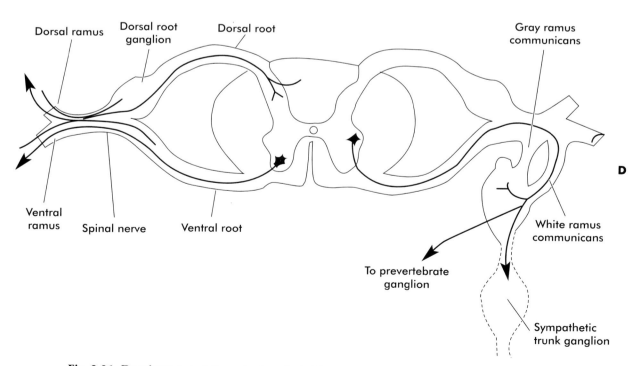

D

Dorsal ramus   Dorsal root ganglion   Dorsal root

Gray ramus communicans

Ventral ramus   Spinal nerve   Ventral root

White ramus communicans

To prevertebrate ganglion

Sympathetic trunk ganglion

Fig. 2-36. Development of the spinal cord. **A,** The walls of the neural tube expand as cells proliferate and migrate. **B,** The sulcus limitans demarcates the boundaries between alar and basal plates. **C,** The basal plate gives rise to the motor sections of the cord, the ventral and lateral horns. The alar plate gives rise to the sensory portions of the cord, the dorsal horns. **D,** Schematic drawing of the principal components of the mature spinal cord.

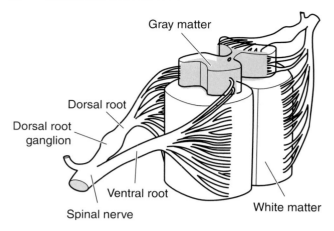

Fig. 2-37. Sensory and motor fibers of the spinal cord are encased in a connective tissue sheath to form "mixed" spinal nerves.

Up until the middle of the second week, the cells of the ectoderm are equipotential. That is, any particular cell is equally capable of developing into neurons, glia, or epithelial cells. Between the second and third weeks, neural induction occurs. This is a complex biochemical interaction between the ectoderm and underlying mesoderm that results in medial and dorsal cells of the ectoderm being committed to the development of neural tissues. The induced medial and dorsal cells begin to proliferate more rapidly than neighboring cells, and they form the precursor of the nervous system, the neural plate (Fig. 2-31). Because of continued local proliferation, a prominent neural groove and accompanying neural folds are observable by day 20. The most lateral cells of the neural plate eventually form the neural crest (Fig. 2-32). At day 21 the neural folds begin to fuse to create the neural tube (Fig. 2-33). By day 24 the neural tube and lateral neural crest are clearly distinct (Fig. 2-34).

The neural tube gives rise to the CNS. Cell types derived from the neural tube include neurons, astrocytes, oligodendrocytes, and ependymal cells (specialized neuroepithelial cells derived from cell lining the neural tube). The microglial cells of the CNS are derived from the mesoderm. The neural crest generates most of the peripheral nervous system, including most of the cranial nerves and 31 pairs of spinal nerves. Cell types derived from the neural crest include neurons and Schwann cells.

The cells that constitute the wall of the primitive neural tube are known as neuroepithelial cells, and they are divided into pseudolayers (Fig. 2-35). The ependymal/ventricular zone, located closest to the lumen of the tube, contains proliferating cells. The outer marginal zone contains the extended outer processes of cells. When the cells of the ependymal layer lose their ability for further mitosis, they migrate

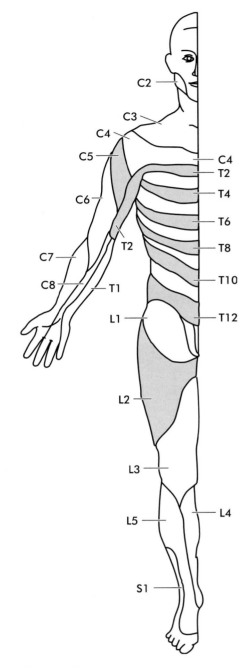

Fig. 2-38. Sensory dermatomes and major nerves for ventral body surface.

away from the lumen to form the intermediate mantle layer. These cells then differentiate into neurons. Some cells migrate into the mantle layer before they lose the ability to undergo mitosis, and they differentiate into glia. Unlike neurons, glial cells retain their ability to proliferate throughout life.

Spinal cord. The spinal cord, the main conduit for transmission of information to and from the brain, demonstrates a reasonably simple pattern of develop-

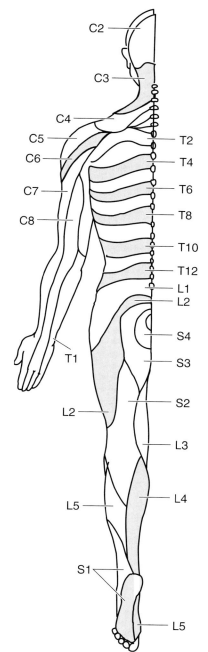

Fig. 2-39. Sensory dermatomes and major nerves for dorsal body surface.

of the spinal cord, which contain the cell bodies of lower motor neurons.

As the cord continues to develop, the lumen of the tube becomes very narrow, leaving only the central canal. Some cells of the ependymal layer do not migrate to the mantle layer. Instead, they become ependymal cells that form a one-cell-thick layer around the central canal. A characteristic feature of ependymal cells is a thin, hairlike projection (cilium) oriented toward the lumen of the canal.

During the development of the peripheral nervous system (PNS), cells migrate from the neural crest to form various peripheral ganglia, the most notable of which are the ganglia of the sympathetic and para-sympathetic divisions of the autonomic nervous system. Neurons migrate to specific locations according to biochemical interactions with the local environment, other neurons, and glia. The establishment of synaptic contacts between cells is generally quite specific and governed by complex interneuronal interactions.

Neural crest cells also form the sensory ganglia of some of the cranial nerves and the dorsal root ganglia of spinal nerves. Neural crest–derived cells of dorsal root ganglia differentiate into sensory neurons. As part of the differentiation process, the sensory neurons send out two axonal-like processes. One projects to the developing cord via the dorsal root, while the other innervates the sensory periphery (skin). Often the two axonlike processes fuse to form a single T-shaped process.

The lateral and ventral horns of the spinal cord contain cells that originate from the neural tube. These cells mostly differentiate into motor neurons that send axonal fibers toward muscles and glands via the ventral roots. The outgoing motor fibers are typically encased in connective tissue along with incoming sensory fibers to form "mixed" spinal nerves (Fig. 2-37). Despite the fact that lower motor neurons are derived from the neural tube, they are considered part of the peripheral nervous system. They are myelinated by Schwann cells, not oligodendrocytes.

Near the periphery the spinal nerves divide into ventral and dorsal rami, which each contain both sensory and motor fibers. At some levels of the cord rami communicans connect spinal nerves with the ganglia of the autonomic nervous system. There are 31 pairs of spinal nerves—8 cervical nerves, 12 thoracic nerves, 5 lumbar nerves, 5 sacral nerves, and 1 coccygeal nerve (this is absent in about 50% of the population). A skin region innervated by a particular spinal nerve is known as a dermatome. Figs. 2-38 and 2-39 show the relationship between dermatomes and spinal nerves.

Brain. The brain develops from the rostral, cephalic end of the neural tube. By the fourth embryonic week,

ment and organization (Fig. 2-36). The mantle layer of the neural tube matures into the gray matter of the cord, whereas the marginal layer becomes the white matter of the cord. The developing neural tube can be divided into alar and basal plates, with the sulcus limitans demarcating the boundary between the two. The dorsally located alar plate develops into the dorsal horn of the spinal cord. Dorsal aspects of the spinal cord are mostly involved in sensory function. The basal plate develops into the lateral and ventral horns

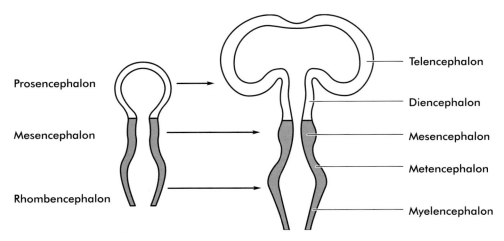

Fig. 2-40. The brain develops from the caudal end of the neural tube. Initially there are three swellings of the tube, the primary brain vesicles. As development continues, five secondary vesicles are apparent.

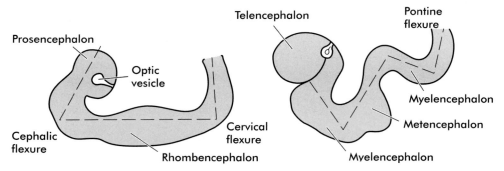

Fig. 2-41. Disproportionate proliferation of cells at certain levels gives rise to the brain flexures.

even before the neural tube has closed completely, three swellings known as the three primary brain vesicles are apparent at the cephalic end of the tube (Fig. 2-40). The prosencephalon develops into the forebrain, the mesencephalon develops into the midbrain, and the rhombencephalon develops into the hindbrain. Soon after development of the primary vesicles, the continued proliferation of cells causes the development of midbrain (cephalic) and cervical flexures (Fig. 2-41). Following this, the prosencephalon divides into the telencephalon and diencephalon, while the rhombencephalon divides into the metencephalon and myelencephalon. The pontine flexure then forms, and the five secondary vesicles begin to develop into various brain structures.

The lumen of the neural tube shrinks down to leave only the central canal at the level of the spinal cord. It expands to form a series of interconnected chambers — the ventricular system — at the level of the brain (Fig. 2-42). The ventricular system is filled with cerebrospinal fluid (CSF) that bathes the interior of the brain. The ventricular system is contiguous with

the spinal canal. Through a series of foramina, CSF generated by the choroid plexus of the lateral and third ventricle flows into the subarachnoid space, which covers the surface of the entire central nervous system (Fig. 2-43).

For the most part, the development of brain cells is similar to that of spinal cord cells. Initially, there are ventricular and marginal zones with migrating cells forming an intermediate zone. In the telencephalic region of the brain, which gives rise to the cerebral hemispheres, two additional zones are seen. There is a subventricular zone, where some cell types proliferate, and also the cortical plate, formed by cells that have migrated past the mantle and marginal layers (Fig. 2-44).

In general, large cells are produced first, with small cells being produced late in development. Cells are added to the cortical plate in an inside-out fashion, with new cells migrating past older cells. The cortical plate ultimately forms the cerebral cortex. Various telencephalic nuclei arise from the mantle layer, with subcortical white matter being associated with the

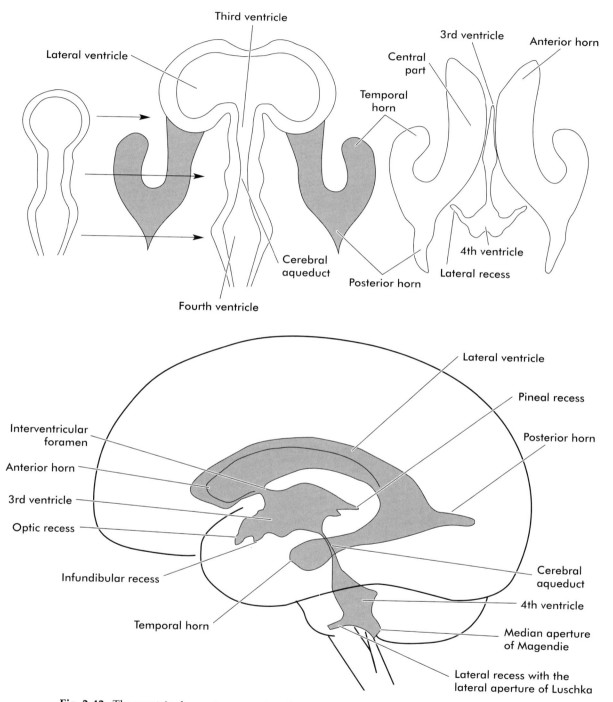

Fig. 2-42. The ventricular system, a series of internal, interconnected fluid-filled chambers, develops from the lumen of the neural tube.

marginal layer. The development of the cerebellum (also illustrated in Fig. 2-44) is rather complex.

Table 2-1 summarizes the relationships between mature brain structures and their embryonic origins. The medulla, pons, and midbrain constitute the brainstem. The brainstem serves several important functions. For example, it contains a number of relay nuclei and neural circuits that transmit information between higher brain regions and the spinal cord. The brainstem also contains relay nuclei for several cranial nerves. Several nuclei of the pons and medulla are involved in the regulation of respiration and blood pressure. Much of the brainstem has a reticular core of intertwined gray and white matter. The integrated action of the midbrain, pontine, and medullary reticular core (the reticular formation) regulates the level of cortical arousal (Fig. 2-45).

Myelencephalon. The medulla oblongata extends up from the first cervical spinal nerve to the pontine flexure. Two important nuclei found in the lower medulla are the nucleus cuneatus and the nucleus gracilis (Fig. 2-46). These nuclei are located dorsally and are sometimes referred to as the dorsal column nuclei. They are relay nuclei of the somatosensory system that receive touch and pressure information from the ipsilateral skin. The neurons of these nuclei give rise to internal arcuate fibers that cross the midline and ascend to the ipsilateral thalamus as a fiber tract known as the medial lemniscus.

The most prominent medullary nucleus, the inferior olive, is involved in motor control functions (Fig. 2-47). The olive receives collateral input from the dorsal column nuclei and oculomotor centers in the brainstem and indirectly from the cerebral cortex (through the red nucleus). It gives rise to climbing fibers, one of the major sources of input into the cerebellum. Climbing fibers cross the midline, linking each inferior olive with the contralateral cerebellum.

The medullary pyramids can be seen on the ventral surface of the medulla. The pyramids are composed of the axons of motor fibers descending from motor and supplementary cortex. These descending fibers decussate at the medullary level (Fig. 2-48).

Five of the twelve pairs of cranial nerves exit the brain at the medullary level (Fig. 2-49). The most caudal nerve, nerve XII, is the hypoglossal nerve. This motor nerve is concerned mostly with movement of the tongue. Nerve XI, the accessory nerve, has cranial and spinal divisions. The cranial division is concerned with movement of the pharynx and larynx, while the

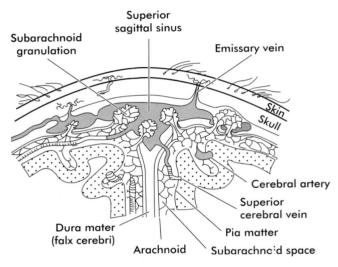

Fig. 2-43. Cerebrospinal fluid produced in the ventricles flows in the subarachnoid space.

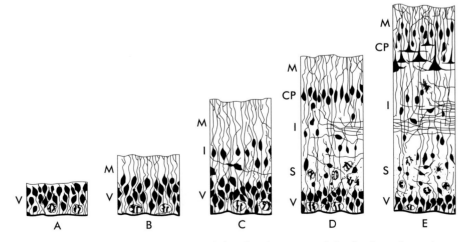

Fig. 2-44. Semidiagrammatic drawing of the development of the basic embryonic zones and the cortical plate. *V*, Ventricular/ependymal zone; *M*, marginal zone; *I*, intermediate zone; *S*, subventricular zone; *CP*, cortical plate. (From Sidman RL, Rakic P: Brain Res 62:1-35, 1973.)

spinal division controls some of the proximal musculature of the head and shoulders. Cranial nerve X, the vagus nerve, is a mixed nerve containing both sensory and motor fibers. The vagus has both efferent and afferent connections to the larynx, it plays a role in taste sensation from the tongue, and it has parasympathetic branches involved in the control of the abdominal and thoracic viscera, including the heart. Nerve IX, the glossopharyngeal, is also a mixed nerve. It is involved in movement of the pharynx and taste sensation from the posterior third of the tongue. Nerve VIII, the vestibulocochlear nerve, leaves the brainstem just above the medulla. It is a sensory nerve involved in both auditory and vestibular function.

The dorsal portion of the pons is similar in structure to the medulla. Descending motor and ascending sensory tracts pass through a reticular core that also contains the nuclei of three of the cranial nerves. Cranial nerve VII, the facial nerve, is a mixed nerve. It innervates the facial musculature and carries taste sensation from the anterior two thirds of the tongue. Nerve VI, the abducens, is a motor nerve that innervates the lateral rectus muscle of the eye. Cranial nerve V is the trigeminal nerve. It is a mixed nerve involved in movements of the jaw and sensation from the teeth and skin of the face.

Metencephalon. The ventral portion of the pons provides for connections between each cerebral hemisphere and the contralateral cerebellar hemisphere. Pontine nuclei receive input from each of the cerebral lobes and give rise to a large number of pontocerebellar fibers that enter into the cerebellum through the massive middle cerebellar peduncle (Fig. 2-50). Most of these fibers, but not all, cross the midline before

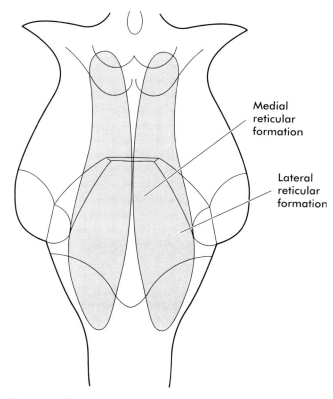

Medial reticular formation

Lateral reticular formation

Fig. 2-45. The brainstem reticular formation plays an important role in cortical arousal. It receives collateral input from both ascending and descending fiber tracts, and it sends projections up to higher brain levels and down into the spinal cord.

Table 2-1. Divisions of the nervous system

Primitive brainstem divisions	Mammalian brain divisions	Portion of fully developed brain	Behavioral division
Prosencephalon (frontbrain)	Telencephalon (endbrain)	Neocortex Basal ganglia Limbic system Olfactory bulb Lateral ventricles	Forebrain
	Diencephalon (between brain)	Thalamus Epithalamus Hypothalamus Third ventricle	Brainstem
Mesencephalon (midbrain)	Mesencephalon (midbrain)	Tectum Tegmentum Cerebral aqueduct	
Rhombencephalon (hindbrain)	Metencephalon (across brain)	Cerebellum Pons Fourth ventricle	
	Myelencephalon (spinal brain)		Spinal cord

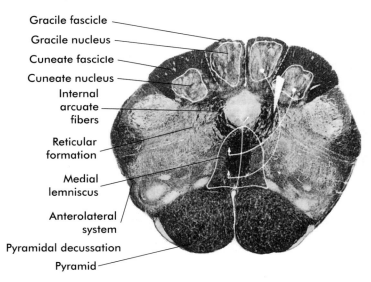

Gracile fascicle

Gracile nucleus

Cuneate fascicle

Cuneate nucleus

Internal arcuate fibers

Reticular formation

Medial lemniscus

Anterolateral system

Pyramidal decussation

Pyramid

Fig. 2-46. The nuclei cuneatus and gracilis are important relay nuclei for somatosensation. Located at the lower medullary level, their output fibers cross the midline (as the internal arcuate fibers) and ascend contralaterally as the medial lemniscus. This section was prepared with a myelin stain, so white matter fiber tracts appear dark while gray matter regions containing cell bodies appear light. (From Martin JH: Neuroanatomy: text and atlas, Norwalk, CT, 1989, Appleton & Lange.)

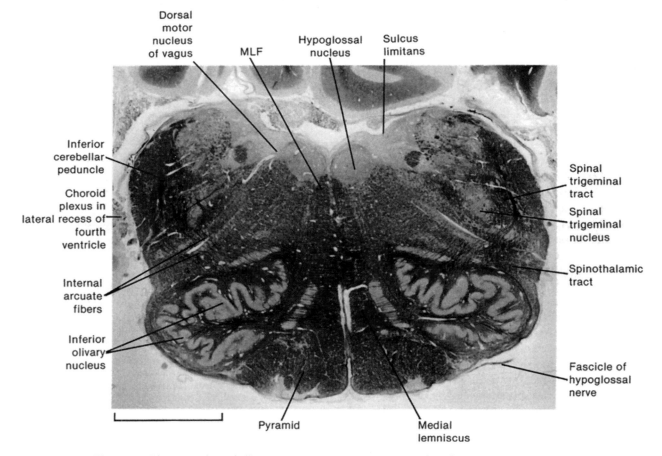

Dorsal motor nucleus of vagus

MLF

Hypoglossal nucleus

Sulcus limitans

Inferior cerebellar peduncle

Choroid plexus in lateral recess of fourth ventricle

Internal arcuate fibers

Inferior olivary nucleus

Spinal trigeminal tract

Spinal trigeminal nucleus

Spinothalamic tract

Fascicle of hypoglossal nerve

Pyramid

Medial lemniscus

Fig. 2-47. The rostral medulla contains many important nuclei, the most prominent of which is the inferior olive, located in the dorsolateral portions of the section. (From Nolte J: The human brain: an introduction to its functional anatomy, ed 3, St Louis, 1993, Mosby.)

entering into the cerebellum, where they project mostly to the cerebellar hemisphere.

The cerebellum is an exceptionally large structure in the human brain. It is a phylogenetically old structure that receives ascending input from most of the sensory systems and descending input from the cerebral

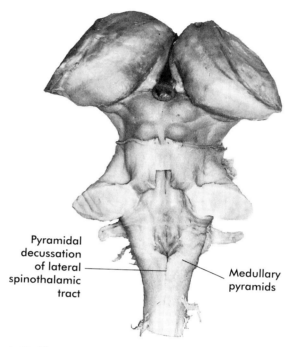

Fig. 2-48. The medullary pyramids are formed by descending motor fibers of the lateral corticospinal tract that arises from motor and supplementary motor areas. The fibers cross the midline (decussate) at the medullary level. (From DeArmond SJ, Fusco MM, Dewey MM: Structure of the human brain: a photographic atlas, ed 3, New York, 1989, Oxford University Press.)

cortex. The surface of the cerebellum is marked by numerous narrow folds that increase the cortical surface area. The cerebellum is attached to the brainstem by three pairs of peduncles that contain afferent and efferent fibers. Afferent fibers come from several sources, including the inferior olivary cortex, pontine nuclei, vestibular fibers, and spinocerebellar tract. Deep cerebellar nuclei provide the main output of the system. Output projections include those to the red nucleus, pontine nuclei, vestibular nuclei, and ventral lateral and ventral anterior thalamus.

The cerebellum is particularly important in sensory-motor integration and coordination, although the precise function of the cerebellum varies from one part to the next, according to its interconnectivity with the rest of the nervous system. For example, those portions of the cerebellum receiving sensory input from the vestibular system help to maintain balance and equilibrium. The cerebellum plays an important role in the control of muscle tonus, especially in relationship to locomotion, postural reflexes, and nonstereotyped behaviors. Lesions of the cerebellum cause a number of significant deficits. Impairments of equilibrium, posture, and skilled motor activity are common. Normally smooth movements often become jerky, rapid movements are slowed, and target-directed movements often miss their mark.

Mesencephalon. The mesencephalon develops into the midbrain. Like the rest of the brainstem, the midbrain has a reticular core with some discrete nuclei. Two important nuclei of this reticular core are the locus coeruleus and the raphe. The locus coeruleus, located at the base of the midbrain and caudal

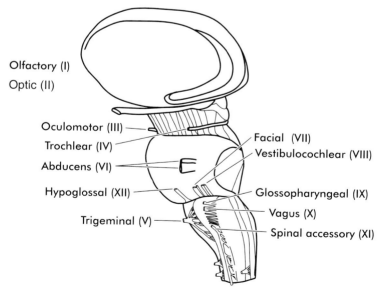

Fig. 2-49. Lateral view of the brainstem showing the exit points for cranial nerves III to XII. Cranial nerves I and II exit the central nervous system at higher levels.

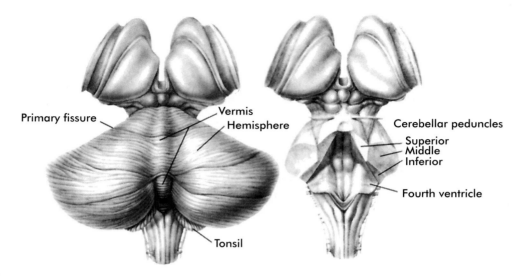

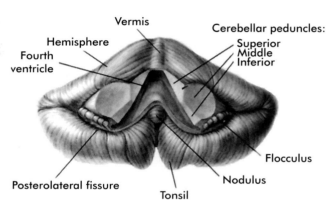

Fig. 2-50. The cerebellar peduncles link the cerebellum to the brainstem. (From Martin JH: Neuroanatomy: text and atlas, Norwalk, CT, 1989, Appleton & Lange.)

pons, gives rise to at least five noradrenergic fiber tracts that project throughout the diencephalon and telencephalon (Fig. 2-51). Midline raphe cells give rise to serotonergic projections that likewise project throughout the brain (Fig. 2-52). These serotonergic and noradrenergic fibers play an important role in the regulation of arousal, conscious state, and sleep.

The tectum forms the dorsal aspect of the mesencephalon. The tectum is composed mainly by two structures, the inferior and superior colliculi (Fig. 2-53). The inferior colliculus is important in auditory information processing. The superior colliculus is involved in visual processing, especially in relationship to the visual guidance of eye movements.

The ventral portion of the mesencephalon, the tegmentum, contains several nuclei, including two very important motor nuclei, the red nucleus and the substantia nigra (Fig. 2-54). The red nucleus gives rise to descending rubrospinal fibers, and it has reciprocal

connections with motor cortex and the cerebellum. The substantia nigra is part of a system of interconnected subcortical nuclei collectively referred to as the basal ganglia. It receives input from several telencephalic nuclei including the caudate and putamen. The substantia nigra is subdivided into the pars compacta and pars reticularis. The pars compacta is one of the main sources of dopamine-containing fibers. The main output connections of the substantia nigra are to the ventral anterior and ventral lateral nuclei of the thalamus. Degeneration of the substantia nigra (especially pars compacta) is prominent in parkinsonism, a motor disorder characterized by a resting tremor and difficulty in the initiation of movement.

Cranial nerve IV, the trochlear nerve, leaves the mesencephalon from the dorsal aspect. The trochlear nerve innervates the superior oblique muscles of the eye. Cranial nerve III, the oculomotor nerve, exits ventrally.

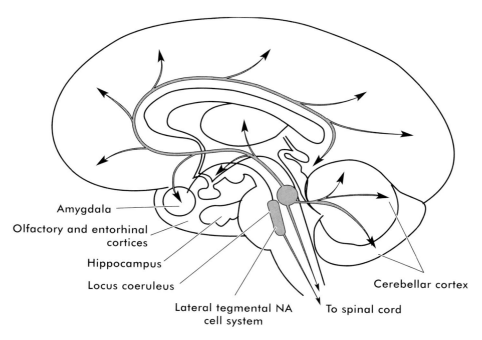

Amygdala

Olfactory and entorhinal
cortices

Hippocampus

Locus coeruleus

Lateral tegmental NA
cell system

To spinal cord

Cerebellar cortex

Fig. 2-51. The reticular core of the mesencephalon contains the locus coeruleus, which sends noradrenergic projections throughout the brain.

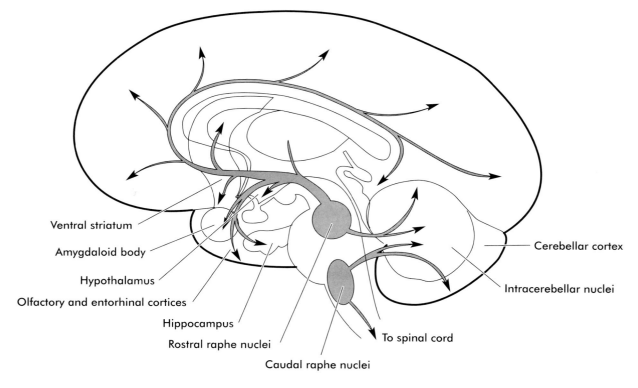

Ventral striatum

Amygdaloid body

Hypothalamus

Olfactory and entorhinal cortices

Hippocampus

Rostral raphe nuclei

Caudal raphe nuclei

To spinal cord

Cerebellar cortex

Intracerebellar nuclei

Fig. 2-52. The reticular core of the mesencephalon contains the raphe nuclei, which send serotonergic projections throughout the brain.

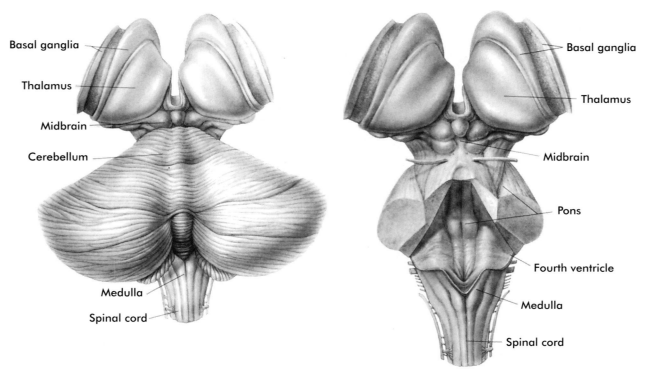

Fig. 2-53. The superior and inferior colliculi of the mesencephalic tectum are located underneath the cerebellum, on the dorsal surface of the brainstem. (From Martin JH: Neuroanatomy: text and atlas, Norwalk, CT, 1989, Appleton & Lange.)

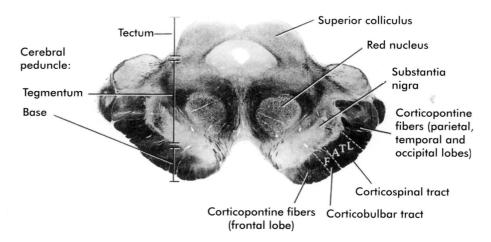

Fig. 2-54. Myelin-stained transverse section through the midbrain showing two very important motor nuclei, the red nucleus and the substantia nigra. The descending corticospinal tracts show somatotopic organization. *F*, Face; *A*, arm; *T*, trunk; *L*, leg. (From Martin JH: Neuroanatomy: text and atlas, Norwalk, CT, 1989, Appleton & Lange.)

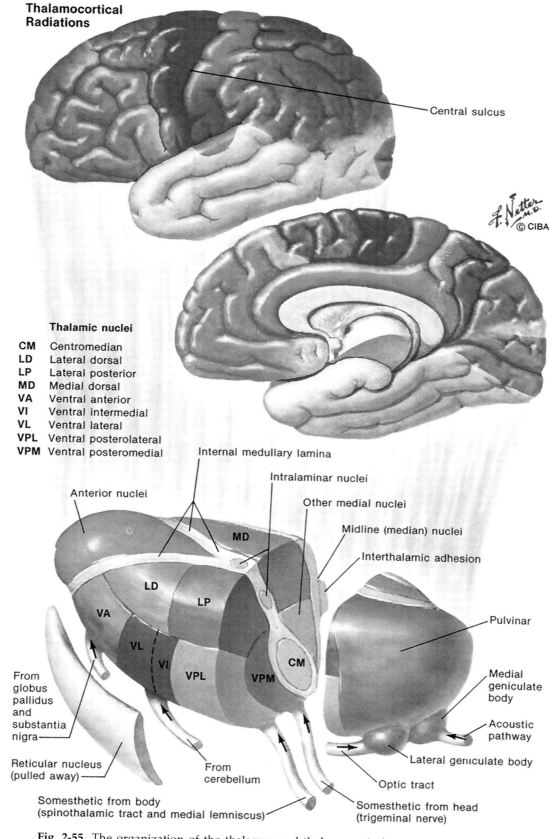

Thalamocortical Radiations

—Central sulcus

Thalamic nuclei

CM	Centromedian
LD	Lateral dorsal
LP	Lateral posterior
MD	Medial dorsal
VA	Ventral anterior
VI	Ventral intermedial
VL	Ventral lateral
VPL	Ventral posterolateral
VPM	Ventral posteromedial

Internal medullary lamina

Intralaminar nuclei

Other medial nuclei

Midline (median) nuclei

Interthalamic adhesion

Anterior nuclei

MD

LD

LP

VA

VL

VI

VPL

VPM

CM

Pulvinar

Medial geniculate body

Acoustic pathway

Lateral geniculate body

Optic tract

From globus pallidus and substantia nigra

Reticular nucleus (pulled away)

From cerebellum

Somesthetic from body (spinothalamic tract and medial lemniscus)

Somesthetic from head (trigeminal nerve)

Fig. 2-55. The organization of the thalamus and thalamocortical projection zones. (From Netter FH: The CIBA collection of medical illustrations, Vol 1: Nervous system; Part I: Anatomy and physiology, West Caldwell, NJ, 1983, CIBA Pharmaceutical.)

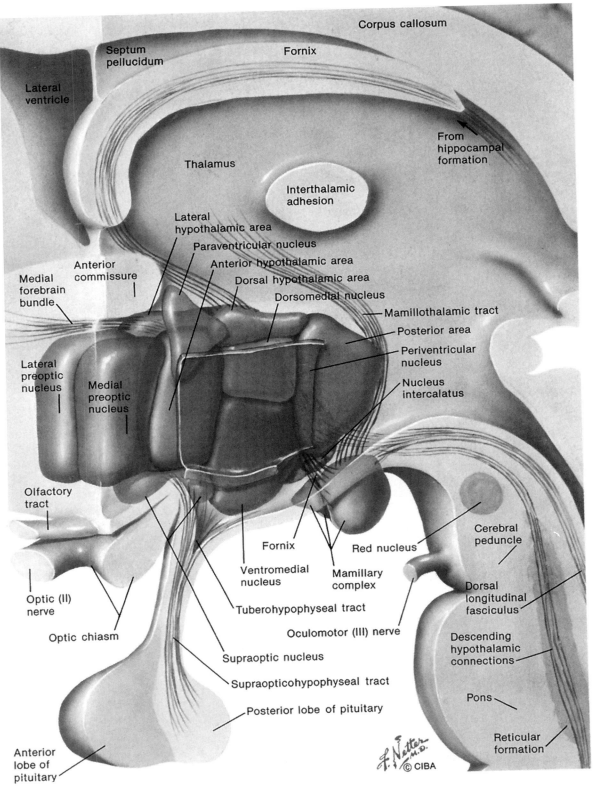

Fig. 2-56. Schematic reconstruction of the hypothalamus, which is composed of many small nuclei that are involved in the regulation of neuroendocrine functions and motivational behavior. (From Netter FH: The CIBA collection of medical illustrations, Vol 1: Nervous system; Part I: Anatomy and physiology, West Caldwell, NJ, 1983, CIBA Pharmaceutical.)

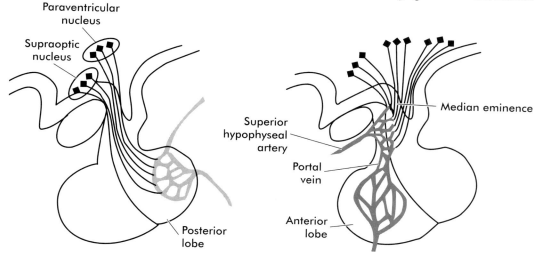

Fig. 2-57. The hypothalamus regulates the release of hormones from the pituitary by direct neural pathways and indirect neurovascular coupling. **A,** The paraventricular and supraoptic nuclei send axons that release oxytocin and vasopressin onto capillaries of the posterior lobe of the pituitary. **B,** Cells of the middle hypothalamic nuclei send projections that secrete releasing and inhibiting factors into the median eminence of the hypophyseal portal system. The portal system carries these substances to the anterior pituitary where they regulate the release of various hormones.

Diencephalon. The diencephalon forms the central core of the cerebrum. The largest diencephalic structure is the thalamus, which is actually a collection of small nuclei (Fig. 2-55). Six separate nuclear groups can be identified in the thalamus of each hemisphere. These are the (1) anterior group, (2) lateral group, (3) medial group, (4) intralaminar nuclei, (5) midline nuclei, and (6) reticular nucleus. There are two basic types of thalamic nuclei, relay (specific) nuclei and diffuse-projecting (nonspecific) nuclei. Relay nuclei convey information between particular subcortical regions and restricted portions of the cerebral cortex. Diffuse projecting nuclei receive many converging sources of input and give rise to diffuse cortical projections.

The relay nuclei are particularly important in mediation of perception, control of voluntary movement, emotional responses, and language. All of the senses, with the exception of olfaction, relay information to the cortex by way of one of the specific sensory nuclei. The lateral geniculate nucleus receives input from retinal ganglion cells and projects to primary visual cortex. The medial geniculate receives auditory input through the inferior colliculus. It projects to the auditory cortex. The ventral posterior lateral and ventral posterior medial nuclei relay touch, pressure, pain, and temperature information to primary somatosensory areas.

Two thalamic nuclei are involved in motor information processing. The ventral lateral nucleus receives input from the cerebellum, the substantia nigra, and the telencephalic nuclei of the basal ganglia. It projects to primary motor cortex. The ventral anterior nucleus receives input from the basal ganglia and sends projections to premotor areas.

Several thalamic nuclei are involved in more cognitive functions such as emotion, memory, and motor planning. For example, the anterior nucleus receives input from the mamillary bodies through the mamillothalamic tract. It projects to the cingulate gyrus. This pathway, from the mamillary bodies to the anterior thalamus to the cingulate cortex, is part of Papez's circuit, a neural pathway believed to be important in the modulation of emotion. The medial dorsal nucleus of the thalamus projects extensively to prefrontal cortex, including the orbitofrontal regions. This nucleus receives input from prefrontal cortex, other thalamic nuclei, and a variety of subcortical structures including the amygdala, pallidum, and reticular formation. The lateral dorsal group of thalamic nuclei, consisting of the pulvinar, lateral dorsal nucleus, and lateral posterior nucleus, possesses extensive reciprocal connections with parietal, occipital, and temporal cortex. It is believed that these nuclei play an important role in complex visual and language functions.

Some thalamic nuclei appear to be involved in arousal-related functions. The reticular nucleus surrounds the thalamus and is traversed by fibers connecting the thalamus and cerebral cortex. These fibers establish synaptic contacts with reticular neurons that send projections to other thalamic nuclei and the midbrain reticular formation. The intralaminar nuclei of the thalamus are characterized by a strong projection to the striatum and diffuse projections to widespread areas of the cerebral cortex.

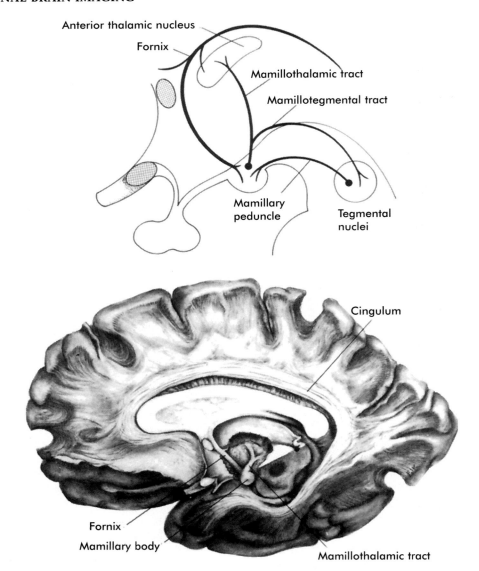

Fig. 2-58. Connections of the mamillary body. **A,** Highly schematic drawing of main input and output connections. **B,** Blunt dissection from medial side showing major input and output pathways. (From Heimer L: The human brain and spinal cord, functional neuroanatomy and dissection guide, New York, 1983, Springer-Verlag.)

Fibers projecting between the thalamus and cerebral cortex compose part of the internal capsule, which also contains axonal fibers projecting from cortex to other subcortical nuclei, the brainstem, and the spinal cord.

The hypothalamus, like the thalamus, is a collection of small nuclei (Fig. 2-56). Hypothalamic nuclei play an important role in regulation of the autonomic nervous system and motivational behaviors. Hypothalamic function is intimately linked with the pituitary gland, which has important neuroendocrine functions. The hypothalamus is often divided into three zones: anterior/periventricular, middle, and posterior. The periventricular zone, which borders the third ventricle, is particularly important in neuroendocrine

function. Two of the most prominent nuclei of this group are the suprachiasmatic and paraventricular nuclei. The suprachiasmatic nucleus receives direct input from the retina and plays an important role in establishing circadian rhythms and visual modulation of neuroendocrine functions. The paraventricular nucleus, together with the supraoptic nucleus, sends a dense projection of vasopressin and oxytocin-releasing fibers into the posterior lobe of the pituitary gland (Fig. 2-57, *A*). These substances are involved in the regulation of blood pressure and blood volume. The preoptic region of the hypothalamus is involved in temperature regulation. It also contains neurons that synthesize gonadotropin releasing hormone (GnRH) and project to the median eminence, where

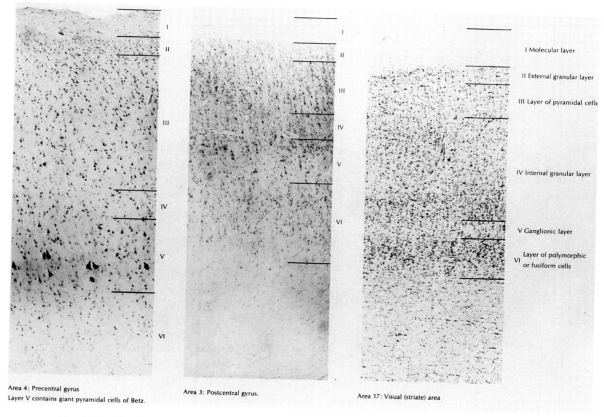

Fig. 2-59. Nissl-stained sections through various cortical regions show the diversity of cortical cytoarchitecture. (From DeArmond SJ, Fusco MM, Dewey MM: Structure of the human brain: a photographic atlas, ed 3, New York, 1989, Oxford University Press.)

the primary capillaries of the hypophyseal (pituitary) portal system are located. Through the portal circulation, GnRH is believed to influence the release of reproductive hormones by the pituitary.

The middle hypothalamic region contains several nuclear zones that project to the median eminence. The infundibular nucleus, ventromedial nucleus, and nearby portions of the basal hypothalamus give rise to a diffuse projection system that terminates on the hypophyseal portal vessel system (Fig. 2-57, *B*). This provides a neurovascular link between the hypothalamus and anterior pituitary. Neurons of the infundibular region play an important role in the regulation of the release of prolactin and growth hormone by the pituitary. The ventromedial nucleus receives input from the amygdala, which is part of the telencephalic limbic system. This nucleus is important in the regulation of appetite and other consummatory behaviors.

The dominant structures of the posterior zone are the mamillary nuclei. They receive a major input from the telencephalic hippocampus through the fornix. Additional input is derived from the tegmentum. The mamillary bodies send projections to the thalamus and tegmental nuclei (Fig. 2-58). They are considered part

of the limbic system, and they are involved in emotive, motivational, and mnemonic functions.

The diencephalon also includes the subthalamus (a motor relay nucleus of the basal ganglia system) and to the poorly understood epithalamus. The largest structure of the epithalamus is the pineal body, which is believed to play a role in the organization and regulation of circadian rhythms.

Cranial nerve II, the optic nerve, enters the diencephalon immediately behind the optic chiasm, where fibers from the nasal retinae decussate. Embryologically, the retina is derived directly from the diencephalon, and the optic nerve is myelinated by oligodendroglia.

Telencephalon. The most anterior of the secondary brain vesicles is the telencephalon. Telencephalon gives rise to the mostly unmyelinated fibers of cranial nerve I, the olfactory nerve; the neocortex of the cerebral hemispheres; several large, internally located nuclei of the basal ganglia system; and the limbic system.

The neocortex of the human brain is only 1.5 to 3.0 mm thick, but its large surface area of over 2000 cm^2 makes it man's most distinguishing feature. This

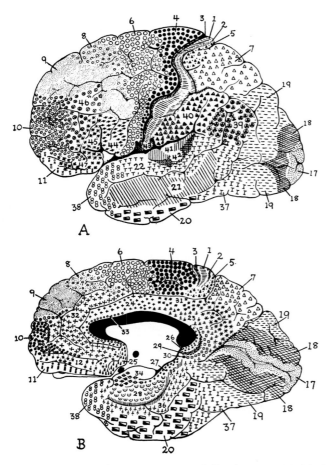

Fig. 2-60. Cytoarchitectonic map of Brodmann. (Modified from Brodmann K: Vergleichende Lokalisationslehre der Grosshimrinde in ihren Prinzipien dargestellt auf Grund des Zellenbaues, Leipzig, 1909, Barth.)

large surface area is achieved by convolution of the cortical surface into a pattern of sulci and gyri. There is considerable variability in sulcal and gyral patterns between individuals, and even some variability between the two cerebral hemispheres. The brain is typically divided into five lobes: frontal, parietal, temporal, occipital, and internal limbic. Some of the most prominent cortical landmarks are the longitudinal fissure, which divides the two cerebral hemispheres; the central sulcus, which divides parietal somatosensory cortex from frontal motor cortex; and the lateral (sylvian) sulcus, which demarcates the upper margin of the temporal lobe. Figs. 2-29 and 2-30 showed the locations of some of the larger, least variable sulci and gyri of the human brain.

The cortex of the cerebral hemispheres is a six-layered mixture of cell bodies and local fibers that varies in size and configuration from one cortical region to the next. Fig. 2-59 illustrates some of the diversity in cortical lamination and cytoarchitectonic patterns. In general, the upper four cortical layers receive input projections from other cortical areas, the brainstem, and subcortical nuclei (e.g., basal ganglia and thalamus), whereas the lower two layers are output projection layers. Layer 4 is the main recipient of thalamic input and it is particularly prominent in primary sensory areas. Layer 5 is particularly prominent in the motor cortex, where it contains large pyramidal Betz cells that give rise to a portion of the descending pyramidal motor tract.

The best known cytoarchitectonic map of human cerebral cortex is that derived by Brodmann (1909).[28] Brodmann identified approximately 50 neuroanatomically distinct cortical regions, shown in Fig. 2-60. The cytoarchitectonic diversity of the brain is coupled to the brain's functional diversity. Indeed, functional

Table 2-2. Selected Brodmann's areas

Lobe	Name	Number	Location
Frontal	Primary motor area	4	Precentral gyrus, paracentral lobule
	Premotor area, supplementary motor area	6	Superior and middle frontal gyri, precentral gyrus
	Inferior portion = frontal eye field	8	Superior and middle frontal gyri
	Broca's area	44,45	Opercular and triangular parts of inferior frontal gyrus
Parietal	Primary somatosensory area; S1	3,1,2	Postcentral gyrus, paracentral lobule
	Somatosensory association area	5,7	Superior parietal lobule
	Angular gyrus	39	Inferior parietal lobule
	Supramarginal gyrus	40	Inferior parietal lobule
Occipital	Primary visual area; V1	17	Banks of calcarine sulcus
	Visual association area; V2, V3, V4, V5	18,19	Surrounding 17
Temporal	Primary auditory area; A1	41	Superior temporal gyrus
	Auditory association area; A2	42*	Superior temporal gyrus
	Auditory association area; posterior portion = Wernicke's area	22	Superior temporal gyrus

*Considered part of the primary auditory cortex by many authors.

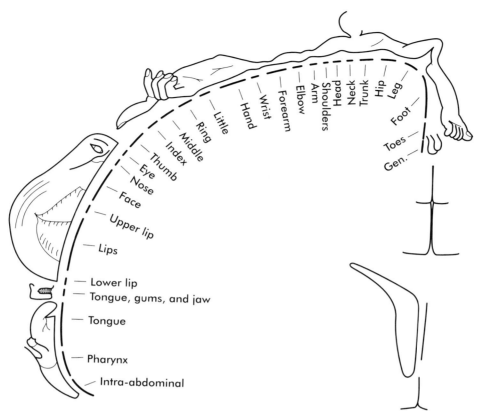

Fig. 2-61. Orderly representation of the body surface in primary somatosensory cortex as shown in this coronal section through the postcentral gyrus. (Adapted from Penfield W, Rasmussen T: The cerebral cortex of man: a clinical study of localization of function, New York, 1950, Macmillan.)

differentiation of brain regions closely follows neuroanatomic differentiation. For example, areas 3 and 17 show remarkably different neuroanatomy, and they are involved in processing very different types of information (somatosensory versus visual). Table 2-2 provides some data on the functional properties of the best characterized Brodmann areas.

One of the key functional properties of cerebral cortex is its columnar organization. In many regions of the brain, small cell columns (perpendicular to the cortical surface) form functional units, with the functional properties shifting between columns. For example, primary somatosensory cortex, in particular Brodmann's area 3b, displays an orderly topographic representation of the body surface (Fig. 2-61). By passing a microelectrode perpendicular to the cortical surface, the activity of brain cells can be recorded. Near the inferior region of the postcentral gyrus, the recorded cells respond selectively to tactile stimulation of the face. The hand representation is found about halfway up the gyrus, while the foot representation is on the upper medial surface.

Extensive sets of fibers interconnect various cortical areas (Fig. 2-62). There are three basic types of projections: short, long, and interhemispheric. Short fibers interconnect cortical columns and also link nearby gyri. Longer connections link one lobe to another. Interhemispheric fiber tracts, known as commissures, link the two hemispheres. The largest of the forebrain commissures is the corpus callosum. Most callosal fibers link homotopic regions that connect identical regions between the hemispheres. However, some significant heterotopic projections link different cortical areas interhemispherically. The cortex is also linked extensively with subcortical areas such as the thalamus, basal ganglia, and subcortical nuclei of the limbic system.

The basal ganglia system plays a particularly important role in the initiation and control of movement. The telencephalic portion of the basal ganglia is divided into lenticular and caudate nuclei (Fig. 2-63). The lenticular nuclei are the putamen and the globus pallidus. The caudate and putamen are collectively referred to as the corpus striatum.

Understanding the function of the basal ganglia is complicated because the system contains multiple feedback loops. On the basis of connectivity, the nuclei of the basal ganglia can be divided into three catego-

Cerebral Cortex: Localization of Function and Association Pathways

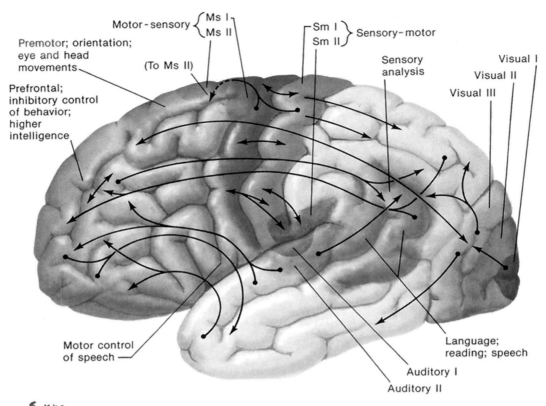

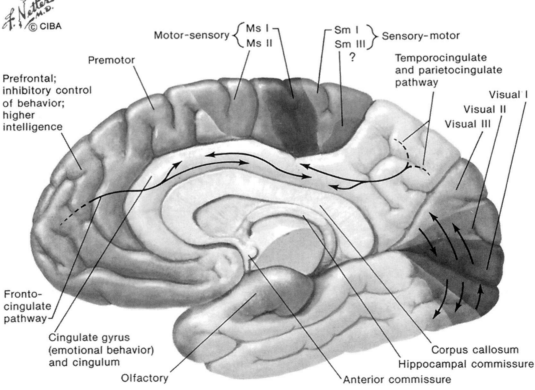

Fig. 2-62. Short- and long-range projections between cortical areas. (Adapted from Netter FH: The CIBA collection of medical illustrations, Vol 1: Nervous system; Part I: Anatomy and physiology, West Caldwell, NJ, 1983, CIBA Pharmaceutical; **B** to **D**, from Kolb B, Whishaw IQ: Fundamentals of human neuropsychology, San Francisco, 1980, WH Freeman.)

Continued.

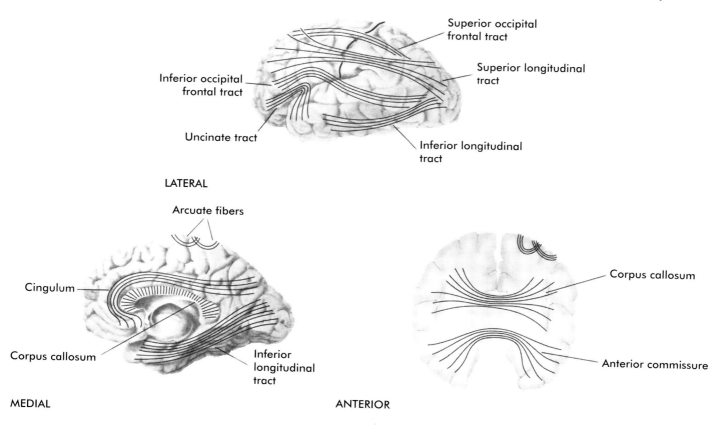

Fig. 2-62, cont'd.

ries: (1) input nuclei, which receive afferents from regions other than the basal ganglia, (2) output nuclei, which have efferent connections that leave the basal ganglia, and (3) intrinsic nuclei, which interconnect elements of the basal ganglia. The putamen, caudate nucleus, and nucleus accumbens are the major input nuclei. The three output regions are the internal segment of the globus pallidus, the ventral pallidum, and the pars reticulata component of the substantia nigra. There are four intrinsic regions: the external segment of the globus pallidus, the subthalamic nucleus, the pars compacta division of the substantia nigra, and the ventral tegmental area.

The main input to the system is derived from the cerebral cortex and the intralaminar centromedian nucleus of the thalamus. The centromedian nucleus is heavily innervated by projections from the pars compacta division of the substantia nigra. The output of the basal ganglia is directed to the ventral anterior, ventral lateral, and dorsal medial nuclei of the thalamus. These nuclei project to premotor and prefrontal cortical regions.

There are four principal input-output loops through the basal ganglia. As shown in Fig. 2-64, these are (1) the sensory-motor loop, (2) the oculomotor loop, (3) the association loop, and (4) the limbic loop.

The sensory-motor loop plays an important role in the control of skeletal musculature. The oculomotor loop is important in the control of the extraocular muscles. The functions of the association and limbic loops are poorly understood. The association loop is suspected to be involved in spatial memory and the evaluation of behavior. The limbic loop may subserve certain emotional functions.

Disorders of the basal ganglia are characterized by difficulty in the initiation of movement, appearance of uncontrolled abnormal movements, and changes in muscle tone, the exact manifestations depending on the dysfunctional subsystems. Table 2-3 provides the characteristic features of some of the most common disorders of the basal ganglia.

The limbic system comprises a number of cortical and subcortical structures, including the hippocampus and amygdala (Fig. 2-65). The limbic system plays an important role in monitoring the body's internal state. It also plays key roles in the regulation of emotions and in the storage and retrieval of memories.

The hippocampal formation consists of (1) the hippocampus proper, (2) the dentate gyrus (a long narrow gyrus joined side to side to the hippocampus), and (3) the subiculum.

The hippocampal cortex is three-layered allocortex

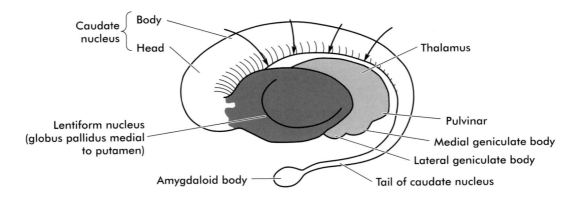

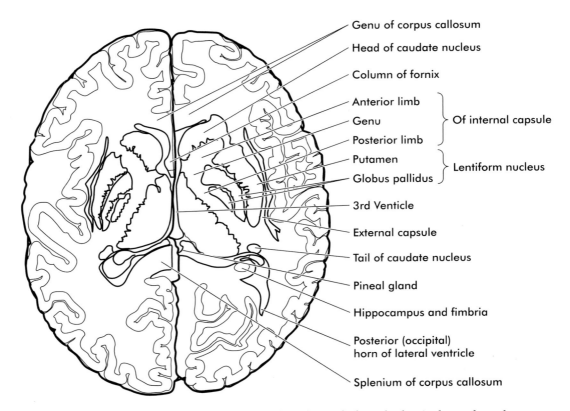

Fig. 2-63. The basal ganglia contains several nuclei, including the lenticular and caudate nuclei. **A,** Lateral view showing C-shape of caudate. **B,** Transverse sections through basal ganglia showing relationships to other telencephalic and diencephalic structures.

(in contrast to six-layered neocortex of the rest of the cerebral hemispheres). The dominant input to the hippocampal formation is along the perforant path that arises from multimodal entorhinal cortex of the parahippocampal gyrus (Fig. 2-66, *A*). Fibers of the perforant path project to the dentate gyrus, where densely packed granule cells give rise to mossy fibers that project to pyramidal cells located in the CA3 region of the hippocampus (Fig. 2-66, *B*). CA3 cells send collateral axons to CA1 pyramidal cells. CA1 connects with the subiculum. The subiculum gives rise to the output connections of the hippocampal forma-

tion. Some cells of the subiculum project back to the entorhinal cortex, whereas others give rise to the fornix, the dominant output pathway of the hippocampus. The fornix projects through the septal area to the diencephalic mamillary bodies.

There are three subdivisions of the amygdala (Fig. 2-67). The corticomedial division receives input from the olfactory system and it is believed to influence appetitive behaviors through the connections of the stria terminalis to the ventromedial nucleus of the hypothalamus. The basolateral division of the amygdala has reciprocal connections with several

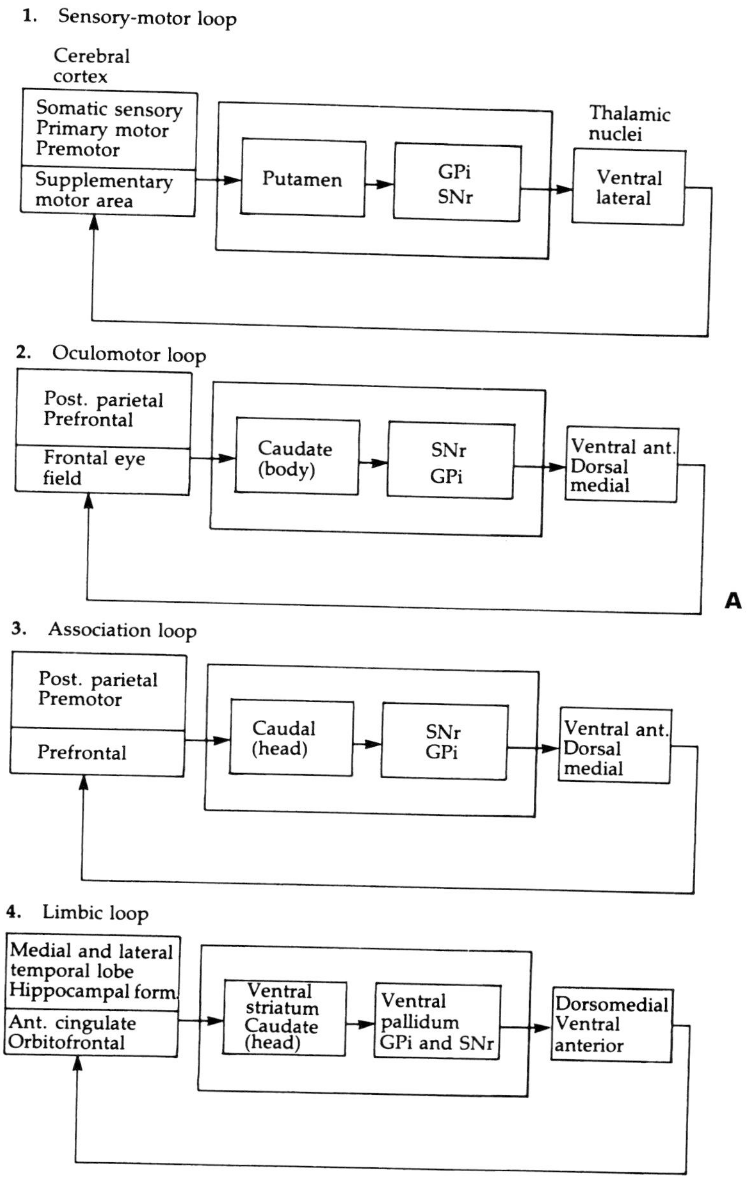

Fig. 2-64. A, Block diagrams of the four principal input-output loops of the basal ganglia: (1) sensory-motor loop, (2) oculomotor loop, (3) association loop, and (4) limbic loop. *GPi,* Globus pallidus internal segment; *SNr,* substantia nigra pars reticulata.

Continued.

cortical regions, including the medial prefrontal, orbital, temporal, and cingulate areas. Output projections from the basolateral nucleus go mostly to the dorsomedial nucleus of the thalamus and also to the nucleus accumbens. The central nucleus of the amygdala receives input from brainstem relay nuclei involved in processing sensory information from the viscera. Its output is to hypothalamic nuclei and also to several brainstem nuclei.

FUNCTIONAL SUBSYSTEMS[7,8,11,29-35]

It should be fairly obvious from the preceding discussion that the brain is organized into func-

tional subsystems, according to connectivity patterns. Overall, the brain consists of multiple serial pathways, working in parallel and with modest interactions between processing modules. The anatomy, physiology, and biochemistry of these interactive systems provide the ultimate substrate of the brain-code, and it is specification of these functional interactions that is the real goal of most neuroimaging studies.

Much of what is currently known about sensory, motor, and cognitive subsystems has been derived from invasive anatomic and physiologic studies, and studies of the neurologic and neuropsychologic con-

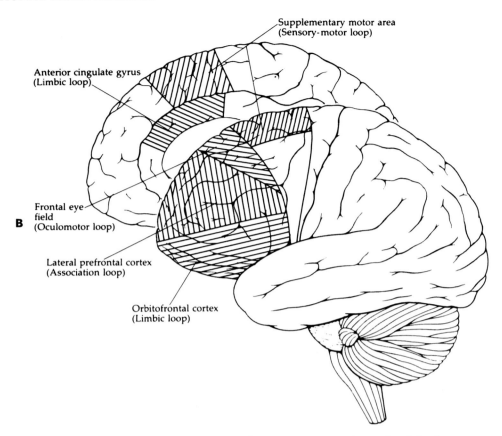

Supplementary motor area
(Sensory-motor loop)

Anterior cingulate gyrus
(Limbic loop)

Frontal eye
field
(Oculomotor loop)

B

Lateral prefrontal cortex
(Association loop)

Orbitofrontal cortex
(Limbic loop)

Fig. 2-64, cont'd.   B, Approximate cortical projection zones for each of the loops. (From Martin JH: Neuroanatomy: text and atlas, Norwalk, CT, 1989, Appleton & Lange.)

sequences of brain damage. A brief review of these systems and relevant clinical observations will provide a valuable foundation for evaluating neuroimaging methods designed for further noninvasive elucidation of the brain-code.

Somatosensory System[36-38]

Sensory processing modules are more thoroughly understood than motor and cognitive modules, and they provide several important insights into the basic organization of functional subsystems. The first element of a sensory processing module is a receptor element that transduces environmental energy into neural energy. There are several types of somatosensory stimuli, including pressure, vibration, heat, and pain. Different neuronal elements (some associated with specialized epithelial cells) are involved in transducing each. It is noteworthy that perceptual encoding of stimulus type by sensory systems is mostly achieved via a concept known as the labeled line. That is, modality is encoded by what specific neuronal elements are active and not by a particular temporal pattern of activity in nonspecific cells. For example, certain neurons encode vibratory information. Regardless of how they are stimulated (e.g., by artificial application of an electric current), the basic perception

is one of vibration. The line from those neurons is perceptually labeled as encoding vibration.

There are two main projection streams in the somatosensory system, each composed of several labeled lines. One stream, the dorsal column–medial lemniscal system, is involved in the processing of tactile, vibratory, and proprioceptive information. The other stream, the anterolateral spinothalamic system, carries pain and temperature information.

The primary sensory neurons of the dorsal column system (Fig. 2-68) have their cell bodies in the dorsal root ganglia. Sensory fibers enter the spinal cord through the dorsal root. Fibers from the lower part of the body ascend ipsilaterally in the fasciculus gracilis, while fibers from the upper body ascend in the fasciculus cuneatus. These fibers synapse in the dorsal column nuclei of the medulla. The dorsal column nuclei contain second-order neurons that send projections across the midline where, as the medial lemniscus, they ascend to the ventral posterior lateral nucleus of the thalamus. The dorsal column nuclei also relay somatosensory information to the cerebellum. Sensation from the face is carried by the trigeminal nerve to the pontine trigeminal nucleus, which gives rise to bilateral projections to the ventral posterior medial nuclei of the thalamus.

Table 2-3. Disorders of the basal ganglia

Disorder	Pathophysiology	Chemical changes	Clinical manifestations	Treatment
Parkinson's disease	Degeneration of the nigrostriatal pathway, raphe nuclei, locus coeruleus, and motor nucleus of vagus	Reduction in dopamine, serotonin, and norepinephrine	Slowly progressing disease, third most common neurologic disease (affects 5 million Americans); about 15% of patients have first-degree relative with disease; mean age of onset is 58 years; findings are tremor at rest (3-6 beats/sec), cogwheel rigidity, bradykinesia, and postural reflex impairment	L-DOPA with or without peripheral DOPA decarboxylase inhibitor Anticholinergic agents: trihexyphenidyl (Artane) or benztropine (Cogentin), others
Huntington's disease	Degeneration of intrastriatal and cortical cholinergic neurons and GABA-ergic neurons	Reduction in choline acetyltransferase and glutamic acid decarboxylase activities and GABA	Progressive disease with associated dementia and death within 15 to 20 years; about 10,000 cases in United States; autosomal dominant; onset at any age but usually in adulthood; findings are chorea, decreased tone (sometimes), and dementia	No specific therapy; dopamine antagonists (phenothiazine, butyrophenones) useful to control chorea; so far GABA agonists not effective
Ballismus	Damage to one subthalamic nucleus, often caused by acute vascular accident	No data	Most severe form of involuntary movement disorder known; tends to clear up slowly	Neuroleptics (butyrophenones)
Tardive dyskinesia	Alteration in dopaminergic receptors causing hypersensitivity to dopamine and its agonists	Normal cerebrospinal fluid and homovanillic acid (acid metabolite of dopamine) levels	Iatrogenic disorder caused by long-term treatment with phenothiazine or butyrophenones; abnormal involuntary movements, especially of face and tongue, usually temporary but can be permanent	Stop offending drug; reserpine

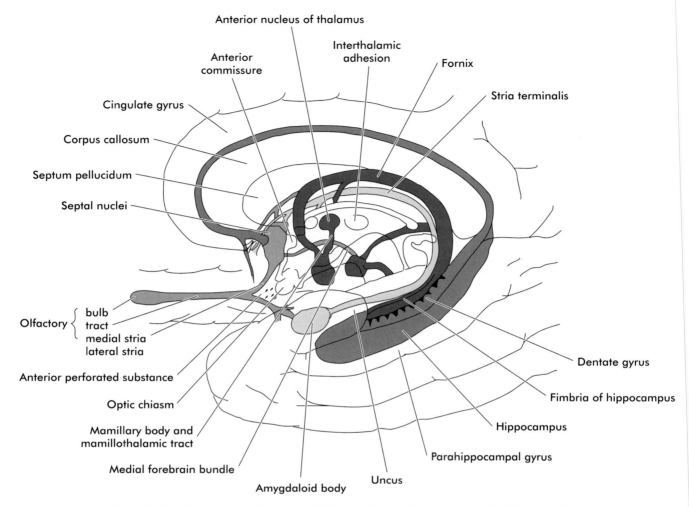

Anterior nucleus of thalamus

Interthalamic adhesion

Anterior commissure

Fornix

Stria terminalis

Cingulate gyrus

Corpus callosum

Septum pellucidum

Septal nuclei

Olfactory { bulb / tract / medial stria / lateral stria

Anterior perforated substance

Optic chiasm

Mamillary body and mamillothalamic tract

Medial forebrain bundle

Amygdaloid body

Uncus

Parahippocampal gyrus

Hippocampus

Fimbria of hippocampus

Dentate gyrus

Fig. 2-65. The limbic system is closely affiliated with the rhinencephalon (which is involved in olfaction). The main structures of the limbic system are the amygdala, hippocampus, parahippocampal gyrus, fornix, mamillary bodies, anterior nucleus of the thalamus, and cingulate gyrus.

The thalamic nuclei contain tertiary relay neurons that project to layer IV of the primary somatosensory cortex (S-I) of the postcentral gyrus. The projection fibers maintain topographic order. Fibers from the leg project to superior and medial areas of the postcentral gyrus, while fibers from the hand project to middle regions of the gyrus.

The cortical area devoted to processing information from each body region is disproportionate to the size of the body region. For example, more cortex is devoted to processing information from the hand and face than is devoted to the entire back. This reflects both the high number of fibers coming from these regions and additional cortical magnification, which is believed to reflect the importance of precise processing of functional data from these regions.

The postcentral gyrus can be divided into three cytoarchitectonic regions: Brodmann's areas 1, 2, and 3. Area 3 is further subdivided into areas 3a and 3b (Fig.

2-69). These different regions are involved in the processing of different types of somatosensory information. Area 1 processes data from rapidly adapting skin receptors. Area 2 is intimately involved in the processing of proprioceptive information from deep tissue receptors encoding pressure and joint position. Area 3a processes data from deep tissue muscle stretch receptors. Area 3b, the most important region for processing tactile information, receives information from both slowly and rapidly adapting skin receptors.

Primary somatosensory cortex projects to several brain regions. Layer VI sends modulatory feedback projections to the ventral posterior lateral and medial nuclei of the thalamus. Layer V sends projections to the basal ganglia, brainstem, and spinal cord. Layers II and III give rise to the main output of S-I. Some fibers project to the secondary somatosensory cortex (region S-II), which is located along the inferior bank of the postcentral gyrus. Other fibers project anteriorly to

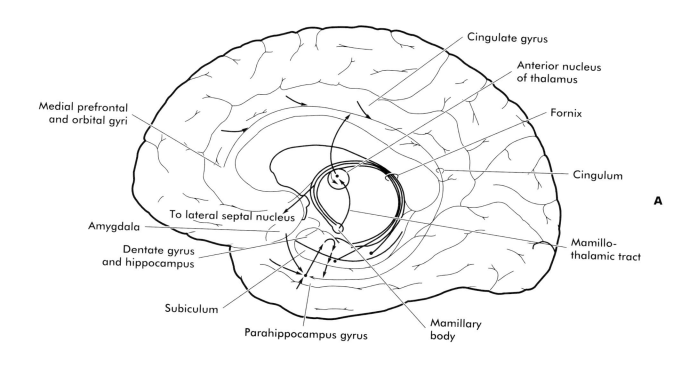

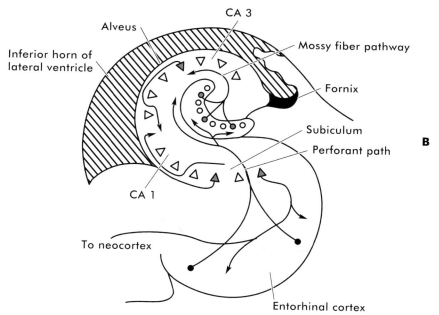

Fig. 2-66. A, Afferent and efferent projections of the hippocampus. **B**, Intrinsic connections of the hippocampal formation. (**A**, from Martin JH: Neuroanatomy: text and atlas, Norwalk, CT, 1989, Appleton & Lange; **B**, from Heimer L: The human brain and spinal cord, functional neuroanatomy and dissection guide, New York, 1983, Springer-Verlag.)

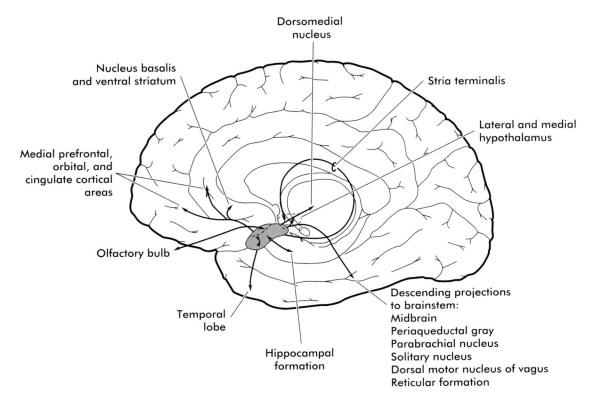

Fig. 2-67. Input and output connections of the amygdala.

motor cortex (Brodmann's area 4), while still others proceed posteriorly to the posterior parietal association cortex of Brodmann's area 5. The S-I area also gives rise to commissural fibers that cross the midline in the body of the corpus callosum. Most fibers project homotopically to S-I, whereas others project heterotopically to contralateral S-II. Secondary somatosensory cortex gives rise to projections to several regions, including entorhinal cortex and posterior insular cortex.

The functional properties of somatosensory cortical neurons become more complex as one moves farther up the processing stream, away from primary somatosensory cortex. For example, individual cells in the 3b hand representation respond best to tactile stimulation within a very restricted region of the hand surface, whereas cells in area 5 demonstrate larger receptive fields (i.e., they respond to stimulation within a larger area of the hand surface). Some cells in area 5 display complex receptive field properties such as directional selectivity for stimuli moving across the hand surface[39] (Fig. 2-70). Areas S-II and the posterior insular cortex are believed to play an important role in somatic memory and recognition of objects by touch.

Primary sensory neurons conveying pain and temperature information also have their cell bodies in the dorsal root ganglia. Pain information is carried by both unmyelinated C fibers and small-diameter, lightly myelinated A-delta fibers. C fibers are activated by high-intensity mechanical, thermal, or chemical stimulation, and they are believed to mediate long-lasting, burning-type pain. A-delta fibers respond primarily to noxious heat and mechanical stimuli. Their activity is believed to be the peripheral substrate of sharp, prickling pain. Fig. 2-71 illustrates the central projection pathways for pain and temperature.

At present, details about the cortical processing of pain are scarce, although neuroimaging studies (especially PET, see subsequent chapters) are beginning to provide some insights.

Auditory and Vestibular Systems[40]

The auditory system is a complex system designed for precise characterization of sound intensity and pitch. A series of mechanical elements, the middle ear ossicles, transmit sound-related vibratory energy from the eardrum to the oval window, where vibrations are set up in the fluid media of the cochlea (Fig. 2-72). The organ of Corti, located on the upper surface of the basilar membrane of the cochlea, contains specialized hair cells that act as the neural transducers in this system. Oscillations of the basilar membrane produce an activating shearing force on the cilia of the hair cells.

The mechanical properties of the basilar membrane are such that high-frequency sounds cause oscillations at the base of the membrane, near the oval window, whereas low-frequency sounds cause oscillations at the apex. This imparts tonotopic organization to the

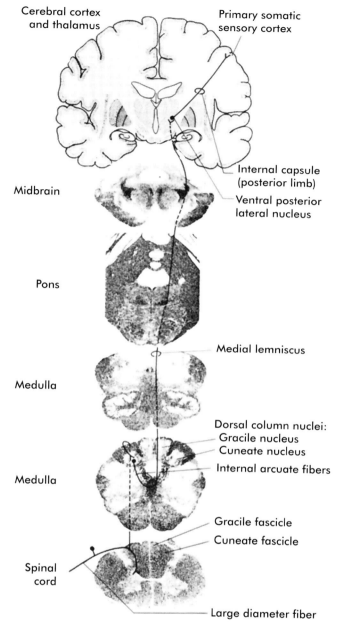

Fig. 2-68. The dorsal column–medial lemniscus somatosensory pathway for touch, pressure, and proprioception. (From Martin JH: Neuroanatomy: text and atlas, Norwalk, CT, 1989, Appleton & Lange.)

hair cells along the organ of Corti. Cells at the apex encode low-frequency sounds, and cells at the base, high-frequency sounds.

When hair cells are activated, they release neurotransmitters that activate the peripheral axons of the cells of the spiral ganglia that innervate them. The central projections of the spiral ganglia cells form the cochlear branch of cranial nerve VIII, the vestibulocochlear nerve. Fig. 2-73 provides the details of the central projection pathway to primary auditory cortex of the transverse temporal (Heschl's) gyrus, Brod-

mann's area 41. The tonotopic organization of the primary auditory projection fibers is maintained throughout the projection pathway. Neurons deep along Heschl's gyrus respond best to high-frequency tones while neurons close to the lateral margin of the gyrus respond best to low-frequency tones. Primary auditory cortex projects to several association regions, including Brodmann's area 22 and Wernicke's area. These are located along the dorsal and lateral aspects of the superior and middle temporal gyri. Transcallosal projections are also prominent.

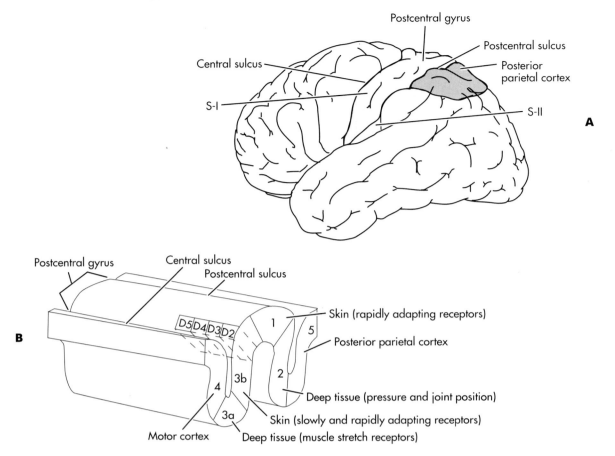

Fig. 2-69. A, Primary somatosensory cortex is located at the postcentral gyrus. **B,** This area is divided into several Brodmann's areas that process different types of somatosensory information.

Continued.

It is noteworthy that several complex auditory computations take place at subcortical nuclei early in the auditory processing pathway. Of particular note is the role of the superior olivary complex in computations related to sound localization.

The vestibular apparatus, located in the inner ear along with the cochlea, includes the semicircular canals, the utricle, and the saccule (Fig. 2-72). Specialized hair cells, similar to those found in the cochlea, are the receptor cells for the vestibular system. These cells are innervated by the distal process of neurons located in Scarpa's ganglia. The centrally projecting axons of these neurons form the vestibular division of cranial nerve VIII. Fig. 2-73 illustrates the central pathways of the vestibular system. The brainstem vestibular nuclei contain the critical circuitry for several vestibular reflexes, including the very important vestibular-oculomotor reflexes. The cortical representation for vestibular function is poorly defined, but on the basis of connectivity, the relevant cortical region is believed to be located in the parietal lobe just caudal to primary somatosensory cortex.

Gustatory and Olfactory Systems[41]

Gustatory receptors are clustered in the taste buds that are located on the tongue, palate, pharynx, larynx, and epiglottis. Three different cranial nerves—VII, IX, and X—participate in taste sensation. The afferent fibers of these nerves enter the brainstem solitary tract and terminate in the solitary nucleus. Fig. 2-74 illustrates the central projection pathways. The parvocellular portion of the ventral posterior medial nucleus of the thalamus relays taste information to the frontal operculum and anterior insular cortex. It is noteworthy that even though tongue tactile and taste receptors are inter-

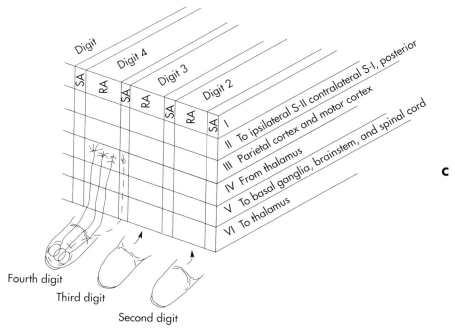

Fig. 2-69, cont'd. C, Area 3B shows somatotopic organization and columnar organization (for both body site and slowly adapting [*SA*] and rapidly adapting [*RA*] input pathways). Different cortical layers interconnect with different sites. (Adapted from Kandel ER, Schwartz JH: Principles of neuroscience, ed 2, New York, 1985, Elsevier Science Publishing.)

mingled at the periphery, the central processing pathways are very different, with different cortical regions subserving touch and taste sensation from the tongue.

The primary olfactory neurons, which are located in the olfactory epithelium, have a bipolar configuration. The peripheral fiber has chemosensitive terminals that respond to the chemical constituents of specific odors. The centrally projecting fibers form the olfactory nerve and synapse on neurons of the olfactory bulb. Some local processing and encoding of olfactory information are executed within the bulb.

The output cells of the bulb, mitral and tufted cells, give rise to the olfactory tract. The tract has five discrete projection zones, shown in Fig. 2-75. Projections to the amygdala are believed to be particularly important in the integration of visceral functions and in processing the emotional context and consequences of olfactory stimuli. Projections to the piriform cortex and entorhinal cortex are believed to be important in olfactory perception, as are the projections from entorhinal cortex to the orbitofrontal olfactory area. The entorhinal projections may also be an important substrate for defining the mnemonic significance of some olfactory stimuli.

Visual System[42-44]

There are two types of primary receptive cells in the visual system, both of which are specialized epithelial cells. One type of photoreceptor, known as a rod, is extremely sensitive to low-level illumination. Rods are believed to form the receptor substrate of night vision. The second type of photoreceptor, the cone, responds at higher levels of illumination. Cones are believed to be particularly important in object vision. There are three types of cone (red, green, and blue), each containing different photopigments that convey specific spectral sensitivities. As a result, cones are highly important in color vision.

Beyond the photoreceptors, the retina contains many cell types engaged in extensive preprocessing of visual data prior to their leaving the eye. Retinal ganglion cells are the output cells of the eye. There are three types of retinal ganglion cells: W, X, and Y. X cells have medium-size cell bodies and narrow dendritic fields. They are particularly important in fine spatial and color vision. The axons of X cells are slowly conducting, and they project to the parvocellular layers of the lateral geniculate nucleus of the thalamus. Y cells have large cell bodies, large dendritic arborizations, and very rapidly conducting axons. Y cells

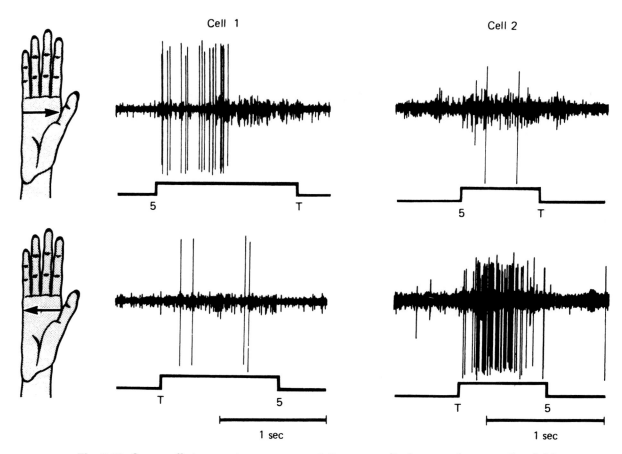

Fig. 2-70. Some cells in somatosensory association areas display complex receptive field properties including directional selectivity. Extracellular recordings from two cells with different selectivities are shown. (Adapted from Costanzo RM, Gardner EP: J Neurophysiol 43:1319-1341, 1980.)

project to the magnocellular layers of the lateral geniculate, and they are believed to be particularly important in the processing of visual motion. W cells have small cell bodies but very extended dendritic trees that receive input from an extended area of photoreceptors. These cells have slowly conducting axons that project mostly to the superior colliculus.

Ganglion cell axons leave the eye to form the optic nerve. At the optic chiasm, fibers originating from the nasal hemiretinae of each eye decussate to project to the contralateral side of the brain. Fibers from the temporal hemiretinae continue to project ipsilaterally. Because of the optics of the eye, objects in the right visual world form images on the nasal hemiretinae of the right eye and temporal hemiretinae of the left eye. All information from the right visual field is relayed to the contralateral left hemisphere. The converse situation is also true.

Anatomically separate pathways mediate visual perception and visual reflexes and orienting responses (Fig. 2-76). The tectum, in particular the superior colliculus and pretectal nuclei, receives input mainly from W cells. This midbrain pathway is particularly

important in mediating oculomotor reflexes and orienting the head and body to visual stimuli. Additional inputs to the region include those from primary visual cortex and the spinal cord. Efferents of the optic tectum project to pontine oculomotor centers and the lateral posterior and pulvinar nuclei of the thalamus. These thalamic nuclei project to association areas of the occipital, parietal, and temporal lobes.

The pathway to primary visual cortex mediates the perception of form, movement, and color. The axonal fibers of X and Y retinal ganglion cells project to the lateral geniculate nucleus (LGN) of the thalamus. The LGN is a six-layered structure (Fig. 2-77). The two innermost layers (1 and 2) contain large magnocellular relay neurons, whereas the four outermost layers contain small parvocellular cells. Y cells project to the magnocellular layers, whereas X cells project to parvocellular layers. The integrity of projections from each eye is maintained, the ipsilateral and contralateral eye projecting to different LGN laminae.

The axons of LGN output neurons form the optic radiations, which proceed to the primary visual cortex (Brodmann's area 17), located along the cal-

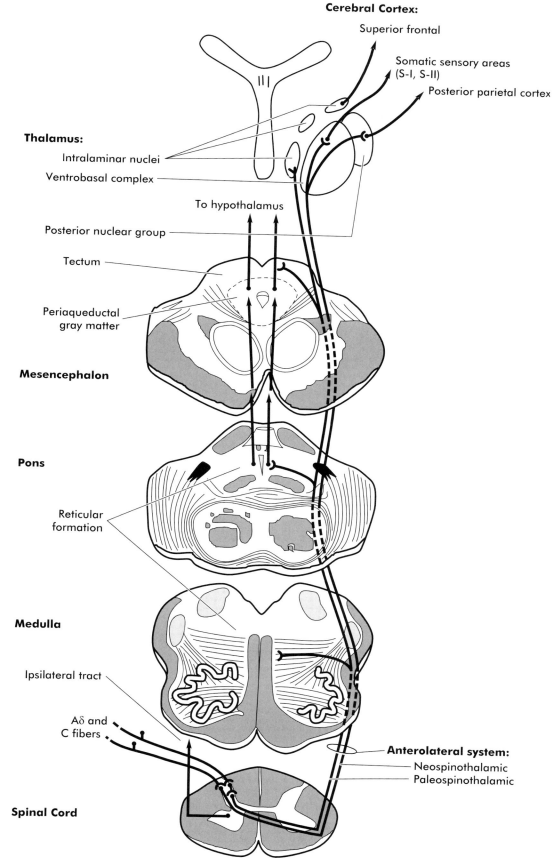

Fig. 2-71. Anterolateral spinothalamic somatosensory pathway for pain and temperature.

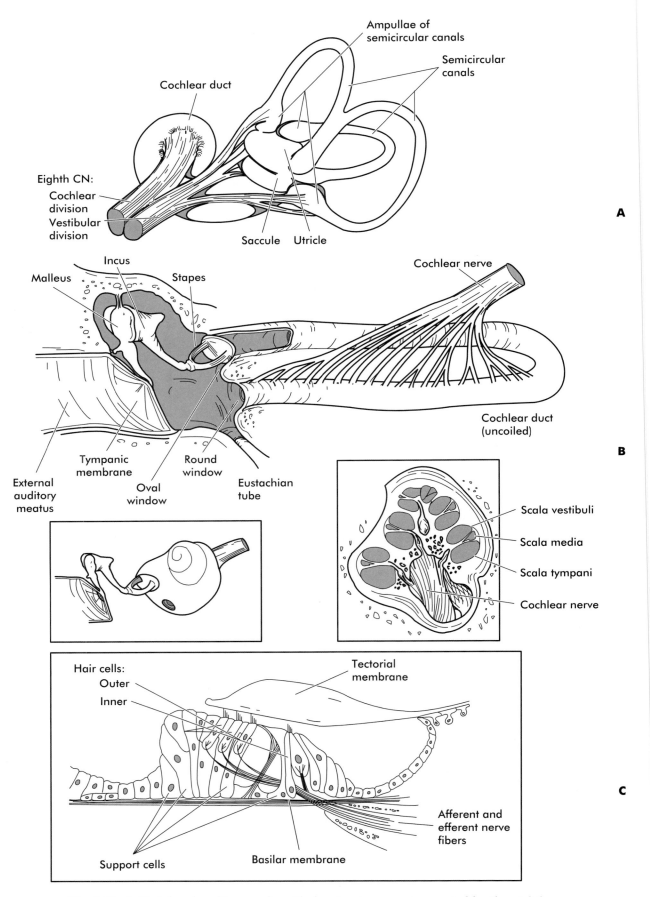

Fig. 2-72. A, Peripheral auditory and vestibular structures are innervated by the eighth cranial nerve. **B,** The middle and inner ear with straightened-out schematic view of the cochlea. **C,** Expanded view of section through the cochlear duct illustrating the organ of Corti.

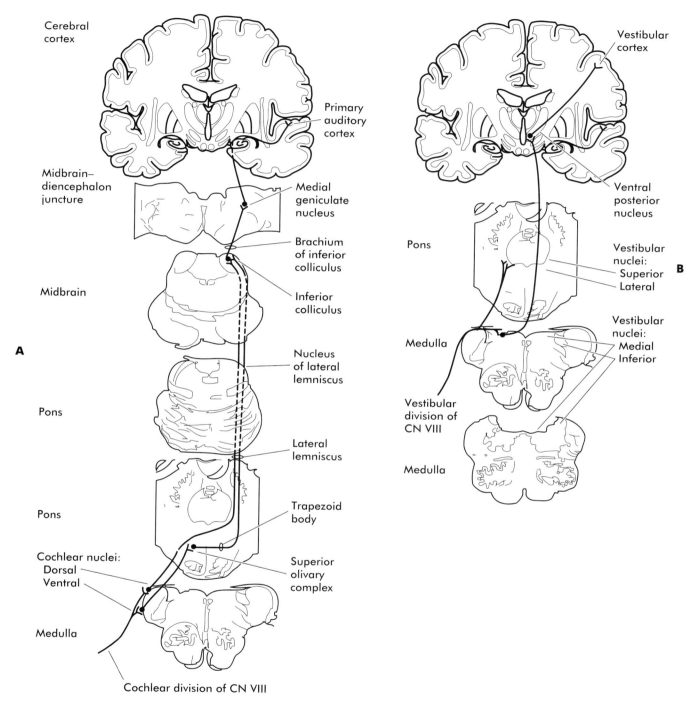

Cerebral cortex

Primary auditory cortex

Midbrain–diencephalon juncture

Medial geniculate nucleus

Brachium of inferior colliculus

Midbrain

Inferior colliculus

A

Nucleus of lateral lemniscus

Pons

Lateral lemniscus

Pons

Trapezoid body

Cochlear nuclei: Dorsal Ventral

Superior olivary complex

Medulla

Cochlear division of CN VIII

Vestibular cortex

Ventral posterior nucleus

Pons

Vestibular nuclei: Superior Lateral

B

Medulla

Vestibular nuclei: Medial Inferior

Vestibular division of CN VIII

Medulla

Fig. 2-73. A, Central projections of the auditory system. **B**, Central projections of the vestibular system.

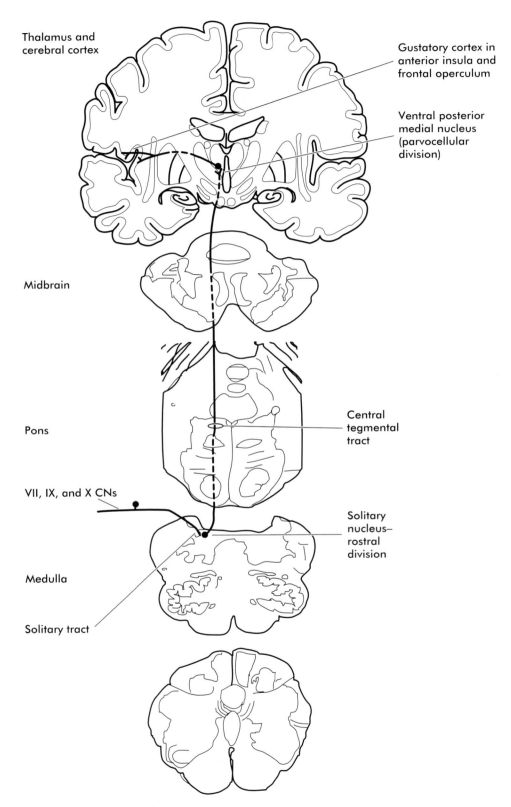

Thalamus and cerebral cortex

Gustatory cortex in anterior insula and frontal operculum

Ventral posterior medial nucleus (parvocellular division)

Midbrain

Pons

Central tegmental tract

VII, IX, and X CNs

Solitary nucleus– rostral division

Medulla

Solitary tract

Fig. 2-74. Central projections for gustatory system.

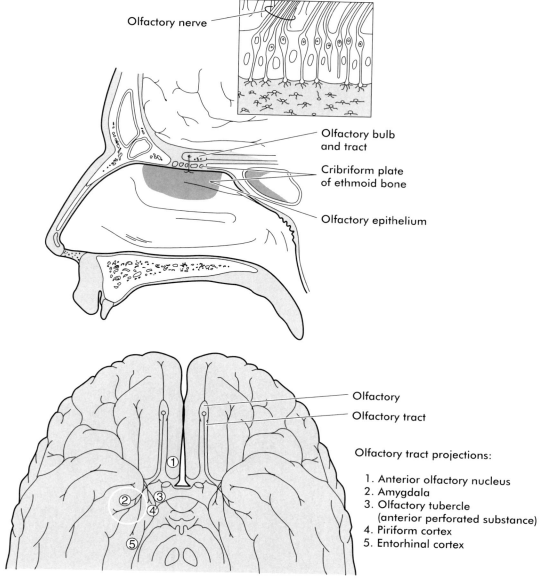

Fig. 2-75. A, Primary olfactory neurons are located in the olfactory epithelium in the nasal cavity. **B,** Central projections for olfaction.

carine fissure of the occipital lobe. Just as primary somatosensory cortex demonstrates somatotopy, primary visual cortex demonstrates retinotopy. That is, there is an orderly representation of the retina (and hence, visual space) at the cortical level (Fig. 2-78). The separation between ipsilateral and contralateral eye projections is also maintained as alternating ocular dominance columns (Fig. 2-79). Cells located along the margins of ocular dominance columns often show responsivity to both eyes. That is, binocular interactions begin to take place in primary visual cortex.

Retinal ganglion cells, LGN cells, and area 17 cells in layer IV (the primary thalamic projection zone) re-

spond best to small spots of light at particular points in visual space. The receptive field properties of visual neurons become increasingly complex as one moves up in the cortical hierarchy. For example, cells of the visual cortex in layers other than IV demonstrate orientation selectivity. That is, they respond best to a bar of light with a particular orientation. Several columns of cells are devoted to processing data from each region's space, and there is an orderly representation of orientation selectivity as one moves from one column to the next. Indeed, for each region's space, there is a slab of visual cortex (known as a hypercolumn) that contains a complete set of orientation columns and a pair of ocular dominance columns (Fig.

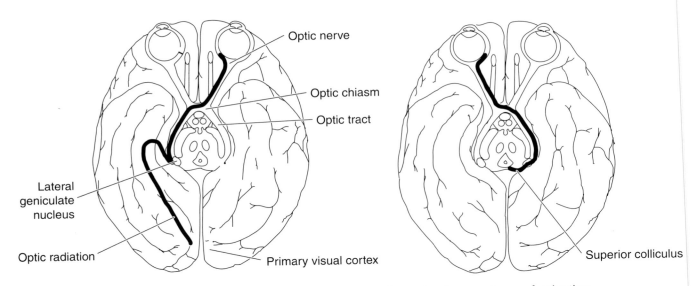

Fig. 2-76. Separate visual projection pathways mediate visual perception and orienting responses. Visual reflexes and orienting responses are regulated through the optic tectum (*left*), whereas perception is mediated by the geniculostriate pathway (*right*).

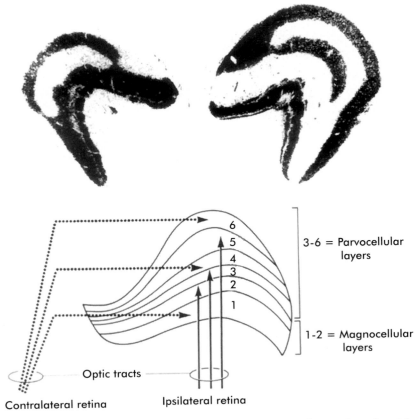

Fig. 2-77. The lateral geniculate nucleus is the main thalamic relay nucleus for vision. It is a six-layered structure. Each layer receives input from the contralateral or ipsilateral eye, with little intermixing. The innermost two layers contain large cells and are preferentially innervated by the fibers of Y-type retinal ganglion cells. The four outer layers have small cells innervated by the fibers of X-type retinal ganglion cells. (From Martin JH: Neuroanatomy: text and atlas, Norwalk, CT, 1989, Appleton & Lange.)

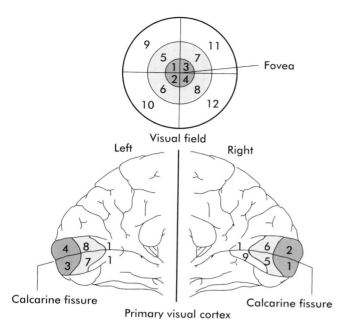

Fig. 2-78. Primary visual cortex located along the calcarine sulcus demonstrates retinotopic organization.

2-80). Within the hypercolumn there are some regions that are particularly sensitive to color properties and others particularly sensitive to movement. Pathways for the processing of color and form, on the one hand, and motion, on the other hand, begin to diverge at higher cortical levels.

Primary visual cortex sends projections to (1) subcortical nuclei including the superior colliculus and thalamus, (2) contralateral visual cortex (through the splenium of the corpus callosum), and (3) visual association area V2 (Brodmann's area 18). Most of what is known about the physiology and anatomy of processing in higher visual areas has been derived from work with Macaque monkeys. A schematic of some of the most important interconnected cortical elements is shown in Fig. 2-81. After area V3, there is a divergence of the processing stream into a temporal component and a parietal component. The temporal processing stream is particularly concerned with processing color and form information. The parietal stream is mostly concerned with processing information on visual motion and on extracting information on the spatial positions of objects. A large portion of

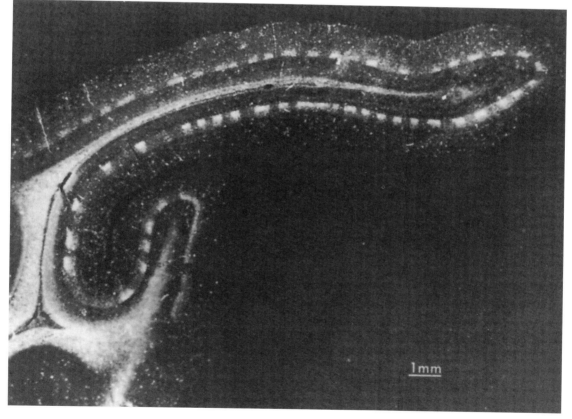

Fig. 2-79. This darkfield autoradiograph of the primary visual cortex in an adult monkey demonstrates the thalamic input to the cortex. Tritiated proline and fucose had been injected into the ipsilateral eye 2 weeks prior to histology. The section, cut through cortical layer IV, demonstrates alternating projection zones from the ipsilateral (*light*) and contralateral (*dark*) eye. (From Hubel DH, Weisel TN: Proc R Soc Lond [Biol] 198:1-59, 1977.)

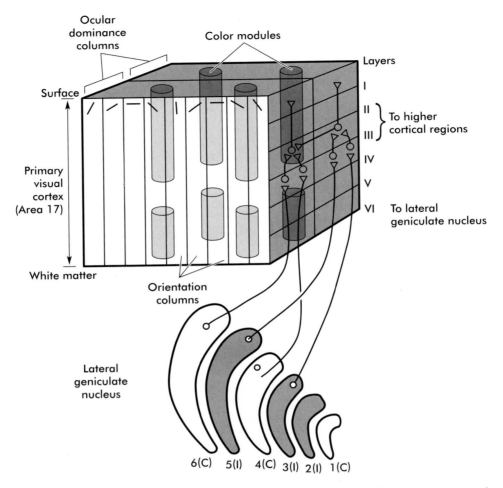

Fig. 2-80. The basic module of visual information processing for each location in space is the hypercolumn. It consists of a complete set of orientation columns and a pair of ocular dominance columns.

the primate brain is devoted to the processing of visual information, a testament to the importance of this function to survival of the organism. At high-level visual association areas of the brain, the properties of neurons can become quite specific. For example, some cells in the temporal lobe are preferentially stimulated by visual images of a hand, whereas others are selective for facelike stimuli.

Motor System[45-47]

Motor control is achieved via a complex series of interactions among the cortex, basal ganglia, thalamus, cerebellum, and brainstem nuclei. The nervous system has three classes of descending pathways: (1) motor control pathways, (2) sensory modulation pathways, and (3) autonomic nervous system control pathways. Motor control pathways originate in the cerebral cortex and brainstem, and they ultimately convey information to neurons that innervate the skeletal musculature. Sensory modulation pathways also originate in the cortex and brainstem, but they term-

inate on interneurons in the dorsal horn. The descending pathways that regulate functions of the autonomic nervous system mostly originate in the hypothalamus and they terminate on brainstem and spinal cord parasympathetic and sympathetic nuclei.

The major descending pathways involved in motor control are summarized in Table 2-4. The lateral corticospinal tract and the rubrospinal tract are pathways that play the most important roles in the control of voluntary limb movements. Fig. 2-82 illustrates the descending projections. The lateral corticospinal tract is the major control pathway. Its descending upper motor neuron fibers originate from the primary motor cortex of the precentral gyrus (Brodmann's area 4) and supplementary motor regions in Brodmann's area 6 (Fig. 2-83). The precentral gyrus demonstrates topographic organization (Fig. 2-84), with electrical stimulation of a particular point on the cortical surface eliciting activity in a small muscle group.

The rubrospinal tract originates in the magnocellular division of the midbrain red nucleus. The

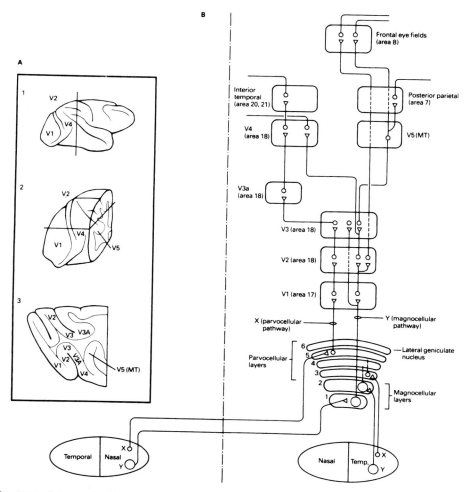

Fig. 2-81. Schematic diagram of the visual projections from the retina to visual cortical areas, as determined by neuroanatomic studies with macaque monkeys. After area V3, the cortical stream bifurcates into temporal and parietal pathways. The temporal pathway is believed to be mostly concerned with color and object detail, whereas the parietal stream is mostly concerned with movement and localization of objects in visual space. (Adapted from Van Essen DC: Annu Rev Neurosci 2:227-263, 1979.)

normal functioning of the rubrospinal tract is not well understood, but it is a clinically important pathway because it is thought to subserve some residual voluntary motor function after damage to the lateral corticospinal tract.

Four medially descending pathways control axial and girdle musculature: (1) the ventral corticospinal tract, (2) the reticulospinal tracts, (3) the vestibulospinal tracts, and (4) the tectospinal tract (Fig. 2-85). These pathways demonstrate bilateral organization, in contrast to the contralateral organization of the rubrospinal and lateral corticospinal tracts.

The ventral corticospinal tract originates in motor and supplementary motor cortex. There are two separate reticulospinal tracts, one originating in the pons, the other in the medulla. They descend predominantly in the ipsilateral spinal cord and help to regulate posture and locomotion. The tectospinal tract,

originating in the deep layers of the superior colliculus, is believed to participate in the coordination of head movements with eye movements, through control of the muscles of the neck, shoulder, and upper trunk. The lateral vestibulospinal track originates in Deiters' nucleus. It is an ipsilateral projection system believed to play a role in the maintenance of balance. The medial vestibulospinal tract arises from the medial vestibular nucleus and is involved in the control of musculature that mediates head position.

Primary motor cortex receives input from several brain regions, including the thalamus (which provides a link to the basal ganglia and cerebellum), supplementary and premotor areas, and somatosensory cortex. The subcortical interactions were discussed in previous sections on the cerebellum and basal ganglia, and they are summarized in Fig. 2-86. Fig. 2-87 shows some of the cortical components believed to be

Table 2-4. Projection systems and the function of the spinal cord

Tract	Site of origin	Decussation	Spinal cord column	Site of termination	Function
Cerebral cortex					
Corticospinal lateral	Areas 6,4,1,2,3,5,7	Crossed-pyramidal	Lateral	Dorsal horn, lateral intermediate zone, ventral horn	Sensory control, voluntary movement (limb muscles)
Ventral	Areas 6,4	Uncrossed*	Ventral	Medial intermediate zone, ventral horn	Voluntary movement (axial muscles)
Corticobulbar	Areas 6,4,1,2,3,5,7	Crossed and uncrossed†	Brainstem only	Cranial nerve sensory and motor nuclei, reticular formation	Sensory control, voluntary movement (cranial muscles)
Brainstem					
Rubrospinal	Red nucleus (magnocellular)	Ventral tegmentum	Lateral	Lateral intermediate zone and ventral horn	Voluntary movement, limb muscles
Vestibulospinal					
Lateral	Deiters' nucleus (lateral vestibular nucleus)	Ipsilateral*	Ventral	Medial intermediate zone and ventral horn	Balance
Medial	Medial vestibular nucleus	Bilateral	Ventral	Medial intermediate zone and ventral horn	Head position/neck muscles
Reticulospinal					
Pontine	Pontine reticular formation	Ipsilateral*	Ventral	Medial intermediate zone and ventral horn	Involuntary movement, axial and limb muscles
Medullary	Medullary reticular formation	Ipsilateral*	Ventrolateral	Medial intermediate zone and ventral horn	Involuntary movement, axial and limb muscles
Tectospinal	Deep superior colliculus	Dorsal tegmentum	Ventral	Medial intermediate zone and ventral horn	Coordinates neck with eye movements

*While these tracts descend ipsilaterally, they terminate on interneurons that decussate in the ventral commissure and thus influence axial musculature bilaterally.
†The projections to the hypoglossal nucleus are crossed, those to the part of the facial nucleus that innervates upper facial muscles are bilateral, and those to the lower facial muscles are contralateral. Projections to the trigeminal motor nucleus are bilateral.

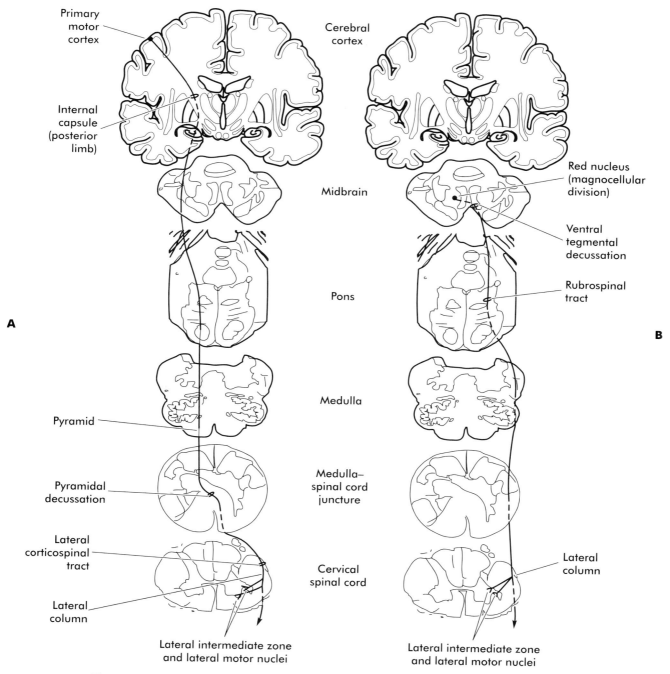

Fig. 2-82. Descending motor projections for control of voluntary movement. **A**, Lateral corticospinal tract; **B**, rubrospinal tract.

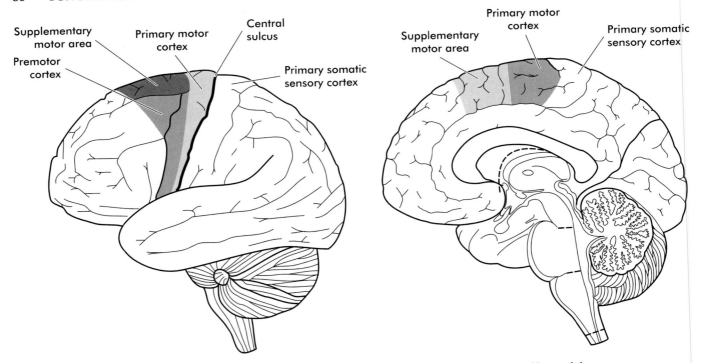

Fig. 2-83. Lateral and medial view showing cortical areas that give rise to the fibers of the lateral corticospinal tract.

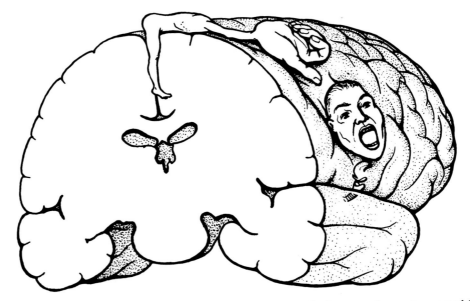

Fig. 2-84. Primary motor cortex, like other primary cortical areas, shows topographic organization. (From Carpenter MB: Human neuroanatomy, ed 7, Baltimore, 1976, Williams & Wilkins.)

involved in the planning of voluntary movements. Premotor cortex is especially important in reaching behaviors and sensory guidance of movements. Supplementary motor cortex is especially active in the execution and planning of complex sequential movements. Parietal areas are believed to provide spatial information for targeted movements.

Cognitive Systems[48-50]

Most of what is known about cognitive systems in the brain has been extrapolated from data on the cognitive consequences of brain damage and, more recently, from neuroimaging studies (especially PET) of normal subjects performing cognitive tasks. These cognitive maps are undergoing constant updating

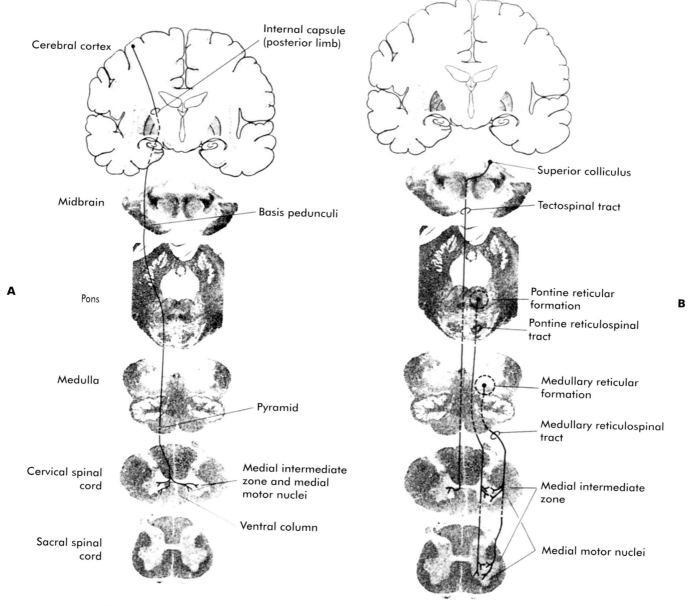

Fig. 2-85. Descending pathways for control of axial and girdle musculature. **A,** Ventral corticospinal tract; **B,** reticulospinal and tectospinal tracts.

Continued.

and revision so only the dominant regions involved in the most studied cognitive processes will be summarized here. Of particular interest are subsystems subserving language, event-memory, and emotions, because these are compromised in a wide range of clinical conditions.

The dominant cortical regions involved in linguistic processing are fairly well defined (Fig. 2-88). Broca's area, located in the inferior frontal operculum, is particularly important in language production. In contrast, Wernicke's area is important in understanding language and in imparting meaning to speech. Lesions of these and related regions can produce language disturbances known as aphasias. Some of the clinical characteristics of various aphasic syndromes are summarized. Damage to the angular gyrus can disrupt visual-verbal processes (such as object naming and reading), as illustrated in Fig. 2-89. Subcortical areas including the basal ganglia and pulvinar are also believed to be important in linguistic function.

One of the most important observations in neuropsychology is that the two cerebral hemispheres do not play equivalent roles in the support of language.

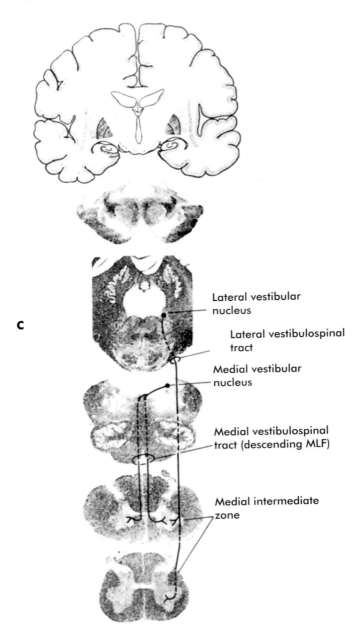

C

Lateral vestibular nucleus

Lateral vestibulospinal tract

Medial vestibular nucleus

Medial vestibulospinal tract (descending MLF)

Medial intermediate zone

Fig. 2-85, cont'd. C, Vestibulospinal tracts. (From Martin JH: Neuroanatomy: text and atlas, Norwalk, CT, 1989, Appleton & Lange.)

In the majority of the population the left hemisphere is dominant for language function. That is, whereas damage to inferior frontal cortex on the left produces a severe nonfluent aphasia, comparable damage on the right results in little impairment. Structural asymmetries, particularly in the planum temporale, are believed to be part of the neuroanatomic basis for this type of hemispheric specialization (Fig. 2-90).

There are many different types of memory, ranging from simple habituation to memory for skilled movements (e.g., how to drive a car) to memory for specific events (e.g., a recently heard phone number). Differ-ent neuronal mechanisms and systems subserve each. Clinically, disruption of event-memory is the most common form of memory disturbance.

Structures of the limbic system are particularly important in event memory. For example, bilateral damage to the hippocampus and its projection path-ways can cause severe amnestic syndromes. Fig. 2-91 illustrates the interconnectivity of regions involved in visual event-memory. Fig. 2-92 shows a comparable circuit consisting of the main structures believed to participate in tactile learning. Note the modality-specific and nonspecific parts of these circuits. It is presumed that long-term memories are stored in cellular networks within modality-specific association areas, but this has yet to be demonstrated conclusively.

The neural substrates of emotion are complex, involving interactions between cortical and subcortical regions including the limbic system and hypothala-mus. Of particular note are several cortical areas shown in Fig. 2-93.

CEREBRAL VASCULATURE[51,52]
Arterial Supply

The principal source of nourishment for the ner-vous system is glucose. Through glycolysis and the associated tricarboxylic acid cycle, glucose is metabo-lized and energy is generated and stored in the form of adenosine triphosphate (ATP). The nervous system does not store glucose in appreciable amounts, so even short-term disruption of the availability of glucose can severely disrupt brain processes. Glucose and oxygen are delivered to the brain through the cerebrovascular system. Disorders of brain vasculature are one of the most significant causes of neural dysfunction, so an understanding of vascular anatomy is important. Also, as described later, several neuroimaging techniques take advantage of the fact that changes in the synaptic activity of a region induce changes in regional cerebral blood flow.

The vertebral and carotid arteries supply blood to the central nervous system (Fig. 2-94). The inter-nal carotid arteries provide the anterior circula-tion while the vertebral arteries supply blood for the posterior circulation. At the level of the medulla, the right and left vertebral arteries merge to form the basilar artery, which ascends along the ventral surface of the brain.

The brainstem receives blood from the posterior circulation. Three cerebral arteries supply blood to the diencephalon, basal ganglia, and cerebral hemi-spheres. Two of these, the anterior and middle cerebral arteries, derive from the anterior circulation, whereas the third, the posterior cerebral artery, receives blood from the posterior circulation. The anterior and posterior circulation systems are interconnected at two locations: (1) on the ventral surface of the diencepha-

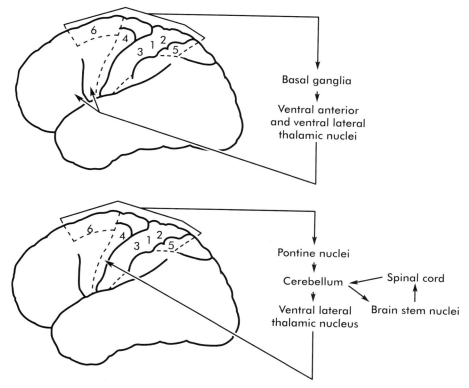

Fig. 2-86. Schematic of cortical interactions with basal ganglia and cerebellum in the control of movement.

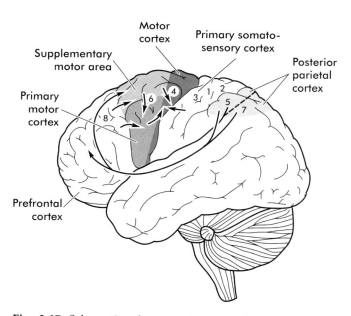

Fig. 2-87. Schematic of some of the cortical interactions believed to be critical in the planning of voluntary movements. Although the arrows are unidirectional, the interconnecting pathways are all reciprocal.

lon, where branches of the carotid and basilar arteries form an anastomotic network of arteries known as the circle of Willis (Fig. 2-94), and (2) at the terminal ends of the cerebral arteries, on the convexity of the cerebral cortex.

Fig. 2-94 shows the derivation of the three cerebral arteries. Fig. 2-95 shows their projections on the lateral and midsagittal surfaces. The anterior cerebral artery supplies blood to the dorsal and medial portions of the frontal and parietal lobes and also to the anterior portions of the hypothalamus. The middle cerebral artery has an exceptionally large projection zone. It courses along the surface of the insular cortex and the inner opercular surfaces of the frontal, temporal, and parietal lobes before emerging on the lateral convexity to supply lateral aspects of the frontal, temporal, and parietal cortical regions. The posterior cerebral artery supplies the occipital lobes, thalamus, and caudal hypothalamus. Branches from the internal carotid and each of the three cerebral arteries supply the basal ganglia. Fig. 2-96 shows the arterial territories in axial and coronal cross sections. Fig. 2-97 shows the full complexity and density of the arterial circulation.

Venous Drainage

Venous drainage of the spinal cord and caudal medulla is achieved by a direct route to the systemic circulation. In contrast, most cerebral structures are

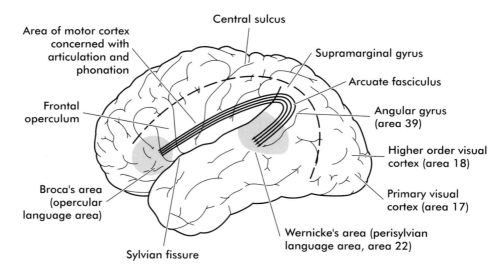

Fig. 2-88. Schematic showing the location of cortical regions responsible language. (Adapted from England MA, Wakley J: Color atlas of brain and spinal cord: an introduction to normal neuroanatomy, St. Louis, 1991, Mosby.)

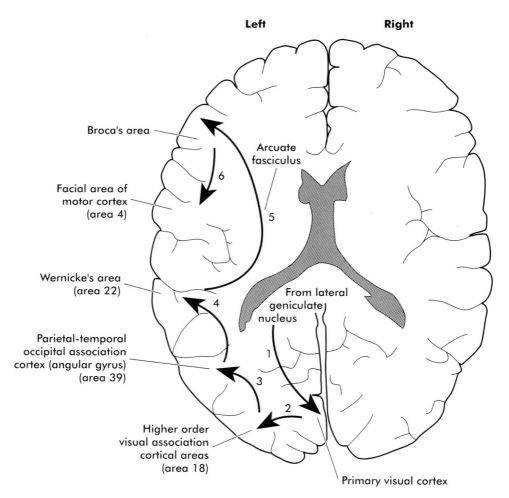

Fig. 2-89. Schematic of putative pathway for naming of visual objects.

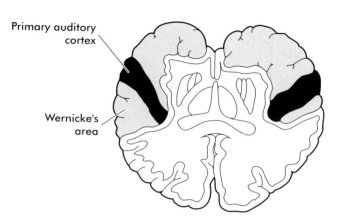

Primary auditory cortex

Wernicke's area

Fig. 2-90. The two cerebral hemispheres are asymmetric. The planum temporale contains Wernicke's area and is generally larger in the left cerebral hemisphere. This is believed to be one of the neuroanatomic substrates of left hemisphere specialization for language.

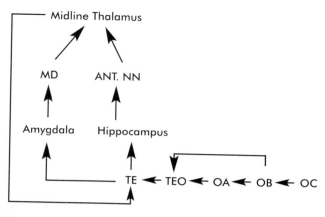

Fig. 2-91. The proposed pathway for visual event–memory involves an interaction between visual areas and the limbic system. *OC*, Primary visual cortex of the occipital lobe; *OB* and *OA*, prestriate visual association areas of the occipital lobe; *TEO* and *TE*, visual association areas of the temporal lobe; *MD*, medial dorsal nucleus of the thalamus; *ANT NN*, anterior nucleus of the thalamus. (Adapted from Mishkin M: Phil Trans R Soc Lond [B101] 298:85-95, 1982; from Roland PE: Brain activation, New York, 1993, Wiley-Liss.)

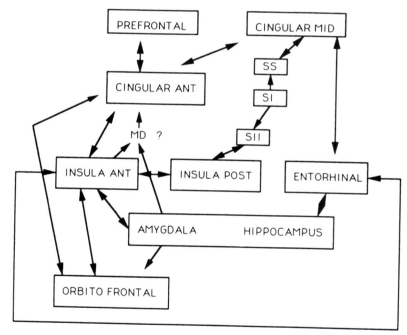

Fig. 2-92. Putative neural circuit for regulation of tactile learning. (From Roland PE: Brain activation, New York, 1993, Wiley-Liss.)

drained by veins that empty into dural sinuses. The dural sinuses are a collection of large channels located between layers of dura mater, one of three membranous coverings of the central nervous system. These sinuses function as low-pressure channels through which venous blood flows back to the systemic circulation.

Venous drainage of the cerebral hemispheres is provided by superficial and deep veins (Fig. 2-98).

The superficial veins arise from the cortex and underlying white matter and drain into the superior sagittal and straight sinus. The superior sagittal sinus runs along the midline of the cranial cavity at the superior margin of the falx cerebri formed by dura in the interhemispheric fissure (Figs. 2-99 and 2-100). The great cerebral vein of Galen collects venous blood from many smaller deep veins and drains into the straight sinus.

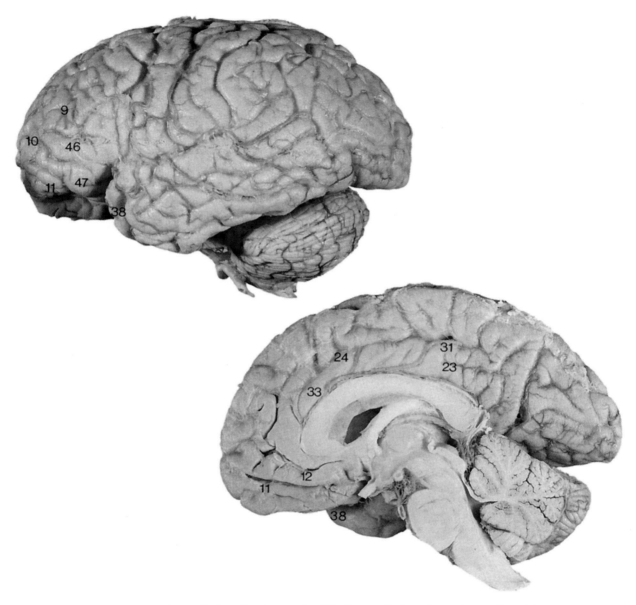

Fig. 2-93. Cortical areas believed to be involved in the regulation of emotion. (Adapted from England MA, Wakley J: Color atlas of brain and spinal cord: an introduction to normal neuroanatomy, St Louis, 1991, Mosby.)

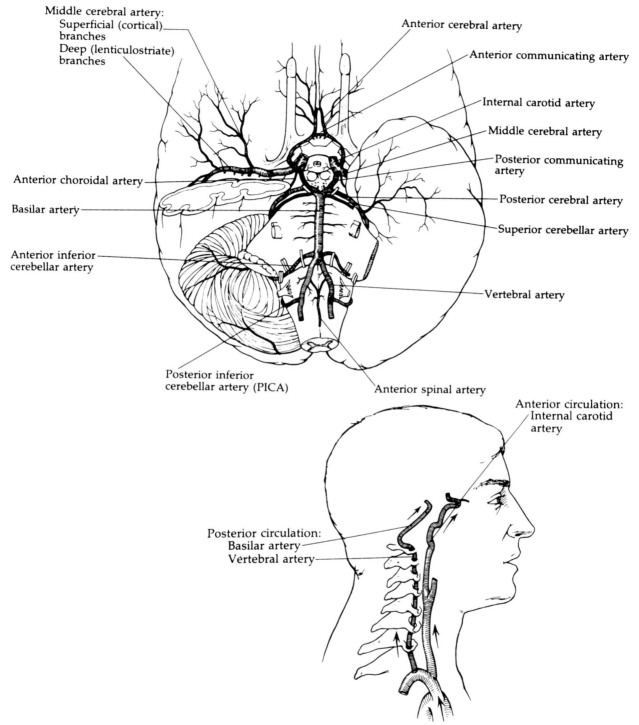

Fig. 2-94. Anterior and posterior divisions of cerebral circulation arise from the carotid and vertebral arteries. (From Martin JH: Neuroanatomy: text and atlas, Norwalk, CT, 1989, Appleton & Lange.)

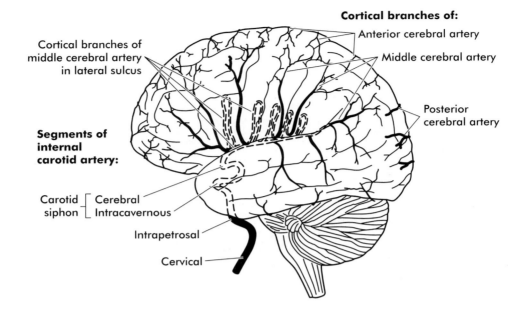

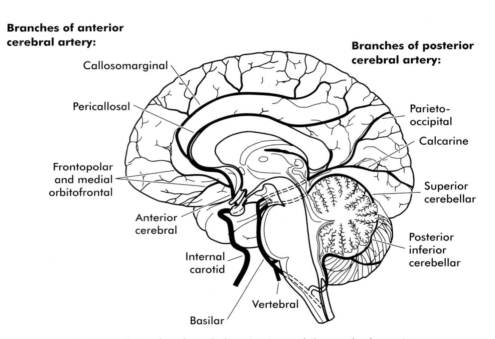

Fig. 2-95. Lateral and medial projections of the cerebral arteries.

Regulatory Mechanisms

Mean cerebral blood flow is regulated by changes in arterial pressure and cerebral flow resistance. Arterial pressure is regulated by circulatory reflexes that are mediated by specialized receptors (baroreceptors) located in the aortic arch and carotid sinuses. The firing rate of baroreceptors is a function of blood pressure. When the pressure is high, the baroreceptor reflex causes inhibition of sympathetic adrenergic efferents to the cardiovascular system and reflex stimulation of the vagus nerve. These actions lead to

a decrease in pressures. When the pressure is low, these same mechanisms provide for up-regulation of the pressure.

Several factors modulate cerebral flow resistance. One factor is blood viscosity, a function of the concentration of red blood cells. Vasoconstriction induced by the sympathetic adrenergic system can also regulate blood flow, especially in hypertensive states.

Local metabolic factors also influence blood flow. Decreases in pH or oxygen concentration cause vasodilation and an increase in blood flow, as does an

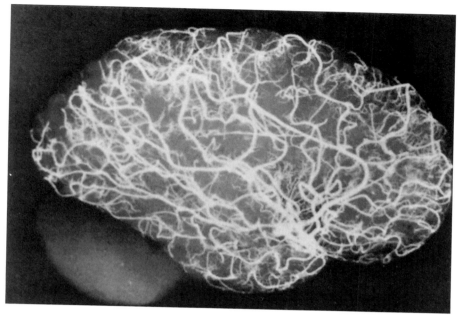

Fig. 2-96. Roentgenogram of a fresh cadaver brain where the anterior, middle, and posterior cerebral arteries have been injected with a radiopaque material. (Courtesy Dr. Harry A. Kaplan; from Carpenter MB: Human neuroanatomy, ed 7, Baltimore, 1976, Williams & Wilkins.)

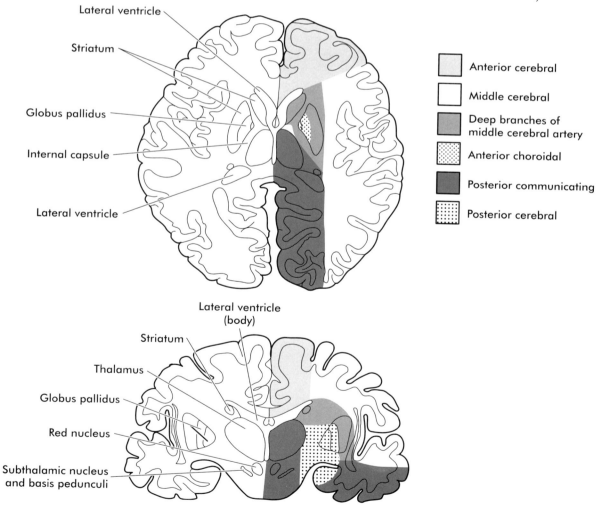

Fig. 2-97. Transverse and coronal sections showing territories of various cerebral arteries.

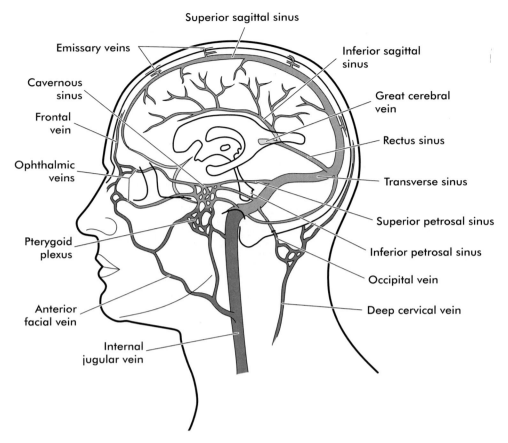

Fig. 2-98. Venous system of the brain. (From Carpenter MB: Human neuroanatomy, ed 7, Baltimore, 1976, Williams & Wilkins.)

increase in local carbon dioxide concentration. Increases in the local concentration of potassium ions and adenosine may also cause vasodilation.

Coupling of Neurophysiologic Activity with Cerebral Metabolism and Blood Flow

The sodium-potassium pump of neurons is the dominant consumer of energy within neurons. The activity of the pump is regulated by several factors, including intracellular sodium concentration. Postsynaptic activation of cells, therefore, leads to an increase in pump activity and an increase in energy/glucose demand. Hence, the regional cerebral metabolic rate is closely coupled to the regional synaptic activity. When the metabolic rate and demand for glucose rise, the metabolic blood flow regulatory mechanisms described above cause an increase in regional cerebral blood flow. Regional blood flow is thus indirectly coupled to the level of regional neural activity. Several neuroimaging techniques (PET being the most notable) take advantage of this observation. Using positron-emitting compounds such as O15 water, regional blood flow can be measured. As described in subsequent chapters, through a comparison of stimulated and nonstimulated conditions, determining those brain regions that show stimulation-induced changes in blood flow is relatively straightforward. To the extent that this accurately reflects changes in regional cerebral metabolic rate and the underlying neuronal activity, this is a powerful method for assessing brain function.

FUNCTIONAL NEUROIMAGING

After a discussion of methods for noninvasive imaging of brain structure, the remaining chapters in this book will focus on a detailed discussion of techniques for noninvasive imaging of brain function, with an emphasis on methodologic considerations, and clinical applications.

From the preceding discussion on the structure and function of the nervous system, it should be apparent that there are three basic functional neuroimaging strategies. One strategy directly monitors brain electrophysiology by measuring the electrical potential distribution caused on the scalp surface (EEG) or by measuring the neuromagnetic fields generated by intracellular currents (MEG). The major advantages of this strategy are (1) their completely noninvasive

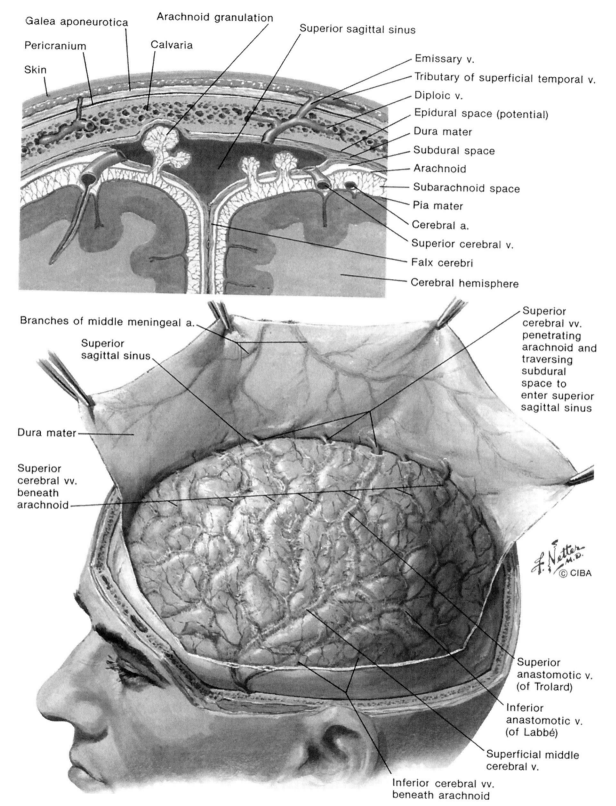

Fig. 2-99. Spaces between sheaths of dura mater form the venous sinuses. (From Netter FH: The CIBA collection of medical illustrations, Vol 1: Nervous system, Part I: Anatomy and physiology, West Caldwell, NJ, 1983, CIBA Pharmaceutical.)

Continued.

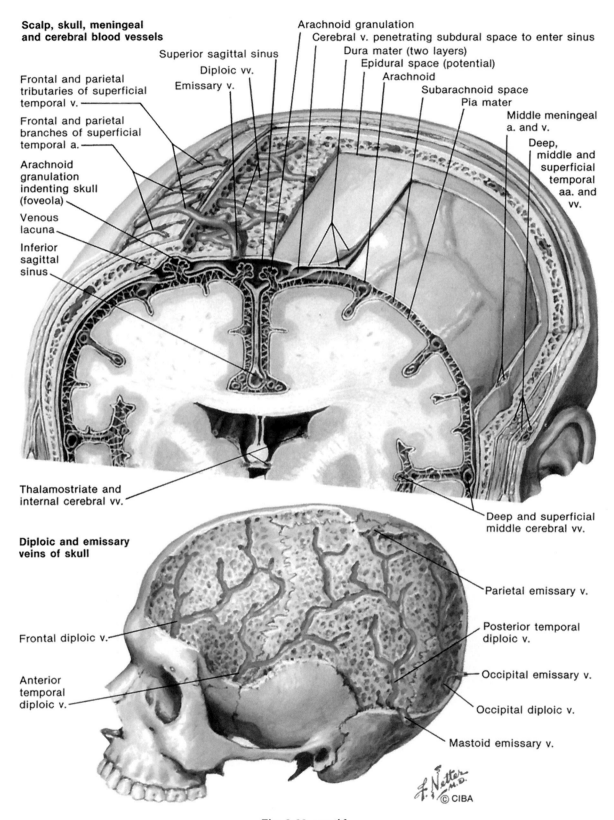

Scalp, skull, meningeal and cerebral blood vessels

Arachnoid granulation

Cerebral v. penetrating subdural space to enter sinus

Superior sagittal sinus

Diploic vv.

Emissary v.

Dura mater (two layers)

Epidural space (potential)

Arachnoid

Subarachnoid space

Pia mater

Frontal and parietal tributaries of superficial temporal v.

Frontal and parietal branches of superficial temporal a.

Arachnoid granulation indenting skull (foveola)

Venous lacuna

Inferior sagittal sinus

Middle meningeal a. and v.

Deep, middle and superficial temporal aa. and vv.

Thalamostriate and internal cerebral vv.

Deep and superficial middle cerebral vv.

Diploic and emissary veins of skull

Parietal emissary v.

Posterior temporal diploic v.

Occipital emissary v.

Occipital diploic v.

Mastoid emissary v.

Frontal diploic v.

Anterior temporal diploic v.

Fig. 2-99, cont'd.

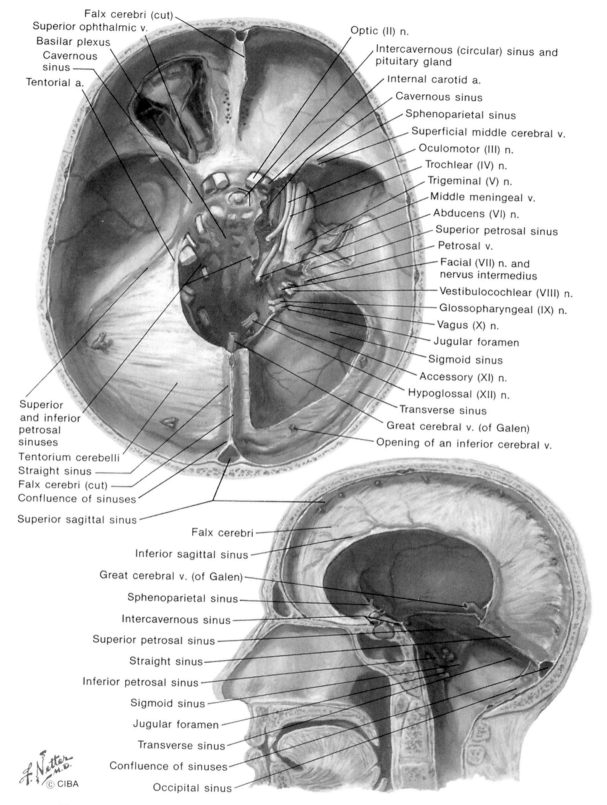

Fig. 2-100. Locations of venous sinuses. (From Netter FH: The CIBA collection of medical illustrations, Vol 1: Nervous system, Part I: Anatomy and physiology, West Caldwell, NJ, 1983, CIBA Pharmaceutical.)

nature, (2) the direct measurement of the physiologic events of interest, and (3) the excellent temporal resolution. The major drawback of this method is the difficulty in spatial localization of the neural populations of interest. When many brain regions are active in synchrony, electromagnetic inverse modeling procedures quickly become intractable.

The second strategy monitors regional cerebral metabolic rate. This strategy, employed by PET and SPECT, provides for good spatial localization of active regions. However, the strategy is an indirect one. It generally involves introduction of radioactive tracers, and it provides poor temporal resolution of brain activity, a critical disadvantage in trying to decipher the brain-code.

The third neuroimaging strategy monitors the local cerebral blood flow and volume. This strategy, employed by PET and FMRI, provides good spatial localization of active regions. However, the thing being measured—blood flow—is at least two steps removed from the thing of interest—electrophysiologic activity. Caution is therefore demanded in the interpretation of data using this strategy, especially when assessing patient populations where disease or medication can alter the coupling between regional metabolism and regional blood flow. Nevertheless, in certain situations these techniques can be very powerful.

As illustrated in the following chapters, these considerations can be used to help decide which technique, or combination of techniques, is most appropriate for clinical evaluation of specific patient populations. It is a significant achievement, in the fourth year of the decade of the brain, that through an integration of structural and functional neuroimaging techniques, elucidation of the brain-code during normal function and disease may now be possible.

REFERENCES

1. Blakemore C: Mechanisms of the mind, Cambridge, 1977, Cambridge University Press.
2. Sperry RW: Neurology and the mind brain problem, Am Sci 40:291-312, 1952.
3. Cook ND: The brain code, London, 1987, Methuen.
4. Spurzheim JG: Phrenology, or the doctrine of the mind, London, 1825, Knight.
5. Peters A, Palay SL, Webster HdeF: The fine structure of the nervous system: the neurons and supporting cells, Philadelphia, 1976, Saunders.
6. Bullock TH, Orkand R, Grinnell A: Introduction to nervous systems, San Francisco, 1977, Freeman.
7. Carpenter MB: Human neuroanatomy, ed 7, Baltimore, 1976, Williams & Wilkins.
8. Singer SJ, Nicholson GL: The fluid mosaic model of the structure of cell membranes, Science 175:720-724, 1972.
9. Ochs S: Axoplasmic transport and its relation to other nerve functions, New York, 1982, Wiley.
10. Bunge RP: Glial cells and the central myelin sheath, Physiol Rev 48:197-251, 1968.
11. Kandel ER, Schwartz JH: Principles of neuroscience, ed 2, New York, 1985, Elsevier Science Publishing.
12. Hodgkin AL: The conduction of the nerve impulse, Springfield, IL, 1964, Charles C Thomas.
13. Kandel ER, editor: Handbook of physiology. Vol 1: The nervous system. part 1, Bethesda, MD, 1977, American Physiological Society.
14. Eccles JC: The physiology of the synapse, Berlin, 1964, Springer.
15. Mata M, Fink DJ, Gainer H, et al: Activity-dependent energy metabolism in rat posterior pituitary primarily reflects sodium pump activity, J Neurochem 34(1):213-215, 1980.
16. Regan D: Human brain electrophysiology, New York, 1989, Elsevier.
17. Halliday AM, editor: Evoked potentials in clinical testing, London, 1993, Churchill Livingston.
18. Lindsley DB: Average evoked potentials—achievements, failures, and prospects. In Donchin E, Lindsley DB, editors: Average evoked potentials. methods. results and evaluations, Washington DC, 1969, NASA.
19. Hughes JR: EEG in clinical practice, Boston, 1982, Butterworth.
20. Lewine JD: Clinical electroencephalography and evoked potentials. In Orrison WW Jr, editor: Functional brain imaging, St Louis, 1995, Mosby.
21. Lewine JD: Magnetoencephalography and magnetic source imaging. In Orrison WW Jr, editor: Functional brain imaging, St Louis, 1995, Mosby.
22. Hari R, Ilmoniemi RJ: Cerebral magnetic fields, CRC Crit Rev Biomed Engineer 14:93-126, 1986.
23. Williamson SJ, Kaufman L: Analysis of neuromagnetic signals. In Gevins AS, Redmond A, editors: Handbook of electroencephalography and clinical neurophysiology, vol 1: Methods and analysis of brain electrical signals, Amsterdam, 1987, Elsevier.
24. Hari R: The neuromagnetic method in the study of the human auditory cortex. In Grandori F, Hoke M, Romani GL, editors: Auditory evoked magnetic fields and electric potentials, Basel, Switzerland, 1990, Karger.
25. Lewine JD: Neuromagnetic techniques for the noninvasive analysis of brain function. In Freeman SE, Fukushima E, Greene ER, editors: Noninvasive techniques in biology and medicine, San Francisco, 1991, San Francisco Press.
26. Cowan WM: The development of the brain, Sci Am 241:112-133, 1979.
27. Jacobson M: Developmental neurobiology, ed 2, New York, 1978, Plenum Press.
28. Brodmann K: Vergleichende Lokalisationslehre der Grosshirnrinde in ihren Prinzipien dargestellt auf Grund des Zellenbaues, Leipzig, 1909, Barth.
29. Netter FH: The CIBA collection of medical illustrations. Vol 1: Nervous system. Part 1: Anatomy and physiology, West Caldwell, NJ, 1983, CIBA Pharmaceutical.
30. Martin JH: Neuroanatomy: text and atlas, Norwalk, CT, 1989, Appleton & Lange.
31. Heimer L: The human brain and spinal cord. functional neuroanatomy and dissection guide, New York, 1983, Springer-Verlag.
32. Nolte J: The human brain: an introduction to its functional anatomy, ed 3, St Louis, 1993, Mosby.
33. DeArmond SJ, Fusco MM, Dewey MM: Structure of the human brain: a photographic atlas, ed 3, New York, 1989, Oxford University Press.
34. Kolb B, Whishaw IQ: Fundamentals of human neuropsychology, San Francisco, 1980, Freeman.
35. England MA, Wakely J: Color atlas of the brain and spinal cord: an introduction to normal neuroanatomy, St Louis, 1991, Mosby.

36. Iggo A, Andreas KH: Morphology of cutaneous receptors, Annu Rev Neurosci 5:1-31, 1982.

37. Mountcastle VB: The view from within: pathways to the study of perception, Johns Hopkins Med J 136:109-131, 1975.

38. Iggo A, editor: Handbook of sensory physiology. Vol 2: somatosensory system, New York, 1973, Springer.

39. Costanzo RM, Gardner EP: A quantitative analysis of responses of direction-sensitive neurons in somatosensory cortex of awake monkeys, J Neurophysiol 43:1319-1341.

40. Darian-Smith I, editor: Handbook of physiology, Section 1: The nervous system. Vol Ill: Sensory processes, Bethesda, MD, 1984, American Physiological Society.

41. Finger TE, Silver WL, editors: The neurobiology of taste and smell, New York, 1987, Wiley.

42. Hubel DH, Wiesel TN: Brain mechanisms of vision, Sci Am 241:150-162, 1979.

43. Van Essen DC: Visual areas of the mammalian cerebral cortex, Annu Rev Neurosci 2:227-263, 1979.

44. DeYoe EA, Van Essen DC: Concurrent processing streams in monkey visual cortex, TINS 11:219-226, 1987.

45. Brooks VB: The neural basis of motor control, New York, 1986, Oxford University Press.

46. Ito M: The cerebellum and neural control, New York, 1984, Raven Press.

47. Brooks VB, editor: Handbook of physiology. Section 1: The nervous system. Vol II: Motor control, Bethesda, MD, 1981, American Physiological Society.

48. Damasio AR, Geschwind NR: The neural basis of language, Annu Rev Neurosci 7:127-147, 1984.

49. Mishkin M: A memory system in the monkey, Phil Trans R Soc Lond [B] 298:85-95, 1982.

50. Plum F, editor: Handbook of physiology. Section 1: The nervous system; Vol V. Higher functions of the brain, Bethesda, MD, 1981, American Physiological Society.

51. Meyer JS, editor: The anatomy and pathology of cerebral vasculature, New York, 1975, Spectrum.

52. Roland P: Brain activation, New York, 1993, Wiley.

Clinical Brain Imaging: Computerized Axial Tomography and Magnetic Resonance Imaging

William W. Orrison, Jr.
John A. Sanders

The introduction of computerized axial tomography (CAT or CT) and magnetic resonance imaging (MRI or MR) into the field of brain imaging has resulted in dramatic improvements in the evaluation of suspected intracranial abnormalities. These two techniques now comprise the majority of clinical brain images generated throughout the world. In order to appreciate the clinical significance of functional imaging of the brain and evaluate the need for or effectiveness of this latest evolution in brain imaging, it is necessary to have a basic understanding of current diagnostic techniques. Although a comprehensive review of this topic is beyond the scope of this text, a limited review is presented. It is intended to introduce the topic of modern clinical brain imaging as influenced by CT and MR. This includes the dramatic impact that CT particularly has demonstrated regarding other imaging modalities. Detailed presentations of the other important diagnostic methods including FMRI, PET, SPECT, MSI, MRS, and EEG are given in subsequent chapters. The commonality in processing the images from each of these methods is presented here.

Although the mathematics involved in actually presenting the pictures from each of the functional imaging methods has been known for many years, it was the initial application in CT that introduced most of the recent advances in image processing and made these techniques so clinically applicable. In addition, for the most part, each of these methods remains dependent on CT and/or MR not only to identify locations of potential intracranial pathology but also to provide the most reasonable assumptions regarding probable etiologies. Therefore CT and MR occupy a central, essential, and currently irreplaceable position in the field of diagnostic brain imaging in spite of the many exciting and promising emerging functional techniques.

Although CT scanning has been available as a diagnostic method for less than one-quarter of a century, there have been remarkable advances in this technology and it remains one of the essential elements of neurodiagnosis. Technologic advances in CT have been accompanied by extraordinary improvements in image quality and system capability. Not only have there been dramatic improvements in the quality of CT images, but there have also been almost unbelievable advances in scan time, spatial resolution, contrast resolution, image artifacts, and radiation exposure. Historically, CT scan systems have been labeled according to "generation." The first generation CT scanners were rotate, translate-type systems that required a complete rotation about the head for both the x-ray tube and the detectors at each slice location. Second generation CT scanners applied multiple x-ray tubes and detectors in order to decrease scan time. Third generation CT scanners further improved on this concept by using a 360-degree continuous sweep of the x-ray tube and the detector array. Fourth generation CT scanners allowed for the x-ray source to sweep around a stationary detector array, further decreasing image time; fifth generation CT scanners utilize electron beam technology to further improve on scan time and image quality. The result of these dramatic improvements in CT technology translates directly into patient care on a daily basis, with scan times decreasing from minutes to seconds.

CT SCANNER COMPOSITION

The essential components of a CT scanner include the gantry, x-ray source, detection system, computer, and display network.[1] The gantry is typically a "donut" structure surrounding a table that extends into the "donut hole" (see Fig. 1-8). Within the gantry are the x-ray source and the x-ray detection system. The x-ray source is usually an x-ray tube or multiple x-ray tubes that move around the patient being scanned. The x-ray detection system may also move around the patient or consist of multiple stationary detectors. The configuration of the x-ray tube and the detector system is such that a thin slice or planar volume of tissue is evaluated. The x-ray beam is collimated or restricted to a thin volume. This offers the advantage of decreasing the superimposition of adjacent tissues and virtually eliminates the scatter effects found in conventional radiographic examinations. The computer system uses a mathematical technique (algorithm) to reconstruct the radiographic data. This CT algorithm is generally a filtered backprojection method that allows for the analysis of the information obtained from the thin column x-rays. The angle of the scan is changed and the amount of radiation attenuation from multiple angles around the patient enables calculation of the attenuation occurring at specific points within the patient. The scan angle is constantly changed so that new information is backprojected and averaged. Computer analysis and digital storage are then accomplished. The display system usually employs a high-resolution television monitor for immediate evaluation and subsequent storage on computer disk, magnetic tape, or laser disk. The final images are often transferred to traditional x-ray film using direct photographic or laser processing.[1-3]

MAGNETIC RESONANCE OR MAGNETIC RESONANCE IMAGING

Magnetic resonance imaging (MRI) represents a recent and dramatic advance in neurodiagnostic imaging. This noninvasive anatomic/pathologic imaging technique utilizes magnetic fields and radiofrequency (RF) energy to manipulate atomic nuclei. The scanner itself may appear similar in many respects to a CT machine; however, the two pieces of equipment are quite different (see Fig. 4-4). The objective of MRI, like CT, is to produce cross-sectional images in which there is significant contrast between tissues of interest. MRI, however, unlike CT, depends on the physical phenomenon of spinning subatomic particles of nuclei. The most commonly used nucleus in MRI is that of hydrogen (which is a single proton) because of its relatively strong signal and natural abundance in biologic tissues. Most of these protons are associated with water and, to a lesser extent, fat. When placed in a strong magnetic field, these protons behave like tiny bar magnets and tend to orient in a direction along the magnetic field (see Fig. 4-7).

In MRI a large current is passed through a low-resistant and typically superconducting coil to generate the main magnetic field. Currents through smaller coils provide the additional fields used for imaging. It is also possible to use permanent magnets or electromagnets to generate the main magnetic field. Magnetic fields in clinical MRI use vary from approximately 0.02 to 4.0 T. The earth's average magnetic field is 5×10^{-5}

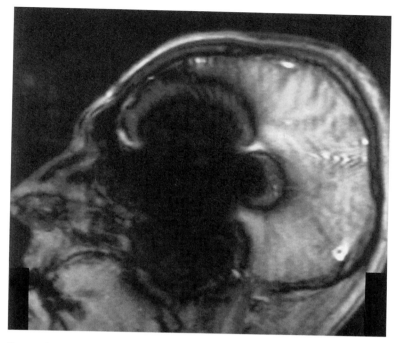

Fig. 3-1. Coronal T1-weighted sagittal scout MR demonstrating marked metallic artifact from an intracranial aneurysm clip. The patient was carefully removed from the MR scanner without incident. Compare to a normal sagittal MR in Figs. 3-2 and 3-3, *A.*

T. Therefore these magnetic fields are, in general, extremely strong when compared to the earth's magnetic field. The higher field strength magnets are associated with a very strong pull on metal objects, and it is important to remember that metal objects taken into many MRI scan rooms can become lethal projectiles. Additional sources of patient insult include metallic objects that may be in contact with the patient and can heat during the scanning process, resulting in skin burns; damage to stimulating devices such as pacemakers; and movement of implanted surgical material such as aneurysm clips. Placement of a patient with a ferromagnetic intracerebral aneurysm clip into a high magnetic field can be fatal[4] (Fig. 3-1).

After the patient has been placed within a strong magnetic field, the next step is to introduce an RF field in order to add small amounts of energy to the protons aligned within the magnetic field. The result of this RF input is to change the orientation of the protons within the magnetic field. Effective transfer of energy occurs as a "resonance" specific to both the nuclei (i.e., protons) studied and the precise magnetic field strength surrounding it. A specially RF-shielded room is required to eliminate interference from outside radio sources.

Upon termination of the RF excitation, the protons are free to return to their normal orientation in the field and to give up all of the energy they have absorbed. This returned RF energy can be detected by a receiver coil or antennae (see Figs. 4-13 and 4-14).

Through the use of a preparation sequence of small magnetic field gradients and RF pulses, the location of the nuclei in 3-D space, as well as the information about its surrounding environment, can be encoded into the return signal. The excitation and detection process is repeated enough times to uniquely encode each part of the object. Computer processing of the set of signals provides the final image(s) of the spatial distribution of nuclei within the object (Fig. 3-2).

Although MRI represents one of the most sophisticated and detailed central nervous system evaluations possible, there are limitations to this technique. A wide variety of artifacts exist, with the most common being patient motion (Fig. 3-3). Additional artifacts that may occur include flow from arterial pulsation, venous blood flow, and cerebrospinal fluid (CSF) movement. Metallic artifacts may also significantly distort image quality (see Fig. 3-1). Wraparound artifact, also referred to as aliasing, occurs when the diameter of the object being imaged exceeds the field of view (Fig. 3-4). The truncation artifact can be identified as a number of multiple or recurrent rings located at areas of abrupt transition in signal intensity. In spite of these and additional artifacts that may plague MRI studies, this technique remains the most sensitive and one of the most widely used diagnostic modalities. Knowledge of these artifacts prevents misinterpretation of images, and they rarely preclude the use of MR as a neurodiagnostic method in individual patients.[2]

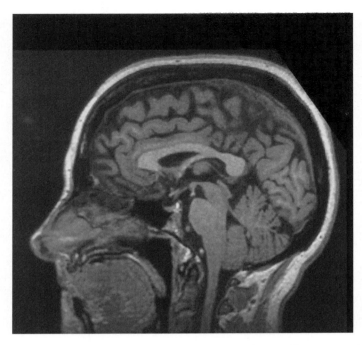

Fig. 3-2. Normal sagittal T1-weighted MR demonstrating the excellent anatomic definition available with MR. Compare to Fig. 3-1, which demonstrates the significant loss of information from metallic artifact.

Projection Reconstruction: CT, MR, SPECT, and PET

X-ray computed tomography (CT), positron emission tomography (PET), single photon emission computed tomography (SPECT), and nuclear magnetic resonance imaging (MRI) all fall in the general imaging class of reconstruction of the object from their projections. Tomography refers to the creation of images in slices or sections. A knowledge of the basic technique of making a planar image or tomogram from traditional x-rays dates to the early 1900s. This concept was based on the fact that if one plane or section of the body is kept fixed while the x-ray source and the film are moved, an unblurred image of the section of interest will result. During planar tomography, the patient remains motionless and the x-ray tube and cassette are moved in opposite directions. Although various methods of tomography are available, including complex motion tomography (in which the x-ray tube and cassette move in patterns such as elliptical or figure-of-eight), all of these techniques result in structures outside the plane of interest being included even though blurred. Additional shortcomings of the technique include images of low contrast, because all of the tissue contributes to the image, and radiation doses that can be significant[2,5] (Fig. 3-5).

Computed tomography is a form of x-ray examination in which a planar volume or slice of the body is studied. By collimating or limiting the x-ray to a thin beam, there is a decrease in the superimposition of tissues problematic in planar tomography. This thin collimation also limits the scatter effects that accompany traditional x-ray examinations. In nuclear medicine studies such as PET and SPECT, the radiation source results from radionuclides distributed within the body, typically following an intravenous injection. MR imaging is based on the density or concentration of protons in body tissues. Although the detection of differences in proton density utilized by magnetic resonance techniques is not based on x-ray attenuation, the computer processing of the data is similar to that used in CT. (The details of MR image acquisition are discussed in Chapter 4.)

Even though the tomographic capability of nuclear medicine was demonstrated as early as 1958 by Kuhl, and again in 1966 by Kuhl and his colleagues for brain scanning, it was not until the advent of x-ray CT that the most significant advances in all aspects of computed tomographic imaging began.[6-8]

The description of x-ray CT by Hounsfield in 1973 set the stage for remarkable advances in many areas of medical imaging.[8] It is the same basic technologic approach used for x-ray CT that enables the tomographic images of such modalities as MR, PET, and SPECT, all of which come under the general imaging class of reconstruction of an object from their projections. A projection is most commonly visualized as a shadowgram obtained by illuminating an object by

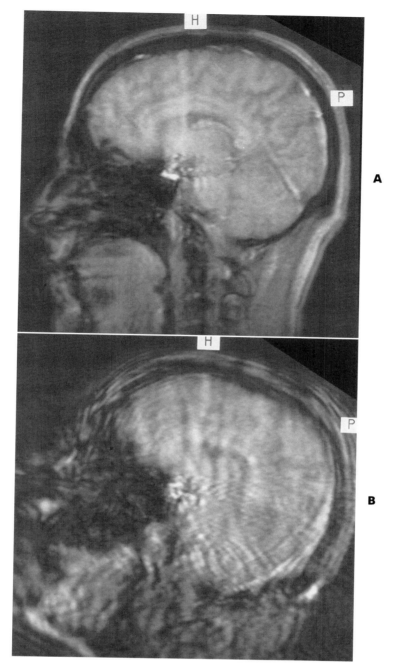

Fig. 3-3. A, Routine "scout" midline sagittal MR obtained for localization purposes. **B,** Same patient "localizer" image with motion artifact (compare to **A**).

penetrating radiation, typically in the x-ray wavelength range. For a complex object such as the head, a large number of structures will contribute to the total absorbance of the penetrating x-rays. From an x-ray point of view, an object is just a spatial distribution of attenuation coefficients.

For plane film radiography, a two-dimensional set of parallel paths is measured from one angle. For most CT systems, only a one-dimensional set of paths is measured at a time (Fig. 3-6). For simplicity, one can consider the case of two-dimensional images and slices to which the "tomography" part of CT refers. By rotating either the source-detector or the object and repeating the x-ray measurements, a set of shadowgrams or projection views from multiple angles can be obtained. The goal of the reconstruction process is to obtain an accurate estimation of the imaged object from the measured set of projections.

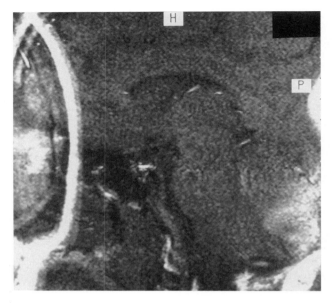

Fig. 3-4. "Localizer" midline sagittal image using a small field of view and resulting in significant aliasing or "wraparound" artifact. Compare to Fig. 3-3, *A*.

Radon Transform

Projection reconstruction is conveniently described mathematically in terms of the Radon transform, named for the Austrian mathematician who developed the formalism in 1917 while working on gravitational problems.[9] Radon showed mathematically that a two- or three-dimensional object could be reconstructed from an infinite set of projections taken from multiple angles. The initial application of the Radon transform was in astronomy, prior to its adoption by medicine during the development of x-ray CT.

The set of all projections from the different angles makes up the Radon transform of the object. For the first generation of CT scanners, the absorbance of a pencil-shaped x-ray beam would be recorded as the source and detector translated together across the length of the object (Figure 3-6). After this recording, the apparatus would be rotated to the next angular increment and the measurement repeated.

Therefore each projection through the object, at a given angle, is a line integral along the beam path. This projection is recorded along a line perpendicular to

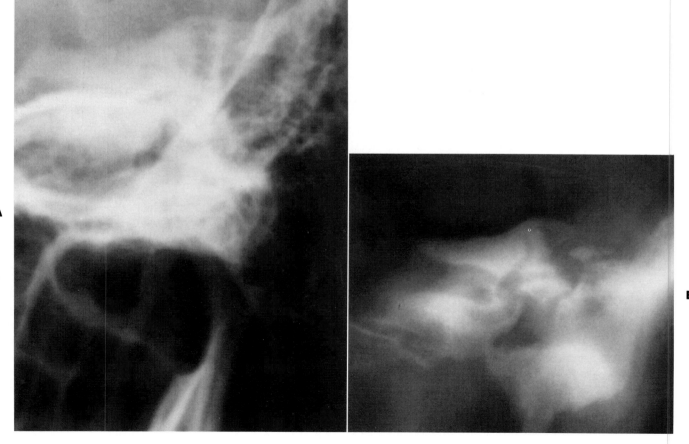

Fig. 3-5. A, AP radiograph of the temporal bone. **B,** Tomographic image of the temporal bone demonstrating markedly improved anatomic detail (compare to **A**).

the direction of the given angle (Fig. 3-7). The total of all projections at different angles is the Radon transform of the object. Each point in the Radon transform of the object represents a line integral through the object. The overall objective is to determine the original object spatial density distribution from a "sufficient" set of projections, that is, to find the corresponding inverse Radon transform. In practice, only estimates of the actual transform can be made since there are only a finite number of projections available. Furthermore, even though film-recorded x-ray is thought of as being continuous, these computed techniques use measurements recorded from a finite number of detectors or detector increments. Having collected a discrete set of numbers, the estimated image will also be a discrete set, or array, of numbers.

Backprojection

Backprojection is the oldest and simplest projection reconstruction method. This method has been likened to drawing the floor plan of a house by looking in the windows.[5] Even though we may only be able to look into the house from the outside, by circling the house and looking into each window, we can draw a reasonable plan. Of course, the more windows, the easier it will be to construct an accurate representation. Although no longer used in its most basic form, this method continues to serve as the fundamental basis of several more effective procedures currently employed in image reconstruction.

At any point along a recorded projection, the value of the absorbance is a summation of all the absorbance contributions along the path. The easiest assumption to be made about the nature of this pattern of absorbances is that it is uniform along the path. This is equivalent to assuming that the object is completely homogeneous and that the attenuation arises equally from all points along the path.

In this case, the values along the projection are "backprojected" into a pixel grid the size of the image field-of-view (FOV). Using the known values of the projection angle and the distance along the projection, the measured attenuation is divided up equally among the pixels along the measurement beam path. As shown in Fig. 3-8, a dense point recorded along a single projection will therefore show up as a dense strip through the pixel grid.

This process is repeated for each of the acquired projections. Since the backprojected values at each pixel location are summed over all of the projections, this method is occasionally referred to as the summation method. As shown in Fig. 3-9, a dense point in the object will now be identified by the intersection of the dense strips from all of the projections. After several projections, the reconstructed appearance of a point object will have a star-shaped appearance. After many projections the appearance of a single dense point in the object will be a circularly symmetric shape, as shown in Fig. 3-10.

The backprojection procedure reconstructs an image in which each point in the "actual" image is blurred by this pattern, and this 2-D profile is referred to as the point-spread-function (PSF) for the reconstruction process. Ideally, each point in the actual image would be reconstructed only to a single point in the reconstructed image (no spreading among neighboring pixels). The PSF characterizes a fundamental error in the reconstruction process that prevents an entirely perfect production of an image of the object.

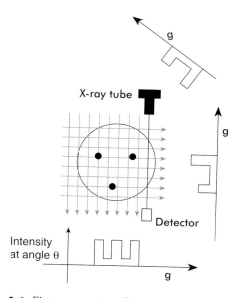

Fig. 3-6. First generation CT scanning procedure.

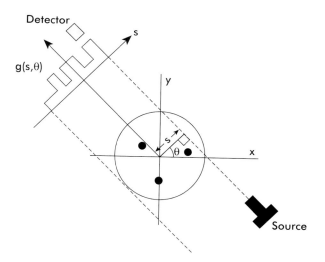

Fig. 3-7. Radon transform geometry. The object is some function of spatial (x,y) coordinates, and the radon transform is the set of linear absorbance measurements made at all angles g(s,o).

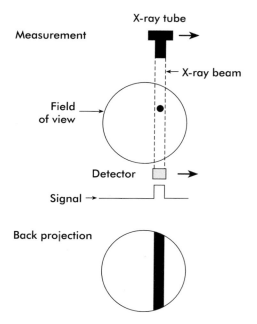

Fig. 3-8. The dense point between the x-ray tube and the detector appears as a dense strip through the pixel grid on backprojection.[122]

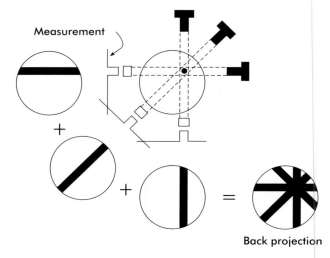

Fig. 3-9. Summation of different individual backprojections results in a spoke pattern or star-shaped appearance.[122]

The output blurred image can be considered as being the actual image merged with the PSF characteristic of the reconstruction process. The convolution operation is the mathematic description of the process of taking an uncorrupted image and methodically working pixel by pixel and row by row, applying the PSF blurring to each pixel. While projection reconstruction using simple backprojection is relatively easy to understand and implement, a method is required that reconstructs the actual, and not a blurred, image.

Iterative Methods

One approach to a more accurate projection reconstruction relies on computer methods to repeatedly examine estimated object distributions. Iterative techniques are based on using the computer to make successive approximations through repeated calculations, each time trying to successively derive better approximations to the attenuation coefficient in each voxel. An arbitrary set of attenuation values is used at the start, and repeated corrections are made until the calculated pattern of attenuation coefficients gives patterns that are the same as those measured.

These procedures basically guess at the actual image, compute the pattern of data that would be collected from this guess, and compare this data pattern with the actually measured patterns. Based on the characteristics of the comparison differences, a change is made to the estimated image and the projection data are recomputed to see if the predicted patterns are closer to the measured patterns.

The nature of the changes made to the estimate based on the comparison results characterizes the differences between iterative methods. Iterative least squares techniques (ILST) update the whole estimated matrix simultaneously, algebraic reconstruction techniques (ART) update along a ray, and simultaneous iterative reconstruction techniques (SIRT) update a point at a time.

These methods are not commonly used in practice, in part because they cannot proceed until after the complete data set has been acquired, but also because the multiple iterations can take a long time and, while often successful, the estimation process may not ever converge to the true image.

Filtered Backprojection

Because the image obtained by backprojection is not the actual image but a blurred version, the backprojection operation does not provide the true inverse Radon transform of the image. In order to obtain the actual image, one must pass the blurred image through a 2-D filter designed to blur the image with a PSF that is the inverse of that in Fig. 3-10, thereby cancelling the PSF pattern from the backprojection step. This combined processing is called "filtered backprojection" and does give the desired inverse Radon transform. Because of potential difficulties in designing an appropriate and stable 2-D inverse filter for the backprojected image, the order of filtering and backprojection is often reversed. The process is commonly referred to as "convolution backprojection" if the filtering step is performed directly on the projections and "filtered backprojection" if the filtering is performed on Fourier-transformed versions of the projections. Convolution backprojection is the most com-

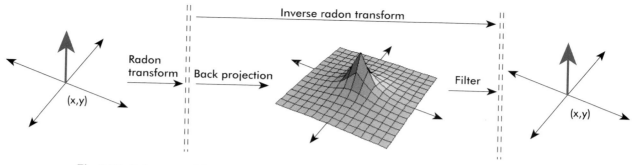

Fig. 3-10. Point spread function representing the blurring of each image point in an image reconstructed using simple backprojection.

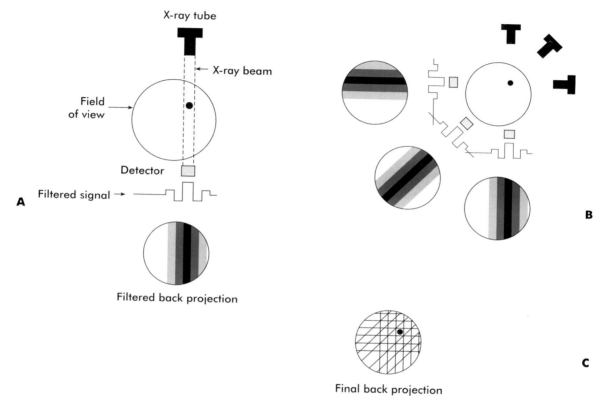

Fig. 3-11. A, Filtered backprojection technique that involves an initial backprojection with negative and positive components, followed by **B,** different projections being filtered and backprojected. **C,** The final backprojection is a summation that results in improved definition, since the alternating positive and negative components cancel out the spoke of star-shaped pattern of simple backprojection. (See Fig. 3-9.)[122]

monly employed method of performing projection reconstruction.

Since the filtering is applied to the data prior to backprojection, its shape is not simply related to the shape of the backprojection PSF of Fig. 3-10. The pattern of the projection to be backprojected will be modified to have additional positive and negative parts that, when backprojected and added with the rest of the filtered and backprojected projections, leads to cancellation of the blurring beyond the actual location of a point (Fig. 3-11).

The filter to apply to the projections prior to backprojection must be modified from the theoretical value to avoid amplifying the noise inherent in measured projections. Therefore the final PSF after the entire reconstruction process will be much improved, but still not ideal, and the effectiveness with which different manufacturers select an appropriate compromise filter contributes to differences in image quality between instruments.

Once a design has been selected, it is applied to the projected data using a convolution algorithm, prior to

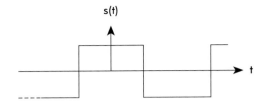

$$s(t)$$

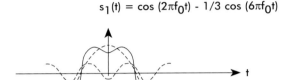

$$s_1(t) = \cos(2\pi f_0 t) - 1/3 \cos(6\pi f_0 t)$$

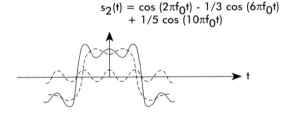

$$s_2(t) = \cos(2\pi f_0 t) - 1/3 \cos(6\pi f_0 t) + 1/5 \cos(10\pi f_0 t)$$

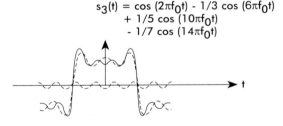

$$s_3(t) = \cos(2\pi f_0 t) - 1/3 \cos(6\pi f_0 t) + 1/5 \cos(10\pi f_0 t) - 1/7 \cos(14\pi f_0 t)$$

Fig. 3-12. Fourier transform of a square wave function.[123]

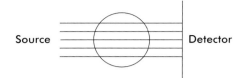

(a) Parallel beam

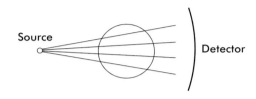

(b) Fan beam

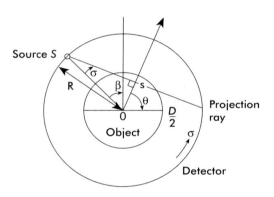

(c) Fan beam geometry

Fig. 3-13. Projection data acquisition.[124]

the backprojection step. Alternatively, the filtering can be readily implemented using the basic Fourier transform property that a convolution operation with two functions (the projection and the filter) is equivalent to a simple multiplication of the Fourier transforms of both the functions. The resulting product can be inverse Fourier transformed to give the filtered projection ready for backprojection.

Fourier Reconstruction

The Fourier transform (FT) reflects the concept that any function, pattern, or variation of a quantity in time or space can be considered as being composed of a sum of periodic sine and cosine waves having an appropriate pattern of amplitudes of each sine or cosine frequency (Fig. 3-12). The Fourier transform of the function provides the corresponding listing, at each frequency increment, of the amplitudes (and phases) of the periodic components that sum up to give that function. The concept is readily extended to multiple dimensions, and the 2-D Fourier transform of an image represents the decomposition of spatial frequency components making up the intensity patterns in the input image. The richness of this approach and the availability of fast Fourier transform (FFT) computer algorithms for conveniently obtaining forward and inverse transforms have helped this type of analysis become commonly employed throughout science and engineering. Another way to obtain the inverse Radon transform is by using Fourier reconstruction methods.

This method depends on the "projection theorem," which states that a one-dimensional Fourier transform of a projection is equivalent to the values that would occur along a one-dimensional line through the full two-dimensional Fourier transform of the object (see Fig. 4-48). This line in the Fourier transform passes

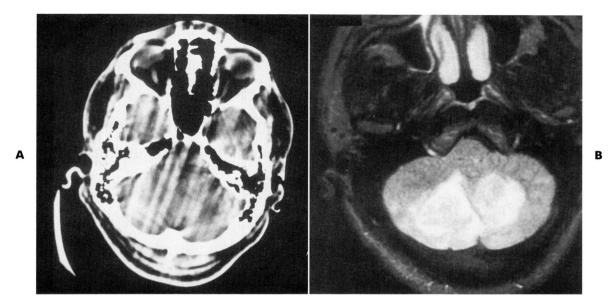

Fig. 3-14. A, CT scan at the skull base demonstrating artifacts that obscure the visualization of the posterior fossa structures. **B,** T2-weighted MRI through the posterior fossa in the same patient demontrating abnormal signal intensity from a posterior fossa neoplasm. Compare with **A** and note that the MR scan is relatively artifact-free compared to the CT scan.

radially through the center of the frequency coordinate system and will be at an angle determined by the angle at which the projection was taken. This is illustrated in Fig. 4-48 and means that one can essentially obtain a 2-D Fourier transform by taking 1-D Fourier transforms of each of a set of measured projections. This 2-D Fourier transform data will be available along the radial lines determined by the set of measured projections. As shown in Fig. 4-49, all that is required to reconstruct an object is to take the inverse 2-D Fourier transform (IFT) of the available data.

The FFT algorithms implement forward and inverse Fourier transforms in a very efficient manner but require the input data to be on a regular grid. The IFT can be performed on the radial data but not efficiently so an interpolation step is usually employed to convert the data along radial lines to the rectangular grid. For x-ray CT, this interpolation requirement for Fourier reconstruction is generally more computationally expensive (and introduces more error) than direct convolution filtering, so convolution (or filtered) back-projection is generally used rather than Fourier reconstruction.

Fan Beam Geometry

Third and fourth generation CT machines avoid the slow mechanical translation of the source/detector assemblies that is a feature of earlier instruments. These systems use only rotational motion around the object and employ a fan-shaped beam of divergent x-rays from a single source to rapidly obtain each projection. This situation requires modifications to the reconstruction geometry (Fig. 3-13).

The processing for parallel beam projections has been highly developed, so one approach to fan-beam reconstruction involves reordering the acquired data set into a set that would be obtained from parallel (or nearly parallel) projections. Since a ray in a fan beam acquisition corresponds to some ray that would occur in a parallel beam situation, the data can be readily reordered to form the parallel beam data set. This approach then requires two steps: data preprocessing to form a parallel beam data set and application of a normal reconstruction algorithm.

Another alternative, and the one more often employed, is to derive the reconstruction algorithms directly in terms of this modified geometry. This avoids the preprocessing steps and permits more rapid reconstruction, but at the cost of additional complexity. Additional information on these methods is available in references 10 and 11.

CLINICAL APPLICATIONS OF CT AND MR

Despite the fact that there are tremendous advantages to newer techniques such as CT and MRI, these procedures are not entirely without risk and require consideration prior to use. CT and MRI remain among the most costly of the diagnostic procedures, and economic factors are also important considerations. Appropriate use of neuroimaging methods requires a thorough knowledge

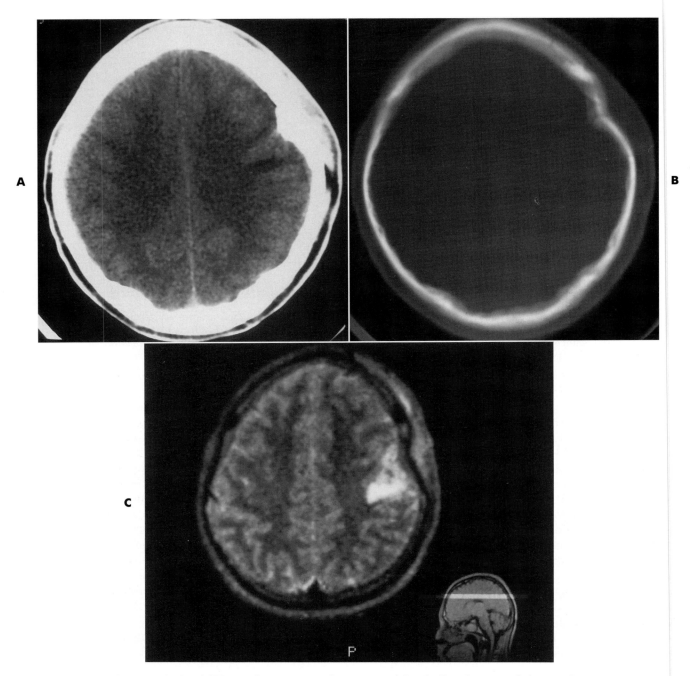

Fig. 3-15. **A,** Axial CT scan demostrating depression of the skull with minimal abnormality identifiable within the brain substance. **B,** "Bone windows" of this same CT scan demonstrating the depressed skull fracture that is obvious by CT. **C,** T2-weighted MR (TR 2000, TE 105) demonstrating the depressed contour of the skull but with poor definition of the fracture as compared to the "bone windows" on CT. Note the marked abnormality in the brain substance identified as increased signal intensity that is not well defined on the CT scans. This case demonstrates the complementary nature of CT and MR.

of the patient's clinical condition, the suspected diagnosis, and the appropriate use of contrast agents. Contrast agents for both CT and MRI are effective primarily because of a breakdown in the blood-brain barrier and/or increased vascularity of lesions. MRI is superior in the evaluation of particular parts of the brain that are difficult to see with CT because of bone artifacts. This is especially true when assessing areas near the foramen magnum, cerebellopontine angles, posterior fossa, and inferior temporal lobes. Owing to the increased thickness of the base of the skull, CT artifacts are common in these

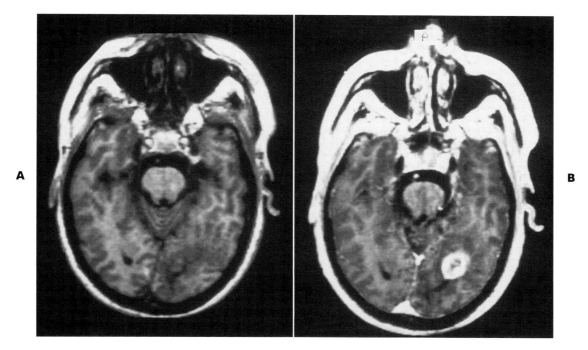

Fig. 3-16. A, Axial T1-weighted MR demonstrating minimal abnormality. **B,** Axial T1-weighted MR following the administration of gadolinium demonstrating strikingly abnormal contrast enhancement in this patient with metastatic disease.

regions and MRI offers the advantage of artifact-free visualization (Fig. 3-14). However, MRI is not suitable for some patients because of claustrophobia, motion, and presence of intracranial aneurysm clips or pacemakers. In addition, there are frequently limits on patient size and patient condition, such as requirements for extensive monitoring equipment and assisted ventilation. Metal artifacts from prior surgery or injury can entirely negate the diagnostic value of MRI in some cases (see Fig. 3-1). In general, MRI is more sensitive than CT, yet MRI is frequently a less specific diagnostic method. For example, acute hemorrhage may be more readily diagnosed by CT than MRI; skull fractures are also better diagnosed by CT. These methods can be complementary in that CT may best demonstrate fractures while MRI will often show disease within the brain that is not readily visualized by CT (Fig. 3-15).

CONTRAST AGENTS

In general, intravenous contrast agents are administered in CT and MR to enhance areas of abnormality that may be otherwise difficult or impossible to detect. These agents are also used to enhance the definition of lesions that are identified and to better characterize the exact nature of such lesions. Contrast agents are primarily effective secondary to a breakdown in the blood-brain barrier and as a result of increased vascularity in pathologic tissue. Therefore, when contrast enhancement is present it provides additional

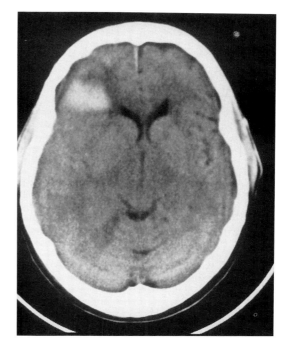

Fig. 3-17. Axial CT scan of a focal intracerebral hemorrhage.

information to the diagnostician not available on the noncontrasted image (Fig. 3-16). Contrast can be problematic, and it is important to remember that because contrast turns pathology "white" on images using conventional methods of display, pathology that is white before contrast administration can be mistaken for abnormal enhancement. On CT this is particularly true of hemorrhage (Fig. 3-17). CT contrast agents, like all commonly employed radiographic contrast agents, utilize substances with a high electron density to absorb x-rays and thus produce a "contrast" effect. These are typically iodinated agents and are given in a dosage of about 40 grams of iodine for a cranial CT study.[2,12,13]

Currently, MR contrast primarily involves the use of relatively nontoxic paramagnetic agents such as gadolinium diethylenetriamine pentaacetic acid (Gd-DTPA, gadopentetate dimeglumine). Unlike CT contrast agents, MR contrast enhancement is produced secondary to the alterations these agents produce in the local magnetic environment. The contrast is not directly observed, but their magnetic effect on nearby hydrogen nuclei enables the enhancement to occur. These paramagnetic substances act as relaxation centers for other nuclei in the local microenvironment and shorten the magnetic relaxation times of the surrounding hydrogen nuclei. Although these types of agents have a physiologic distribution and excretion similar to the radiographic contrast agents, MR is generally a more sensitive method of detection of contrast requiring dosages in the range of one-twentieth that of CT. Standard doses for intravenous administration range generally from 0.1 mmol/kg to 0.3 mmol/kg.[2,14,15]

CT AND MR IN CENTRAL NERVOUS SYSTEM DISEASE

The clinical utility of CT and MR includes application to virtually all causes of central nervous system (CNS) disease. The value of a "normal" examination is difficult to estimate since the decrease in clinic visits, in physician's and other health care professionals' time, and possibly in patient concern are all nearly impossible to accurately determine. In all probability, most negative studies significantly improve the care of patients and the effectiveness of the health care provider. Positive studies, however, receive the most attention, and the value of a given imaging system is, in general, based on its ability to detect CNS pathology. There are several disease categories of the CNS for which the use of CT and MR has proved essential. These include neoplasms, infections, cerebrovascular disease, head trauma, intracranial hemorrhage, and white matter disease.

NEOPLASMS

Annually, approximately 40,000 individuals within the United States develop brain tumors, which may result in paralysis, dementia, seizures, and death.[16] The high worldwide incidence of brain tumors makes this a problem for all countries. CT and MR play such an essential role in the care of these patients that one

or both of these modalities have become available for the management of intracranial masses in nearly all parts of the globe.

The evaluation of intracranial neoplasms involves CT and/or MRI; in fact, it would be hard to imagine attempting to adequately manage patients with intracranial masses at the current standard of care without at least one of these techniques. The general characteristics applied to intracranial neoplasms on CT and MRI include (1) mass effect, (2) edema, (3) abnormal contrast enhancement, (4) hemorrhage, and (5) calcification[2,17-26] (Fig. 3-18). Mass effect is frequently identified as effacement of cortical sulci, midline shift, ventricular displacement, and evidence of brain herniation. Edema is a common characteristic of neoplasms and is identifiable on both CT and MRI scans. The CT scan appearance typically shows decreased attenuation or low density, and on MRI there is decreased signal intensity on T1-weighted images and increased signal intensity on proton density and T2-weighted images (Fig. 3-19).

Neoplasms, in general medical terminology, are usually considered as being in the broad categories of "benign" or "malignant." Although these terms are used in the final description of intracranial neoplasms, they are remarkably absent from the general schemes used to define neoplasms of the central nervous system viewed by neuroimaging techniques.[27] This results partly from the fact that, until recently, the location of an intracranial neoplasm was far more important than the cell type of the neoplasm. Regardless of the most benign "nature" of a neoplasm, when located in a vital part of the brain it can be devastatingly incapacitating or even fatal. As a result, many intracranial neoplasms are considered to "behave" in a malignant manner even if histologically "benign." It is primarily the availability of functional brain imaging that has changed the traditional management approach to intracranial masses including neoplasms in this regard. Even malignant neoplasms that were previously thought to be unresectable because of their close anatomic relationship to vital areas of brain function are now being successfully resected without residual neurologic dysfunction (see Chapter 9). This is not because these neoplasms are less "malignant" but rather because their location is not as closely related to "vital" brain regions as would be anticipated from traditional neuroanatomic/functional predictions. Although the variations in these neuroanatomic/functional predictions in "normal" subjects are generally minor, there may be major alterations in the location of brain function in the face of pathology or developmental abnormalities (see Chapter 9).

Although many brain neoplasms remain relatively untreatable, the number of lesions in this category continues to decline, and the rate of improved treat-

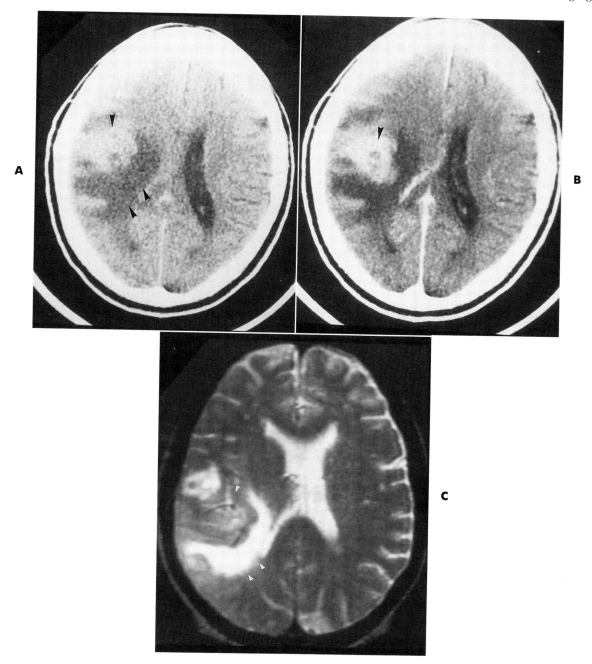

Fig. 3-18. A, Axial CT in a patient with a high-grade glioma demonstrating abnormal increased density from hemorrhage and/or calcification (*arrow*) with adjacent edema (*arrows*) resulting in mass effect on the cortex and lateral ventricle. **B,** Following the administration of intravenous contrast there is abnormal contrast enhancement (*arrow*). **C,** Axial T2-weighted MR (TR 2500, TE 80) demonstrating variable signal intensity in the region of the neoplasm (*arrow*) with surrounding edema (*arrows*).

ment has been accelerated by an improved understanding of the brain's functional capacities. This includes the capability of altering the location of important functional regions or displaying a significant degree of "plasticity." It is therefore necessary to remember that the traditional imaging classifications of neoplasms are extremely important for the under-

standing of a reasonable differential diagnosis; the degree of "malignancy" as classified by histologic methods will in all probability increase in significance. Unfortunately, there is no generally accepted histologic classification system for central nervous system neoplasms.[27]

The two most important criteria for evaluating the

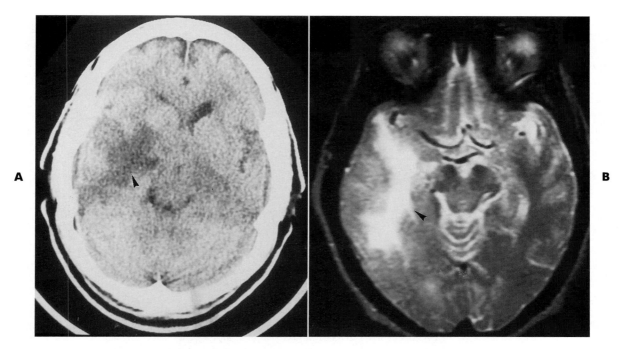

Fig. 3-19. A, Axial CT scan demonstrating decreased attenuation (*arrow*) from edema. **B,** Axial T2-weighted MR (TR 2500, TE 80) demonstrating abnormal increased signal intensity from edema (*arrow*).

images of intracranial neoplasms are the location of the mass and the age of the patient.[27] The location of an intracranial neoplasm is in general initially described as either intraaxial or extraaxial.[2] Intraaxial implies that the neoplasm is within the substance of the brain, and extraaxial indicates that the mass is outside the actual brain but usually closely related. Extraaxial masses frequently arise from the tissues that support the brain, such as the meninges. At times, these extraaxial masses minimally involve the brain, and at other times they may compress the brain, invade the brain, or induce reactions such as edema within the substance of the brain. In general, the more invasive the neoplasm, whether intraaxial or extraaxial, the more likely it is to be malignant and difficult to treat.

Intraaxial neoplasms include types referred to as astrocytomas, oligodendrogliomas, ependymomas, and lymphomas, with gliomas comprising the most common types of brain neoplasms and representing about 50% of all intracranial neoplasms. The three most common types of glioma are the astrocytoma, the oligodendroglioma, and the ependymoma. Astrocytomas represent the majority of gliomas (75%) and have several histologic forms. These neoplasms are usually histologically described and given a number to grade the degree of malignancy. Eventually, these "infiltrating" neoplasms are commonly fatal and therefore behave in a "malignant" fashion even when relatively "low-grade," without treatment.[2,27-29]

The "benign" or "low-grade" astrocytoma is graded as a grade II by the World Health Organization (WHO) system and as a grade 1 or grade 2 by the older but still used "Kernohan" system. These tumors represent about 15% of the gliomas and are difficult to distinguish from the next higher grade or anaplastic astrocytoma. It is possible for a patient with this type of neoplasm to have a long survival, but even with surgical treatment half of these tumors go on to become a higher grade. Patients generally survive for 5 to 10 years and commonly die from the resulting higher grade neoplasm. Exceptions do happen, with some patients surviving for significantly longer or shorter time periods.[2,27,30]

Low-grade astrocytomas are typically isodense or slightly hypodense on noncontrast CT. There may be areas of calcification in as many as one-fourth of these neoplasms. Although mass effect and edema can be present, these changes are often absent. Contrast enhancement is frequently minimal or absent. In fact, these neoplasms can be extraordinarily difficult to diagnose by CT, and MR may be required in order to suggest the diagnosis[2,27,31] (Fig. 3-20). The low-grade astrocytoma is usually hypointense or isointense relative to brain tissue on T1-weighted MR but is typically hyperintense on proton density and T2-weighted sequences. As on CT, mass effect, edema, and contrast enhancement are often minimal or absent (see Fig. 3-20). However, as the tumor degenerates to

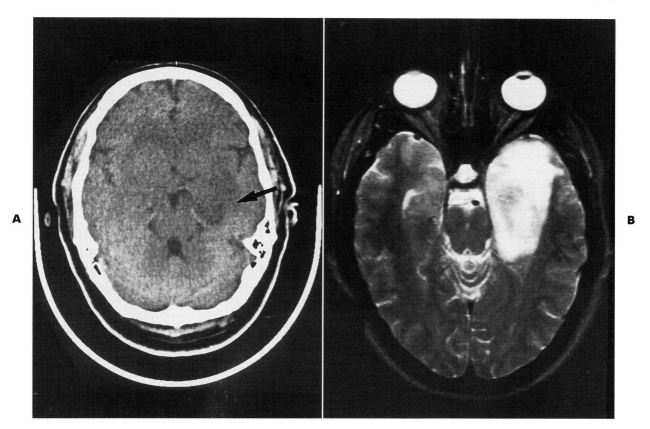

Fig. 3-20. A, Axial CT scan demonstrating a focal area of minimal decreased attenuation (*arrow*). **B,** Axial T2-weighted MR (TR 2500, TE 90) in the same patient demonstrating markedly abnormal increased signal intensity from a low-grade astrocytoma.

a higher grade, contrast enhancement is more common, and this can be used as one marker of disease progression.[2,27,32-34]

Approximately 25% of gliomas are anaplastic or grade III by the WHO definition. These are called grade 3 by the Kernohan system and represent the next level of malignancy after low grade. These neoplasms are significantly more malignant, with an average survival of only 2 years. These tumors usually look much more aggressive on imaging, exhibiting edema, mass effect, and contrast enhancement on both CT and MR. Anaplastic neoplasms are much more obvious on non–contrast-enhanced CT with mixed density, and an irregular margin of contrast enhancement is frequently seen on CT and MR (Fig. 3-21). The MR without contrast demonstrates hypointensity and/or isointensity, but when hemorrhage is present the signal can vary to hyperintensity. The T2-weighted sequences demonstrate abnormal hyperintensity, but again this can be variable, especially when hemorrhage and/or necrosis is present. In addition, a surrounding rim of increased signal from edema is common[2,27,31-34] (Fig. 3-21).

The grade IV WHO or grade 4 Kernohan astrocytoma is better known as the glioblastoma multiforme, because of its highly variable appearance on both gross and microscopic inspection. This is also reflected in its highly variable appearance on both CT and MR. Characterized by areas of necrosis, increased vascularity, hemorrhage, irregular margins, mass effect, and edema, it is the most malignant of the glial tumors. Unfortunately, this is the most common of the astrocytomas, representing about half of these neoplasms, and it has a typical survival of less than 15 months. These tumors frequently have CNS metastases but rarely metastasize outside the CNS. The CT and MR images reflect the pathologic state of these tumors, with highly variable patterns of density on CT and intensity on MR. Contrast enhancement, although also highly variable, is usually striking[2,27,31-34] (Fig. 3-22).

Most metastatic cancer to the CNS occurs within the brain parenchyma or presents as an intraaxial mass. Metastatic disease represents 15% to 30% of all intracranial tumors and is most frequently from primary neoplasms of the lung and breast. Additional sources include melanoma as well as neoplasms of the GI and GU tracts. CT may demonstrate single or multiple areas of hypodensity, isodensity, or hyperdensity. Hemorrhage is common. Contrast enhancement is usually present and intense but can vary

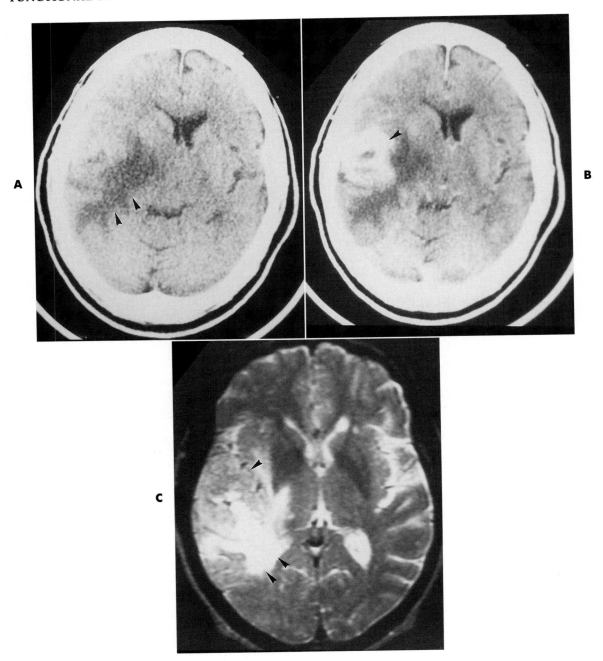

Fig. 3-21. A, Axial CT scan demonstrating mass effect and edema from a grade 3 astrocytoma (*arrows*). **B,** Following the administration of intravenous contrast there is abnormal contrast enhancement (*arrow*). **C,** Axial T2-weighted MR (TR 2500, TE 80) demonstrating abnormal signal intensity within the area of neoplasm (*arrow*) and markedly abnormal increased signal intensity from surrounding edema (*arrows*).

significantly, particularly following treatment with steroids, chemotherapy, and radiation. Enhancement patterns on both CT and MR include homogeneous, nonhomogeneous, ring, and a total lack of enhancement. The MR signal prior to contrast is also variable, particularly when the lesions are hemorrhagic. Increased signal on T1 weighting can be due to hemorrhage or, in the case of melanoma, can occur in the

absence of hemorrhage secondary to the T1 shortening effect of melanin. However, most metastases will be isointense or hypointense on T1, with increased signal on more heavily T2-weighted images[2,27,31,35-40] (Fig. 3-23).

Extraaxial neoplasms can occur in a variety of locations, and the differential diagnosis is highly dependent on which of these exact locations is

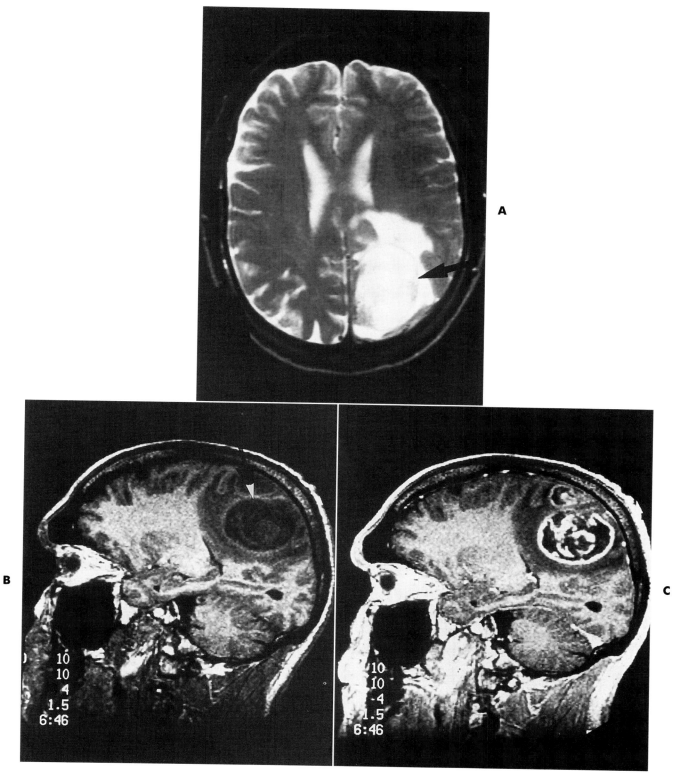

Fig. 3-22. A, Axial T2-weighted MR (TR 2500, TE 90) demonstrating a large posterior parietal mass with surrounding edema (*arrow*). **B,** T1-weighted MR without contrast demonstrating the large mass to be of predominantly decreased signal intensity (*arrow*). **C,** Sagittal T1-weighted MR after gadolinium administration, which demonstrates peripheral and irregular central contrast enhancement in this patient with a glioblastoma multiforme.

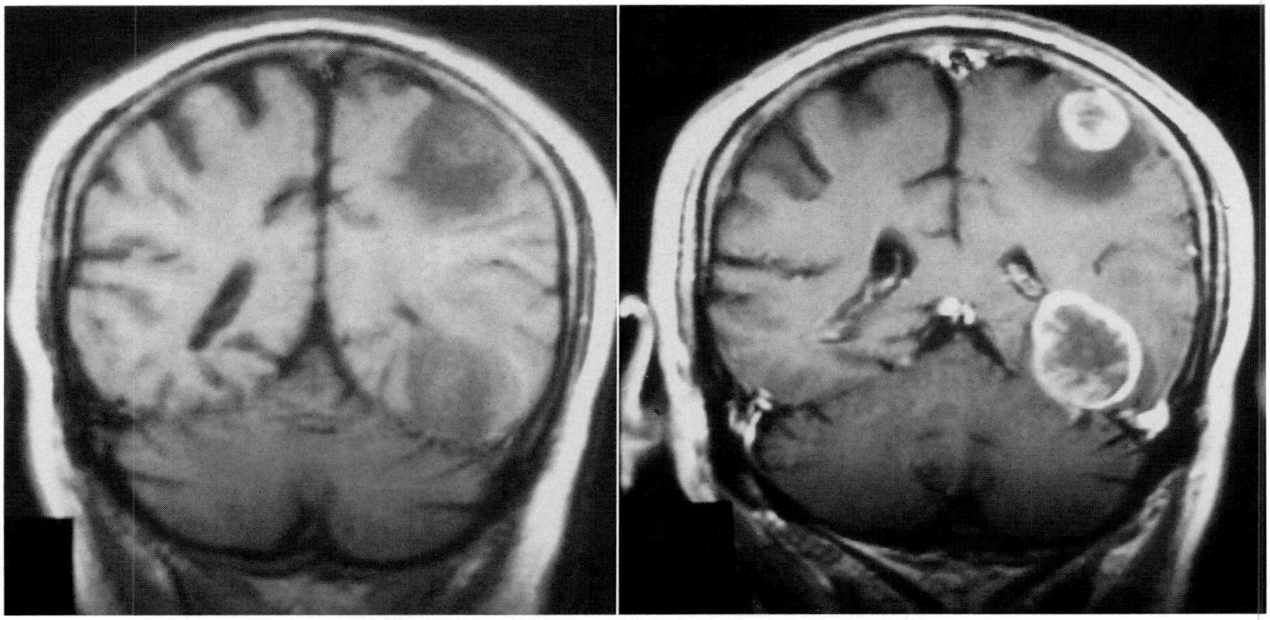

Fig. 3-23. A, Coronal T1-weighted MR (TR 800, TE 15) demonstrating focal areas of abnormal signal intensity from metastatic disease. **B,** Coronal T1-weighted MR (TR 800, TE 15) following the administration of gadolinium demonstrating abnormal contrast enhancement from metastatic disease.

involved. Meningiomas represent the most common nonglial primary brain tumor and are typically found extraaxially. The majority of meningiomas are dura-based, extraaxial neoplasms in a supratentorial location. These tumors represent 15% of all intracranial neoplasms and their locations include, but are not limited to, the parasagittal convexity, lateral convexity, olfactory groove, sphenoid ridge, posterior fossa, tentorium, and intraorbital and intraventricular sites. Patient outcome is, in general, directly related to the location of the neoplasm, and following surgical resection, these neoplasms tend to have a favorable prognosis. Meningiomas are usually well circumscribed and isodense to hyperdense on noncontrast CT, with isointensity common on all pulse sequences on MR. Calcification may contribute to the hyperdensity on CT, since about one fourth of these neoplasms are seen to calcify.

Hyperostosis of the adjacent bone may be minimal or striking. Following contrast administration there is typically intense and homogeneous enhancement on both CT and MR. This is variable, but some enhancement is virtually always present. Edema is common but not necessarily related to the size of the meningioma. Mass effect on the adjacent cortex is the rule, with "inward buckling" of the white matter often visible. A "mushrooming margin" may be a sign of a more aggressive histology; however, even the most benign of these tumors may have poorly defined borders[2,27,41-46] (Fig. 3-24). An exhausting array

of the more unusual and rare neoplasms of the CNS includes both intraaxial and extraaxial presentations. To some extent, the presentation of each of these less typical tumors is generally weighed against the likelihood that the mass represents one of the more common neoplasms, perhaps with an uncommon presentation. The final differential diagnosis of a CNS mass will depend on the location, age of the patient, distinguishing features of the tumor, and appearance on various imaging studies. Using current techniques, a list of the most likely etiologies can be given in a reasonable order of probability. However, it is important for all health care providers involved in the use or interpretation of these imaging studies to remember that we are basically working with "differential scopes" and not "microscopes." The overconfidence that a "typical" presentation of any mass can create is frequently shattered by the realization that a different etiology was in fact the cause of a given patient's difficulty. As our imaging technology increases in sophistication, it is increasingly important to remember that these studies have serious limitations and that we must continue to recognize the uniqueness of each patient and his/her condition. Put more simply, a brain tumor is not a brain tumor is not a brain tumor, and, more important, each person's brain is capable of remarkably different physiologic and functional responses to the presence of pathology that may directly affect treatment options.

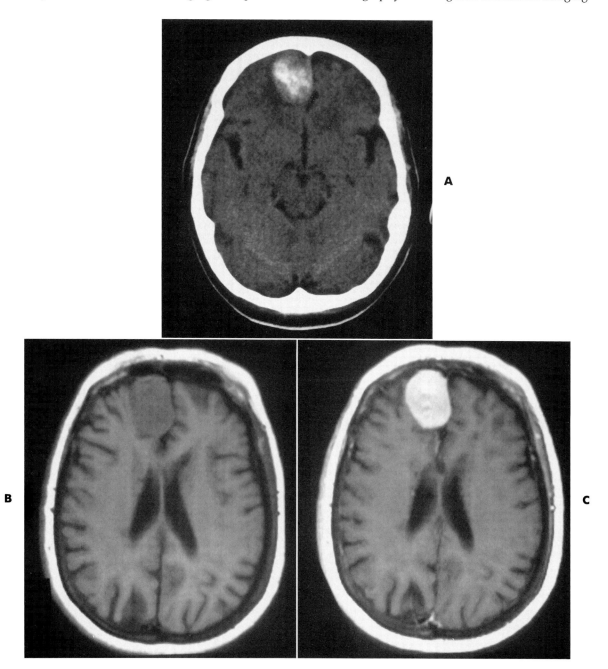

Fig. 3-24. A, Axial CT scan of the brain demonstrating a high-density (calcified) extraaxial mass. **B**, Axial T1-weighted MR (TR 600, TE 15) demonstrating a relatively isointense extraaxial mass. **C**, T1-weighted MR (TR 600, TE 15) after gadolinium administration demonstrating intense abnormal contrast enhancement in this extraaxial meningioma.

INFECTIONS

CNS infections may be the result of a direct extension from adjacent disease in the paranasal sinuses, middle ear, mastoids, soft tissues, orbits, or cranial nerves. In addition, such infections can be introduced from more remote sources as a result of penetrating trauma or by secondary hematogenous spread from distant organs. These infections may be limited to brain conditions such as encephalitis, meningitis, or brain abscesses. CNS infections can also represent one manifestation of a more systemic infectious disorder such as acquired immunodeficiency syndrome (AIDS). Regardless of the nature of the CNS infection, it is important to recognize the possibility of an infectious etiology on brain images, since these disorders are frequently amenable to therapy and early intervention may often be the key to a favorable clinical outcome.

Encephalitis represents a diffuse inflammatory process of the brain that can be caused by a variety of agents and includes bacterial, fungal, parasitic, and viral infections. The most common causes of encephalitis are viral, and one of the most common types of viral encephalitis in patients who are not immunocompromised is herpes simplex virus type 1. These patients may present a difficult clinical picture with fever, headache, confusion, disorientation, seizures, or various levels of coma.

The CT scan early in the disease may show no significant abnormality or a mild decrease in density in the temporal lobes with or without mass effect. Contrast administration may show linear, patchy, ringlike, or cortical enhancement. Over time, hemorrhage is typical and highly suggestive of herpes. MR is more sensitive than CT in the early stages of herpes simplex encephalitis and will frequently demonstrate changes of edema with increased signal on proton density and T2-weighted sequences. These changes are typically seen in the temporal lobes and extend to the insular cortex with sparing of the basal ganglia. Enhancement does not usually occur early, but more extensive changes, including abnormal contrast enhancement and hemorrhage, accompany disease progression[2,47-49] (Fig. 3-25).

Although viral infections occur in immunocompromised patients and commonly include the human immunodeficiency virus (HIV), the most common opportunistic infection in AIDS is toxoplasmosis. This type of infection is caused by *Toxoplasma gondii*, an obligate intracellular parasite. Diffuse encephalitis can occur, but more commonly focal lesions of cerebritis or abscess formation are identified. Focal areas of inflammatory change within the brain are generally referred to as cerebritis, and as these areas progress to central necrosis with a surrounding membrane, the term "abscess" is used to describe the lesion. In cerebritis, the CT scan will show a focal area of decreased density, and following contrast infusion there is little enhancement in the initial stages. An increase in enhancement occurs with progression of the inflammatory process. MR will show similar changes with focal areas of abnormal increased signal on proton density and T2-weighted images and central or patchy enhancement after contrast administration (Fig. 3-26). As the central area of cerebritis becomes necrotic and liquefies, a surrounding membrane with increased vascularity is typically formed. This is reflected on the CT and MR images as a focal area of CSF density or intensity centrally surrounded by an enhancing rim. This "ring enhancement" pattern is typical but not diagnostic of abscess, with *Streptococcus* being one of the more common infective organisms (Fig. 3-27). The

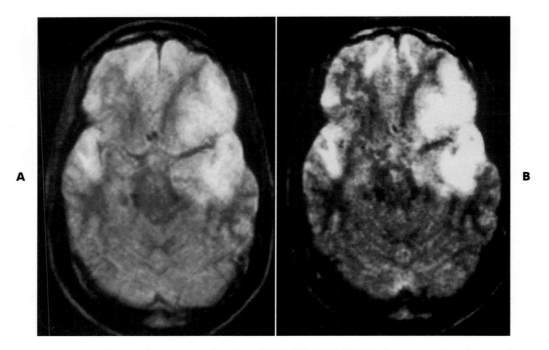

Fig. 3-25. A, Proton density–weighted axial MR (TR 2000, TE 45) demonstrating abnormal increased signal intensity in the frontal and temporal lobes from herpes simplex encephalitis. **B,** Axial T2-weighted MR (TR 2000, TE 105) also demonstrating abnormal signal intensity from herpes simplex encephalitis.

causes of a ring-enhancing pattern on CT or MR include abscess, primary or metastatic neoplasm, lymphoma, resolving hematoma, thrombosed aneurysm or arteriovenous malformation, infarction, sar-

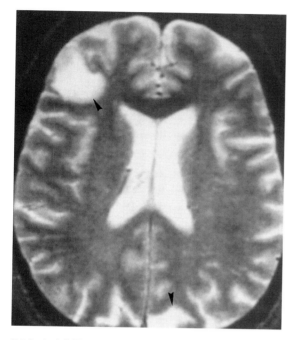

Fig. 3-26. Axial T2-weighted MR (TR 2500, TE 80) demonstrating focal areas of abnormal increased signal intensity (*arrows*) from toxoplasmosis in a patient with AIDS.

coidosis, and multiple sclerosis[2,47,48,50-52] (Fig. 3-28).

The most common form of CNS infection is meningitis. Meningitis is usually viral or bacterial; however, fungal and parasitic forms occur as well. The clinical presentation of a patient with meningitis includes headache, fever, stiff neck, confusion or disorientation, and a positive cerebrospinal fluid analysis. CT may reveal increased density in the subarachnoid spaces prior to contrast infusion, presumably resulting from increased vascularity with meningeal inflammation. Following the administration of contrast there may be intense cortical enhancement. MR can be more sensitive than CT in the diagnosis of meningitis, with T1-weighted sequences demonstrating poorly defined subarachnoid spaces prior to contrast and intense enhancement of these spaces following contrast infusion (Fig. 3-29). Half of the adult patients diagnosed with meningitis will develop complications, which may include ventriculitis, subdural effusion, subdural empyema, cerebritis, abscess formation, infarction, and hydrocephalus[2,47,53-55] (Fig. 3-30).

CEREBROVASCULAR DISEASE

Cerebrovascular disease is a common entity, representing the third leading cause of death in the United States. Cerebrovascular disorders primarily affect patients over the age of 55 and are most frequently related to atherosclerotic disease. In general, cerebrovascular disorders related to ischemia include

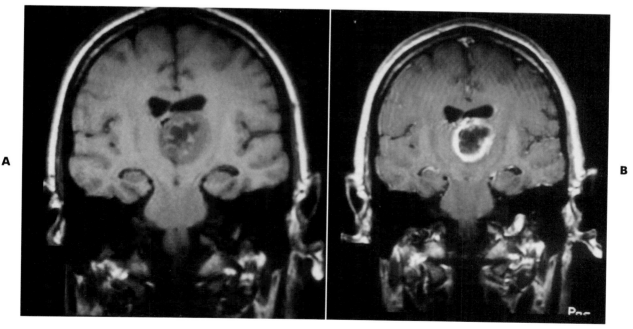

Fig. 3-27. A, T1-weighted coronal MR (TR 700, TE 15) prior to the administration of gadolinium demonstrating a midline predominantly decreased intensity mass. **B,** Coronal T1-weighted MR (TR 700, TE 15) following the administration of gadolinium demonstrating a ring-enhancing mass in this patient with a streptococcal abscess.

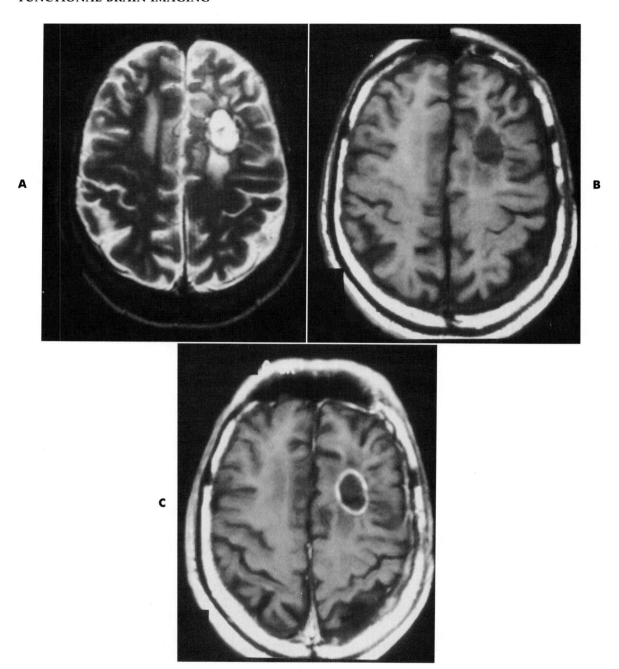

Fig. 3-28. **A**, Patient with a known resolving hematoma, which on axial T2-weighted MR (TR 2500, TE 90) demonstrates abnormal increased signal intensity. **B**, Noncontrasted T1-weighted MR (TR 600, TE 15) demonstrates decreased signal intensity consistent with an area of encephalomalacia from prior hemorrhage. **C**, Contrast-enhanced T1-weighted MR (TR 600, TE 15) demonstrating ring enhancement in this resolving hematoma.

subclinical disease without symptoms, transient ischemic attack (TIA), reversible ischemic neurologic deficit (RIND), stroke in progress, and completed stroke.[56]

The patient who presents with signs or symptoms consistent with cerebral ischemia, particularly stroke, typically is evaluated by a noncontrast CT. This enables the rapid assessment of possible hemorrhage and will usually suffice to exclude other major disorders that may mimic stroke[57] (Fig. 3-31). The MR evaluation of a patient with suspected cerebral ischemia has been shown to be more sensitive than CT.[58-60] The MR appearance of a completed stroke is usually of increased signal intensity on T2- and proton density–weighted images, with relative decreased signal on T1-weighted sequences. The MR examina-

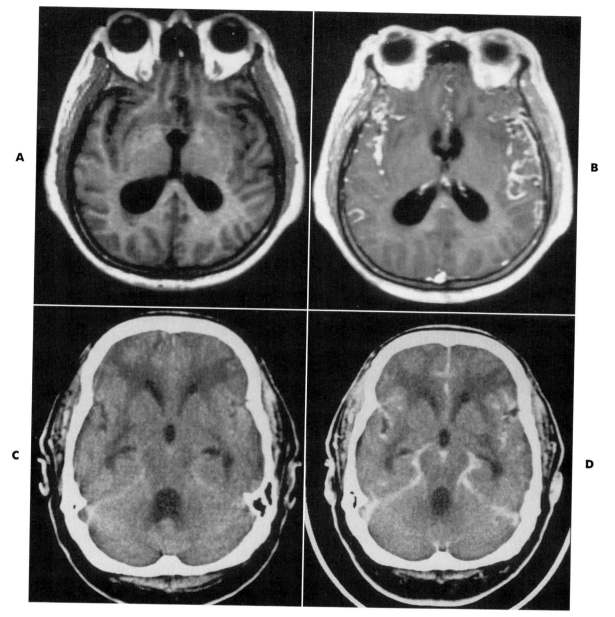

Fig. 3-29. A, T1-weighted MR prior to the administration of gadolinium demonstrating a slight increase in ventricular size. **B,** Postgadolinium enhanced T1-weighted MR demonstrating markedly abnormal contrast enhancement in the meninges in this patient with meningitis. **C,** Axial CT scan without contrast demonstrating abnormal increase density in the subarachnoid spaces and the basilar cisterns. **D,** Following intravenous contrast administration, the axial CT scan demonstrates diffuse abnormal contrast enhancement involving the meninges over the surface of the brain and in the basal cisterns. There is evidence of early obstructive hydrocephalus.

tion may show changes in the brain within the first 2 to 4 hours of an acute stroke; on lower field strength scanners or with diffusion techniques, these changes may be observed within minutes[61,62] (Fig. 3-32).

Gadolinium administration may improve the detection, dating, and grading of cerebral infarction (Fig. 3-33). Four types of MR contrast enhancement in cerebral infarction have been described, including intravascular, meningeal, transitional, and parenchymal.[63] Intravascular enhancement and meningeal enhancement may be the earliest signs of cerebral infarction and can typically be seen within the first 48 hours following the acute event. Parenchymal enhancement is not expected to be identified for the first 1 to 2 days and will typically be present by the end of the first week.[63-66] This enhancement is primarily

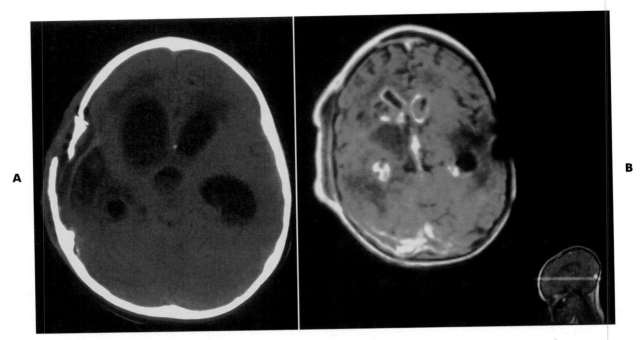

Fig. 3-30. A, Axial CT scan demonstrating postoperative changes and marked hydrocephalus. **B,** Axial T1-weighted MR following the administration of gadolinium demonstrating abnormal contrast enhancement within the walls of the ventricles from ventriculitis. The metallic artifact is secondary to shunt placement performed following the CT scan *A.*

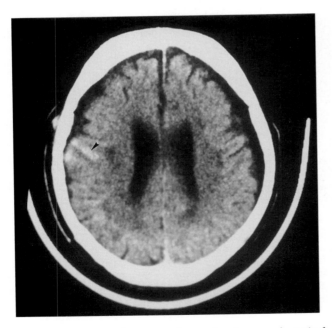

Fig. 3-31. Axial CT demonstrating a focal area of cortical hemorrhage in this patient with an acute hemorrhagic cerebral infarction *(arrow).*

secondary to blood-brain barrier breakdown, and a variety of patterns of contrast enhancement may be seen. These include cortical or subcortical gyriform enhancement, wedge-shaped enhancement, or more diffuse enhancement. Contrast enhancement is gen-

erally most obvious at the second week and may show a noticeable decrease in the T2 and proton density MR changes, with contrast enhancement being the primary means of demonstrating the area of infarction.[63-67]

TRAUMA

Traumatic brain injury occurs more than 2 million times each year in the United States. Economic costs of traumatic brain injury have been estimated to exceed $25 billion annually.[16] CT and MRI are both valuable in the evaluation of acute head trauma. These modalities may be complementary in many instances, and the availability of both modalities at the time of acute head trauma may be necessary for complete diagnosis. The traumatic changes identifiable by CT and MRI include edema, contusion, hemorrhage, hematoma, shearing injury, and fracture.

Brain edema is commonly classified as vasogenic, cytotoxic, and interstitial. Vasogenic edema is considered the most common and is attributable to blood-brain barrier breakdown. This is the type of edema most commonly seen in trauma but may also be associated with primary brain neoplasms, metastases, hemorrhage, infarction, and inflammation. Vasogenic edema represents a leakage of fluid from within the cellular structures of the brain and may be seen as thin linear projections into the adjacent white matter from the area of abnormality (Fig. 3-34). On the other hand, cytotoxic edema is an increase in the intra-

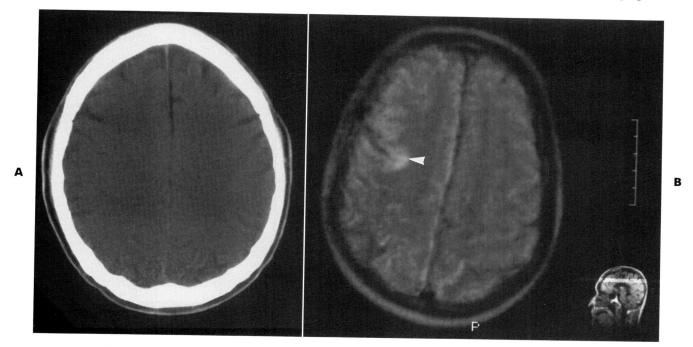

Fig. 3-32. A, CT scan of a patient with an acute cerebral infarct that demonstrates no significant abnormality. **B,** Axial proton density–weighted MR (TR 2000, TE 45) demonstrating an abnormal area of increased signal intensity (*arrow*) in this patient with an acute cerebral infarction.

cellular water content considered to be secondary to ischemia or anoxia. A failure of the cellular sodium pump allows an increase in intracellular sodium and water content. This process may be reversible upon return of an adequate oxygen supply to the involved brain. Interstitial edema represents an increase in CSF in the paraventricular interstitial spaces. This type of edema is generally related to an elevated intraventricular pressure and may be identified on MRI as a high-intensity margin around the ventricles.[2,68-70]

Shearing injuries or deep white matter injuries are frequently identified and may result from rapid rotational forces. The lack of uniformity between white and gray matter leads to different degrees of rotation of these tissues and thus results in injury at the junction of gray and white matter interfaces. Although these injuries may be identified with CT, MRI appears to be much more sensitive[71-75] (Fig. 3-35).

Focal abnormalities in the posttraumatic brain are often identified and frequently represent cerebral contusions. These contusions may be multiple and usually can be found in the anterior temporal, frontal, and occipital regions. Contusions are identified as areas of increased density or hemorrhagic change by CT, and MRI will demonstrate a focal area of abnormal signal intensity (Fig. 3-36). Additional findings that may be present on CT and MRI include subdural and epidural hematomas (Fig. 3-37). Subarachnoid hemor-

rhage and intraventricular hemorrhage may also be present[2,73,74] (Fig. 3-38).

Hemorrhage

The causes of intracranial hemorrhage include trauma, aneurysms, arteriovenous malformations, hypertension, neoplasms, collagen vascular diseases, amyloid angiopathy, venous thrombosis, and coagulopathies. The proper identification of intracranial hemorrhage is important in the diagnosis and management of patients with acute and chronic intraparenchymal hematomas.

Hemorrhage secondary to head trauma may be seen in the subarachnoid space or identified as areas of hemorrhagic contusion with actual hematoma formation (Fig. 3-39). In general, acute hemorrhage is readily diagnosed by CT. The areas of increased density usually stand out strikingly, and CT is a rapid and accessible means of managing these frequently seriously ill patients. Spontaneous subarachnoid hemorrhage (SAH) occurs somewhat commonly, and CT is diagnostic in the vast majority of cases (see Fig. 3-38). However, a normal CT does not entirely rule out the possibility of SAH, which may still be present in up to 20% of negative CT scans performed within the first 48 hours after hemorrhage. Over time, the accuracy of the CT examination declines, until minimal evidence of SAH is expected at 1 week.[2,76,77]

An intracranial aneurysm can be demonstrated in

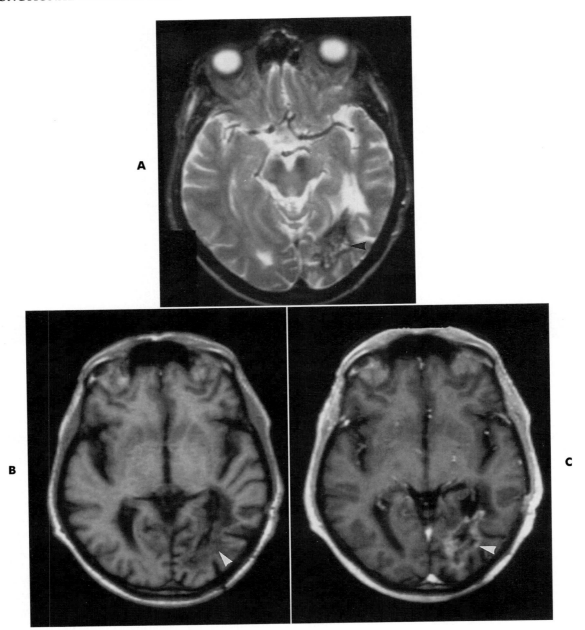

Fig. 3-33. A, Axial T2-weighted MR (TR 2500, TE 90) demonstrating a hemorrhagic infarction (*arrow*). **B,** Axial T1-weighted MR (TR 10, TE 4, FA 10) demonstrating a focal area of decreased intensity in the area of cerebral infarction (*arrow*). **C,** Axial T1-weighted MR (TR 10, TE 4, FA 10) demonstrating peripheral cortical contrast enhancement in this cerebral infarction (*arrow*).

about three fourths of the patients who present with SAH, and a small number will be secondary to arteriovenous malformation (AVM). In the remaining cases, the cause of the SAH is often undetermined. The SAH that occurs as a result of an intracranial aneurysm may collect in CSF spaces near the location of the aneurysm, and this finding can be of assistance in performing additional diagnostic tests such as angiography (Fig. 3-40). MR angiography may be diagnostic in some cases; however, routine angiography is still

considered the "gold standard" for the evaluation of suspected intracranial aneurysms[2,76-78] (Fig. 3-41).

Arteriovenous malformations (AVMs) are the most common type of vascular malformations of the brain. These malformations involve a direct communication between arteries and veins. Associated clinical problems include headache, hemorrhage, seizures, cerebral ischemia, and infarction. CT and MR may demonstrate abnormally enlarged blood vessels and focal atrophy (Fig. 3-42). Edema and mass effect are seldom encoun-

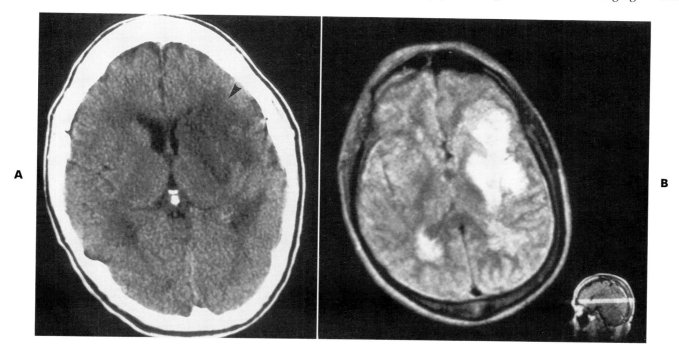

Fig. 3-34. A, CT scan following acute head trauma demonstrating severe edema from intracerebral contusion (*arrow*). **B,** Axial proton density–weighted MR (TR 2000, TE 45) demonstrating abnormal increased signal intensity from cerebral edema as a result of head injury.

tered unless there has been a recent associated hemorrhage.[2,76,77]

Hemorrhage resulting from hypertension is most often seen in elderly patients and occurs most frequently in areas of the basal ganglia and internal capsule (Fig. 3-43). Although there is common involvement of the lateral putamen, hemorrhage in the caudate nucleus, thalamus, brainstem, or cerebellum may also be identified secondary to hypertension.[2,69]

Many published studies have described the MR appearance and evolution of intracranial hemorrhages. There are areas of disagreement in the literature, particularly related to the expected temporal MR appearance of hemorrhage. A common pattern in the appearance of intraparenchymal hemorrhage is identifiable when consideration of the field strength of the MR scanner is included. Understanding the temporal patterns in the appearance of hemorrhage can aid in the interpretation of the complex magnetic resonance images of intraparenchymal hemorrhage. The following designations have been used to describe the time periods after the onset of hemorrhage[80]:

hyperacute—less than 24 hours
acute—1 day to 1 week
subacute—an *early* period from 2 weeks to 1 month, and a late period from 2 weeks to 1 month
chronic—longer than 1 month

In general, on T1-weighted images a hemorrhagic lesion in the *hyperacute* stage is seen as an area of subtle

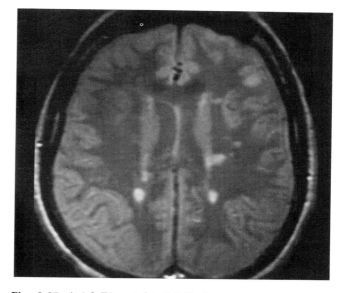

Fig. 3-35. Axial T2-weighted MR demonstrating multiple areas of deep shearing injury in this patient who was involved in a motor vehicle accident.

hyperintensity to isointensity, with T2-weighted images showing a more significant initial hyperintensity. There is a rapid decrease in intensity to mildly hypointense during the *acute* period (1 to 7 days). On T2-weighted sequences the initial hyperintensity decreases to hypointensity within the first 24 to 48 hours (Fig. 3-44). T2-weighted images remain markedly

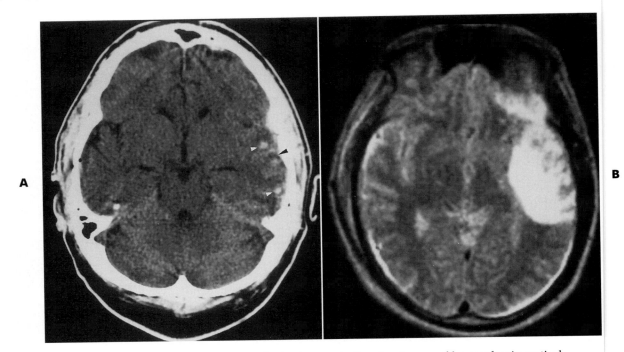

Fig. 3-36. **A,** Axial CT scan of the brain demonstrating focal areas of hemorrhagic cortical contusions (*arrows*). **B,** Axial MR scan obtained immediately following the CT scan in **A,** which demonstrates a large area of contusion and small bilateral subdural hematomas.

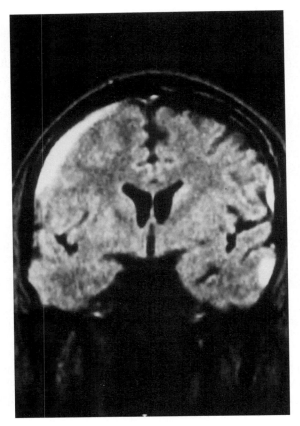

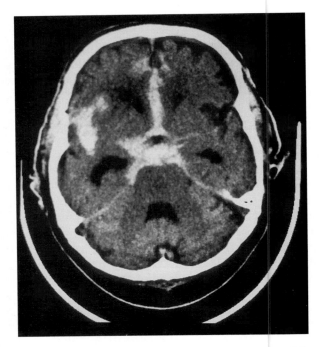

Fig. 3-38. Axial CT scan of the brain demonstrating diffuse subarachnoid hemorrhage (white) and evidence of early obstructive hydrocephalus.

Fig. 3-37. Coronal T1-weighted MR demonstrating bilateral extraaxial fluid collections with high signal from subdural hematomas.

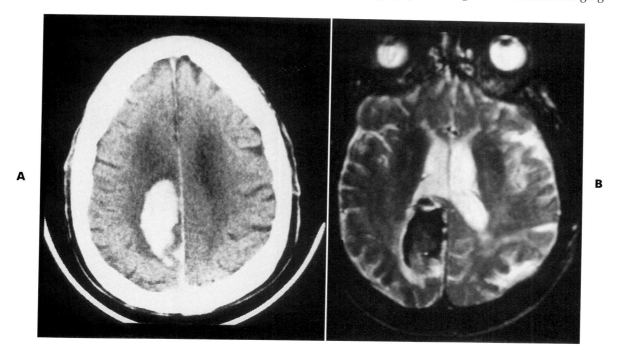

Fig. 3-39. A, Axial CT scan demonstrating an acute hematoma. **B,** Axial T2-weighted MR (TR 2500, TE 90) demonstrating decreased signal intensity in acute hemorrhage (compare to **A**).

hypointense during the *acute* and *early subacute* period, becoming entirely hyperintense by the end of the second to third week. On T1-weighted imaging in the *subacute* period (1 week to 1 month), the hemorrhage gradually returns to hyperintensity, starting from a bright rim and extending inward so that the entire lesion is hyperintense by approximately the first to second week (Fig. 3-45). In the *chronic* stage (longer than 1 month), hemorrhage starts as a hyperintense lesion with a rim of decreased signal surrounding it (Fig. 3-46). This lesion gradually decreases in intensity, becoming hypointense consistent with encephalomalacia on T1. Throughout the *chronic* period T2-weighted images remain hyperintense with a rim of significant hypointensity. This appearance is also consistent with hemorrhage reabsorption and encephalomalacia. These patterns appear to be relatively consistent for hemorrhage on T1- and T2-weighted images and are seen at all field strengths. As the strength of the field increases, the patterns of change are more gradual and show more detail.[80]

The variability in appearance of hemorrhage suggests that a single appearance cannot be considered absolutely diagnostic any time after the onset. The variability observed in intracranial hemorrhage also suggests that a variety of factors may be involved in the pattern of evolving hematomas. Several factors have been proposed to contribute to the MR appearance of hemorrhage. These factors include a variable rate of deoxyhemoglobin and methemoglobin forma-

tion, clot matrix formation and retraction, increased red blood cell (RBC) concentration caused by settling and packing, and changes in intracellular protein concentration resulting from changes in RBC hydration. These factors have the potential to significantly alter the MR appearance of individual hemorrhages and thus introduce variation from the expected temporal pattern of hemorrhage.[80]

Paramagnetic compounds such as deoxyhemoglobin and methemoglobin alter the MR appearance of an area by decreasing the T1 and/or T2 relaxation times. Shortening the T2 and T1 relaxation times results in an increase in image intensity on T1-weighted spin echo images and a decrease in image intensity on a T2-weighted spin echo image, particularly at higher field strengths (> 0.5 T).[80-82] The loss of extracellular fluid around the RBCs that occurs when blood settles and clots could attenuate and possibly eliminate these effects, even at high field strengths.[80,83] The evolution of the hemorrhage and the formation of these paramagnetic forms of hemoglobin may occur at variable times depending on the location and nature of the hemorrhage and the state of the surrounding tissue.[80]

T1 and T2 relaxation times may also decrease by processes that increase the extracellular protein concentration in the area of the hemorrhage. Such processes include clot matrix formation and retraction as well as RBC packing and concentration.[80,84,85] These processes have been shown to shorten T1 and T2 relaxation times, with a more pronounced re

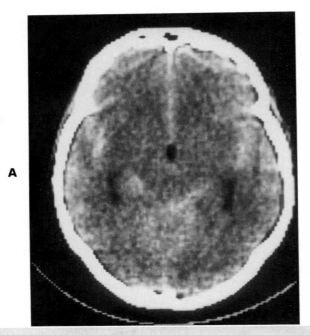

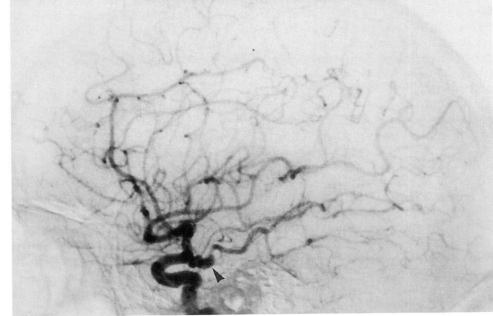

Fig. 3-40. **A**, Axial CT scan demonstrating diffuse subarachnoid hemorrhage with abnormal increased density in the subarachnoid spaces. **B**, Lateral subtraction angiographic film demonstrating a posterior communicating artery aneurysm (*arrow*).

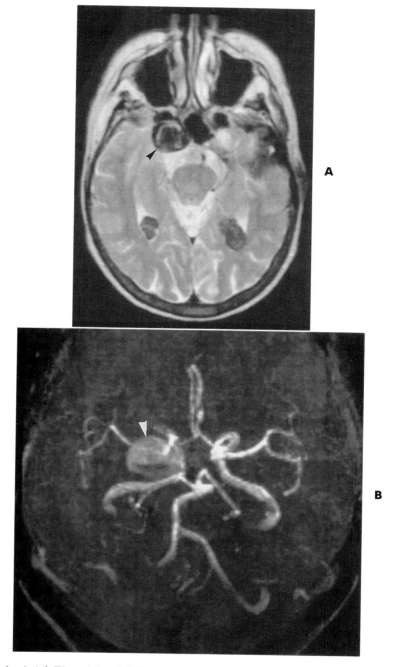

Fig. 3-41. A, Axial T2-weighted MR (TR 3460, TE 93) demonstrating abnormal signal intensity and flow void within an aneurysm (*arrow*). **B,** Magnetic resonance angiogram demonstrating abnormal signal intensity within an aneurysm (*arrow*). (Case courtesy of Dr. Thomas Carlow.)

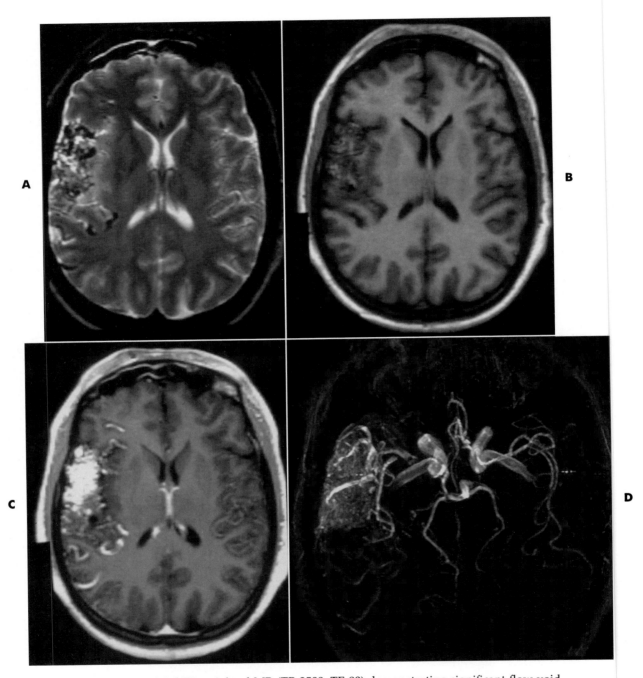

Fig. 3-42. A, Axial T2-weighted MR (TR 2500, TE 90) demonstrating significant flow void in a large arteriovenous malformation. **B,** Axial T1-weighted MR demonstrating focal areas of flow void in arteriovenous malformation. **C,** Axial T2-weighed MR following the administration of gadolinium demonstrating markedly abnormal contrast enhancement in a large arteriovenous malformation. **D,** Axial magnetic resonance angiogram demonstrating abnormal increased vascularity in a large arteriovenous malformation.

duction in T2 than in T1 at both low and high field strengths.[80,86,87]

Fluctuations in RBC hydration may inversely cause a decrease in intracellular protein concentration. These changes in RBC hydration have the ability to produce a profound increase or decrease in T2 relaxation times (particularly at low and intermediate field strengths) and may dominate image contrast on both T1- and T2-weighted spin echo scans.[80,88] Although the lack of an entirely consistent pattern in the appearance of hemorrhage on MR makes the diagnosis more difficult, an understanding of the factors involved can facilitate the identification of hemorrhage by MR. The marked variability that is observed in hemorrhages can be explained in part by the multiple factors of time, biochemical change, and structural alterations in the evolving hematoma.[80]

WHITE MATTER DISEASE

Our understanding of white matter diseases of the brain has been dramatically improved by the advent of MR. It was not until clinical MR became generally available that its impact on this category of disease could be appreciated. Currently, both normal and abnormal conditions of white matter are far better delineated by MR than by any other imaging modality.

Traditionally, white matter disease has been divided into dysmyelinating diseases and demyelinating "myelinoclastic diseases."[89-94] The dysmyelinating diseases are, in general, considered a group of disorders in which there is an absence of normal myelin formation, a delay of myelin formation, or a disturbance in myelin maintenance. Although dysmyelinating diseases are generally considered conditions in which there is an abnormality in the enzymatic, biochemical, or physical condition of myelin, it is possible to see features of both dysmyelination and demyelination simultaneously. This is particularly likely in conditions where a metabolic defect may be present, which causes increased susceptibility to the demyelinating process.[89-92]

Demyelinating or myelinoclastic diseases are conditions primarily affecting the white matter of the brain. This may involve the myelin sheath and/or the oligodendrocyte that produces the myelin. The term "demyelinating disease" is usually in reference to a presumption that normally formed myelin has been subsequently subjected to a condition that results in its loss. Demyelinating diseases are commonly referred to as primary or secondary. The category of primary demyelinating diseases is restricted to those processes that destroy the myelin sheath, tend to spare other parts of the nervous system (such as nerve cells and supporting structures), and demonstrate a relative lack of wallerian degeneration.[89,91,92]

Secondary demyelination refers to conditions that

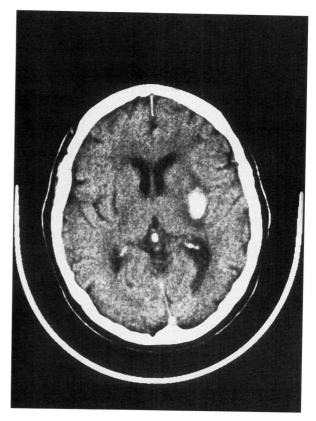

Fig. 3-43. Axial CT scan demonstrating the typical appearance of a hypertensive hemorrhage.

may result in a loss of myelin and includes ischemia, anoxia, infection, toxic agents, and diseases of unknown etiology that frequently demonstrate white matter lesions. When the term "white matter disease" is used in reference to secondary demyelinating processes, this category could include most diseases of the central nervous system.[89-95] As the etiology of the demyelinating diseases is identified, some authors prefer to remove them from the category of white matter disease and place them in a category such as infection.[92] The difficulty with this approach is that it results in a constantly changing list of diseases, and at any given time, there may be a significant difference in opinion regarding etiology. A variety of classification systems for white matter disease have been proposed.[89-97] Regardless of the classification system used, there will be significant difficulties since our understanding of white matter disease is constantly changing.

The normal development of the white matter through the process of myelination is dynamic; it occurs from the fifth fetal month and may continue throughout life, with the normal developmental myelination of the brain extending at least late into the second decade.[93,94,98,99] Myelination proceeds from

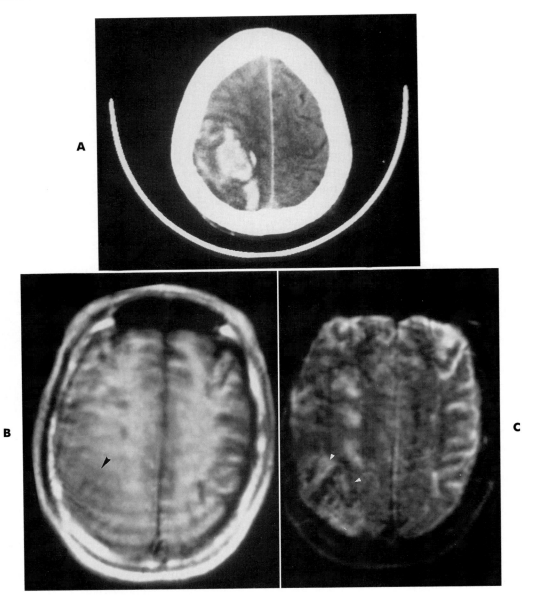

Fig. 3-44. A, Axial CT scan demonstrating acute intracerebral hemorrhage. **B,** Axial T1-weighted MR (TR 600, TE 15) demonstrating relatively isointense signal in the area of hemorrhage (*arrow*) with some focal areas of increased signal. **C,** T2-weighted MR (TR 2500, TE 90) demonstrating focal areas of abnormal increased signal intensity and some areas of abnormal decreased signal intensity (*arrows*) in this acute hemorrhage (evaluated by 1.5 T MR).

the brainstem to the cerebellum, basal ganglia, and cerebral hemispheres, with the general pattern reflecting a caudal to cephalad progression. In addition, there is a dorsal to ventral progression within brain regions. The occipital areas of the cerebral hemispheres myelinate initially, the frontal regions later; the dorsal brainstem myelinates early, with the corticospinal tracts of the ventral brainstem also myelinating later. The process of brain myelination proceeds rapidly until approximately 2 years of age, with a

marked reduction in the process of myelination after the third and fourth decades.[94]

The developing white matter is best identified on T1-weighted images until approximately 6 months of age, with heavily weighted T2 images preferred from 6 to 18 months. T2-weighted images using a TR of 2500 to 3000 msec and a TE of approximately 70 to 100 msec are preferred in children being evaluated with MR (Fig. 3-47). Since myelination is identified differently on T1-weighted images than on T2-

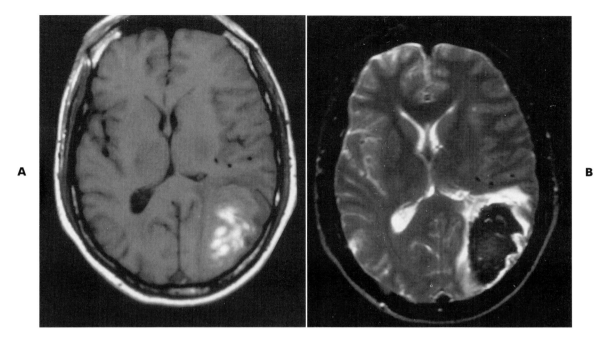

Fig. 3-45. A, Axial T1-weighted MR (TR 648, TE 15) demonstrating abnormal increased signal intensity in an area of acute to subacute hemorrhage. **B**, Axial T2-weighted MR (TR 2380, TE 80) demonstrating a focal area of relatively decreased signal intensity with a surrounding rim of abnormal increased signal intensity caused by edema in this acute to subacute hemorrhage.

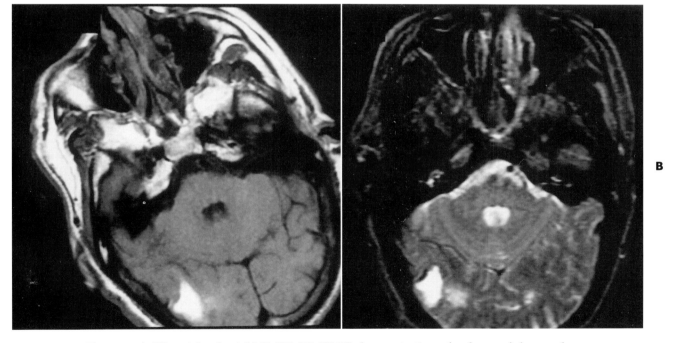

Fig. 3-46. A, T1-weighted axial MR (TR 650, TE 20) demonstrating a focal area of abnormal increased signal intensity in subacute to chronic hemorrhage. **B**, T2-weighted MR (TR 2800, TE 100) demonstrating focally abnormal increased signal intensity in a subacute to chronic hematoma.

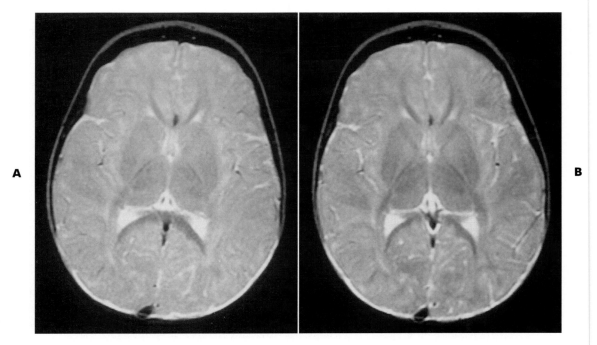

Fig. 3-47. A, Axial T2-weighted MR (TR 2800, TE 100) in a 12-month-old infant (compare to **B**). **B,** Axial T2-weighted MR (TR 2800, TE 110) performed at the same time as **A.** Note the difference that going from a TE of 100 in **A** to a TE of 110 in **B** makes in the appearance of the white matter.

weighted images and at different times, there is some overlap in the evaluation process using these pulse sequences.[93,94,98,99] Factors such as marked prematurity, significant variations in gestational age at birth, and conditions such as CNS insults or nutritional factors may play important roles in the "normal" myelination process.

It appears that the "normal" brain will demonstrate minimal changes on MR from approximately 24 months of age until midlife. Clearly, conditions begin to develop in the fourth or fifth decade that can be detected in the white matter of the central nervous system of "normal" individuals.[100-103] These "white matter changes of aging" complicate the interpretation of MR images since the degree of these changes varies considerably in the normal population.[103] These white matter changes have been described to be (1) focal areas of demyelination, (2) regions of ischemic change, (3) dilated Virchow-Robin spaces, and (4) unidentifiable on pathologic specimens.[100-103] During the interpretation of MR images, it is important to realize that these changes can occur in "normal" populations. The clinical history and an internal reference for acceptable norms are required (Fig. 3-48).

Developmental Delay

Congenital anomalies such as holoprosencephaly, encephalocele, cerebral or cerebellar aplasia, and hypoplasia may be associated with a lack of normally developed white matter. These changes occur between 5 and 8 weeks of gestation. Conditions such as microencephaly and colpocephaly or porencephaly may also involve areas of decreased myelination. These conditions as well as hypoplasia or aplasia of the corpus callosum are expected to occur between 2 and 6 months of gestational age. Hypomyelination and retarded myelination more typically occur between 7 months of gestation and 1 year of age[104] (Fig. 3-49).

A possible cause of delayed myelination during the perinatal period is an anoxic or ischemic injury. There is some overlap in the evaluation process using these pulse sequences. The MR findings in perinatal anoxic-ischemic insult appear to depend on the age at the time of injury and are frequently represented by changes in the normal pattern of myelination or brain maturation.[105,106] Congenital anomalies may explain the findings often attributed to birth anoxia, and it is important to evaluate MR scans for congenital anomalies when birth asphyxia is suspected.[107] Pathologic correlation with CT scanning in perinatal asphyxia has been valuable in the detection of supratentorial hemorrhage; however, white matter lesions have correlated rather poorly.[108] Pathologic correlation with white matter disease in MR is significantly more promising.[100-102]

Anoxic-ischemic insults at approximately 24 to 26 weeks of gestational age result in enlarged ventricular trigones and minimal periventricular gliosis. Insults at

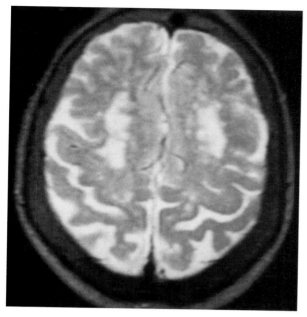

Fig. 3-48. Axial T2-weighted MR (TR 2000, TE 80) demonstrating bilateral abnormal increased signal intensity in the white matter of this 84-year-old normal volunteer.

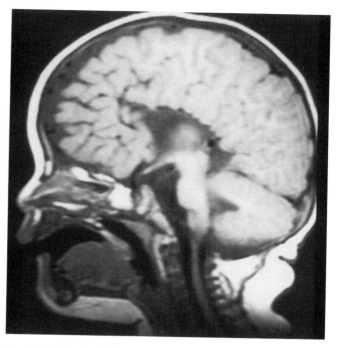

Fig. 3-49. Sagittal T1-weighted MR (TR 600, TE 20) in a patient with agenesis of the corpus callosum. Compare to Fig. 3-2.

28 to 34 weeks demonstrate variable ventricular dilatation with identifiable periventricular gliosis. At approximately 36 weeks of gestation, anoxic-ischemic injury results in mild cortical or subcortical atrophy, with gliosis including the deep white matter and periventricular regions. Full-term infants demonstrate cortical and subcortical gliosis, with atrophy predominately in the watershed regions. At 44 to 46 weeks of age anoxic-ischemic injury results in cortical and subcortical watershed gliosis with atrophy and relative sparing of the immediate periventricular area.[105] Severe anoxic-ischemic injury results in hypoxic damage and gliosis in the basal ganglia region, which will predominately involve the head of the caudate nucleus, lentiform nuclei, and thalamus. Prior to MRI this "status marmoratus" was visible only at pathology. Magnetic resonance can demonstrate the findings of severe asphyxia in the perinatal period as focal areas of increased signal intensity on T2-weighted images.[94]

In term infants, the "watershed areas" are located in two primary regions: between the middle and posterior cerebral arteries as is traditionally identified in adults, and between the anterior and middle cerebral arteries, with the anterior watershed area more sensitive in infants than adults. This parasagittal distribution of "watershed" represents the most sensitive area for anoxic-ischemic injury in term infants.[94] The brain of the term infant is also different from the fetus in that the more mature brain responds to injury with gliosis while the immature fetal brain responds with liquefaction. Hypoxic injury will result in parasagittal or

"watershed" infarcts in the term infant with eventual gliosis or brain scarring. In the early neonatal period these injuries will best be defined on T1-weighted images; with increasing age these lesions will be better defined by more T2-weighted sequences[94,96,105-108] (Fig. 3-50).

Toxic agents such as maternal cocaine abuse can result in fetal ischemic change identifiable on MR as periventricular increased signal on T2-weighted images.[94] CNS infections involving the fetus are unique in that they result in damage to the developing brain. The age of the fetus at the time of insult may be more important than the infectious process. Infections that occur during the first two trimesters will most frequently result in congenital malformations, while those that occur during the third trimester are more likely to be identified as areas of brain injury. Conditions such as cytomegalovirus, toxoplasmosis, herpes simplex virus, and rubella are commonly associated with various degrees of CNS abnormality resulting from fetal infection[109] (Fig. 3-51).

Dysmyelinating Disease (Leukodystrophies)

Metachromatic leukodystrophy results in diffuse abnormal myelination of the cerebral hemispheres and most commonly occurs as a late infantile condition. This disease will frequently present with a disturbance in gait. There is rapid progression to involvement of speech with intellectual deterioration and death in

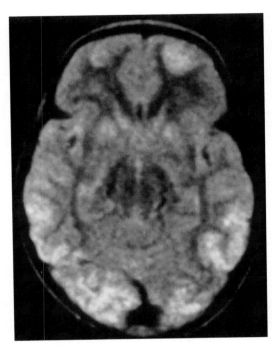

Fig. 3-50. Axial T2-weighted MR (TR 2000, TE 105) in a young child with recent severe hypoxia resulting in abnormal areas of increased signal intensity in the cerebral cortex and basal ganglia.

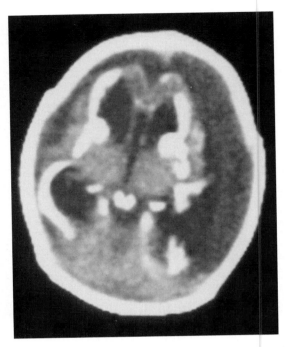

Fig. 3-51. Axial CT scan of an infant who suffered an intrauterine infection with resulting calcifications and loss of brain substance.

approximately 4 years. A juvenile form is identified, with neurologic onset between 5 and 7 years of age and a slower progression. Rarely, this disease can be identified in adults with an organic brain syndrome and progressive neurologic impairment. All types of metachromatic leukodystrophy are the result of a deficiency in the activity of arylsulfatase A. MR in metachromatic leukodystrophy demonstrates abnormal increased signal intensity on T2-weighted images, with decreased signal intensity on T1 and accompanying progressive atrophic change[110,111] (Fig. 3-52).

Krabbe's disease (globoid cell leukodystrophy) begins in early infancy (less than 6 months of age) and is characterized by spasticity and irritability. There is rapid progression to a flaccid state and death within a few years. This disease is a result of a deficiency of galactocerebroside beta-galactosidase.[110,112] As with other disorders of white matter, increased signal intensity on T2-weighted images is expected in the white matter.

Canavan's disease (spongiform leukodystrophy) also begins at less than 6 months of age but may present in the first few weeks of life. This autosomal recessive disorder is secondary to a lack of N-acetylaspartylase and results in hypotonia, macrocephaly, and seizures. Death is common in the first 2 years of life. MR reveals diffuse increase signal intensity on T2-weighted images in the white matter.[110,113]

Alexander's disease (fibrinoid leukodystrophy) can present within the first few weeks of life. This disease is manifested by macrocephaly and progressive spastic quadriparesis, with death in infancy or early childhood. MR again shows diffuse abnormal increase signal on T2 and decreased signal on T1. Early in the disease changes may be identified primarily in the frontal lobes, with severe atrophy of the corpus callosum late in the disease.[110,114,115]

Pelizaeus-Merzbacher disease is an X-linked leukodystrophy that may be seen clinically in the first weeks of life. Cerebellar symptoms, including markedly abnormal eye movements, are characteristic, with progressive neurologic deterioration to death in adolescence or early adulthood. The MR findings are similar to those of a newborn brain with relative lack of myelination.[110,116]

Adrenal leukodystrophy is a sex-linked recessive disorder of childhood characterized by CNS demyelination and adrenal insufficiency. The typical childhood adrenal leukodystrophy will present in a male between 4 and 8 years of age and is clinically manifested by behavioral disorders, dementia, and visual or hearing impairment. Adrenal insufficiency may follow these CNS symptoms, with death occurring in several years. Adrenomyeloneuropathy presents in young adulthood in families with childhood adrenal leukodystrophy. This condition is also X-linked recessive and is the second most common form of the adrenal leukodystrophy–adrenomyeloneuropathy complex.

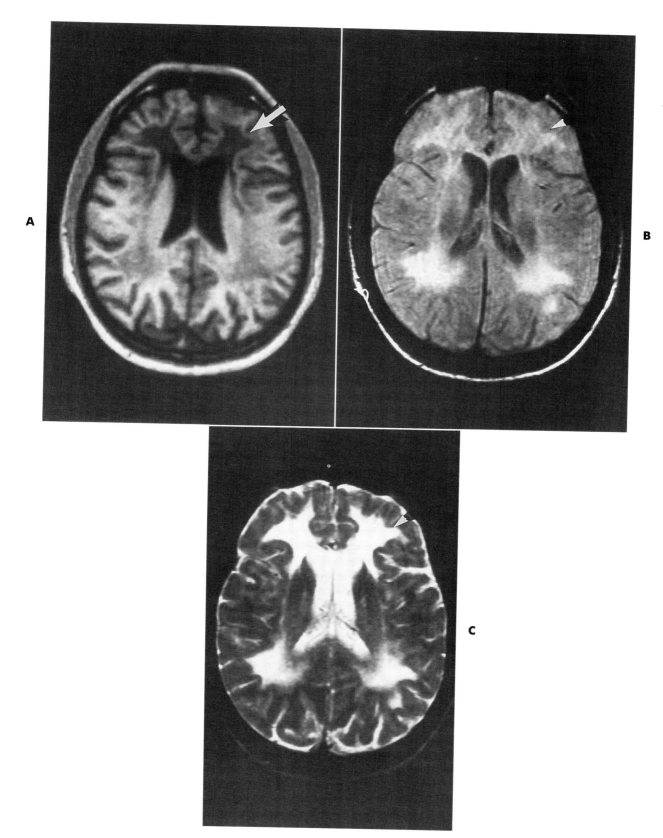

Fig. 3-52. **A,** Axial T1-weighted MR (TR 10, TE 4, FA 10) demonstrating focal areas of abnormal decreased signal intensity in the periventricular white matter in this patient with metachromatic leukodystrophy. **B,** Axial proton density MR (TR 2500, TE 22) demonstrating markedly abnormal increased signal intensity in the periventricular white matter. **C,** T2-weighted MR (TR 2500, TE 90) demonstrating markedly abnormal increased signal intensity in the periventricular white matter in this patient with metachromatic leukodystrophy.

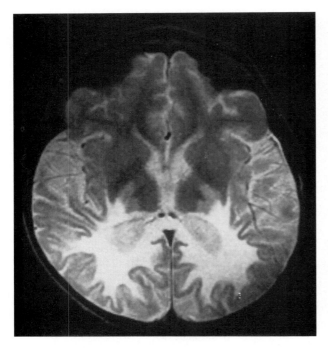

Fig. 3-53. Axial T2-weighted MR (TR 2500, TE 80) demonstrating markedly abnormal increased signal intensity in the periventricular white matter posteriorly in this patient with adrenoleukodystrophy.

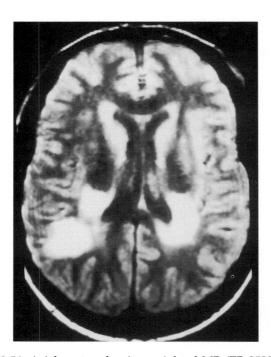

Fig. 3-54. Axial proton density–weighted MR (TR 2500, TE 22) demonstrating markedly abnormal increased signal intensity in the periventricular and subcortical white matter in this patient with multiple sclerosis.

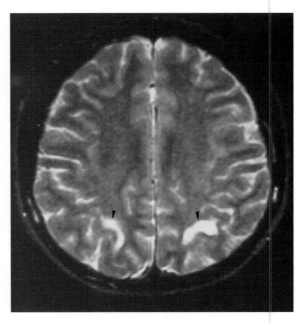

Fig. 3-55. Axial T2-weighted MR (TR 2500, TE 80) demonstrating focal areas of abnormal increased signal intensity in the posterior subcortical white matter in this patient with Navajo neuropathy (*arrows*).

Neonatal adrenal leukodystrophy is the least common form and is autosomal recessive. These infants usually live for a very short period of time. Neonatal adrenal leukodystrophy has not been described in families exhibiting childhood adrenal leukodystrophy or adrenomyeloneuropathy. Patients with adrenal leukodystrophy or adrenomyeloneuropathy demonstrate excessive amounts of very-long-chain fatty acids (VLCFAs) in the Schwann cells and adrenocortical cells. MR may demonstrate areas of abnormal increased signal intensity of T2-weighted images and decreased signal intensity of T1-weighted images particularly in the occipital white matter. Atrophy of the spinal cord may also be present[117] (Fig. 3-53).

Demyelinating Disease (Myelinoclastic)

Multiple sclerosis (MS) is the most common form of demyelinating condition. The clinical presentation is variable and includes acute episodes of focal neurologic deficits, with exacerbations and remissions quite common. The clinical course may be quite variable, from vague symptoms over several months or years to a very rapid onset. Pathologically, multiple focal areas of demyelination varying in size are identified throughout the white matter of the central nervous system. MS plaques are typically identified adjacent to the lateral ventricles and may also be found in the cortical and deep gray matter. MR will demonstrate focal areas of abnormal increased signal intensity on T2-weighted imaging in the periventricular region,

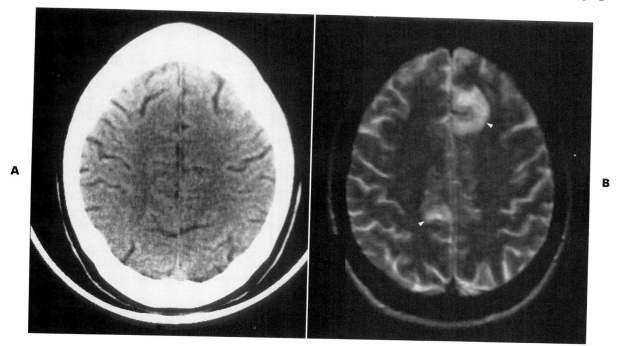

Fig. 3-56. **A,** Axial CT scan demonstrating no definite abnormality and interpreted as normal in this patient with AIDS. **B,** Axial T2-weighted MR (TR 2500, TE 90) demonstrating abnormal areas of increased signal intensity (*arrows*) in the subcortical white matter that were not identified on the CT scan (see **A**).

brainstem, and cerebellar white matter. These abnormal areas of increased signal intensity may also be identified in the subcortical white matter, internal capsule, and temporal lobe white matter. The initial presentation may involve a few scattered lesions or occasionally an isolated focus of abnormal signal intensity[110] (Fig. 3-54).

Navajo Neuropathy

Navajo neuropathy is a hereditary sensorimotor disease that may present in early childhood as an autosomal recessive condition. This disease was originally described as a severe peripheral neuropathy; however, severe CNS white matter changes similar to the leukodystrophies have been described[118] (Fig. 3-55).

Secondary Demyelination

Viral infections may result in severe white matter demyelination as a result of the primary effects of the virus or by viral-induced immune complexes. Progressive multifocal leukoencephalopathy (PML) occurs in immunocompromised individuals and is frequently identified in patients with the acquired immunodeficiency syndrome (AIDS). PML is caused by infection with the DNA papovavirus and results in focal areas of demyelination within the CNS. MR demonstrates multiple focal or confluent areas of abnormal increased signal intensity within the white matter of the

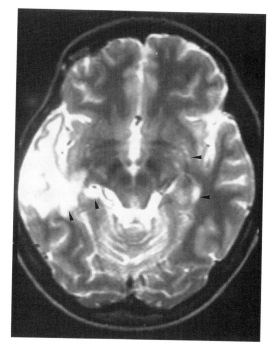

Fig. 3-57. Axial T2-weighted MR (TR 2500, TE 90) demonstrating focal abnormal increased signal intensity secondary to radiation (*arrows*) in this patient treated with maximum radiation therapy following resection of a high-grade glioma.

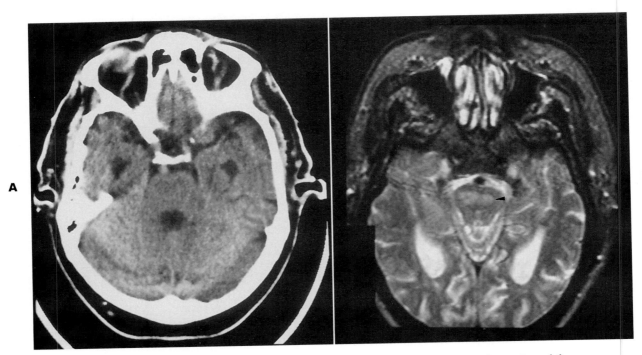

A

B

Fig. 3-58. **A,** Axial CT scan demonstrating focal decreased attenuation in the region of the central pons in this patient with central pontine myelinolysis. **B,** Axial T2-weighted MR (TR 2500, TE 90) demonstrating focal abnormal increased signal intensity in the central pons (*arrow*) in this patient with central pontine myelinolysis. Compare to **A** and note the difficulty in identifying this abnormality on CT.

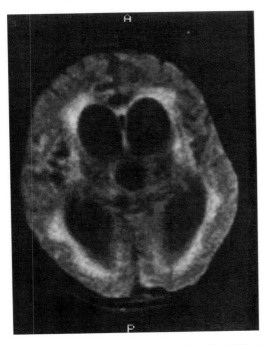

Fig. 3-59. Proton density–weighted MR (TR 2000, TE 30) demonstrating hydrocephalus with focal periventricular abnormal increased signal intensity secondary to trans-ependymal flow of CSF.

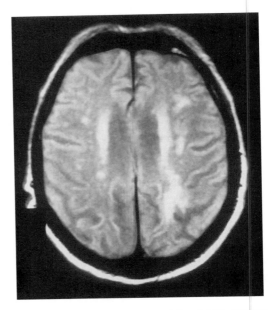

Fig. 3-60. Axial proton density–weighted MR (TR 2500, TE 90) demonstrating periventricular and subcortical white matter changes in an elderly patient.

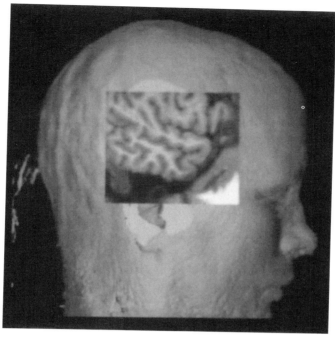

Fig. 3-61. Three-dimensional reconstruction MR of the skin's surface with a "window" revealing the MR image of the underlying brain.

CNS. Similar white matter changes may also be identified as a result of primary AIDS virus infection (Fig. 3-56). Acute disseminated encephalomyelitis (ADE) may present within 1 week after exposure to varicella or influenza. MR will again demonstrate focal abnormalities in the white matter of the CNS. Subacute sclerosing panencephalitis (SSPE) occurs following exposure to the measles virus and may be delayed by as much as 6 years. MR will demonstrate focal abnormalities of increased signal intensity of T2-weighted images in the CNS white matter.[47]

Toxic conditions may result in severe white matter changes. Radiation effects may be seen as focal or diffuse abnormal increased signal intensities on intermediate and T2-weighted images (Fig. 3-57). Subcortical arteriosclerotic encephalopathy and anoxia may also result in abnormal increased signal intensity in the periventricular and subcortical white matter on T2-weighted images. Electrolyte abnormalities and alcohol have been associated with osmotic myelinolysis (OM), which may involve primarily the pons in central pontine myelinolysis (CPM). Extrapontine myelinolysis (EPM) is found in approximately 50% of osmotic myelinosis cases. Central pontine myelinolysis is characterized by a focus of demyelination identified as abnormal increased signal intensity on T2-weighted images in the pons[110,119,120] (Fig. 3-58).

Conditions Affecting White Matter

A variety of conditions may affect the white matter, including primary or secondary neoplasms, encepha-

litis, abscess, infarction, and the edema associated with these conditions. Hydrocephalus has also been demonstrated to result in changes within the periventricular white matter [121] (Fig. 3-59). Dilated Virchow-Robin spaces and enlarged perivascular spaces may contribute to increased signal intensity in the regions of the white matter of the CNS.[102,104]

Adult White Matter Lesions

A common clinical problem that occurs in the interpretation of MR scans is the adult with single or multiple focal areas of abnormal increased signal intensity in the white matter of the CNS. The differential diagnosis of this finding includes ischemia, demyelination, dilated Virchow-Robin spaces, primary or metastatic neoplasm, shearing injury, and idiopathic change (Fig. 3-60). The judicious use of MR contrast will assist in the differentiation of primary and secondary neoplasms with clinical information frequently required to further narrow the differential. Since these white matter changes can occur in the "normal" population, it is equally important to consider the possibility that they may be of little or no clinical significance[103] (see Fig. 3-48).

White matter disease of the central nervous system may be the result of developmental delay, dysmyelinating or demyelinating conditions, secondary demyelination, and a variety of other conditions that can affect these areas of the brain. Although white matter changes may be nonspecific, the recognition of these white matter changes is important. MR is currently the diagnostic procedure of choice for the evaluation of possible white matter disease.

Possible Future Directions

The technologic breakthroughs that have occurred in CT and MR have been so phenomenal that it is hard to predict further advances in this technology. Nonetheless, scientists and manufacturers who work in these areas continue to make remarkable improvements in this already significantly advanced equipment. These include improved spatial resolution, decreased scan times, and computerized assistance for analysis of results. As we continue to observe the remarkable speed and accuracy of this technology, 3-D imaging and virtual reality imaging emerge (Fig. 3-61). Although it is impossible to demonstrate in 2-D pictures, holography is becoming an increasingly viable imaging tool. These "holographic x-rays" literally stand off the page; the viewer can place a pointer or other object within the image in space. This type of real-time interaction can be taken into the operating room and can also be used for review with physicians and patients. It is also possible for surgeons in the operating room to view 3-D or holographic images through specialized glasses or head gear as they operate in real time on the patient. Virtual reality technology enables the surgeon to literally observe the 3-D images obtained on a patient and superimpose these images on the patient as he or she operates. This type of technology may revolutionize the approach to surgery in the future and dramatically improve both patient outcome and the length of hospitalization required for elaborate surgical procedures. CT and MR currently provide the images used by these advanced presentation modalities. It appears that CT and MR will continue to play a vital role in the evaluation of CNS disease. The exquisite anatomic detail provided by these imaging techniques provides the infrastructure for functional imaging of the brain.

REFERENCES

1. Goodenough DJ, Weaver KE: A decade of progress in computed tomography, Diagn Imaging 211-217, 1985.
2. Orrison WW: Introduction to neuroimaging, Boston, 1989, Little, Brown, pp 65-234.
3. Brooks RA, Di Chiro G: Theory of image reconstruction in computed tomography, Radiology 117:561-572, 1975.
4. Klucznik RP, Carrier DA, Pyka R et al: Placement of a ferromagnetic intracerebral aneurysm clip in a magnetic field with a fatal outcome, Radiology 187:855-856, 1993.
5. Croft BY: Single-photon emission computed tomography, St Louis, 1986, Mosby.
6. Kuhl DE: Rotational scanning of the liver, Radiology 71:875-876, 1958.
7. Kuhl DE et al: Transverse section and rectilinear brain scanning with Tc-99m pertechnetate, Radiology 86:822-829, 1966.
8. Hounsfield GN: Computerized transverse axial scanning (tomography): Part I. Description of a system, Br J Radiol 46:1016-1022, 1973.
9. Radon J: On the determination of functions from the integrals along certain manifolds, Mathematische-Physische Klasse 69: 262-277, 1917.
10. Herman GT, Lakshminarayanan AV, Naparstek A: Convolution reconstruction techniques for divergent beams, Comput Biol Med 6:259-271, 1976.
11. Herman GT: Image reconstruction from projections—the fundamentals of computerized tomography, New York, 1980, Academic Press.
12. Norman D, Stevens EA, Wing SD et al: Quantitative aspects of contrast enhancement in cranial computed tomography, Radiology 129:683-688, 1978.
13. Latchaw RE, Gold LHA, Tourje EJ: A protocol for the use of contrast enhancement in cranial computed tomography, Radiology 126:681-687, 1978.
14. Runge VM, Schaible TF, Goldstein HA et al: Gd-DTPA: clinical efficacy, RadioGraphics 8(1):147-158, 1988.
15. Runge VM, Wood ML, Kaufman D et al: Gd-DTPA: future applications with advanced imaging techniques, RadioGraphics 8(1):161-179, 1988.
16. Rose CF, editor: World neurology, Official Newsletter of the World Federation of Neurology 8(1), 1993.
17. Davis DO: CT in the diagnosis of supratentorial tumors, Semin Roentgenol 12(2):97-108, 1977.
18. Weistein MA, Modic MT, Pavlicek W, Keyser CK: Nuclear magnetic resonance for the examination of brain tumors, Semin Roentgenol 14(2):139-147, 1984.
19. Potts DG, Abbott GF, von Sneidern JV: National Cancer Institute study: evaluation of computed tomography in the diagnosis of intracranial neoplasms. III. Metastatic tumors, Radiology 136:657-664, 1980.
20. Graif M, Bydder GM, Steiner RE, Nierdorf FP: Contrast-enhanced MR imaging of malignant brain tumors, AJNR 6:855-862, 1985.
21. Schörner W, Laniado M, Niendorf HP et al: Time-dependent changes in image contrast in brain tumors after gadolinium-DTPA, AJNR 7(6):1013-1020, 1986.
22. Claussen C, Laniado M, Schorner W, Neindorf HP: Gadolinium-DTPA in MR imaging of glioblastomas and intracranial metastases, AJNR 6:669-674, 1985.
23. Lee BCP, Kneeland JB, Cahill PT, Deek MD: MR recognition of supratentorial tumors, AJNR 6:871-878, 1985.
24. Russell EJ, Geremia GK, Johnson CE et al: Multiple cerebral metastases: detectability with Gd-DTPA-enhanced MR imaging, Radiology 165(3):609-617, 1987.
25. Thomson JLG: Computerized axial tomography and the diagnosis of glioma: a study of 100 consecutive histologically proved cases, Clin Radiol 27:431-441, 1976.
26. Brant-Zawadzki M, Badami JP, Mills CM et al: Primary intracranial tumor imaging: a comparison of magnetic resonance and CT, Radiology 150:435-440, 1989.
27. Raushning W: Brain tumors and tumorlike masses: classification and differential diagnosis. In Osborn A, editor: Diagnostic neuroradiology, St Louis, 1994, Mosby, pp 401-522.
28. McCormack BM, Miller DC, Budzilovich GN et al: Treatment and survival of low-grade astrocytoma in adults 1977-1988, Neurosurgery 31(4):636-642, 1992.
29. Hoshino T, Rodriguez LA, Cho KG et al: Prognostic implications of the proliferative potential of low-grade astrocytomas, J Neurosurg 69:839-842, 1988.
30. Philippon JH, Clemenceau SH, Fauchon FH et al: Supratentorial low-grade astrocytomas in adults, Neurosurgery 32:554-559, 1993.
31. Davis DO: CT in the diagnosis of supratentorial tumors, Semin Roentgenol 12(2):97-108, 1977.
32. Weinstein MA et al: Nuclear magnetic resonance for the examination of brain tumors, Semin Roentgenol 14(2):139-147, 1984.

33. Graif M et al: Contrast-enhanced MR imaging of malignant brain tumors, AJNR 6:855-862, 1985.
34. Schorner W, Laniado M, Niendorf HP et al: Time-dependent changes in image contrast in brain tumors after gadolinium-DTPA, AJNR 7(6):1013-1020, 1986.
35. Edelhoff JC, Ross JS, Modic MT et al: MR imaging of metastic GI adenocarcinoma in brain, AJNR 13:1221-1224, 1992.
36. Potts DG, Abbott GF, von Sneidern JV: National Cancer Institute study: evaluation of computed tomography in the diagnosis of intracranial neoplasms. III. Metastatic tumors. Radiology 136:657-664, 1980.
37. Davis JM, Zimmerman RA, Bilaniuk LT: Metastases to the central nervous system, Radiol Clin North Am 20:417-435, 1982.
38. Deck MDF, Messina AV, Sackett JF: Computed tomography in metastatic disease of the brain, Radiology 119:114-120, 1976.
39. Healy ME, Hesselink JR, Press GA et al: Increased detection of intracranial metastases with intravenous Gd-DTPA, Radiology 165(3):619-624, 1987.
40. Hesseling JR, Healy ME, Press GA et al: Benefits of Gd-DTPA for MR imaging of intracranial abnormalities, J Comput Assist Tomogr 12 (2):266-274, 1988.
41. Servo A, Porras M, Jaaskelainen J et al: Computed tomography and angiography do not reliably discriminate malignant meningiomas from benign ones, Neuroradiology 32:94-97, 1990.
42. New PF, Hesselink JR, O'Carroll CP, Kleinman GM: Malignant meningioma: CT and histologic criteria, including a new CT sign, AJNR 3:267, 1982.
43. Escourolle R, Piorier J, Bruinstein LJ: Manual of basic neuropathology, Philadelphia, 1971, Saunders.
44. Slager UT: Basic neuropathology, Baltimore, 1970, Williams & Wilkins.
45. Elster AD, Challa VR, Gilders TH et al: Meningiomas: MR and histopathologic features, Radiology 170:857-862, 1989.
46. Kaplan RD, Coon S, Drayer BP et al: MR characteristics of meningioma subtypes at 1.5 Tesla, J Comput Assist Tomogr 16:366-371, 1992.
47. Osborn A: Infections of the brain and its lining. In Osborn A, editor: Diagnostic neuroradiology, St Louis, 1994, Mosby, pp 671-715.
48. Davidson HD, Steiner RE: Magnetic resonance imaging in infections of the central nervous system, AJNR 6:499-504, 1985.
49. Demaerel PH, Wilms G, Robberecht W et al: MRI of herpes simplex encephalitis, Neuroradiology 34:490-493, 1992.
50. Rovira MJ, Post MJD, Bowen BC: Central nervous system infections in HIV-infected persons, Neuroimaging Clin North Am 1:179-200, 1991.
51. Revel M-P, Gray F, Brugieres P et al: Hyperdense CT foci in treated AIDS toxoplasmosis encephalitis: MR and pathologic correlation, J Comput Assist Tomogr 16:372-375, 1992.
52. Jensen MC, Brant-Zawadski M: MR imaging of the brain in patients with AIDS: value of routine use of IV gadopentetate dimeglumine, AJR 160:153-157, 1993.
53. Harris TM, Edwards MK: Meningitis, Neuroimaging Clin North Am 1:39-56, 1991.
54. Chang KH, Han MH, Roh JK et al: Gd-DTPA-enhanced MR imaging of the brain in patients with meningitis: comparison with CT, AJNR 11:69-76, 1990.
55. Pfister H-W, Feiden W, Einhaupl K-M: Spectrum of complications during bacterial meningitis in adults, Arch Neurol 50:575-581, 1993.
56. Gautier JC, Pullicino P: A clinical approach to cerebrovascular disease, Neuroradiology 27:452-459, 1985.
57. Weisberg LA, Nice CN: Intracranial tumors simulating the presentation of cerebrovascular syndromes, Am J Med 63:517-524, 1977.
58. Bradley WG, Waluch V, Yadley RA et al: Comparison of CT and MR in 400 patients with suspected disease of the brain and cervical spinal cord, Radiology 152:695-702, 1984.
59. Sipponen JT, Kaste M, Ketonen L et al: Serial nuclear magnetic resonance (NMR) imaging in patients with cerebral infarction, Radiology 151:829-835, 1984.
60. Chaney RK, Taber KH, Orrison WW et al: Magnetic resonance imaging of intracerebral hemorrhage at different field strengths, Neuroimaging Clin North Am 2(1):25-51, 1992.
61. Chien D, Kwong KK, Gress DR et al: MR diffusion imaging of cerebral infarction in humans, AJNR 13:1097-1102, 1992.
62. Bizzi A, Righini A, Turner R et al: MR of diffusion slowing in global cerebral ischemia, AJNR 14:1347-1354, 1993.
63. Elster AD, Moody DM: Early cerebral infarction: gadopentetate dimeglumine enhancement, Radiology 177:627-632, 1990.
64. Virapongse C, Mancuso A, Quisling R: Human brain infarcts: Gd-DTPA-enhanced MR imaging, Radiology 161:785-794, 1986.
65. Imakita S, Nishimura T, Naito H et al: Magnetic resonance imaging of human cerebral infarction: enhancement with Gd-DTPA, Neuroradiology 29:422-429, 1987.
66. Imakita S, Nishimura T, Yamada N et al: Magnetic resonance imaging of cerebral infarction: time course of Gd-DTPA enhancement and CT comparison, Neuroradiology 30:372-378, 1988.
67. Elster AD: MR contrast enhancement in brainstem and deep cerebral infarction, AJNR 12:1127-1132, 1991.
68. Fishman RA: Brain edema, N Engl J Med 293:706, 1975.
69. Bradley WG: Pathophysiologic correlates of signal alterations. In Brant-Zawadzki M, Normal D, editors: Magnetic resonance imaging of the central nervous system, New York, 1987, Raven Press, pp 23-41.
70. Bradley WG, Kortman KE: Cranial MRI: Current clinical applications. In Lee SH, Rao KCVG, editors: Cranial computed tomography and MRI, ed. 2, New York, 1987, McGraw-Hill.
71. Zimmerman RA et al: Head injury: early results of comparing CT and high-field MR, AJNR 7:757-764, 1986.
72. Zimmermaan RA, Bilaniuk LT, Gennerall T: Computed tomography of shearing injuries of the cerebral white matter, Radiology 127:393-396, 1978.
73. Gentry LR, Godersky JC, Thompson BH: Traumatic brain stem injury: MR imaging, Radiology 171(1):177-187, 1989.
74. Gentry LR, Godersky JC, Thompson BH: MR imaging of head trauma: review of the distribution and radiopathologic features of traumatic lesions, AJNR 9:101-110, 1988.
75. Gentry LR, Godersky JC, Thompson B et al: Prospective comparative study of intermediate-field MR and CT in the evaluation of closed head trauma, AJR 150:673-682, 1988.
76. Modest LM, Binet EF: Value of computed tomography in the diagnosis and management of subarachnoid hemorrhage, Neurosurgery 3:151-156, 1978.
77. TerBrugge K, Rao KCVG, Lee SH: Cerebral vascular anomalies. In Lee SH, Rao KCVG, editors: Cranial computed tomography and MRI, ed. 2, New York, 1987, McGraw-Hill.
78. Bjorkesten G, Halonen V: Incidence of intracranial vascular lesions in patients with subarachnoid hemorrhage investigated by four-vessel angiography, J Neurosurg 23:29-32, 1965.
79. Weisberg LA: Computerized tomography in intracranial hemorrhage, Arch Neurol 36:422-426, 1979.
80. Chaney RK, Taber KH, Orrison WW et al: Magnetic resonance imaging of intracerebral hemorrhage at different field strengths, Neuroimaging Clin North Am 2(1):25-51, 1992.
81. Seidenwurm D, Meng T, Kowalski H et al: Intracranial hemorrhagic lesions: evaluation with spin-echo and gradient-refocused MR imaging at 0.5 and 1.5 T, Radiology 172:189-194, 1989.
82. Hesseling JR, Healy ME, Dunn WM et al: Magnetic resonance imaging of hemorrhagic cerebral infarction, Acta Radiol (Suppl) 369:46-48, 1986.
83. Thulborn KR, Waterton JC, Matthews PM et al: Oxygenation dependence of the transverse relaxation time of water protons

in whole blood at high field, Biochim Biophys Acta 714:265-270, 1982.

84. Blackmore CC, Francis CW, Bryant RG et al: Magnetic resonance imaging of blood and clots in vitro, Invest Radiol 25:1316-1324, 1990.

85. Hayman LA, Taber KH, McArdle CB et al: The importance of clot formation in MR of blood on spin echo intracranial hematomas, AJNR 10:1155-1158, 1989.

86. Hecht-Leavitt C, Gomori JM, Grossman RI et al: High-field MRI of hemorrhagic cortical infarction, Clin Radiol 39:131-139, 1988.

87. Nose T, Enomoto T, Hyodo A et al: Intracerebral hematoma developing during MR examination, J Comput Assist Tomogr 11(1):184-187, 1987.

88. Fabry ME, Eisenstadt M: Water exchange across red cell membranes: II. Measurement by nuclear magnetic resonance T1, T2, and T12 hybrid relaxation. The effects of osmolarity, cell volume and medium, J Mem Biol 42(4):375-378, 1978.

89. Escourolle R, Poirier J: Pathology of the central nervous system; demyelinating diseases, Man Basic Neuropathol, 128-135, 1973.

90. Mendes JH, Kinsbourne M, Batzdorf U et al: Textbook of child neurology; heredodegenerative diseases, Philadelphia, 1974, Lea & Febiger, pp 101-113.

91. Merritt HH, Moses HL, Moses L: A textbook of neurology; diseases of the myelin sheath, ed 6, Philadelphia, 1979, Lea & Febiger, pp 767-824.

92. Adams RD, Victor M: Principles of neurology; multiple sclerosis and allied demyelinative diseases, New York, 1981, McGraw-Hill, pp 647-663.

93. Holland BA: Diseases of white matter: magnetic resonance imaging of the central nervous system, New York, 1987, Raven Press, pp 259-278.

94. Barkovich AJ: Pediatric neuroimaging; metabolic and destructive brain disorders, New York, 1990, Raven Press, pp 35-75.

95. Leestma JE: Forensic neuropathology, New York, 1988, Raven Press, pp 137-156.

96. Nowell MA, Grossman RI, Hackney DB et al: MR imaging of white matter disease in children, AJR 151: 359-365, 1988.

97. Poser CM: Disease of the myelin sheath. In Minckler J, editor: Pathology of the nervous system, New York, 1968, McGraw-Hill, pp 767-821.

98. Barkovich AJ, Kjos BO, Jackson DE et al: Normal maturation of the neonatal and infant brain: MR imaging at 1.5T, Radiology 166:173-180, 1988.

99. Deitrich RB, Bradley WG, Zaragoza EJ et al: MR evaluation of early myelination patterns in normal and developmentally delayed infants, AJNR 9:69-76, 1988.

100. Braffman BH, Zimmerman RA, Trojanowski JQ et al: Brain MR: pathologic correlation with gross and histopathology. 1. Lacunar infarction and Virchow-Robin spaces, AJNR 9:621-628, 1988.

101. Braffman BH, Zimmerman RA, Trojanowski JQ et al: Brain MR: pathologic correlation with gross and histopathology. 2. Hyperintense white-matter foci in the elderly, AJNR 9:629-636, 1988.

102. Elster AD, Richardson DN: Focal high signal on MR scans of the midbrain caused by enlarged perivascular spaces: MR-pathologic correlation, AJR 156:157-160, 1991.

103. Hunt AL, Orrison WW, Yeo RA et al: Clinical significance of MRI white matter lesions in the elderly, Neurology 39:1470-1474, 1989.

104. Knaap MS, Valk J: Classification of congenital abnormalities of the CNS, AJNR 9:315-326, 1988.

105. Barkovich AJ, Truwit CL: Brain damage from perinatal asphyxia: correlation of MR findings with gestational age, AJNR 11:1087-1096, 1990.

106. Kjos BO, Umansky R, Barkovich AJ: Brain MR imaging in children with developmental retardation of unknown cause: results in 76 cases, AJNR 11:1035-1040, 1990.

107. Naeye RL, Peters EC, Bartholomew M et al: Origins of cerebral palsy, AJDC 143:1154-1160, 1989.

108. Flodmark O, Becker LE, Harwood-Nash DC et al: Correlation between computed tomography and autopsy in premature and full-term neonates that have suffered perinatal asphyxia, Radiology 137:93-103, 1980.

109. Barkovich AJ: Pediatric neuroimaging: Vol I: Infections of the nervous system, New York, 1990, Raven Press, pp 293-325.

110. Osborn AG: Inherited metabolic, white matter, and degenerative diseases of the brain. In Osborn A, editor: Diagnostic neuroradiology, St Louis, 1994, Mosby, pp 716-781.

111. Demaerel P, Faubert C, Wilms G et al: MR findings in leukodystrophy, Neuroradiology 33:368-371, 1991.

112. Jardim LB, Giugliani R, Fensom AH: Thalamic and basal ganglia hyperdensities: a CT marker for globoid cell leukodystrophy? Neuropediatrics 23:30-31, 1992.

113. Brismar J, Brismar G, Gascon G et al: Canavan disease: CT and MR imaging of the brain, AJNR 11:805-810, 1990.

114. Shah M, Ross JS: Infantile Alexander disease: MR appearance of a biopsy-proved case, AJNR 11:1105-1106, 1990.

115. Clifton AG, Kendall BE, Kingsley DPE et al: Computed tomography in Alexander's disease, Neuroradiology 33:438-440, 1991.

116. Silverstein AM, Hirsh DK, Trobe JD et al: MR imaging of the brain in five members of a family with Pelizaeus-Merzbacher disease, AJNR 11:495-499, 1990.

117. Snyder RD, King JN, Keck GM et al: MR imaging of the spinal cord in 23 subjects with ADL-AMN complex, AJNR 12:1095-1098, 1991.

118. Williams KD, Drayer BP, Johnsen SD et al: MR imaging of leukoencephalopathy associated with Navajo neuropathy, AJNR 11:400-402, 1990.

119. Ho VB, Fitz CR, Yoder CC et al: Resolving MR features in osmotic myelinolysis (central pontine and extrapontine myelinolysis), AJNR 14:163-167, 1993.

120. Miller GM, Baker HL Jr, Okozaki H et al: Central pontine myelinolysis and its imitators: MR findings, Radiology 168:795-802, 1988.

121. Bradley WG, Whittemore AR, Watanabe AS et al: Association of deep white matter infarction with chronic communicating hydrocephalus: implications regarding the possible origin of normal-pressure hydrocephalus, AJNR 12:31-39, 1991.

122. Morgan CL: Basic principles of computed tomography, Baltimore, 1983, University Park Press, pp 109, 120.

123. Brigham EO: The fast Fourier transform, Englewood Cliffs, NJ, 1974, Prentice Hall, p 5.

124. Jain AK: Fundamentals of digital image processing, Englewood Cliffs, NJ, 1989, Prentice Hall, p 465.

Magnetic Resonance Imaging

John A. Sanders

Despite its widespread use as a medical imaging modality, magnetic resonance imaging (MRI) is a remarkably recent technologic development. Few technologies have moved so rapidly, evolving from the first crude demonstration to clinically useful, multi-million dollar commercial instruments present at most modern medical centers. This progress has taken place in only 20 years, and the pace shows little sign of slowing. If there had been any time where a plateau of achievement appeared to have been reached, that notion was quickly dispelled by the next break-through. In addition to dramatic reductions in required examination time, the types of diagnostically useful information available from biomedical magnetic resonance continues to expand. A number of exciting functional magnetic resonance imaging (FMRI) techniques for functional brain localization have emerged, and the potentials of angiographic (MRA) techniques for flow measurement and spectroscopic (MRS) techniques for biochemical measurement continue to be explored. While its early predicted potential for routine and easy cancer screening has not yet been realized, MRI has certainly not been disappointing.

To some extent, MRI benefitted tremendously by arriving after computed tomography (CT) scanning had been developed and was being widely used. Early MRI technology, hardware, and software borrowed heavily from existing CT capabilities. Almost 10 years of experience reading tomographic images prepared radiologists for the similar images obtained from the early MRI systems. The development of CT systems established mechanisms by which new and rapidly expanding technologies could be both accepted and efficiently employed. It has also been fortunate that MRI does not directly compete with CT in many radiologic applications.

Clinical MRI technology demonstrates a great deal of maturity, despite ongoing advancements. Particularly in neurologic work, the diagnostic utility of MRI has been indisputably established. The development of commercial systems reflects this through continuing trends toward market stratification and specialization. Early MRI systems closely followed the advancement of the art, which generally meant employing systems of the highest field strengths and the most capabilities.

Current systems are increasingly tailored toward more specific applications, economic structures, and siting requirements. Imaging systems are even more specialized, with specific implementations for neurologic, cardiac, interventional, and extremity work likely to become more available.

Clinical systems using 1.5 T magnetic fields (Fig. 4-1) are still considered to be the high-end, high-field machines, with some able to run at 2.0 T. The flexibility built into these systems supports the latest in sequence development and application. Particularly effective for high-resolution neurologic work, these systems represent a platform for advanced users, research sites, or facilities that want an extra measure of ability to employ the latest procedures as they are developed.

Midfield machines (Fig. 4-2), with fields ranging from 0.5 to 1.0 T, currently make up the largest part of the instrument market. This is the result of continual improvements to image quality to the extent that the results rival those produced by high-field imagers. These systems are designed for easy and efficient clinical practice with an emphasis on consistency, throughput, convenient siting, and user interface. While the sophistication of midfield imagers approaches that of high-field systems, the implementation is geared toward efficient patient studies rather than flexibility.

A number of systems (Fig. 4-3) operate at low and ultralow field strengths of 0.02 to 0.35 T. Often these systems are relatively inexpensive and have very forgiving siting requirements. The moderate but im-

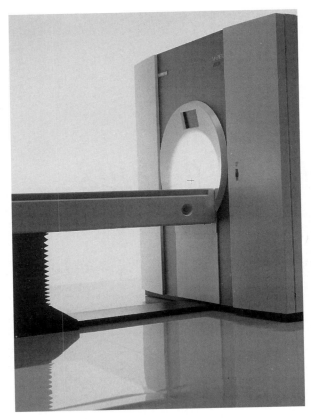

Fig. 4-1. "High field" 1.5 T system. (Courtesy of Siemens Medical Systems, Inc.)

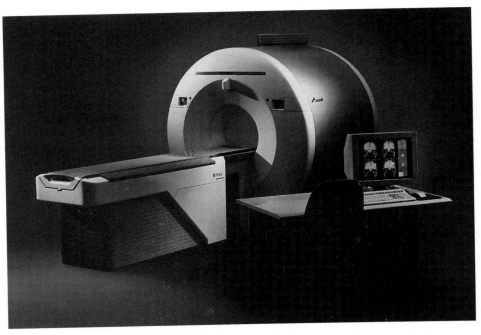

Fig. 4-2. "Mid-field" instrument. (Courtesy of Picker International, Inc.)

proving image quality is appreciated by sites where the highest possible resolution and the most rapid patient throughput are not necessary. These systems often use permanent or resistive magnets that can be designed so patient access is much better than in the higher field superconducting systems. The low field strengths are much safer to use with the metallic and electronic instruments that accompany critically ill patients.

The state of the art in magnet design continues to be extended. Currently, several 4.0 T whole-body instruments are in use for research studies (Fig. 4-4). The engineering required to produce these fields and structurally accommodate the huge forces involved is truly extraordinary. Commercial whole-body systems using 3.0 T fields are also now available. Results using these specialty machines are contributing to several areas of research and have been particularly significant in defining the capabilities of FMRI.

Hardware and software designs continue to be refined and improved, not only for imaging speed but for flexibility in allowing application of new and future pulse sequences. Imaging system design is moving away from isolated devices and toward integration into hospital information networks. Computer hardware is moving in the direction of more standardized platforms (i.e., RISC processors running UNIX) as medical instrument vendors tap into the increasing availability of inexpensive and powerful workstation systems.

As these computer platforms (Fig. 4-5) become more powerful, they are able to more fully support three-dimensional image processing, graphic display, and multimodality data integration. Unfortunately, the current gray scale film-based radiologic practice has not progressed very far, and this medium will soon be a significant bottleneck for efficient data presentation and display of the tremendous amount of information now being produced from these digital imaging modalities.

MR images are somewhat unique in that, to understand the content, many of the details and

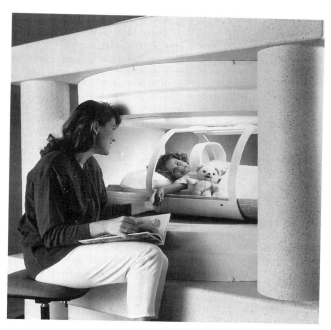

Fig. 4-3. "Ultra-low" field system. (Courtesy of Toshiba America, Inc.)

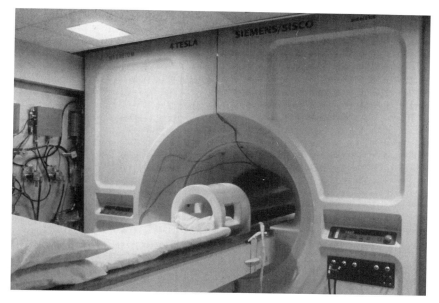

Fig. 4-4. 4.0 T imaging/spectroscopy research instrument. (Courtesy of Kamil Ugurbil, Center for MR Research, University of Minnesota Medical School.)

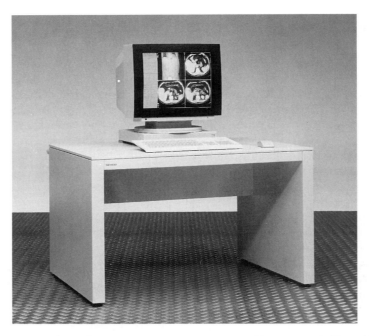

Fig. 4-5. Networked workstation computer systems. (Courtesy of Siemens Medical Systems, Inc.)

parameters used in formation of the image must be considered. The converse of this is also true; in order to obtain diagnostically useful information from a patient imaging study, the appropriate parameters and imaging procedures must be selected and ordered. New FMRI and MRS procedures for brain functional localization exploit the richness of the underlying principles of nuclear magnetic resonance and employ the latest developments in image acquisition and processing. A thorough knowledge of the basic principles of MRI is necessary in order to understand these new techniques. The remainder of this chapter focuses on MRI, relating it, when possible, to CT technology. While related on a fundamental level, a later chapter on MRS will extend the discussion of these principles in order to more thoroughly describe this exciting application.

HISTORY

Physicists Felix Bloch and Edward Purcell independently discovered the phenomenon of nuclear magnetic resonance (NMR) in 1946.[1,2] They observed that transitions could be induced between magnetic spin energy levels of certain nuclei and that the energy required to cause these transitions corresponded to frequencies in the radiofrequency (RF) range. Rapid progress in NMR was made in the next 10 years, during which a theory was developed to explain the observed phenomena of chemical shifts, diffusion, spin-spin coupling, and relaxation processes. With the development of high-resolution NMR spectroscopy,

chemists exploited the chemical shift mechanisms and NMR became established as a primary method of determining the structure of synthetic organic compounds. In 1971, Raymond Damadian showed that an NMR signal could distinguish normal from cancerous tissue on the basis of T1 relaxation characteristics.[3] His 1972 patent proposing an NMR machine for scanning the body to detect disease was one of the first applications of NMR to medicine.[4] Even though the initially anticipated potential of quick and easy screening for cancer has not been fully realized (the relaxation differences between normal and cancerous tissue do not always provide sufficient discrimination), this patent was important in encouraging the early and rapid application of NMR to medicine.

The first published account of NMR imaging was that of a small test object by Paul Lauterbur in 1973.[5] He showed that by trading the homogeneity of the magnetic field (in which the small changes in signal frequency caused by chemical structure are detectable) for a uniformly inhomogeneous field (linear field gradient), one can use the signal frequency to obtain spatial information in the form of one-dimensional projections of the object. By varying the direction of the applied gradient, a set of projections at different angles could be obtained and an image formed using the projection reconstruction methods that were currently in use by x-ray computed tomography (CT). After that, development proceeded rapidly with the completion of the first human NMR scanning machine and the production of the first torso image of a live

Table 4-1. NMR properties of biologic nuclei

Nucleus	Spin quantum number	Resonance frequency at 1 T (MHz)	Natural abundance (%)	Relative sensitivity at constant field
^{1}H	½	42.6	99.98	100
^{2}D	1	6.5	0.0156	1.5×10^{-4}
^{13}C	½	10.7	1.1	1.6×10^{-2}
^{14}N	1	3.1	99.6	1.0×10^{-1}
^{15}N	½	4.3	0.36	3.7×10^{-4}
^{19}F	½	4.4	100.0	83.0
^{23}Na	3⁄2	11.3	100.0	9.3
^{31}P	½	17.2	100.0	6.6
^{35}Cl	3⁄2	4.2	75.4	3.5×10^{-1}
^{39}K	3⁄2	2.0	9.1	4.6×10^{-2}

From Gadian DG: Nuclear magnetic resonance and its applications to living systems, Oxford, 1982, Clarendon Press.

human being in 1977.[6] This was followed by the start of clinical trials in 1980. By 1984, manufacturers worldwide were producing million dollar scanning machines capable of obtaining high-quality images of all parts of the body,[7] primarily for use in specialized clinics. Today, the clinical utility has been established to such an extent that the expensive ($2 million plus) machines are being sold to and used by most major medical centers throughout the world. The field of MRI continues to expand rapidly, and there is a large amount of interest in both academia and industry to continue to develop the enormous potential of this technique.

BASIC PRINCIPLES

A complete understanding of nuclear magnetic resonance can be pursued into very sophisticated math and theory, but the main features can be intuitively understood using a classic mechanics description. This is a distinctive feature about NMR: it is elegantly simple but has a complex and rich foundation. The mathematical model of NMR is based on the Bloch equation, which describes the time dependence of nuclear magnetization in the presence of a magnetic field.

Physical Model

The physical model of NMR starts with the property of certain nuclei called "spin." Nuclei having spin (those with an odd number of protons and/or neutrons) include several that are biologically abundant, such as ^{1}H, ^{13}C, ^{31}P, ^{23}Na, and ^{39}K. Properties of these nuclei are listed in Table 4-1.

Three factors influence the ability to use different nuclei for NMR studies: (1) the percentage of atoms having NMR visible nuclei, (2) the amount of signal given off by a certain number of nuclei, and (3) the number or density of nuclei in biologic systems. For a certain type of atom, defined by the number of protons in the nucleus, there may be differing nuclei available.

The "natural abundance" of certain nuclear species is specified in terms of the percentage of atoms with that particular nucleus type. For example, as indicated in Table 4-1, of all hydrogen atoms, 99.98% have a single proton and no neutrons (^{1}H), 0.016% have a single proton and one neutron (^{2}H = ^{2}D), and 0.004% have single proton and two neutrons (^{3}H).

Some nuclei also give stronger signals than others. Despite the fact that ^{14}N is a large percentage of all nitrogen atoms, the signal from a given number of ^{14}N nuclei is 1000 times smaller than the signal from an equivalent number of protons.

The final consideration is the amount of the particular atom in the biologic system or tissue of interest. In this regard, hydrogen and carbon are by far the most common, and it is indeed unfortunate that ^{12}C, which makes up 98.9% of all carbon atoms, is not NMR visible. While every fluorine atom is ^{19}F, which gives off strong NMR signals, there are few fluorine-containing molecules in most biologic systems.

Modern radiologic procedures are primarily concerned with ^{1}H, which is simply an individual proton, because of its large NMR signal and high natural abundance in biologic systems. While this discussion will focus primarily on proton NMR, much of what applies to protons can be extrapolated to other nuclei since their behavior is similar. Nuclei possessing "spin" are also positively charged, so the spinning motion of the charge induces a local magnetic field, making each nucleus behave like a tiny bar magnet (Fig. 4-6).

This is the first example of induction, a concept that will often arise in NMR. NMR makes use of the duality in which moving charges induce magnetic fields and changing magnetic fields induce voltages that can be used to move charges.

In fact, electrons circulating around the nucleus set up their own magnetic fields and show the characteristics of electron paramagnetic resonance (EPR), which is similar to those of NMR. It is termed "paramagnetic"

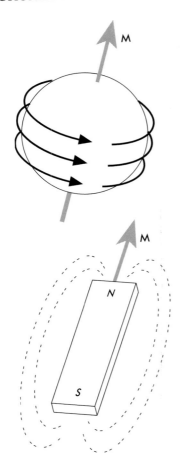

Fig. 4-6. A spinning proton behaves like a tiny bar magnet.

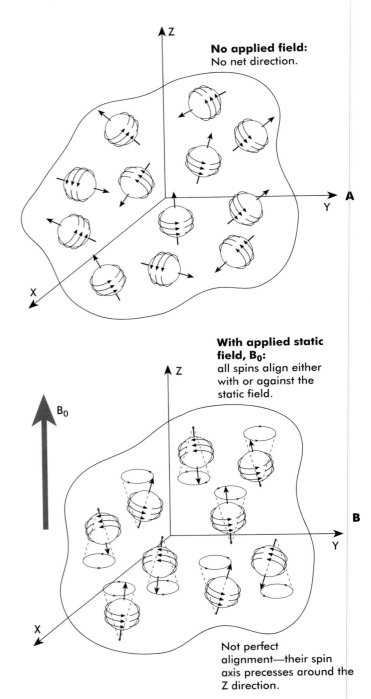

Fig. 4-7. The tiny bar magnets are randomly oriented (**A**) until an external magnetic field is applied (**B**).

because the electron magnetic field is produced only in the presence of an external magnetic field. The term "magnetic resonance" can refer to either NMR or EPR, which is why physicists were somewhat reluctant to drop the "nuclear" part of NMR when the marketing term "magnetic resonance imaging" (MRI) was coined.

These tiny nuclear bar magnets have north and south poles, so the nuclear magnetization has a direction. In the absence of a magnetic field, the individual atoms are randomly oriented and the bulk material has no net magnetization (Fig. 4-7, **A**). However, in an externally applied magnetic field, B_0, many interesting things occur. Like a compass needle, the individual atoms tend to align with an external magnetic field (Fig. 4-7, **B**).

External magnetic fields can be generated by moving charges (a current) in a coil of wire. The multiple loops of certain coils allow the induced magnetic fields from each wire loop to overlap and reinforce each other. The field strengths used in clinical systems range from 0.02 to 2.0 T. Since 1T equals 10,000 gauss (G), these fields range from 200 to 20,000 G. By comparison, the earth's magnetic field is only 0.5 G. The

magnetic field produced is proportional to the amount of moving charge so high currents are needed to produce large field strengths. To avoid the energy use and heat generated by pushing so many charges through the resistance of normal wires, the wires are often kept cooled below the point where they offer no resistance and become "superconducting."

Since each nucleus is spinning, the torque on it produced by the field prevents it from actually

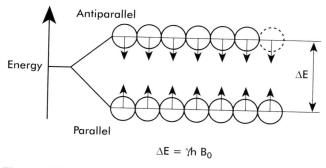

$$\Delta E = \gamma h\, B_0$$

Fig. 4-9. The two orientations of the net nuclei magnetization with respect to the field represent slightly different energy levels. The energy difference is directly proportional to the field strength.

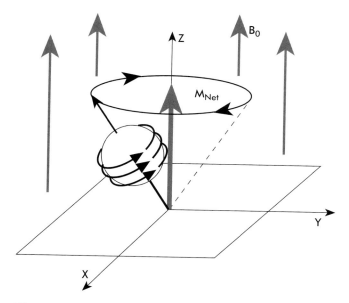

Fig. 4-8. Each spinning nucleus rotates or precesses around the direction of the applied magnetic field.

aligning with the applied magnetic field but instead to "precess," or revolve, around the magnetic field direction, just as a spinning top precesses around the earth's gravitational field (Fig. 4-8). The spin axis of the nucleus traces out a cone around the magnetic field direction. The speed at which the axis rotates around the field direction, the precessional frequency or "Larmor" (resonance) frequency, ω_0, is directly proportional to the field strength, B_0

$$\omega_0 = \gamma\, B_0 \qquad (4\text{-}1)$$

where γ is a proportionality constant, known as the gyromagnetic ratio, that is fixed for each different type of atomic nuclei. Therefore ^{1}H, ^{13}C, ^{31}P, and so on will rotate at different frequencies in a given magnetic field. Since there is relatively little ^{13}C or ^{31}P present in biologic systems, the strength of their signals is weak. Most of the body is made up of proton-rich water or fat, so proton NMR provides enough signal strength to obtain useful imaging resolutions. The γ for ^{1}H is 4257.43 Hz/G (1 Hz = 1 cycle/sec), so protons will precess at 63.9 MHz in a 1.5 T magnetic field. This corresponds to the low VHF band, or approximately TV channel 3. Table 4-1 lists the gyromagnetic ratios for a number of common nuclei.[8]

Equation 4-1 states that precessional frequency is directly proportional to the magnetic field strength. This is perhaps the single most important concept in MRI and is one from which almost everything else can be derived.

Because the nuclei are precessing so rapidly around the direction of the applied field, one can consider the average direction of its magnetization as being the axis of the cone-shaped precessional path (Fig. 4-8). This

magnetization is aligned in the direction of the applied magnetic field. In fact, quantum mechanics dictates that the magnetization of individual protons must be either aligned in the direction of the applied field or aligned in exactly the opposite but parallel (antiparallel) direction. These two states represent specific energy levels, with the parallel state being lower than the antiparallel state (Fig. 4-9). In other words, it takes a specific amount of extra energy to turn a nucleus that points in the direction of the field around to point in the opposite direction to the field. This extra amount of energy increases with increasing magnetic field strength. For nuclei that are more complicated than a proton, there can be additional possible orientations, depending on the value of the nuclear spin.

The amount of energy required to flip orientations is so small that the normal thermal energy available at room temperature is enough to flip spins between states. The relative number of nuclei (N) in each state can be calculated using the Boltzmann relation

$$\frac{N_{lowerE}}{N_{higherE}} = \exp\left(\frac{\Delta E}{KT}\right) = \exp\left(\frac{\gamma\, hB_0}{KT}\right) \qquad (4\text{-}2)$$

where $\Delta E = \gamma hB_0$ is the energy difference between states, B_0 is the applied field strength, γ is the gyromagnetic ratio for the nucleus, h is Planck's constant, K is Boltzmann's constant, and T is the temperature in degrees Kelvin. One can calculate that in a 1.5 T field at room temperature, there are only 10 extra protons per 1 million in the lower energy parallel state than there are in the higher energy antiparallel state.

An approximate analogy is to consider a table full of compasses (in our case, with each pointing only north or south). If one shakes the table wildly, all of the compasses will randomly and rapidly point to either north or south. However, if one counts up the number of compasses pointing in each direction at some particular moment, there will be slightly more of them pointing north.

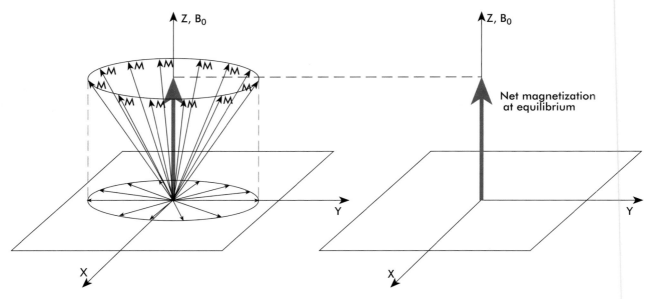

Fig. 4-10. The net longitudinal magnetization is the average orientation of all protons in the sample.

The energy difference between the two orientations is linearly proportional to the applied magnetic field strength. With increasing energy difference, there will be a corresponding increase in the number of extra nuclei in the lower energy state. All of the signals generated in MRI are based on the small difference in the number between the two energy states. These low energy differences between states are one reason why MR techniques tend to be safe but also why they are typically limited by signal strength.

Net Magnetization

All material is made up of a huge number of individual atoms (and atomic nuclei). For example, there are 6.7×10^{22} protons in 1 g of water. With such extremely large numbers, one cannot keep track of individual spins in an object or volume but can only observe the net effects of all the individual spins combined. The sum over all the nuclei in an object volume gives the net magnetization for the object. The description of the net magnetization is based on a coordinate system, with the Z axis being in the direction of the applied magnetic field, as shown in Fig. 4-10. The resting net magnetization is called the equilibrium magnetization or "longitudinal magnetization." Even though a small part of the precessing magnetization of each individual nucleus has a component projecting down into the X-Y plane perpendicular to the Z axis, there is no equilibrium *net* magnetization because the average value or direction of this "transverse magnetization" over all of the nuclei in the sample cancels to zero. The two components of magnetization, transverse and longitudinal (Fig. 4-11), are both parts of the net magnetization

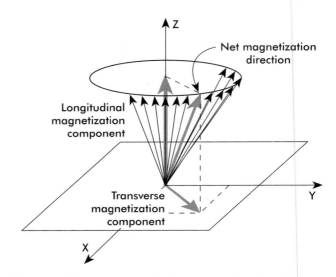

Fig. 4-11. The net magnetization can be described in terms of two components: the longitudinal magnetization in the direction of the Z axis and transverse magnetization as the length of the magnetization in the X-Y plane.

vector and are a convenient way to describe the orientation of net magnetization.

Radiofrequency Magnetic Fields

The proportions of nuclei in the parallel and antiparallel states can be altered by adding enough energy to the nuclei to move them from the lower energy state to the higher energy state. Only with precise tuning to match the energy difference between states does exposure to an oscillating electromagnetic field (at the same radiofrequency wavelength, i.e., 63.9 MHz for a proton in a 1.5 T field) achieve the most

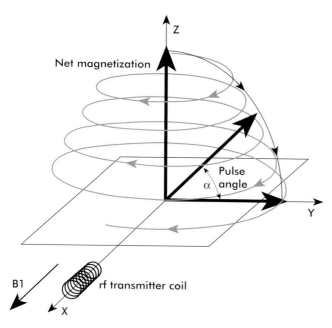

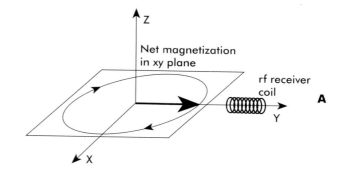

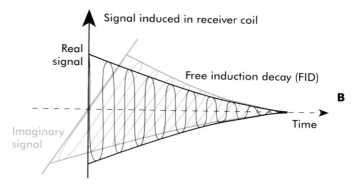

Fig. 4-12. Radiofrequency (RF) energy changes the direction of the net magnetization. The net magnetization will also precess around the direction of an applied RF magnetic field.

Fig. 4-13. The receiver coil is sensitive only to magnetization sweeping around in the transverse plane (**A**) and produces the signal that is amplified and recorded (**B**).

efficient transfer of energy. The resonance condition is said to be met when the nuclei absorb at frequencies that are matched to their natural oscillation. An analogy for the energy transfer is pushing a person on a swing. In order to be able to push the swinging person effectively, the person on the ground must time the shoves to the rhythm of the swing. The maximum boost occurs only when the pushes are given in phase and at the same frequency as the moving swing.

The change in the proportions of parallel and antiparallel spins leads to a change in the direction of the net magnetization vector for the object. As energy is absorbed by the population, the number in each state can be equalized, giving no net longitudinal magnetization. If energy is applied long enough, the populations can be inverted, with more spins antiparallel than parallel. One can consider the net magnetization to also precess around this new applied radiofrequency (RF) magnetic field, referred to as "B_1," just as they did around the original (much larger) magnetic field, referred to as "B_0." Equation 4-1 ($\omega_1 = \gamma B_1$) applies for this B_1 magnetic field, and since the B_1 field strengths are much less than B_0, the rotation frequencies are much slower. During this rotation, as shown in Fig. 4-12, the angle from the original equilibrium direction along the Z axis increases with time. By varying the amplitude and duration of the RF exposure, typically given in millisecond pulses, any desired angle can be produced. The RF pulse is usually described by the amount of rotation angle that it produces (e.g., a 45-degree RF pulse produces a 45-degree rotation of

the net magnetization—a 45-degree "flip angle"). For most angles from the equilibrium longitudinal magnetization, there will be a nonzero component of the magnetization (the transverse magnetization) in the X-Y plane. It is this transverse component that gives a detectable signal in NMR, so an RF pulse producing transverse magnetization is often termed an "excitation pulse." A 180-degree pulse completely inverts the longitudinal magnetization (the number antiparallel exceeds the number parallel) without producing any transverse magnetization, and it is called an "inversion pulse."

NMR systems are designed to measure the transverse magnetization, so the receiver coils, which may be the same as those used to apply the RF field, are designed to be sensitive only to the transverse component of the magnetic field. As the magnetization rotates in this plane and sweeps through the sensitive direction of the receiving coils, a small voltage is induced in the coil, causing a current to flow. As the magnetization continues to rotate, the coil detects a rising and falling signal pattern that is amplified and recorded by the receiver electronics (Fig. 4-13). Specific types of coils are designed for measurement of signal from different parts of the body in order to maximize the efficiency of the induction process (Fig. 4-14). The

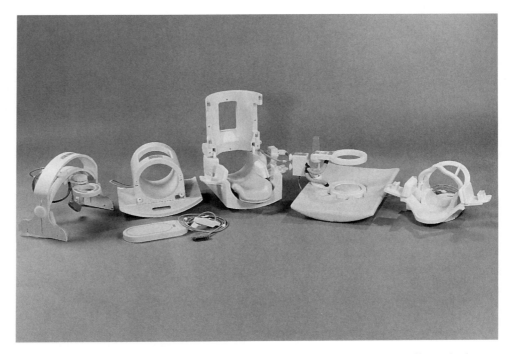

Fig. 4-14. Many different types of specialized receiver coils are available to efficiently detect signals from different parts of the body.

objective of coil design is to have the coil sensitivity be uniform over the sample volume and to have the coil be sensitive only to the transverse component of the rotating magnetic fields.

Since this transverse magnetization rotates so fast (63.9 MHz is 63,900,000 cycles per second, in a 1.5 T field), the first thing that is generally done with the signal is to shift it down in frequency (by the Larmor frequency) to leave a range of frequencies (the "bandwidth") centered at zero frequency (direct current, DC). The signal is "quadrature detected" by using a reference signal 90 degrees out of phase, which produces a complex signal having a "real" and an "imaginary" part.

The most simple NMR experiment is to give a 90-degree excitation pulse to rotate all of the original longitudinal magnetization into the transverse plane where it can be measured. As this transverse magnetization rotates in the X-Y plane at the Larmor frequency, it generates a rising and fading signal in the receiver coil that can be amplified and recorded.

Relaxation Processes

This rotation in the transverse plane does not continue indefinitely once the excitation RF pulse is turned off. When RF energy is no longer being added to the nuclei, they begin to give off the absorbed energy and revert back to their state before the RF pulse. This emission process does not occur instantaneously, and the signal strength, directly related to the

amount of net transverse magnetization, will gradually decay to zero. The molecular environment of the nuclei is reflected in the time variation of signal amplitude as the nuclei return to their equilibrium state following an excitation pulse (Fig. 4-15). This release of energy happens somewhat slowly and occurs in two ways: (1) energy is given up to neighboring molecules in the surrounding environment and is called "spin-lattice" relaxation, and (2) energy is given up to other nearby nuclei and is called "spin-spin" relaxation. Again, for both processes, the frequencies must be matched for the efficient transfer of energy.

Spin lattice relaxation (T1). The spin lattice relaxation is typically considered to be an exponential process described by a "T1" time constant. This relaxation follows the curve shown in Fig. 4-16 and, for a 90-degree excitation pulse, is described by

$$M_z = M_0 \, (1 - e^{-[t/T1]}) \qquad (4\text{-}3)$$

The longitudinal magnetization recovers by $(1 - 1/e)$ or 63% during each time period of T1 milliseconds. After a second T1 period, 63% of what remains would be recovered, so after two T1 periods 86% is recovered (63% from the first period plus 63% of the remaining 37% equals 86% total). Even though this curve (Fig. 4-16) only slowly approaches the original magnetization, it is typically considered to be fully recovered after 5 T1 periods (99.3%). The molecules of the

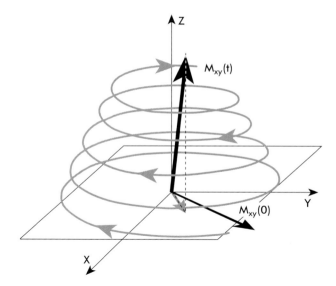

Fig. 4-15. The energy absorbed from the RF pulse is given off by the object as the net magnetization "relaxes" back to its original orientation along the Z axis.

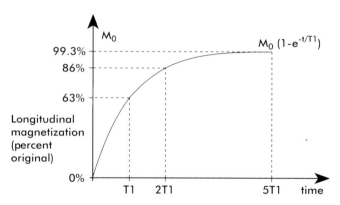

Fig. 4-16. Spin-lattice relaxation, characterized by the T1 time constant, describes the exponential recovery of the equilibrium longitudinal magnetization.

Table 4-2. T1 constants (in msec) at different field strengths

Tissue	0.2	1.0	1.5
Fat	182	241	259
Muscle (skeletal)	372	732	868
Brain—white matter	390	683	786
Brain—gray matter	495	813	921
CSF	1400	2500	3000

From Bottomly PA: Frequency dependence of tissue relaxation times. In Partain CL et al, editors: Magnetic resonance imaging: physical principles and instrumentation, vol 2, Philadelphia, 1988, Saunders.

antiparallel direction will be restored and the net magnetization vector will grow along the Z axis back to the original equilibrium amount.

T1 values for pure water can be up to 5 seconds. Similar environments such as blood or cerebrospinal fluid (CSF) will also be quite long. The water in biologic tissues generally have T1s in the region of 200 to 800 msec. The mid-sized fat molecules move at frequencies near the Larmor frequency and have relatively short T1 values (approximately 50 to 100 msec). Since these motional frequencies are fixed by the surrounding thermal energy, efficient energy transfer at the Larmor frequency depends on the strength of the magnetic field. As shown in Table 4-2, tissue relaxation times will change with changes in magnetic field and generally increase as the magnetic field strength increases.[9]

Spin-spin relaxation (T2). The spin lattice relaxation just discussed only considers the restoration of equilibrium longitudinal magnetization, the length of the magnetization along the Z direction. Spin-spin relaxation is concerned with the loss of net magnetization in the transverse, or X-Y, plane. The loss of transverse magnetization occurs at a different rate than the recovery of longitudinal magnetization. Again this is an exponential process, as shown in Fig. 4-17 and described by

$$M_{XY} = M_0 e^{-(t/T2)} \qquad (4-4)$$

This time the profile is an exponential loss, rather than recovery, that is characterized by a "T2" time constant. After every interval of T2 milliseconds there is 1/e or 37% (100% − 63%) of the magnetization remaining.

In spin-spin relaxation, an excited (flipped to antiparallel) spin can give up its energy not only to surrounding lattice molecules but also to other neighboring nonexcited spins. If this occurs, the numbers in the excited and nonexcited populations (longitudinal magnetization) do not change, but the net transverse magnetization may decrease due to "dephasing." As energy is passed from one spin to another, the spin

surrounding structure ("lattice") are moving and rotating as a result of normal thermal energy. It is this brownian motion that creates local fluctuating magnetic fields at the Larmor frequency and allows the energy to be transferred from the proton and to be dissipated as heat. If the motional frequencies are similar to the Larmor frequency, there is efficient exchange of energy reflected in a short T1 time constant. These motional frequencies depend on the size and shape of the surrounding molecules. It turns out that midsized molecules are often moving at the appropriate frequencies. Small molecules like water move too rapidly for efficient exchange, and large molecules like protein move too slowly. Water bound to large molecules will also move very slowly. Over time, typically 0.05 to 2.0 seconds, the equilibrium situation of slightly more protons in the parallel than

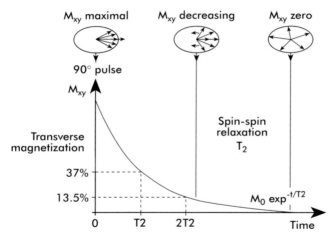

Fig. 4-17. Spin-spin relaxation describes the exponential loss of transverse magnetization after an excitation pulse and is characterized by the T2 time constant.

rotations get out of synchronization, or phase, and the resulting cancellation yields a smaller net magnetization. As shown in Fig. 4-18, any two spins that may have been both pointing in the same direction may now be pointing in opposite directions, giving a zero net direction. Therefore the loss of net magnetization in the transverse plane will always be faster than the longitudinal relaxation (T2 < T1) because of this extra mechanism of cancellation. As shown in Table 4-3, watery environments such as CSF will have relatively long T2s.[10]

Losses in an inhomogeneous field (T2*). Dephasing will also occur if the applied magnetic field environment is nonuniform, since equation 4-1 specifies that the Larmor frequency will also be nonuniform throughout the region. Spins in different parts of the object will be rotating at different frequencies and will quickly lose coherence (become dephased) and have less net transverse magnetization because of the resulting cancellation. This loss of transverse magnetization due to inhomogeneous fields is often much shorter (Fig. 4-19) than the natural T2 signal decay and is characterized by another exponential time constant referred to as "T2*" (pronounced as "T2 star"). The value of this time constant is determined by the technical implementation of the magnetic field and any field inhomogeneity caused by properties of the object itself. Whole-body magnet designs usually produce an approximately basketball-sized center region where the variation in magnetic field varies only within a few parts per million (PPM) of frequency. NMR measurements are only successful if the object is positioned in this homogeneous field region.

Returning to our simple NMR experiment using a 90-degree pulse, we observe that the signal amplitude detected after the RF pulse immediately begins to

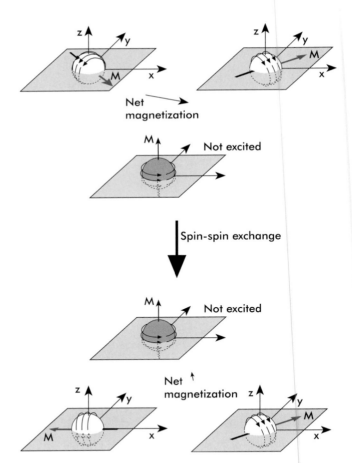

Fig. 4-18. Exchange of excitation energy between spins may result in dephasing and signal loss without a change in the number of excited nuclei.

Table 4-3. T2 constants (in msec) of different human tissues

Tissue	1.0
Fat	85
Muscle (skeletal)	45
Brain—white matter	90
Brain—gray matter	100
CSF	1400

From Heinrichs MA: Magnets, spins and resonances, Erlangen, Germany, 1992, Siemens.

decay with a time constant of T2*. This profile of the signal decay following an excitation pulse is called free induction decay or FID. This FID measures the net transverse magnetization from the entire object. Exploring the characteristics of this type of signal is also taken up in a later chapter on NMR spectroscopy. NMR imaging requires that the detected signal be modified or encoded in a way that signal contributions from different parts of the object can be distinguished.

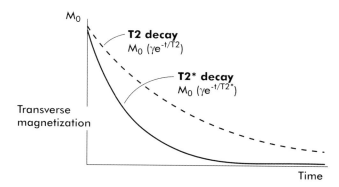

Fig. 4-19. The presence of slight variations in the magnetic field across the object will lead to rapid dephasing of the transverse magnetization at a rate described by the T2* time constant.

Signal Characteristics

There are two aspects to the use of NMR for imaging: (1) spatial encoding of the signals from different parts of the object so they can be distinguished and (2) the characteristics of the information contained within each encoded volume. Before we learn to identify signals from different segments of the object, we need to examine the types of information that can be encoded into each segment and how we can alter this information. Therefore, we will examine these two aspects in the reverse order, first considering the nature of the signals from the object and then discussing how those signals are localized.

If all parts of the object gave identical signals, then the resulting image made from these signals would be uniform and of little interest. However, there are ways to emphasize differences between segments by altering how the NMR measurement is performed.

Returning to the original NMR experiment of a 90-degree RF pulse followed by collection of an FID, no matter how small the region being measured, a biologic object is rarely uniform and will typically provide a signal that comes from several different components. This is because the body is inhomogeneous and is composed, from a proton concentration point of view, of water, fat, and various other components. The other components consist of dissolved metabolites (in millimolar or less concentrations) and large, mostly structural, macromolecules. The signals from each of these components add to give a net single signal from whatever the resolution volume is. This superposition of signals is illustrated in Fig. 4-20 for fat and water. The amount of signal each component contributes to the overall signal depends on the number of protons that are excited and the effects of any relaxation processes in reducing that signal. Thus the overall signal reflects these processes. Differences between different regions of the object reflect these types of influences. The later chapter on spectroscopy

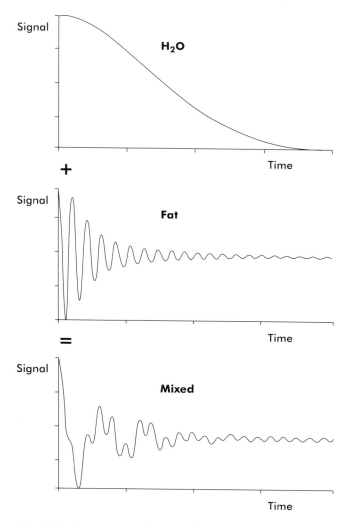

Fig. 4-20. The superposition or addition of signals from each component of the tissue gives the mixed signal that is detected.

is concerned with how to separate and identify these mixtures of component signals.

The density of protons varies little between soft tissues, reflecting the fact that soft tissue is mostly water and that this water content does not vary much (Table 4-4).[11] This is the reason for the lack of contrast observed in soft tissue regions in CT images, and why injected contrast media are commonly required to augment density differences. However, the signals in NMR are also influenced by the relaxation properties, which are described by the T1 and T2 time constants, and these relaxation rates vary significantly from tissue to tissue. NMR instrument settings can be modified to accentuate these differences. The resulting contrast is so dependent on the details of the parameters used that some settings will almost obscure tissue differences while others will bring out dramatic differences between tissues. The appearance of the image must be evaluated with respect to these settings.

Table 4-4. Water content of selected organs

Tissue	Percent water	Percent fat
Brain—gray matter	84-86	5.3
Brain—white matter	68-77	18
Skeletal muscle	79	2.2-3.0
Spinal cord	63-75	2-19
Skin	62	19
Skeleton	28-40	18-25
Cartilage	78	1.3
Adrenals	64	6-26
Thyroid	72-78	—
CSF	99	—
Fat	—	99

From Beall PT, Amley SR, Kosturi SR: Handbook for biomedical applications, New York, 1984, Pergamon.

This is what makes MRI image interpretation more complicated than evaluating CT images, where procedural variability is much less of a consideration.

Pulse Sequences

We shall now examine how the parameter settings interact with the T1 and T2 tissue relaxation characteristics to influence the image appearance and contrast between tissues.

Contrast. Several different models describe image contrast. They are all based on the perception of noticeable differences between brightness (intensity or luminance) levels in an image. While the range in which the human eye can operate spans approximately 10 orders of light intensity, the perceived brightness of an object depends on the intensity of the surroundings. Two objects with different surroundings could have identical intensities (or luminances) but different brightnesses, as shown in Fig. 4-21.

Models of image contrast arise from descriptions of how the eye perceives or detects "just noticeable differences" between an object and its surroundings. This ability to detect subtle intensity differences is typically better at low intensities (i.e., darker image regions) than at higher intensities. This ability is often modeled as the log of the increase in intensity. In digital radiology, one often has the luxury of adjusting the image display (window and level adjustments) to provide an image where the eye is more effective in identifying image differences. In these cases, image contrast is typically described as the difference in intensities divided by the average intensity, with increasing contrast leading to increased conspicuity of image differences.

The problem in MRI is to identify parameter settings that emphasize the inherent differences in tissue properties, primarily the differences in relax-

Fig. 4-21. Two objects with different surroundings can have identical intensities (luminances) but different apparent brightnesses. Image contrast describes the difference of an object's appearance from that of the background.

ation characteristics. This is accomplished by applying a "pulse sequence" of RF events.

T1 sequence parameters. As noted previously, the equilibrium longitudinal magnetization recovers exponentially after a 90-degree RF pulse, following a curve over time described by $(1 - \exp^{[-t/T1]})$, where T1 is a constant factor. At any time, t, after the initial RF pulse, the experiment can be repeated by applying another 90-degree pulse. However, since the longitudinal magnetization may not have fully recovered, that much less magnetization will be affected by the second 90-degree pulse and rotated into the transverse plane for measurement as a FID. For now we will assume that T2* is short and the transverse magnetization decays rapidly. This 90-degree pulse can be repeatedly applied at intervals, called the "repetition time" and denoted by "TR," and after several pulses the processes of excitation and longitudinal recovery will reach a steady state (Fig. 4-22). Imaging sequences typically apply several pulses before collecting data in

Saturation recovery sequence

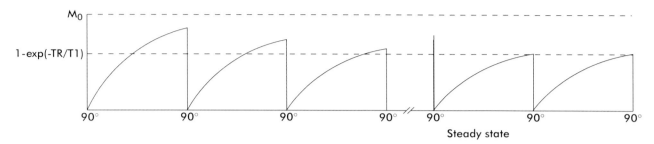

Fig. 4-22. The amount of measurable signal depends on the longitudinal magnetization available at the time of the excitation 90-degree pulse. The time interval between repeated 90-degree pulses, TR, determines how much recovery time is available between each pulse.

order to establish this steady state. At that point, the amount of longitudinal magnetization available for excitation by the 90-degree pulse will directly depend on the amount of time, TR, between pulses: $(1 - \exp^{[-TR/T1]})$. This repetition time parameter can be adjusted to emphasize tissue differences in T1 relaxation rate. The exponential recovery of longitudinal magnetization of two materials with different T1s is shown in Fig. 4-23. One has a T1 of 500 msec (gray matter) and one has a longer T1 of 2000 msec (CSF).

As the graphs show, the amount of magnetization for both of these tissues is similar for very short times and again for longer times, but there are middle TR values where the magnetizations (and signals) from each tissue are quite different. The magnetization difference varies with the choice of TR time and can be set to highlight the maximum difference between tissues. Setting the TR time will emphasize a specific component of the signals from the tissue and any differences in this component between tissues will be apparent. For the example of Fig. 4-23, regions whose components are mostly CSF will appear darker (since there is less signal), and those consisting of mostly gray matter will be brighter.

At longer TR times, all tissue components will have recovered significantly and there will be little intensity or contrast change between tissues. At shorter TR values (approximately 100 to 800 msec), T1 differences will be emphasized and the image is said to be "T1 weighted" or have contrast reflecting primarily T1 differences between the tissues. This type of pulse sequence, consisting of a repeated train of 90-degree RF pulses, is called "saturation recovery" because the spins are saturated by rotating them into the transverse plane and then allowed to recover for a time before repeating the experiment.

If the spins are given a 180-degree pulse, they are said to be inverted since the longitudinal magnetization has been inverted without providing any magnetization (or signal) in the transverse plane. As shown

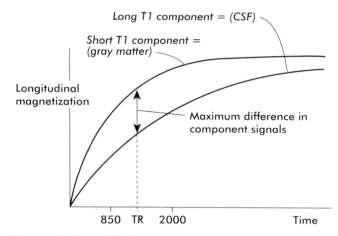

Fig. 4-23. The TR time parameter can be adjusted to emphasize the signals from particular tissue components. The value used is selected to accentuate T1 relaxation differences between tissues.

in Fig. 4-24, the longitudinal magnetization recovers after the pulse but has twice as far to recover, following a curve over time, t, described by $(1 - 2 \exp^{-[t/T1]})$. The longitudinal magnetization along the Z axis recovers without producing any transverse magnetization during the process.

For times soon after the inversion pulse, the longitudinal magnetization is negative, with the length of the vector extending below the zero of the Z axis. It then grows along the positive Z axis, passing through zero (magnetization vector length) on the way. The values typically made into an image are not negative but are instead the nonzero magnitude of the longitudinal magnetization values.

As the longitudinal magnetization recovers, the current value can be measured simply by applying a 90-degree pulse to rotate all current longitudinal magnetization into the transverse plane and provide a signal. The time after the 180-degree inversion pulse to the excitation 90-degree pulse is called the "inversion time" is denoted by "TI," and can be varied to

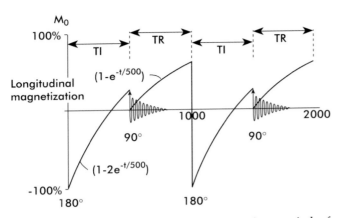

Fig. 4-24. Inversion recovery sequences wait a period of time, TI, after an inversion pulse before measuring the longitudinal magnetization with a 90-degree pulse.

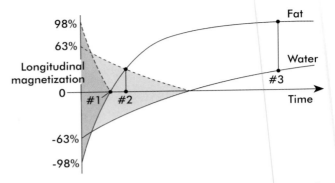

Fig. 4-25. A combination of TI and TR parameters can be used to vary image contrast. Note that images are typically formed from the absolute value of the longitudinal magnetization.

tune T1 contrast. After a time, TR, the 180-degree inversion, TI delay, and 90-degree excitation sequence is repeated.

For two different tissues, say fat and water, one can set a combination of TI and TR to make the fat light and water dark, both the same, or the fat dark and water light. In Fig. 4-25, if the inversion time TI is set at #3, the short T1 component (fat) will be much brighter than the long T1 component of water. Using a TI value of #2 will result in both fat and water being of equal intensity. A setting of #1 is right at the time where the fat longitudinal magnetization is passing through zero and thus will give no signal after the 90-degree pulse and have a dark image appearance. Selecting this value is one way of suppressing unwanted fat signals. This type of sequence is called "inversion recovery" and is specified by TR and TI parameter settings.

Recently developed pulse sequences attempt to avoid waiting for complete T1 recovery by not using a full 90-degree pulse for excitation. The smaller excitation flip angle is used so less longitudinal magnetization is rotated into the transverse plane and needs to recover for the next 90-degree pulse. A full 90-degree pulse converts all of the available longitudinal magnetization into transverse magnetization and leaves no longitudinal magnetization remaining. The use of smaller flip angles exploits the fact that transverse magnetization results from the geometric sine of the flip angle, and the longitudinal magnetization remaining after the pulse is the cosine of the flip angle (Fig. 4-26). Flip angle increases for small angles lead to significant increases in the resulting transverse magnetization while only using small amounts of longitudinal magnetization. At flip angles greater than 45 degrees, the opposite holds: increases in flip angle give smaller increases in transverse magnetization than decreases in longitudinal magnetization. The opti-

mum value of the flip angle, α, for a pulse train depends on the TR of the sequence and the T1 relaxation of the tissue. This optimum value is called the Ernst angle and can be calculated from the equation

$$\cos(\alpha) = \exp\left(-\frac{TR}{T1}\right) \qquad (4\text{-}5)$$

A plot of this angle versus the ratio of TR and T1 is shown in Fig. 4-27. Since TR directly sets the duration of a pulse sequence, the use of smaller angles and shorter TRs allows a significant reduction in imaging time while retaining similar T1 contrast mechanisms as those obtained with 90-degree pulses.

T2 sequence parameters. Tissue T2 relaxation differences can also be used to provide contrast between tissues.

Up to this point, we have only discussed collecting the transverse magnetization as a FID signal immediately after the excitation pulse. This signal decays exponentially at a rate described by the T2* time constant, which reflects the dephasing of the spins by intrinsic T2 spin-spin relaxation mechanisms, as well as dephasing resulting from the inhomogeneous magnetic field. Because T2* is usually significantly shorter than T2, the measurable FID signal is not available for very long.

The effects of this dephasing can be reversed through the use of "spin echoes."[12] A spin echo (SE) is formed by applying a 180-degree pulse at a time τ after the 90-degree excitation pulse. The result of this is that the FID dephasing after the 90-degree pulse is unwound and a measurable "echo" signal forms to a maximum after another τ interval. The time from the 90-degree pulse to the echo maximum is called the echo time and is denoted by TE.

This process works as shown in Fig. 4-28. Immediately after the 90-degree pulse, the magnetization that

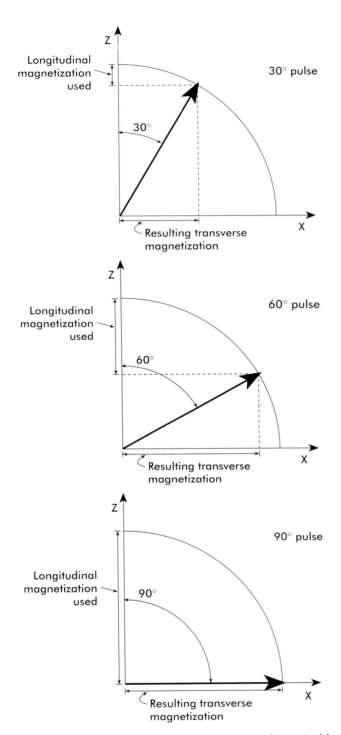

Fig. **4-26.** Low RF rotation angles can produce sizable amounts of transverse magnetization without "using" much longitudinal magnetization.

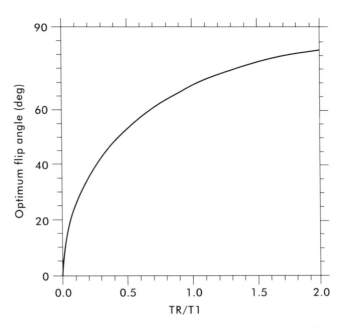

Fig. **4-27.** The Ernst angle is the optimum RF rotation (flip) angle for a given combination of sequence TR and tissue T1. For example, when the ratio of sequence TR to tissue T1 is 1, the Ernst angle will be 68 degrees.

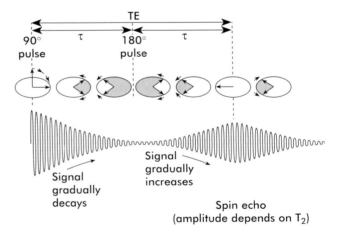

Fig. **4-28.** The 180-degree pulse forms a spin echo signal by inverting the magnetization such that continuing phase accumulation acts to rephase rather than dephase the transverse magnetization.

is now in the transverse plane begins to dephase and signal rapidly decreases as a result of cancellation. At time τ = TE/2, a 180-degree pulse is applied, whereby the entire spin system is "pancake flipped" by the 180-degree rotation. The spins remain in their original inhomogeneous fields throughout the object volume,

but now the phases they accumulate relative to each other act to cancel the phase that was previously acquired. The 180-degree pulse refocuses phase shifts caused by the presence of an inhomogeneous magnetic field. As the separate spin signals become more in phase, the signal becomes greater until complete rephasing occurs at TE = 2τ. Beyond that time the dephasing process repeats itself and acts to reduce the signal. The time of this echo, TE, can be selected by changing the time of application of the 180-degree pulse. Repeated echoes can be formed by reapplying

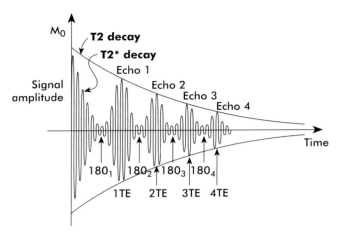

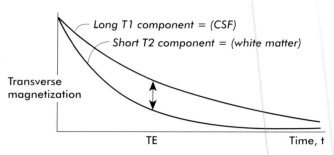

Fig. 4-30. The echo time (TE) can be varied to highlight T2 relaxation differences between tissues.

Fig. 4-29. While the spin echo focuses the dephasing from magnetic field inhomogeneity, it does not refocus dephasing from spin-spin (T2) relaxation, and the signal at the echo time (TE) will be reduced accordingly.

a 180-degree pulse and collecting the signals during the period of peak echo formation.

An additional practical advantage is gained through the use of spin echoes. In order to collect an FID, the system must switch from RF excitation to RF detection very quickly in order to capture the earliest and largest signals. These early signals contain the lowest frequency components of the image that determine overall image intensity. For a two-coil system, where one coil is used for excitation and another is used for detection, this means that the receiver coil must rapidly switch from insensitivity (detuned) to sensitivity. Any residual signal from the excitation pulse may be picked up by the receiving coil and will disrupt the detected signal ("ringing"). Using a single coil for both RF transmission and reception is an even more delicate situation. Delayed collection of echo signals at some time after the excitation avoids these problems.

While the dephasing resulting from magnetic field inhomogeneity is refocused by the formation of spin echoes, the intrinsic T2 dephasing is not recovered and the available signal (Fig. 4-29) decreases according to

$$S(t) = \exp\left[-\frac{t}{T2}\right] \qquad (4\text{-}6)$$

Therefore, the longer one waits to form an echo and collect the signal, the less signal available. The choice of echo time TE is generally made to vary the image contrast based on tissue T2 differences, but another consideration must be the decreasing image signal-to-noise ratio (SNR) with longer TEs.

If two different tissues are considered, one with a long T2 and one with a short T2 (as plotted in Fig. 4-30), one sees that at short postexcitation times the

transverse magnetization and image appearances of both tissues are similar. Likewise, at long TEs the signals are again similar (and low!). As noted for TR and T1 contrast, a value of TE can be chosen so that the signal from each tissue will be very different. In this case, tissues with longer T2s can be made bright relative to tissues with shorter T2. Increasing the TE can add T2 weighting to the image tissue contrast. Spin echoes can be used with most types of excitation pulses and can be combined with both saturation and inversion recovery sequences.

Echoes can be formed without 180-degree RF pulses by using magnetic field gradients to dephase and then rephase the spins. This type of "gradient-recalled echo" is often used in fast imaging sequences where it can produce faster echoes and use less RF power than spin echoes. Upon adding a gradient, which is a small, known, and nonuniform field on top of the large main magnetic field, the spins are quickly dephased and their signals cancel out. By reversing the gradient direction, the dephasing is "unwrapped" (undoing the phase accumulation) and an echo forms at the point where the amount of gradient rephasing balances the amount of dephasing (Fig. 4-31). Adjusting the time of the dephase/rephase gradient balance allows the time of echo formation to be changed. A significant drawback to the use of gradient echoes is that only specific gradient-produced dephasing is rephased by the gradient reversal. Any dephasing resulting from magnetic field inhomogeneities is not rephased, so the signal strength available at the time of the gradient echo is dictated by T2* rather than T2 processes. For fast imaging where the short echo times used are much less than T2*, this is not a very big problem. However, gradient echoes cannot be used at long TEs to obtain heavy T2-weighting because so little signal will remain. While very fast imaging sequences can produce images with good T1 contrast, it is only with the development of "turbo spin echo" techniques that heavily T2-weighted images can be obtained rapidly.

If the imaging parameters use a long TR (providing little T1 weighting) and a short TE (giving little T2

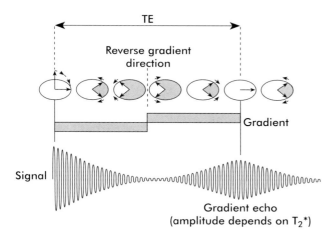

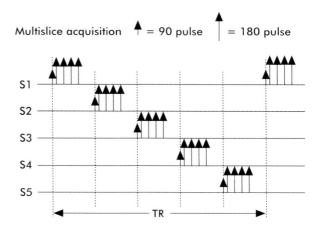

Fig. 4-31. Echo signals can also be formed through gradient reversal. The echo occurs when the areas under the dephasing and rephasing gradients are equal.

Fig. 4-32. For a multislice sequence, the recovery period for one slice can be used to interrogate additional slices. A four-echo sequence is shown.

weighting), a "density-weighted" image results, showing primarily the distribution of protons in the tissue. Image TRs are typically much longer than the TE values, leaving a significant amount of sequence time waiting for T1 recovery. In practice, this time is spent interrogating additional spatial slices. Additional slices can be selected and signals acquired while the longitudinal magnetization of the first slice is recovering. For this basic type of two-dimensional multislice imaging (Fig. 4-32), the number of slices that can be obtained without requiring any additional time is approximately the TR divided by the TE.

Contrast agents. A distinctive feature of MRI is the soft tissue contrast that can be produced through alterations to sequence timing parameters. X-ray CT has long used intraveneous contrast agents in order to increase its limited soft tissue contrast. While a significant departure from the ideal of complete noninvasive diagnosis, the use of MR contrast agents has been demonstrated to be highly effective in improving contrast with pathologic conditions associated with a disrupted blood-brain barrier. The development of alternative contrast agents continues but the use of gadolinium-based compounds is a common part of routine clinical practice.

Unlike x-ray contrast agents, the effects of MRI contrast agents are detected indirectly through local changes in relaxation rates. The paramagnetic substances used, generally metallic ions, have a number of unpaired electrons and therefore a large electronic magnetic moment. Being much greater than the proton magnetic moment, this ion disturbs the local magnetic fields and catalyzes the relaxation of surrounding nuclei. Both T1 and T2 are shortened through direct interactions with water molecules bound to (and exchanging from) ionic binding sites. At

clinical doses, the paramagnetic effect is most apparant with local T1. At high (local) concentrations, water T2 can also be shortened by diffusion in the locally inhomogeneous magnetic fields surrounding the ions.

For a large effect on the tissue relaxation ("relaxivity"), a high number of unpaired electrons are preferred. The commonly used gadolinium ion (Gd^{+3}) has seven unpaired electrons, as compared to chromium (Cr^{+3}) with three and both manganese (Mn^{+2}) and iron (Fe^{+3}) with five. Gadolinium also has a relatively high number of potential water-binding sites. However, like most of these ions, Gd^{+3} is quite toxic as a free ion released from a salt (e.g., from $GdCl_3$) and so must be tightly chelated in stable complexes for safe use. Complexes formed with diethylenetriamine pentaacetic acid (DTPA) satisfy the requirements of not readily dissociating *in vivo* and not disrupting the effectiveness of the relaxation mechanisms. The resulting Gd-DTPA complex uses eight of the nine available coordination sites (Fig. 4-33), leaving one available for water. The chelation also slows the rotation of Gd, increasing the relaxivity. These acid complexes are made soluble in the form of a N- methylglucamine (dimeglumine) salt (Magnevist, Berlex, Wayne, NJ) or a bismethylamide (diamide) salt (Omniscan, Sanofi Winthrop, New York, NY).

These compounds will rapidly (the half-life, $t_{1/2}$, is 3 to 12 minutes) become distributed in the extracellular compartment, and the expected stability of the complex is significantly longer than their renal elimination mechanisms ($t_{1/2}$ of 78 to 96 minutes). The complex will not cross an intact blood-brain barrier and will not accumulate in normal tissues. Pathologic conditions such as abnormal vascularity or neoplasms will allow accumulation of Gd-DTPA, and the local T1 relaxation and image appearance will be dramatically altered (Fig. 4-34). The approximately 0.1 mM/Kg dose is approximately one one-hundredth of the LD_{50} (lethal dose in 50% of subjects),[13] and there is an approximately linear relationship between supplied dose and tissue concentration.[14] While the effects on the relaxation of Gd-DTPA solutions are linear with dose, the change in image contrast with double or triple doses is not necessarily linear.

IMAGE FORMATION

In general, the amplitude of the MR signal represents the transverse magnetization of the signals from the object at some defined point in a sequence of RF

Gd-DTPA

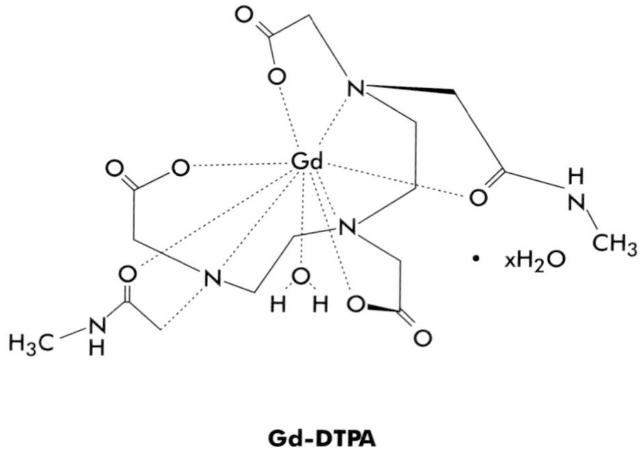

Fig. 4-33. Current FDA-approved contrast agents use diethylenetriamine pentaacetic acid (DTPA) to tightly bind gadolinium (Gd[III]) ions. The unpaired electrons of the Gd^{3+} ion affect local relaxation rates.

and gradient pulses. Additional pulse sequence events can be added to modify the signal so that each region of the object is uniquely identifiable. This process of spatial encoding of the signal is discussed next.

One-Dimensional Frequency Encoding

Gradients. Magnetic field gradients, as mentioned previously, are central to the formation of images using NMR. These are typically small field offsets linearly added and subtracted from the main field. They are produced by having a current move through smaller coils that are configured within the magnet system to give a nearly linear field pattern across the homogeneous volume (Fig. 4-35). This smaller field adds and subtracts with the main field. Within the magnet system there will be three sets of these gradient coils, each orientated in one of the three orthogonal directions. In fact, there may be additional linear and nonlinear gradient coils in the system, and their use for tuning ("shimming") the magnetic field is taken up in the chapter on spectroscopy.

The strength of these gradients depends on the system gradient amplifiers and the coil design, but the maximum linear field strength change per distance is typically around 1 G/cm for clinical whole body imaging systems. That is, for each centimeter along the direction of the gradient, the magnetic field changes by 1 G. This is only a very small offset on top of a "static" field of 1.5 T or 15,000 G. Linear gradients are usually "balanced," meaning that the offset is positive on one side and negative on the other side, with the

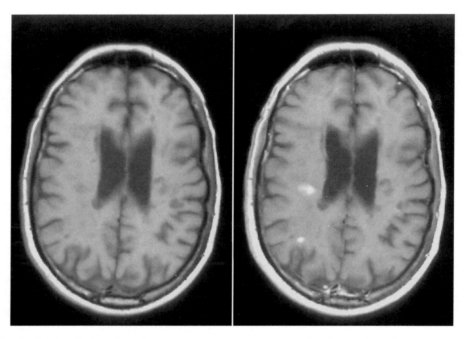

Fig. 4-34. Gadolinium-based contrast agents accumulate in the brain only in areas of disrupted blood-brain barrier and dramatically increase the conspicuity of lesions.

zero point positioned to be in the center of the homogeneous volume. A field gradient can be produced in any arbitrary direction by simultaneously using combinations of all three gradient coils. Another consideration is the gradient "rise time" or how much time is required to turn on and establish a steady gradient. The time required to switch between gradient levels directly influences the speed of the imaging sequences (discussed in more detail later in this chapter).

Referring back to equation 4-1, we know that if the magnetic field varies across the object, so does the Larmor frequency. Applying a linear field gradient, therefore, has the effect of causing each strip of the object to give a signal at a slightly different frequency (Fig. 4-36). Thus the presence of the gradient has "frequency encoded" the object along the direction of the gradient. For each frequency component of the measured signal we can use the known value of the applied gradient strength and direction to calculate which strip of the object the signal is coming from.

As an example, we can consider an object the size of a head, approximately 15 cm wide, positioned in the center of the homogeneous region of the magnet (Fig. 4-37). The desired field-of-view (FOV) is then the ear-to-ear distance. We know that a balanced gradient will give a zero offset in the middle of the head, so the signal frequency there will be the same as that for the main field B_0. We also know that there will be a 7.5 cm distance from the middle to each ear. If a 0.5 G/cm linear gradient is applied from the right ear to the left ear, the right ear will be in a field strength of $B_0 - 3.75$ G (i.e., $B_0 - 0.5$ G/cm $\times$ 7.5 cm) while the left ear will be in a field strength of $B_0 + 3.75$ G.

Using equation 1 and a γ of 4257.43 Hz/G, the frequency at the right ear is $\gamma B_0 - 15,965$ ($\gamma B_0 - \gamma 3.75$ G) and the frequency at the left ear is $\gamma B_0 + 15,965$, so all the signals from the object will fall in a "bandwidth" of 31,930 Hz centered around the "carrier" of

frequency γB_0. For 1.5 T this carrier will be 63,861,450 Hz. As mentioned above, this carrier signal frequency offset is removed during data collection.

Sampling. The digital electronic systems that measure the NMR signals from the object do not continuously record the FID signal but instead acquire "samples" of the signal at specified intervals. The rate of this sampling directly determines the bandwidth of the recorded signal. This can be seen by considering the Nyquist theorem, which requires that at least two samples must be taken per cycle of the signal in order to accurately digitize a signal of some frequency. For our head example, with frequencies of up to $\pm 15,965$ Hz, this means that samples must be taken twice as fast, or 31,930 Hz, or one sample each 31 μsec ($\frac{1}{31,930}$ Hz).

For imaging, the number of samples is taken to be a power of 2 for computational convenience and is typically either $128(2^7)$, 256 (2^8), or 512 (2^9). At 31 μsec

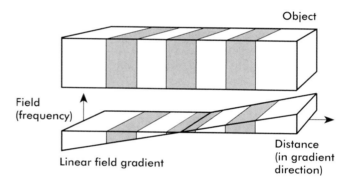

Fig. 4-36. The effect of a field gradient is to cause slices of the object perpendicular to the gradient direction to have the same signal frequency.

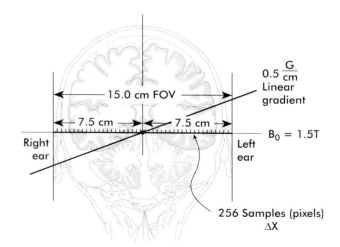

Fig. 4-37. Geometry for the sampling example in the text. The patient is positioned in the center of the homogeneous region of the magnet.

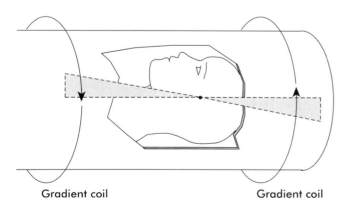

Fig. 4-35. Magnetic field gradients are usually designed to balance at the center of the homogeneous region of the magnet.

each, acquiring 256 samples gives a total collection time of 8.0 msec.

Since there are only 256 samples of the measured signal, there will be only 256 frequency samples in the Fourier transform of the sampled signal. In other words, we have divided our frequency bandwidth of 31,930 Hz into 256 separate segments, with each segment (called a "picture element" or pixel) containing a 125 Hz range (31,930 Hz/256). This value is equal to the value of 1 over the total collection time (1/8.0 MSEC). Since we know the gradient strength used, we can calculate the distance represented by each pixel, which in one dimension represents strips of the object along the gradient direction: 125 Hz/(γ Hz/G × G_x G/cm) = 125 Hz/(4257.43 Hz/G × 0.5 G/cm) = 0.059 cm = 0.59 mm. Each frequency-encoded strip in the X direction (ΔX) will be 0.59 mm wide, which of course is approximately equivalent to the original 15.0 cm ear-to-ear distance divided into 256 strips.

Frequency-encoding parameters. To summarize, there is an interrelationship between these parameters. The sampling rate is directly related to the signal bandwidth, and the total sampling time is directly related to the image resolution. γ and the actual gradient strength in use define the relationship

$$BW_x = \gamma \, G_x \, FOV_x \qquad (4\text{-}7)$$

where BW_x is the (object) signal bandwidth and G_x is the gradient in the X direction. The sampling interval, the "dwell time" Δt, determines the sampling bandwidth, BW_s, and is chosen so BW_s is greater than or equal to BW_x.

From these relations one can see that there are at least three approaches to increase image resolution (reduce ΔX): (1) reduce the FOV, (2) lower the bandwidth, and (3) increase the number of samples. Reducing the FOV requires increasing the gradient by the same factor. Improving the resolution of our head example by more than a factor of 2 will exceed the maximum gradient strength (1 G/cm) available for most scanners.

Reducing the FOV is not always a viable option since reducing it to less than the extent of the object will lead to "wrap" or aliasing of the object signals back into the image, possibly superimposing on top of the desired regions (Fig. 4-38). This occurs when the maximum frequency given off by the object in the gradient is greater than the bandwidth of the receiver determined by sampling. In other words, the sampling is not fast enough (Δt is not small enough) to meet the Nyquist requirement of acquiring two samples per cycle. In these cases any frequency greater than the Nyquist rate (ΔBW) will appear to be detected as BW − ΔBW. The farther the object extends past the FOV defined by the sampling, the more the signal will

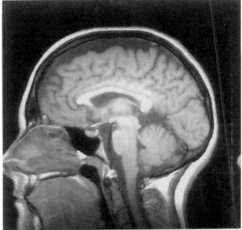

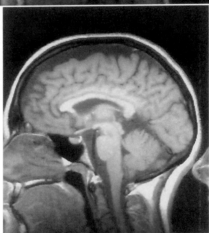

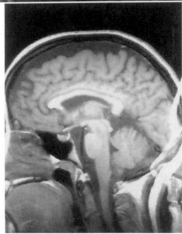

Fig. 4-38. If the signal bandwidth (object extent) is greater than the sampling bandwidth (image FOV), then the excess "wraps" back into the image.

wrap around the opposite edge back toward the image center. One common approach to avoiding wrap in the frequency-encoding direction is to "oversample" the signal, or to double the number of samples within the same total collection time. This decreases Δt by a factor of 2, which results in an increase in the FOV by

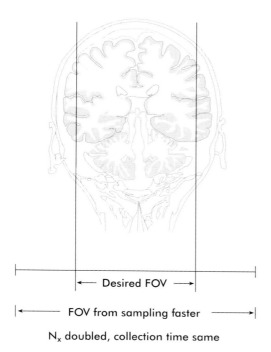

Desired FOV →

|← FOV from sampling faster →|

N_x doubled, collection time same

Fig. 4-39. Oversampling, or taking twice the number of samples in the same period of time, results in a doubled FOV. Only the center section corresponding to the original desired FOV is used.

Resolution volume (voxel)

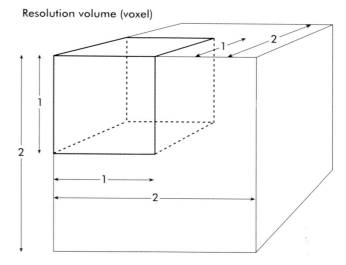

Fig. 4-40. Improving the image resolution by a factor of 2 in one direction while maintaining the same image quality (SNR) requires averaging four repeated measurements. A factor of 2 improvement in all three directions requires 64 ($4 \times 4 \times 4$) repeated measurements.

a factor of 2. Only the middle half of image (as wide as the desired FOV) is then clipped out of the extra wide image (Fig. 4-39), avoiding the wrapped signals.

Lowering the bandwidth corresponds to an increase in the dwell time, Δt, for each sample; this approach will double the required total collection time for obtaining the same number of samples. While decreasing the bandwidth improves the SNR (noise increases as the square root of the bandwidth), increasing the total collection time may not be a practical improvement since the signal strength is simultaneously decaying over time because of the intrinsic T2* processes.

Increasing the number of samples, N_x, while keeping the same dwell time will lead to the same FOV since Δt is unchanged. Again, taking twice the number of samples will cause a doubling of total collection time.

Other than these considerations, there are practical limits to increasing resolution. The number of nuclei contributing to the signal from each frequency-encoded region of the object depends on the density of protons and the size of the region. The major source of noise in MR images is the electronic noise generated in the receiver circuit and the patient. The electronic noise introduced into the system depends on the coil characteristics and the object (patient) with respect to the coil. Reducing the resolution volume directly reduces the SNR ratio.

The imaging time can increase dramatically if image quality (SNR) is maintained while increasing image resolution. In order to uniquely frequency encode all parts of the object, the experiment is typically repeated many times with sufficient time allowed for relaxation recovery of the magnetization. These repeat experiments can be considered to be repeated averages of the same signal, and it is well known that improvements to the SNR only occur as the square root of the number of averages. For example, to double the SNR would require averaging four repeated measurements ($\sqrt{4} = 2$). To double the resolution in two dimensions while maintaining the same SNR, would require 16 (4×4) repeated measurements. To double the resolution in all three directions (Fig. 4-40) while maintaining the same SNR would require 64 ($4 \times 4 \times 4$) times as many measurements, which will typically take 64 times as long as a single measurement.

Two-Dimensional/Three-Dimensional Spatial Encoding

Using a gradient to frequency-encode position can be extended from a one-dimensional case up to a full three-dimensional object. For a 1-D object (extended along a line), each point is associated with a distinct frequency. In 2-D—either a 2-D object or a 2-D slice of a 3-D object—each line perpendicular to the gradient is associated with a distinct frequency. For a complete 3-D object, a single gradient results in each slice of the object being associated with a unique frequency. The complete spatial encoding of the object can be accomplished either by limiting the region being excited ("slice selection") or by using frequency encoding in one direction in conjunction with other methods to encode the remaining directions.

Slice selection. The most common procedure for reducing the dimensionality of the spatial encoding problem is to only expose a limited region of the object to the excitation pulse. Typically, one or several slices of interest through the object are selected for excitation.

The use of a linear field gradient across an object results in the Larmor, or resonance, frequency also varying linearly across the object. If all of the object is excited by a 90-degree pulse, the different frequencies of the returned signal correspond to different parts of the object. This principle can also be used to selectively excite specific regions of the object. This "slice selection" procedure uses an excitation pulse made up of a narrow range of frequencies. The region where these excitation frequencies correspond to the local Larmor frequencies depends directly on both the range of frequencies chosen and the strength of the gradient across the object.

A sinusoidal RF waveform at a single frequency is described by both the height of each peak (the amplitude) and the time interval between each peak of an oscillation cycle (the frequency, in cycles/sec or Hz). The RF waveform can consist of a range of individual frequency signals, with each signal frequency having its own amplitude. The Fourier transform is the mathematical method of decomposing these mixed signals and providing a listing (spectrum) of frequencies and their amplitudes. The range of component frequencies is, in fact, the signal bandwidth, and it is possible to create a signal that consists of only a particular range of frequencies.

If an excitation RF pulse is constructed with a particular bandwidth and irradiates an object in a gradient, only those object regions whose Larmor frequencies correspond to the frequencies of the excitation pulse will absorb energy and will have a transverse magnetization signal. For a given RF excitation bandwidth, the gradient strength can be altered to "spread" those frequencies across different extents of the object. Thus a combination of RF bandwidth, gradient strength, and gradient direction can be found to selectively excite any desired slice region of the object. The relation between these parameters is

$$Thickness_s = \frac{BW_{rf}}{\gamma G_z} \qquad (4\text{-}8)$$

where BW_{rf} should not be confused with BW_{samp} defined by the sampling $(1/\Delta t)$. For example, to excite a 1.0 cm slice of an object that is in a 0.5 G/cm gradient, the bandwidth of the excitation RF pulse must be 2129 Hz $(\gamma \frac{Hz}{G} \times 0.5 \frac{G}{cm})$. However, a significant practical problem is that it is not possible to create a signal with an ideal rectangular frequency profile of the desired

bandwidth. An ideal pulse has all frequencies within the bandwidth of the same amplitude and all of the frequencies beyond the upper and lower limits of zero amplitude. A nonsquare frequency profile that can be implemented directly leads to a nonsquare spatial profile for the slice; typical pulse profiles are actually shaped like that shown in Fig. 4-41. The 180-degree pulse profiles are often worse than 90-degree profiles, but both profiles may be improved through the use of numerically optimized frequency profiles.

Projection reconstruction. X-ray computed tomography (CT), positron emission tomography (PET), single photon emission computed tomography (SPECT), and nuclear magnetic resonance imaging (MRI) all fall in the general imaging class of reconstruction of the object from their projections (Fig. 4-42). This can be considered to be an image restoration procedure that tries to obtain the "actual" image of the object from the available "corrupted" images that were measured. All of these modalities use variations of the Radon transform situation most commonly associated with x-ray CT.

Projection reconstruction is described in terms of the Radon transform, named for the Austrian mathematician who developed the formalism in 1917 while working on gravitational problems.[15] The earliest MRI work used the same approach as CT so we will look at this case first. These concepts can be generalized to 3-D space, but we will begin with the simpler case of 2-D images and slices to which the "tomography" part of CT refers. Each projection through the object, at some angle, θ, is a line integral along lines perpendicular to the direction of θ. The total of all projections at different angles is the Radon transform of the object: $f(x,y) \;-> \; g(s,\theta)$ for the angle θ. The objective is to determine the original object spatial density distribution $f(x,y)$ from the "sufficient" set of projections $g(s,\theta)$—that is, to find the corresponding inverse Radon transform. The density distribution $f(x,y)$ represents any measured property of the object. For x-ray CT, SPECT, and PET, it is the specific density to x-ray absorption. For MRI, it is a modified proton density, where certain characteristics of the density can be emphasized by modifying the pulse sequence timing.

In x-ray CT, it is easy to visualize how a projection is made—just a shadow of the object where the intensity of the projection is proportional to the density of the object. The absorption of x-ray photons is described by the Beer-Lambert law

$$I = I_0 \, exp \, (-\mu D) \qquad (4\text{-}9)$$

where I is the intensity of the beam, initially of intensity I_0, after passing through the object of thickness D. μ is a characteristic of the material and is known as the linear absorption coefficient. Since the bones of the body are quite dense (μ is much larger

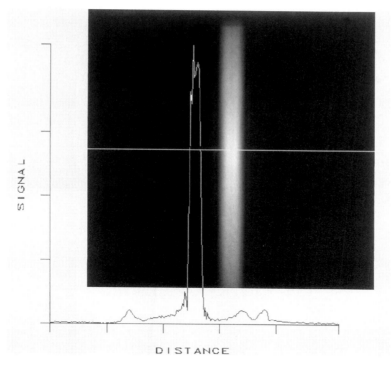

Fig. 4-41. Slice selection excitation pulses do not have ideal rectangular spatial profiles.

than that for air), the "light" or electromagnetic energy having enough strength to penetrate through it must be high, with frequencies in the x-ray range. To effectively form the projection, we want all of the impinging x-ray lines to be parallel when they reach the object. This corresponds to an x-ray source infinitely far away, or, in practice, effective collimation of the beam. The set of projections making up the Radon transform is collected by moving the x-ray source around the object and recording projections from all angles.

In PET or SPECT, the x-rays come from within the body from unstable nuclei attached to chemicals administered to the subject. In the case of PET, these chemicals (e.g., glucose) are transported and metabolized as usual, but when the nuclei decay, a positron (e^+) is emitted that travels only a short distance before it combines with an electron (e^-). This "annihilation" event results in two x-rays shooting off from that point in exactly opposite directions and is detected by sensors surrounding the object. Essentially this gives a projection from the inside out. Using the observation of the two opposite detections along with knowledge of the sensor geometry, the location of the annihilation can be calculated. More detail on SPECT and PET is available in later chapters.

For NMR, we have discussed how a magnetic field gradient will encode all points along the gradient with a distinct signal frequency. The strips of the object perpendicular to the gradient will all have the

same frequency signal. The signals from each strip are indistinguishable and add up to give a single amplitude at that frequency. The 1-D frequency encoding of the object by the gradient thus represents the projection of the object at the angle of the gradient direction. By incrementing the gradient direction through all angles, the Radon transform data set can be filled.

Given the complete Radon transform of the object, the problem is to find the inverse transform. The first approach that comes to mind, and was tried, is to reverse the process and "backproject" all of the intensities into a grid and to then add up the intensities in each grid box. However, this is not the inverse transform, as the artifactual points of Fig. 4-43 indicate. One can show that in the limit of an infinite number of projections at all angles, this backprojection will blur each point in the image by a function that looks like that shown in Fig. 4-44. To get the actual image of f(x,y), one must pass the image through a 2-D filter designed so that its blurring pattern at each point looks like the inverse of that in Fig. 4-44. This is called "filtered backprojection" and does give the desired inverse Radon transform. It is also called "convolution backprojection" if the filtering step is done in the time domain rather than in frequency.

The first NMR image formed in this way was in 1973[5] by PC Lauterbur and is shown in Fig. 4-45. This was shortly followed by the production of full head images in 1980[16] (Fig. 4-46). The quality of modern

X-ray CT

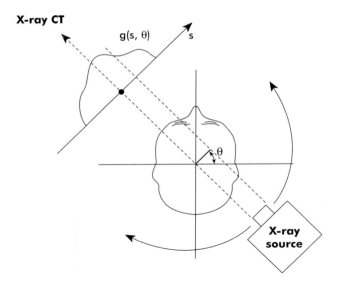

PET

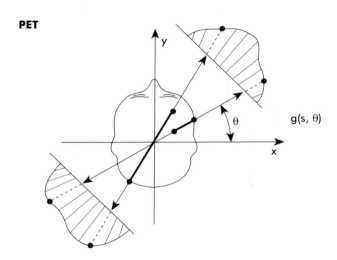

NMR

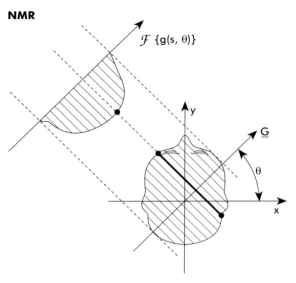

Fig. 4-42. Radon transform geometry for CT, PET, and early MRI.

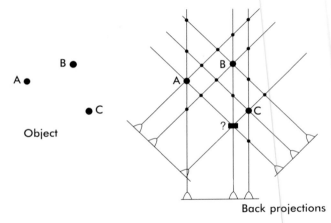

Back projections

Fig. 4-43. The intuitive backprojection summation algorithm does not reconstruct the correct image of an object from the set of projections. (From Jain Anil D: Fundamentals of digital image processing, Englewood Cliffs, NJ, 1989, Prentice Hall, p 441.)

head images (Fig. 4-47) shows the dramatic improvements made to this imaging technology.

Fourier reconstruction. Another way to obtain the inverse Radon transform, one that is more suitable for NMR, is by using Fourier reconstruction. This method depends on the "projection theorem" that says that taking the Fourier transform of a projection is the same as taking a central slice through the full 2-D Fourier transform of the object. This is illustrated in Fig. 4-48 and means that one can essentially obtain a 2-D Fourier transform by taking 1-D transforms of each of a set of projections. This is termed "filling Fourier space," where Fourier space is sometimes referred to as "k" space.

To reconstruct the object f(x,y), all one need do is take the inverse 2-D Fourier transform (IFT). From this slice-by-slice filling process, the data in Fourier space are available on a polar, rather than raster, grid. It is possible to perform a polar IFT, but it is significantly easier to interpolate the available polar data points to points on a rectangular grid in Fourier space and then perform two orthogonal IFTs using a fast Fourier transform (FFT) algorithm (Fig. 4-49). The FFT algorithms implement forward and inverse Fourier transforms in a very efficient manner but require the input data to be on a regular grid. For x-ray CT, the interpolation requirement for the IFT/FFT is generally more computationally expensive than direct convolution filtering, so filtered backprojection is generally used.

Because of the way the projection for NMR is formed, the projection is actually the frequency spectrum along the direction of the gradient. In other words, we directly detect the Fourier transform of the projection and, by the projection theorem, a slice of the

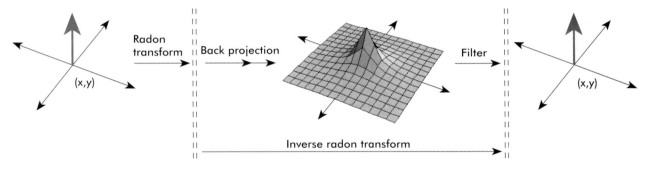

Fig. 4-44. With many projections, backprojection results in each point of the object image being blurred. Passing the image through a filter that corrects for this blurring restores the desired image.

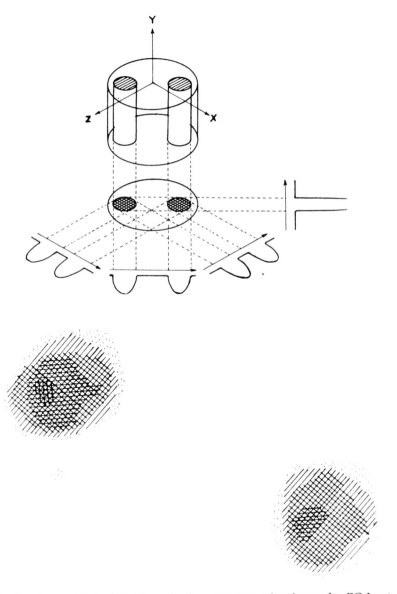

Fig. 4-45. The first published NMR projection reconstruction image by PC Lauterbur in 1973. (From Lauterbur PC: Nature, 242:190-191, 1973.)

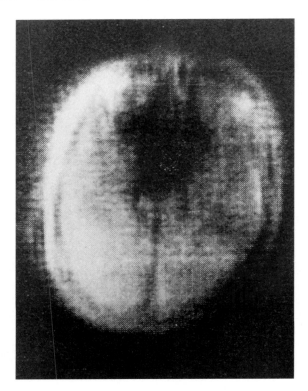

Fig. 4-46. The first published NMR reconstructed image of a head. (From Holland GN, Morre WS, Hawkes RC: J Comput Assist Tomog 69:262-277, 1980.)

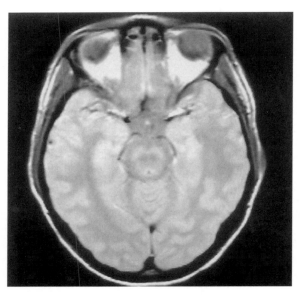

Fig. 4-47. A recent NMR reconstructed image of a head. Although approximately the same weightings are used as in Fig. 4-46, system and sequence improvements have resulted in a better image being produced in less time.

2-D Fourier transform of the object. The detected NMR signals from each gradient direction are directly filling Fourier space (without having to transform the projection); all that is necessary for reconstruction is to interpolate the data onto a rectangular grid and apply the 2-D IFT to get the image of the object.

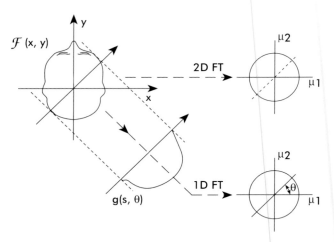

Fig. 4-48. The projection theorem states that the one-dimensional Fourier transform of a projection (at an angle θ) is equivalent to a central line through the two-dimensional Fourier transform (at θ) of the object.

A significant problem with this method is that errors can be introduced when the data are interpolated from polar to rectangular grids in Fourier space. Most methods in use today avoid this by using certain unique features of NMR to obtain data directly on the rectangular grid.

Phase encoding. The detected NMR signal is a complex signal and contains phase as well as magnitude information. The signal phase, as well as frequency, can be used to encode spatial position. Essentially, the same number of projections are taken, but now all the projections are made from one angle with differing amounts of phase twist. In x-ray CT, the phase information is not available so the projections must be taken from different angles.

Instead of rotating the direction of the projections and incrementing the angle θ by varying the amounts of both the X and Y gradients, the X gradient strength is kept constant for all projections while the Y gradient strength is separately varied for each projection. The amount of phase applied is adjusted by varying the Y gradient pulses. Typically, the duration of the pulse is kept constant and the amplitude of the gradient is varied, stepping through a "phase-encoding table" from projection to projection (Fig. 4-50). Thus the information along the X direction is encoded by signal frequency, as before, while the information along Y is encoded by using the signal phase.

The encoding of position with phase can be illustrated by way of an analogy to a group of spins all moving linearly in the same direction and at the same speed (Fig. 4-51). The speed of the spins will be directly related to the magnetic field strength as described in equation 4-1. When there is no field gradient along Y, all of the spins are at the same speed and move together. When a gradient is applied along the Y direction, the travel speed will then depend on the position

Procedure:

1. Take FTs of multiple projections: Fill Fourier space on polar raster:

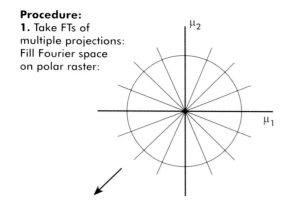

2. Interpolate to rectangular raster

3. Take 2-D IFT

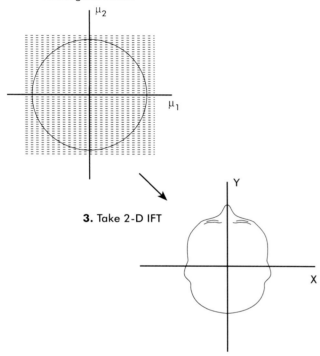

Fig. 4-49. By the projection theorem, the set of Fourier transformed projections are equivalent to a set of polar lines in Fourier space. Interpolating the data to a regular grid allows the use of fast methods for taking the inverse Fourier transform and obtaining the image.

of the spins in that direction, so that the spins farthest from the center will move faster than those nearest the center. When the gradient is removed, the spins go back to all moving at the same rate but are now out of phase by an amount depending on the strength and duration of the gradient that each spin experienced. Realistically, the spin speed reflects rotational speed and not physical displacement, and these stationary spins acquire relative phases as shown in Fig. 4-52.

Phase encoding works by spatially weighting each projection differently each time. An analogous situation occurs when considering the weighting function to be a simple one-row-wide slit in an opaque material covering an image (Fig. 4-53). A single projection

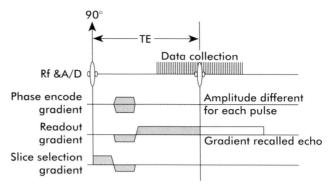

Fig. 4-50. Spatial encoding of a two-dimensional slice typically employs frequency encoding in one direction (X) and phase encoding in the other direction (Y). The constant "readout" gradient during data collection provides the frequency encoding while the set of repeated projections, each with a different phase encoding gradient amplitude, contains the phase encoding.

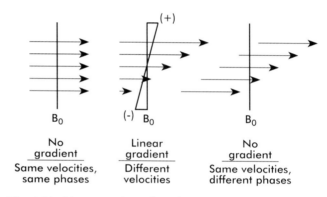

Fig. 4-51. Linear analogy for phase encoding using linear velocities rather than rotational velocites.

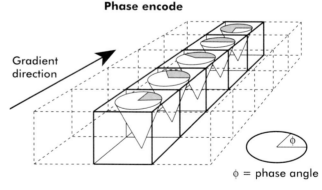

Fig. 4-52. After the phase-encode gradient pulse, the spins in the direction of the gradient have different relative phases depending on the strength and duration of the gradient pulse.

allows only a single line to be observed and recorded. By moving this slit function to a different line and repeating the acquisition, the whole image can be collected after sequentially moving the slit to each row.

Instead of a simple slit profile, the modulation function used in MRI is sinusoid shaped, such that

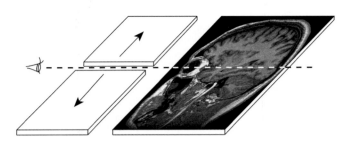

Fig. 4-53. The example modulation function is a simple one-row- wide slit. To obtain the entire image, multiple views must be taken, with the slit being moved to uncover each row.

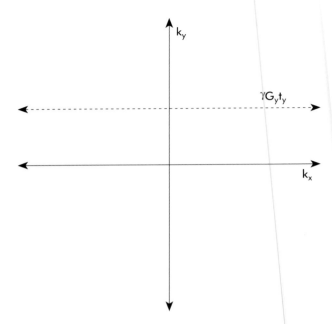

Fig. 4-54. One line in Fourier space is selected by the amplitude and duration of the phase-encoding gradient pulse.

specific spatial frequencies are emphasized — particularly those spaced so that they fall at the peaks of the sinusoid. The spatial frequencies emphasized, corresponding to the positions of sinusoid peaks across the object, are varied from projection to projection. The same number of projections are obtained as there are lines in the desired image.

This modulation is created by applying differing amounts of phase twist (spin warp) during each projection. The maximum gradient strength of the phase-encoding table is specified so that there is 2π of phase shift across the desired FOV: $\gamma\, G_y\, \Delta t\, FOV = 2\pi$. Since each spatial frequency is being directly measured by an appropriately modulated projection, a corresponding line in Fourier (frequency) space is collected for each projection (Fig. 4-54). An increment in the phase-encode table corresponds to an increment to another line in Fourier space. The sampling of the frequency encoding, performed in the same direction for each projection, fills in the data along the line. Once all of the Fourier lines are collected (with all of the data on a rectangular grid), the image can be directly reconstructed by applying Fourier transforms to the data in each direction.

Half-Fourier imaging. A complex number is described by both a real and an imaginary part. For a complex object that consists of only a real (and not an imaginary) part, its Fourier transform has the property of being conjugate symmetric ("hermitian"), which means that a number with a negative imaginary part will be equal to the same number with a positive imaginary part (real + imaginary = real − imaginary). In most circumstances a physical object is purely real and so its data in Fourier space should be conjugate symmetric. This means that the top and bottom parts of the data in Fourier space should be the same. Since we are collecting data directly in Fourier space, it is possible to use this property and generate the lower

half of the lines from the symmetric data collected in the upper half. These "half-Fourier" techniques have the potential of reducing imaging times by a factor of 2 (even 4 if the property is applied along each line). Unfortunately, the practical application of this is limited by the presence of various additive phase shifts that the data pick up from the receiver electronics, gradient-caused eddy currents, RF penetration phase shifts, and other sources (including blood flow and respiratory motion). Most implementations attempt to estimate and correct the data for these unknown shifts by measuring extra lines across the midline before symmetrically filling the remaining missing data. The corrections are not always successful in restoring the data set and the image may contain artifacts; since only half the number of lines of data is acquired, the image signal to noise will decrease accordingly by a factor of $\sqrt{2}$.

Effects of moving spins. Blood flow and other biologic motions result in changes to the detected signal and a corresponding alteration of the image appearance. Two basic flow effects can be considered: (1) motion in the presence of a gradient results in the accumulation of phase shifts relative to stationary spins, and (2) motion perpendicular to the imaging slice regions results in spins having a different magnetization (having seen a different sequence of pulse events) moving into the regions where signals are being measured. These effects can be exploited in the measurement and/or generation of images reflecting this motion, allowing the formation of MR angiographic (MRA) images. In general, MR signals and angiographic images are sensitive only to the velocity of the moving nuclei. In order to obtain a volume or flux flow measurement, the cross-sectional area of the flow must be identified and specified.

Movement of a spin in a magnetic field gradient results in the accumulation of a phase shift relative to the phase of stationary spins. The amount of phase accumulation depends on the direction and velocity of the spins relative to the applied gradient and on the gradient amplitude and duration. The simplest case to consider is that of linear motion of a single spin, with a velocity of V_x for Δt seconds, in the direction of a constant gradient of strength G_x (Fig. 4-55). A stationary spin at location X_0 will have a rotation angle of $\gamma G_x X_0 \Delta t$, which is how fast it is rotating ($\gamma G_x X_0$) times how long it has rotated (Δt). A moving spin starting at X_0 will have moved to a position $X_0 + V_x \Delta t$ after Δt seconds and will have experienced the different (and increasing) magnetic fields of the gradient as it moved. This will result in the accumulation of an extra phase angle of $0.5 \gamma G_x V_x (\Delta t)^2$. This extra phase shift is directly proportional to the velocity and the gradient strength but rapidly increases with the square of the time spent in the gradient.

Since multiple complete rotations cannot be distinguished from single or partial rotations, the gradient strength and duration used in MRA flow-encoding sequences are usually adjusted so that the velocity range of interest does not give more than a 360-degree (one rotation) phase shift. For example, to have the maximum expected velocity of 10 cm/sec accumulate a 360-degree phase shift during a 10 msec gradient pulse, a gradient strength of 0.47 G/cm should be used. For constant velocity flow, this phase shift will be a constant offset to the phase encodings of each phase-encoding projection and will lead to the corresponding image location having an additional phase shift after the Fourier transform. This is the basis of "phase contrast" MRA techniques, since locations without moving spins will have only random (noise) phase shifts while blood flow locations will show specific and coherent phase shifts. Quantitative measurement techniques sum the phase shifts over the area of the vessel to give estimates of flow volume. Many system processes and nonideal responses also lead to signal phase shifts and, thus, to specific patterns in images made of the phase shifts. Most phase-contrast procedures use subtraction of flow-sensitized and flow-desensitized acquisitions to remove the effects of these background phase processes.

If the flow directions change randomly during the measurement (as with diffusion) or are oriented approximately randomly (as with the perfusive flow at the level of the microvasculature), the accumulated phase shifts will also be random and will lead to

1 Dimensional motion case:

One moving spin starting from X_0 . . . . . . Linear velocity:
$X(t) = X_0 + V_x * t$

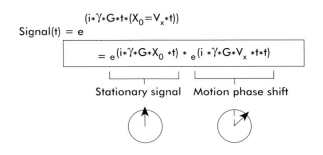

$F1 = \gamma * G * X(t) = \gamma * G * (X_0 + V_x * t)$

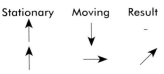

Examples: (if equal numbers)

Fig. 4-55. Motion of spins in the presence of a gradient results in the accumulation of a phase shift relative to that of stationary spins.

cancellation and reduction of the measured signal (Fig. 4-56).

Gradient waveform patterns can be employed to compensate for the motion-caused phase shifts at the time of signal measurement. These "flow compensation" gradients can refocus steady flow (and even linear acceleration) but not the random phase shifts and the associated signal loss from diffusive motions. Spin echo sequences that use symmetric echoes will also result in the compensation of constant velocity phase shifts at the time of every even-numbered echo of the sequence. The gradients applied during each pair of echoes implement a flow-compensating pattern, and this process has been termed "even-echo refocusing."

The common occurrence of pulsatile blood flow or rhythmic respiratory motion results in the appearance of "ghost" artifacts in the image. These repeated copies of the flowing region (or moving surfaces) across the image are the result of periodic velocity components and the associated phase accumulations

DIFFUSION:

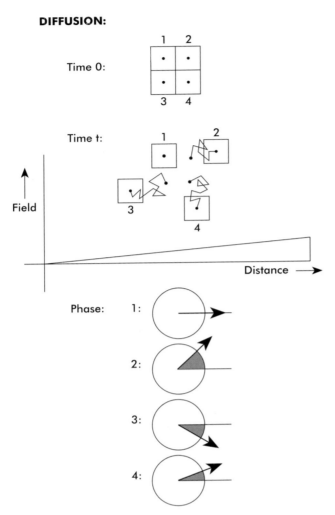

Fig. 4-56. Diffusion in a gradient leads to the accumulation of random phase shifts, which results in the reduction of the measured signal through phase cancellation.

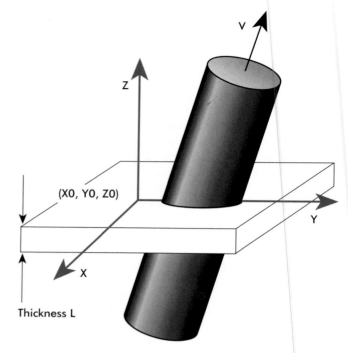

Fig. 4-57. Movement of spins perpendicular to the image slice will cause both the inflow of unsaturated spins and the outflow of excited spins.

from the cyclic nature of these types of motions. The repeat pattern reflects the frequencies of the motion, with single motional frequencies giving distinct repetitions of the ghost subimages while multiple frequencies lead to a smearing of repetitions across the phase-encoding direction.

The motion of spins perpendicular to the image slices causes spins with a different history of previous pulses to move into the imaging region (Fig. 4-57). Often these spins have not been influenced by previous slice selective RF pulses and are "unsaturated" relative to stationary spins. Since they have more longitudinal magnetization available for excitation, they will provide stronger signals than nearby stationary spins. This effect is exploited in "time-of-flight" MRA with bright regions of the image reflecting this inflow of fresh spins. Furthermore, these pulse sequences attempt to reduce or eliminate the signals from stationary spins so that the movement of spins

into the slice will be more apparent. For the relatively fast arterial flows, time-of-flight techniques work well with the thick slabs excited during 3-D imaging sequences because inflowing spins move fast enough to travel across the slab (Fig. 4-58). Slower venous flows will not travel as far and are often imaged using multiple 2-D slice excitations (Fig. 4-59).

Quantitation of this flow is possible if the experiment is performed so that the distance the inflowing spin moves is known. If this appearance is unwanted, the signals from these moving spins can be suppressed through the use of selective saturation pulses ("sat bands") placed adjacent to the image slices of interest, so that any spins moving from these areas and into the imaging region will not produce any signal. In addition to this "flow-related enhancement," there can also be the production of "flow voids" if the velocity of the spins is great enough that most of the excited spins in the selected slice leave the image slice before experiencing the selective inversion (spin echo 180-degree) pulse. The imaging parameters used determine whether these "wash in" and "wash out" effects will lead to a local signal increase or decrease.

CURRENT IMAGING TECHNIQUES

To summarize, the major differences between imaging with NMR and x-ray CT (or optic techniques) are that in NMR (1) the images have complex values

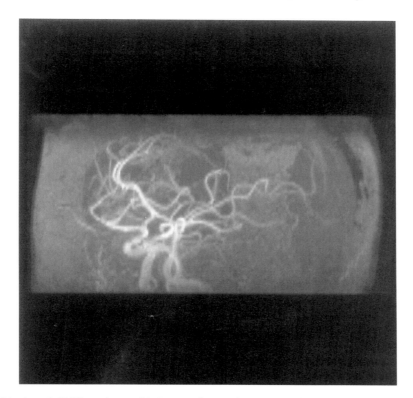

Fig. 4-58. Arterial MR angiographic image obtained using a multiple 3-D slab time-of-flight technique.

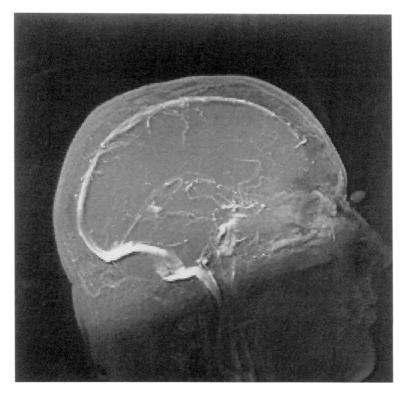

Fig. 4-59. Venous MR angiographic image obtained using a sequential multislice 2-D time-of-flight technique.

(amplitude and phase) for each pixel, (2) the object signals have a "memory" of previously applied pulses (from the pulse sequence), (3) image contrast reflects four mechanisms (T1, T2, and velocity, in addition to density), and (4) the Fourier transform data are directly acquired. Current imaging procedures exploit these differences as opportunities for efficient formation of diagnostically useful images.

"Standard" Methods

Spin echo. Spin echo sequences are still the most commonly used sequences and serve as a reference to describe the image weighting and time requirements of other sequences. As we have seen, spin echo imaging techniques directly acquire a single line in Fourier space for each phase-encoded projection acquired. The gradients in the readout (X) direction are designed to balance at the center of the echo (TE), giving no phase encoding at that time. The amplitude of the phase-encoding gradient selects the Fourier line being acquired.

The corresponding paths in Fourier space are shown in Fig. 4-60 for the cases of both gradients being applied together or separately. The effect of each gradient and the 180-degree RF inversion pulse on the path taken in Fourier space can be seen in these examples. Having both gradients active simultaneously allows the echo times to be made shorter.

Gradient echo. Gradient echo sequences are typically associated with low (less than 90-degree) flip angles. Gradient reversal allows the formation of echo signals without the use of 180-degree RF pulses and are generally employed in sequences desiring short TEs. As mentioned previously, T2* dephasing is not refocused and gradient echoes are not appropriate for use with TEs greater than T2* of the tissue. The quick echo formation, along with the much shorter TRs possible with low flip angles, allows images to be formed rapidly (e.g., 25.6 sec for a 256 line image using a TR of 100 msec). The simple Fourier space path of these sequences is shown in Fig. 4-61, and individual acquisition lines are selected by the amplitude of the phase-encoding gradient.

Since the TR is generally short relative to tissue T2, a significant amount of transverse magnetization remains by the time of the next excitation pulse. There are two general approaches to dealing with this magnetization.

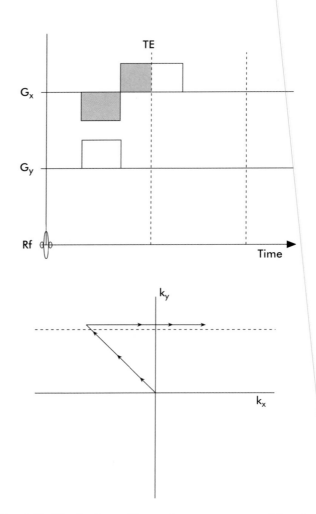

Fig. 4-61. The basic gradient echo sequence provides the data for a single line in Fourier space for each phase-encoding amplitude.

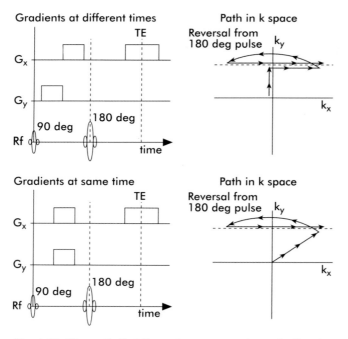

Fig. 4-60. The path that the pulse sequence traces in Fourier space is directly determined by the gradient and RF pulse applied. The path for a spin echo sequence is shown for **A**), separate gradient pulses and **B**), simultaneous gradient pulses.

The approach taken by sequences such as FLASH (Siemens, Fast Low-Angle SHot[17] or SPGR (GE, SPoiled GRASS) is to eliminate all of this magnetization through the use of "spoiler" gradient pulses before the next excitation pulse. This gradient quickly dephases any remaining transverse magnetization, and only the longitudinal magnetization reaches a steady state from the continuing series of excitation pulses. The T1 and T2 contrast mechanisms for FLASH sequences are similar to those of spin echo sequences.

Steady state sequences such as FISP (Siemens, Fast Imaging with Steady-state Precession) or GRASS (GE, Gradient Refocused Acquisition in the Steady-State) sustain the remaining transverse magnetization and, in fact, attempt to make it uniform from pulse to pulse by adding a postcollection gradient pulse to rephase spins by an amount equal to the dephasing caused by the phase-encoding pulse. In these sequences, both the longitudinal and the transverse magnetization reach a steady state and determine the characteristics of the signals obtained. As TR becomes greater than T2* of the tissues, the T2* processes eliminate any transverse magnetization and the signal characteristics approach those of FLASH. For TR less than T2*, the FISP signal is a function of the ratio of T1 to T2*, with T2* weighting increasing with TE and T1 weighting increasing with decreasing flip angle (less starting transverse magnetization).

Fast Imaging Methods

While the reduction in imaging times using low flip angle gradient recalled echoes is substantial, there are always applications that demand more rapid imaging times. Any speed improvement can be applied to increasing the SNR quality of the image data (e.g., by data averaging), improving the resolution of the image data (while maintaining image quality), imaging additional spatial locations, imaging dynamic processes (by repeated acquisitions), obtaining additional types of information (e.g., MR angiographic or spectroscopic), or increasing the number of patients that can be examined. In order to reduce imaging times to less than that required by the low flip angle, gradient echo methods, there are two general approaches: (1) reduce TR and TE along with added preparative pulses to provide contrast, and (2) acquire more than one Fourier line of data after each excitation pulse.

Prepared magnetization methods. As both TR and TE are made shorter and the flip angles are made more shallow, the opportunities for either T1 or T2 contrast mechanisms to influence the signal decrease. During a TR time of 5 to 10 msec, little T1 or T2* relaxation can occur and contribute to image contrast, and the resulting images will primarily reflect only spin density. In order to generate image contrast, an additional

set of "preparation" pulses can be applied before a rapid period of image acquisition.

To generate T1 contrast, a 180-degree pulse is applied to invert the longitudinal magnetization and start it following its relaxation curve back to equilibrium. After a selected amount of time (TI) during the recovery process, a rapid imaging sequence is used to acquire the image data in 300 to 900 msec (Fig. 4-62). This is similar to the inversion recovery sequences described earlier except that with these "turboFLASH" or "snapshot-FLASH" sequences[18,19] the entire image is obtained after a TI interval rather than just one Fourier line. Typically, TIs greater than approximately 300 msec are used so that all of the component signals have recovered past their null point.

T2 contrast can be generated through the use of a spin echo sequence followed by a 90-degree pulse. In this "driven equilibrium" type of sequence (Fig. 4-63), the 90-degree pulse is applied exactly at the TE time (2τ) determined by the 180-degree spin echo pulse (at τ) and will convert any transverse magnetization present at that time into longitudinal magnetization. Tissues having a short T2 do not have as much

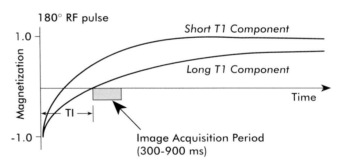

Fig. 4-62. T1 contrast can be obtained with short TR and low flip angle imaging by collecting the entire image after an inversion pulse.

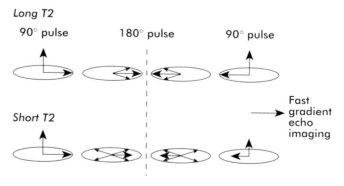

Fig. 4-63. T2 contrast can be obtained by using preparation pulses consisting of a spin echo (90 to 180 degrees) set of pulses, followed by an additional 90-degree pulse to convert any net transverse magnetization back into longitudinal magnetization. This magnetization is then measured by a fast gradient imaging sequence.

transverse magnetization remaining at TE and thus will not provide much longitudinal magnetization for measurement after the 90-degree pulse. A rapid image acquisition then measures the longitudinal magnetization and creates an image reflecting T2 contrast. A spoiling gradient between the preparation and imaging sequences eliminates any residual transverse magnetization left by RF pulse imperfections.

The contrast mechanism of this type of imaging is complicated by tissue relaxation and recovery occurring during image acquisition. Each Fourier space line acquired will have a slightly different intensity. Image parameter changes determining the length of the imaging time will lead to changes in the resulting image contrast. In general, the time of acquisition of the phase-encode lines closest to the center of Fourier space (containing the lowest image spatial frequencies) will determine the primary contrast features of the resulting image.[21]

The variation in intensity among the Fourier space lines effectively results in the data being filtered, with the amount of filtering increasing with long TRs, higher flip angles, and longer collection periods. The artifacts that result include blurring or pronounced edge enhancement.[20-22] Variations in the individual flip angles used in the imaging RF pulse train can be used to obtain uniform Fourier space data intensity[23,24] or any arbitrary signal (filter) response.[25]

Depending on the number of image lines (resolution) required, good quality images can be acquired in 800 to 2000 msec. The hardware requirements for these techniques are less severe than for other high-speed methods, and they are often used for routine clinical examinations.

These techniques can be extended to acquire a full 3-D data set. Sequences such as the T1-weighted MP-RAGE (Siemens, Magnetization Prepared RApid Gradient-Echo)[26] use a separate preparation pulse for each phase-encoded slice of the 3-D data set. In addition to the TI interval, this sequence uses a recovery period, selected by the TR parameter, after the image acquisition and before the next preparation period. High-contrast (T1), full-head image data sets, with millimeter resolution, can be acquired in approximately 6.5 minutes.

Echo planar techniques. Echo planar imaging (EPI) is the standard for ultra-high-speed techniques, despite its being first proposed by P. Mansfield almost 20 years ago.[27,28] With this type of imaging, all of the data for reconstruction of an image is acquired after a single excitation pulse. After the excitation pulse, a series of echoes, each with different phase encoding, are quickly and repetitively refocused and sampled. A constant G_x gradient is applied for the entire time while a large G_y is rapidly switched to repetitively

refocus echo signals (Fig. 4-64). Each echo has a different phase encoding as the result of the time intervals between each echo and selects a different line through Fourier space. Only data from half of Fourier space are acquired. Data are acquired continuously during the generation of the series of echoes.

There are several variants of EPI, primarily distinguished by the particular Fourier space path followed. Commonly implemented are the MBEST (Modulus Blipped Echo-planar Single-pulse Technique[29]) or "Instascan"[30,31] sequences (Fig. 4-65), which have reduced artifacts from field inhomogeneities and blood flow. The oscillating gradient in the read direction sweeps through Fourier space along that axis, and data are acquired throughout both halves of Fourier space. Along the orthogonal axis, the phase-encoding gradient moves the trajectory in discrete steps with each phase-encoding pulse.

With these sequences, a negative gradient lobe first dephases the signal, and then the sampling of the NMR signal starts in the presence of a constant (or blipped) gradient and an oscillating gradient. The

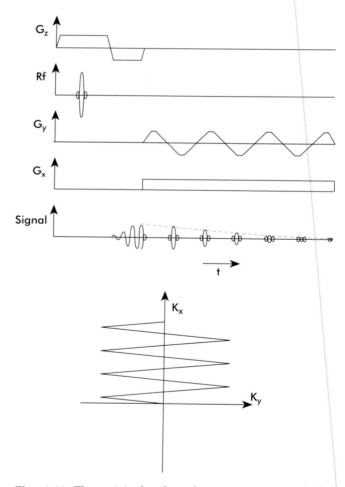

Fig. 4-64. The original echo planar sequence and the corresponding Fourier space path followed.

echo signals are sampled under alternating gradient pulses and, in order to fill the data matrix in the correct order, every other line has to be reversed. Therefore EPI is very susceptible to ghost artifacts if there are small changes in the even and odd echoes.

While these techniques can produce images extremely quickly (30 to 100 msec), they place severe demands on the scanner hardware, and extensive modifications are required for successful implementation. In addition to having data acquisition systems that can accommodate the long data sampling periods, the gradient systems must be able to generate and rapidly switch between large gradient values. Often systems are implemented that allow EPI only along the orthogonal (nonoblique) directions, often being limited to less than all three slice planes, since achieving the required gradient switch rates along the Z axis of the magnet can be technically difficult. Much of the work since the initial demonstration of whole body EPI at 1.5 T[31] has been confined to axial imaging, but additional work has demonstrated the feasibility of nonaxial EPI.[32]

For most standard clinical imaging systems, the maximum gradient strength and switching rate available are approximately 1 G/cm and 2 G/cm per millisecond, respectively. Therefore, on the order of 80 to 100 msec is required to acquire 64 Fourier lines. This is longer than normal tissue T2*, and the lack of signal by the end of collection makes EPI on these conventional systems impractical. The development of new fast-switching gradient systems will allow EPI to become more commonly available on commercial MRI scanners.[33,34] An alternative approach to obtaining the required gradient excursions with existing gradients is to drive the gradient coil so that it produces a continuous sinusoidal gradient pattern[35] (Fig. 4-66). Continuous sampling of this signal results in data being acquired in a nonuniform way in Fourier space, which requires interpolation to a rectangular grid or a generalized transformation for correct image reconstruction. With the proper corrections applied to the data, nonuniform Fourier data patterns can be successfully reconstructed.[35,36]

Because the magnetization is measured after only a single excitation pulse, the effective TR for EPI is

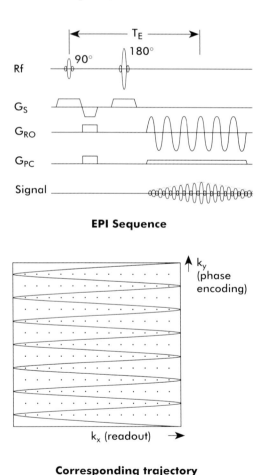

EPI Sequence

Corresponding trajectory

Fig. 4-66. Continuous sampling during sinusoidal gradient patterns results in the collection of nonuniformly spaced data in Fourier space. Methods are available to reconstruct images from this type of data.

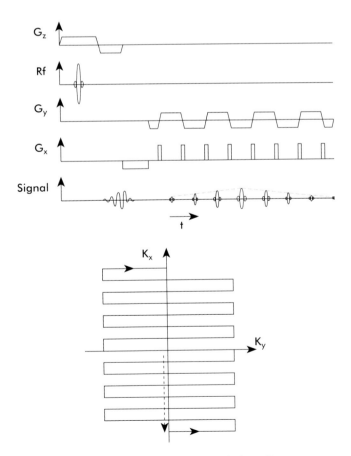

Fig. 4-65. Typical EPI sequences and their Fourier space paths.

infinitely long. The 90-degree excitation pulse makes all of the equilibrium longitudinal magnetization available for spatial encoding and data collection, and these methods are very efficient in terms of SNR even though they lack the data averaging ($\sqrt{N}$) SNR improvement that multiple acquisition sequences enjoy. In addition, these sequences have a relatively large bandwidth, which generally tends to lower the SNR.

There are several difficulties in obtaining successful EPI images. This single acquisition approach uses a long sampling period, approximately 25 to 64 msec, which, considering the signal decay from T2* processes, means that later echoes of the echo train will have very low signal strengths. Since the echo collection time is limited by T2*, for short T2* tissues one has to either acquire less data (reducing the image resolution) or acquire data more rapidly (requiring faster gradient switching). The long collection times require very good magnetic field homogeneity in order to avoid susceptibility artifacts and geometric distortions. The gradient refocusing, rather than RF echo refocussing, makes the sequences prone to these artifacts. Since fat and water have different resonant frequencies, the long readout period also makes the sequence prone to severe chemical shift artifacts. Both of these effects become more pronounced at higher field strengths. Eddy currents generated by such large switched gradients also pose a problem but are typically effectively addressed using actively shielded gradient coil systems that cancel the magnetic gradients outside of the imaging volume.

Some safety concerns are associated with the use of such fast gradient switching times. The rapid changes in magnetic field may approach the threshold for stimulating peripheral nerve activity. Such activity has been reported and investigated.[37-40]

Other data filling patterns (paths) in Fourier space are possible with these techniques, either acquiring all of the data after one excitation, or over a number of excitations. Spiral[41,42] and square spiral Fourier space paths[43,44] have also been demonstrated (Fig. 4-67). A constant linear velocity path shows improved SNR characteristics over constant angular velocity paths by equally weighting all parts of Fourier space. These single excitation gradient waveforms can be implemented with standard gradients, but interleaved multiexcitation acquisition reduces gradient demands, decreases bandwidth, and reduces artifact sensitivity. Spiral readouts also have good flow properties and generate minimal flow artifacts.[45] Square spiral paths preserve most of these advantages while allowing data to be collected directly on a regular grid.

Segmented Fourier space techniques. Given the difficulty in acquiring the full set of Fourier space data after only one excitation, a logical compromise is to

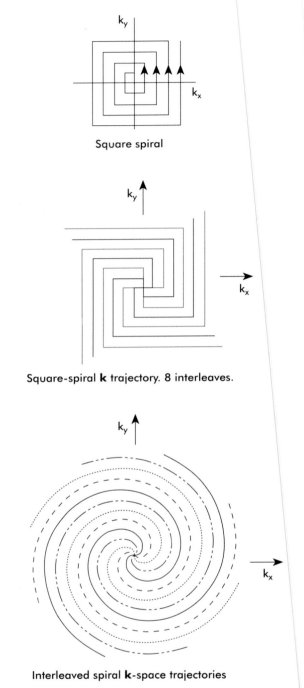

Square spiral

Square-spiral **k** trajectory. 8 interleaves.

Interleaved spiral **k**-space trajectories

Fig. 4-67. Gradient waveforms can be implemented to collect Fourier data along spiral and square-spiral paths. The data set can be collected after either one or several excitations. (Adapted from Meyer CH, Hu BS, Nishimura DG et al: Magn Reson Med 28:202-213, 1992.)

acquire only part of the data after each of several excitations. Thus the requirement of acquiring the data before T2* decay is less severe and the influence of susceptibility artifacts is lessened. Depending on the number of Fourier lines acquired per excitation, these techniques are not much slower than EPI. However, these repeated sequences do not start each excitation with the full equilibrium longitudinal magnetization (as does EPI) unless long TR times are used and the use of low flip angles will produce less transverse magnetization and signal. These sequences put less demand on gradient switching times and are more likely to be successful on standard imaging systems.

With these "segmented" Fourier methods, acquiring image data in several blocks can lead to phase discontinuities in Fourier space and ghost image artifacts in the reconstructed images. These artifacts are particularly severe with sequences that acquire individual blocks of Fourier data and can be lessened by acquiring the data in an interleaved or alternating pattern. These types of discontinuities are harder to avoid at high magnetic fields where T2s are short.

The RARE sequence (Rapid Acquisition with Relaxation Enhancement[46]) is a standard for these techniques. This is a rapid spin echo method that uses a series of RF (180-degree) refocused echoes to acquire more than one line in Fourier space after an excitation. Each echo of the multiecho, Carr-Purcell-Meiboom-Gill (CPMG) echo train[47,48] has a different phase encoding and so imaging times are reduced by a factor of the number of echoes used (Fig. 4-68). In principle, all of the encoded echoes could be acquired after one excitation pulse, but that would require the very rapid generation of the echoes before T2 decay processes eliminate the signal. Typically, a fewer number of echoes are generated and encoded per excitation, providing a corresponding factor of reduction in imaging time. With the exception of fat being very bright, the images obtained are similar to the T2 images produced by conventional spin echo sequences.

An advantage that RARE techniques have over EPI is that the use of RF echoes, rather than gradient echoes, results in the signal decay during collection being determined by T2 rather than the faster T2* processes. Therefore longer collection periods are feasible. Because of the long acquisition times, where only the signals from long T2 components remain, the initial images were heavily T2 weighted. Subsequent development work has reduced the T2 weighting and the associated T2 decay-related artifacts. By reordering the phase encodings, which is equivalent to selecting Fourier space filling patterns, a range of image contrasts can be selected.

The speed of these techniques can be used for acquisition of additional spatial locations, either using a multislice[49] or 3-D acquisition.[50] These high-resolution, T2-weighted data sets previously required an excessive amount of time to acquire using conventional spin echoes.

To reduce RF power deposition of RARE, a lower flip angle can be used for the refocusing RF pulses,

RARE k-spaced trajectory

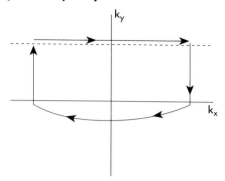

RARE pulse sequence

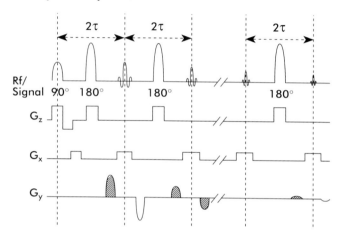

Fig. 4-68. The RARE sequence and its Fourier space trajectory. (Adapted from Melki PS, Jolensz FA, Mulkern RV: Magn Reson Med 26:328-341, 1992.)

which is the basis of FLARE ("Fast Low-Angle RarE"[51]) and even faster U-FLARE ("Ultrafast FLARE"[52]) sequences. RARE serves as the basis for a number of sequence variants referred to as "turbo spin echo," "fast spin echo," or FSE, sequences. The contrast of FSE images can be manipulated by varying TR interval, echo spacing and echo train length.[53] In addition, the phase-encoding order can be modified to adjust the image T2 weighting.[54,55] The time of acquisition of the low frequency (center Fourier lines) strongly determines the overall image contrast.

Fig. 4-69 shows an FSE sequence for two different Fourier space filling patterns that result in different image weightings. Each echo is individually phase encoded, read in the presence of a frequency-encoding gradient, and then phase unwrapped so that the next one can be phase encoded differently. Multiple horizontal lines in Fourier space are acquired within one TR period, with each echo providing a separate line. This sequence uses asymmetric Fourier space filling patterns with additional acquisitions

A

$90°_x$ $180°_y$ $180°_{-y}$ $180°_y$ $180°_{-y}$

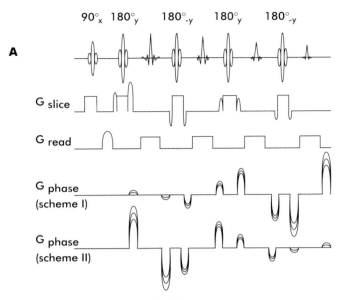

G slice

G read

G phase
(scheme I)

G phase
(scheme II)

Fast Spin-Echo Sequence

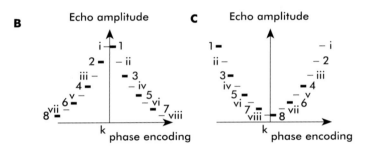

B   Echo amplitude

i ─■─ 1
2 ─■   ─ ii
iii ─   ─■ 3
4 ─■   ─ iv
v ─   ─■ 5
8 ─■ 6 ─■   ─■ vi
vii   ─■ 7 viii

k phase encoding

C   Echo amplitude

1 ─■   ─ i
ii ─   ─ 2
3 ─■   ─ iii
iv ─   ─■ 4
5 ─■   ─ v
vi ─   ─■ 6
7 ─ ─■ vii
viii ─■ 8

k phase encoding

Fourier Space Filling Schemes

Fig. 4-69. A fast spin echo sequence and two potential Fourier space filling patterns. The acquired lines are interleaved to avoid phase discontinuities and ghost artifacts. (Adapted from Zhou X, Cofer GP, Suddarth SA et al: Magn Reson Med 30:60-67, 1993.)

(excitations) filling in the gaps in an interleaved fashion. The pattern of Fig. 4-69, **B** (two-excitation RARE[53]) results in little T2 weighting but has a maximal SNR, since low spatial frequency lines are taken immediately before the signal has a chance to decay. The pattern of Fig. 4-69, **C**,[55] produces images that are heavily T2 weighted, have a lower SNR, and will show edge enhancement artifacts because of the collection of the high-frequency lines with a higher signal strength. Alterations to this filling pattern can be used to control image contrast.[56,57]

The applied phase encoding for each echo can be reversed prior to the next echo or the phase encodings can be allowed to accumulate.[58] Because of the longer collection time, the number of additional slices of a multislice set that can be acquired within the TR period is reduced, so this sequence is best used with a

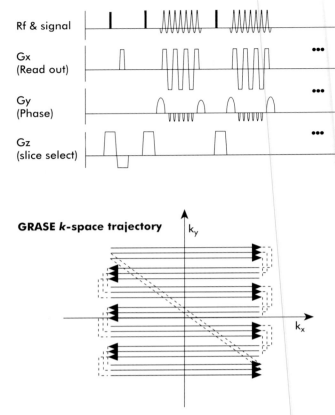

Rf & signal

Gx
(Read out)

Gy
(Phase)

Gz
(slice select)

GRASE k-space trajectory

Fig. 4-70. GRASE sequences form and phase encode gradient echoes between the series of RF echoes in order to obtain Fourier data more rapidly and without increasing RF power deposition. (Adapted from Oshio F, Feinberg DA: Magn Reson Med 26:355-360, 1992.)

small number of spatial slices. Full 3-D sequences can be created by removing the slice selection gradient and adding a phase encoding gradient before the first echo.

Using echoes for phase encoding that have experienced different amounts of T2 decay results in image filtering, particularly in the phase-encode direction. It is possible to use the first echoes (having less T2 weighting) to form a T1-weighted image and use later echoes to form a T2-weighted image. Longer echo trains give more T2 weighting but increase imaging speed by reducing the number of TR-long repeats of the sequence required to fill Fourier space. The use of RF echoes makes these sequences insensitive to susceptibility artifacts, even less so than conventional spin echo sequences.[59,60]

A further refinement of this technique is used in GRASE (GRadient And Spin Echo[61-63]) sequences (Fig. 4-70). The use of selective 180-degree RF pulses to form echoes is slower than gradient reversal switching. This technique alternates between gradient and RF refocusing within the echo train and consequently forms the images faster and with less heat deposition.

By creating multiple, short gradient echo trains between successive 180-degree pulses, the field inhomogeneities and chemical shift effects evolve over the relatively short time between the 180-degree pulses instead of the longer time of the total echo train as in EPI. An RF refocused CPMG (alternating RF directions) echo train is formed, and three or more gradient recalled echoes are created during each RF echo. Therefore the total number of signals per echo train is the product of the number of RF refocused echoes, N_{rf}, and the number of gradient recalled echoes per RF echo N_{gr}. For example, if N_{rf} is 8 and N_{gr} is 3, there will be a total of 24 phase-encoded signals acquired per excitation and the imaging time will be reduced by a factor of 24. The subsequent acquisitions interleave the lines acquired in Fourier space.

The acquired lines must be reordered so that the phase is continuous in Fourier space in order to avoid ghost artifacts. By the use of multiple RF refocusing pulses combined with the Fourier space sampling pattern, the images are not as distorted by inhomogeneity and chemical shift artifacts as those of EPI.

MRI technology is rich and varied, noninvasively providing an enormous range of information. From an established ability to provide high-quality structural information, MR techniques continue to advance and provide other clinically relevant physiologic information as well. New applications include detailed velocity/flow hemodynamic assessments, spectroscopic studies illuminating the details of biochemical status, and functional activation studies for localization and understanding of brain organization and function. In addition, short image acquisition times allow the tracking of dynamic processes, both intrinsic (e.g., cardiac) and introduced (e.g., bolus injections).

The primary limit on the wealth of diagnostic information that can be obtained for each patient is in the amount of patient time required. Approximately 1 hour of MR examination time is the practical limit of patient comfort and cooperation for routine clinical studies. As scan times go down through use of new sequencing techniques, the available examination time can be used to improve the quality of the data or to obtain additional types of data. A range of MR physiologic measurement techniques is poised to fill any reclaimed imaging time. The further refinement of MRA, MRS, and FMRI techniques will allow them to fit into current clinical practice and to routinely provide clinically useful information not practically available by any other method.

REFERENCES

1. Bloch F, Hansen WW, Packard ME: Nuclear induction, Physiol Rev 69:127-128, 1946.
2. Purcell EM, Torrey HC, Pound CV: Resonance absorption by nuclear magnetic moments in a solid, Physiol Rev 64:37-38, 1946.
3. Damadian RV: Tumor detection by nuclear magnetic resonance, Science 171:1151-1153, 1971.
4. Jaklovsky J: NMR imaging: a comprehensive bibliography, Reading, MA, 1983, Addison Wesley.
5. Lauterbur PC: Image formation by induced local interactions: examples employing nuclear magnetic resonance, Nature 242:190-191, 1973.
6. Damadian RV, Goldsmith M, Minkoff L: NMR in cancer: XVI. FONAR image of the live human body, Physiol Chem Phys 9:97-100, 1977.
7. Hoult DI: NMR imaging techniques, Br Med Bull 40:132-138, 1984.
8. Gadian DG: Nuclear magnetic resonance and its application to living systems, Oxford, 1982, Clarendon Press.
9. Bottomley PA: Frequency dependence of tissue relaxation times, In Partain CL, Price RR, Patton JA et al; editors: Magnetic resonance imaging: physical principles and instrumentation, vol 2, Philadelphia, 1988, Saunders, p 1082.
10. Heinrichs MA: Magnets, spins and resonances, Erlangen, Germany, 1992, Siemens Aktiengesellschaft.
11. Beall PT, Amtey SR, Kasturi SR: NMR data handbook for biomedical applications, New York, 1984, Pergamon Press, p 103.
12. Hahn EL: Spin echoes, Physiol Rev 80:580-594, 1950.
13. Weinmann HJ, Brasch RC, Press WR et al: Characteristics of gadolinium-DTPA complex: a potential NMR contrast agent, AJR 142:619-624, 1984.
14. Strich G, Hagan PL, Gerber KH et al: Tissue distribution and magnetic resonance spin lattice relaxation effects of gadolinium-DTPA, Radiology 154:723-726, 1985.
15. Radon J: On the determination of functions from the integrals along certain manifolds, Math-Phys Klasse 69:262-277, 1917.
16. Holland GN, Moore WS, Hawkes RC: Nuclear magnetic resonance tomography of the brain, J Comput Assist Tomogr 4:1-3, 1980.
17. Hasse A, Frahm J, Matthaei D et al: FLASH imaging. Rapid NMR imaging using low flip-angle pulses, J Magn Reson 67:258-266, 1986.
18. Haase A, Matthaei D, Bartkowski R et al: Inversion recovery snapshot FLASH MR imaging, J Comput Assist Tomog, 13:1036-1040, 1989.
19. Hasse A: Snapshot FLASH MRI: applications to T1, T2, and chemical shift imaging, Magn Reson Med 13:77-89, 1990.
20. Mugler JP, Spraggins TA: improving image quality in snapshot FLASH and 3D MP RAGE sequences by employing reordered phase encoding, Abstracts, 9th SMRM Annual Meeting, New York, 1990, p 1310.
21. Holsinger AE, Riederer SJ: The importance of phase-encoding order in ultra-short TR snapshot MR imaging, Magn Reson Med 16:481-488, 1990.
22. Chien D, Atkinson DJ, Edelman RR: Strategies to improve contrast in turboflash imaging: reordered phase in coding a K-space segmentation, J Magn Reson Imaging 1:63, 1991.
23. Stehling MK: Optimized (incremented) rf-angle gradient-echo imaging: ORANGE, Abstracts, 9th SMRM Annual Meeting, New York, 1990, p 459.
24. Wang SJ, Nishimura DG, Macovski A: Multiple-readout selective inversion recovery angiography, Magn Reson Med 17:244-251, 1991.
25. Mugler JP, Epstein FH, Brookeman JR: Shaping the signal response during the approach to steady state in three-dimensional magnetiatio-prepared rapid gradient-echo imaging using variable flip angles, Magn Reson Med 28:165-185, 1992.
26. Mugler JP, Brookeman JR: Three-dimensional magnetization-prepared rapid gradient-echo imaging (3D MP RAGE), Magn Reson Med 15:152-157, 1990.

27. Mansfield P: Multi-planar image formation using NMR spin-echoes, J Phys C Solid State Phys 10:L55, 1977.
28. Mansfield P: Real-time echo-planar imaging by NMR, Br Med Bull 40:187-190, 1984.
29. Ordidge R, Coxon A, Howseman A et al: Snapshot head imaging at 0.5 T using the echo planar technique, Magn Reson Med 8:110-115, 1988.
30. Rzedzian R, Pykett IL: Instant images of the human heart using a new, whole-body MR imaging system, AJR 149:245-250, 1987.
31. Pykett IL, Pzedzian RR: Instant images of the body by magnetic resonance, Magn Reson Med 5:563-571, 1987.
32. Weisskoff RM, Cohen MS, Rzedzian RR: Nonaxial whole-body instant imaging, Magn Reson Med 29:796-803, 1993.
33. Mueller OM, Roemer PB, Park JN et al: A 4-switch GTO speed-up inverter for fast-scan MRI, Abstracts, 11th SMRM Annual Meeting, Berlin, 1992, p 589.
34. Ideler KH, Nowak S, Borth G et al: A resonant multi-purpose gradient power switch for high performance imaging, Abstracts, 11th SMRM Annual Meeting, Berlin, 1992, p 4044.
35. Bruder H, Fischer H, Reinfelder HE et al: Image reconstruction for echo planar imaging with nonequidistant k-space sampling, Magn Reson Med 23:311-323, 1992.
36. Yan H, Braun M: Image reconstruction from Fourier domain data sampled along a zig-zag trajectory, Magn Reson Med 18:405-410, 1991.
37. Cohen MS, Weisskoff RM, Rzedzian RR et al: Sensory stimulation by time-varying magnetic fields, Magn Reson Med 14:409-414, 1990.
38. Budinger TF, Fischer H, Hentschel D et al: Neural stimulation dB/dt thresholds for frequency and number of oscillations using sinusoidal magnetic gradient fields, Abstracts, 9th SMRM Annual Meeting, New York, 1990, p 276.
39. Bourland JD, Nyenhuis JA, Mouchawar GA et al: Human peripheral nerve stimulation from z-gradients, Abstracts, 9th SMRM Annual Meeting, New York, 1990, p 1157.
40. Mansfield P, Harvey PR: Limits to neural stimulation in echo-planar imaging, Magn Reson Med 29:746-758, 1993.
41. Ahn CB, Kim JH, Cho ZH: High speed spinal-scan echo planar NMR imaging—I IEEE Trans Med Imaging MI-5 (1):2-7, 1986.
42. Macovski A, Meyer C: A novel fast-scanning system, Abstracts, 5th SMRM Annual Meeting, Montreal, 1986, p 156.
43. Meyer CH, Macovski A: Square spiral fast chemical shift imaging, Magn Reson Imaging 5:519-520, 1987.
44. Meyer CH, Macovski A, Nishimura DG: Square-spiral fast imaging, Abstracts, 8th SMRM Annual Meeting, Amsterdam, 1989, p 362.
45. Meyer CH, Hu BS, Nishimura DG et al: Fast spiral coronary artery imaging, Magn Reson Med 28:202-213, 1992.

46. Hennig J: RARE imaging: a fast imaging method for clinical MR, Magn Reson Med 3:823-833, 1986.
47. Carr HY, Purcell EM: Effects of diffusion on free precession in nuclear magnetic resonance experiments, Physiol Rev 94:630-638, 1954.
48. Meiboom S, Gill D: Modified spin-echo method for measuring nuclear relaxation times, Rev Sci Instrum 29:688-691, 1958.
49. Hennig J, Friedburg H: Clinical applications and methodological developments of RARE technique, Magn Reson Imaging 6:391-395, 1988.
50. Hennig J, Friedburg H, Ott D: Fast three dimensional imaging of cerebrospinal fluid, Magn Reson Med 5:380-383, 1987.
51. Hennig J: Multiecho imaging sequences with low refocussing flip angles, J Magn Res 78:397-407, 1988.
52. Norris DG: Ultrafast low-angle RARE: U-FLARE, Magn Reson Med 17:539-542, 1991.
53. Mulkern RV, Wong STS, Winalshi C et al: Contrast manipulation and artifact assessment of 2D and 3D RARE sequences, Magn Reson Imaging 8:557-566, 1990.
54. Mulkern RV, Melki PS, Jakab PI et al: Phase-encode order and its effect on contrast and artifact in single-shot RARE sequences, Med Physics 18:1032-1037, 1991.
55. Melki PS, Mulkern RV, Ranych LP et al: Comparing the FAISE method with conventional dual-echo sequences, J Magn Reson Imaging 1:319-326, 1991.
56. Melki PS, Jolensz FA, Mulkern RV: Partial rf echo planar imaging with the FAISE method I: Experimental and theoretical assessment of artifact, Magn Reson Med 26:328-341, 1992.
57. Melki PS, Jolensz FA, Mulkern RV: Partial rf echo planar imaging with the FAISE method II: Contrast equivalence with spin-echo sequences, Magn Reson Med 26:342-354, 1992.
58. Zhou X, Cofer GP, Suddarth SA et al: High-field NMR microscopy using fast spin-echoes, Magn Reson Med 30:60-67, 1993.
59. Jolensz FA: Fast spin-echo technique extends versatility of MR, Diagnostic Imaging June, 79-86, 1992.
60. Jones KM, Mulkern RV, Mantello MT et al: Brain hemorrhage: evaluation with fast spin-echo and conventional dual spin-echo sequences, Radiology 182:53-58, 1992.
61. Feinberg DA, Oshio K: GRASE (gradient and spin echo) imaging: a novel fast MRI technique, Radiology 181:597-602, 1991.
62. Oshio K, Feinberg DA: GRASE (gradient and spin echo) imaging: a novel fast MRI technique, Magn Reson Med 20:344-349, 1991.
63. Oshio K, Feinberg DA: Single-shot GRASE imaging without fast gradients, Magn Reson Med 26:355-360, 1992.

Positron Emission Tomography

Michael F. Hartshorne

Positron emission tomography (PET) has been used as a research tool since the early 1970s. In the past few years it has also been shown to have an increasing potential for application to clinical medicine. PET technology is based on the ability to accurately detect and image positron-emitting radionuclides. This technique consists of intravenously injecting short-lived radionuclides and then imaging the patient in a specialized detector system. By selecting appropriate radiolabeled compounds, PET images can demonstrate biochemical or physiologic processes involved in cerebral metabolism. These labeled compounds contain an isotope that, during its decay, produces a positron that travels no more than a few millimeters before combining with a negative electron. At that point of interaction, two photons are released in opposite directions with sufficient energy to be detected by sensitive detectors positioned around the head. PET, like computed tomography (CT), magnetic resonance imaging (MRI), and single photon emission computed tomography (SPECT), relies on computerized reconstruction procedures to produce tomographic images. In the case of PET, these tomographic images represent the spatial distribution of the radionuclides that have been administered to the subject. It is possible to overlay or imprint the information obtained from PET onto more detailed anatomic images such as MRI or CT for improved anatomic localization of the activity detected.

PET technology has provided the initial "noninvasive" views into the mysteries of the human brain. It was the first technique allowing complete localization of functional responses in humans. It was this approach to a "functional" assessment of brain activity that has supported advances in the areas of functional MR, magnetic source imaging (MSI), and SPECT. Many of the experimental paradigms utilized today in these other functional imaging modalities were developed by PET investigators. Even though many of the details of the coupling between tissue metabolic rate and neuronal electrical activity remain controversial, it is generally accepted that there is a close relationship between local cerebral neuronal activity, cerebral glucose metabolism, and cerebral blood flow. PET studies have not only provided an experimental basis to substantiate such relationships but have also demonstrated the complexities of metabolic changes with neuronal activation, particularly with respect to the role of oxidative respiration.

Landmark PET studies by Marcus Raichle, Peter Fox, and colleagues (discussed below) have led to significant advances in our understanding of the complexities of brain metabolism. For example, it was expected that local cerebral glucose metabolism and cerebral blood flow would increase with an increase in neuronal activity. However, these authors demonstrated that oxygen utilization does not increase in proportion to the large increases in local cerebral blood flow and glucose uptake. These results show that the blood flow increases associated with increased neuronal activity do not occur in response to the requirements of oxidative metabolism. Additional studies have shown that glucose oxidation is nearly maximal during resting conditions. Since nonoxidative glucose metabolism is inefficient in producing energy and the response of oxidative metabolism is limited, these results suggest that neural energy demands may be significantly less than would be anticipated from the large increases in blood flow and glucose uptake that are known to occur with cerebral activation. These types of complex neuronal and metabolic interactions make up the core of the brain-code problem. PET technology offers a unique opportunity, particularly when coupled with electrophysiologic techniques such as electroencephalography (EEG) and magnetoencephalography (MEG), for the neuroscientific community to better understand the complicated interplay between the brain's electrical and metabolic functions. The principles of techniques such as functional MRI (discussed in detail in Chapter 7), to a large extent, build on the work of prior PET investigations.

INSTRUMENTATION AND HISTORY

PET imaging is based on the production and detection of paired 511 keV annihilation photons. Consequently, a scintillator with a high atomic number is needed to achieve the sensitivity to detect these photons. Some systems use collimators in front of the detectors to improve sensitivity, but in principle, none is needed. However, optimal detection and recording of 511 keV photons do require the system to reject any events that do not occur on opposite sides of the brain nearly simultaneously. This ensures that noncoincident events such as scattered or background radiation are not recorded. Because this process is performed by system circuitry, it is sometimes called "electronic collimation."

Time-of-flight (TOF) PET scanners precisely measure the interval between arrival of each annihilation photon, making it possible to calculate the location of the disintegration. Two photons arising in the center of the scanner's field of view arrive simultaneously at the opposing detectors. Two arising close to one detector (and far from its counterpart) arrive at slightly different times. If the exact times of arrival are known, the origin of the positron decay event can be calculated and located in space on the line connecting the two detectors. For TOF scanners, a scintillator with a quick decay of the light pulse, several nanoseconds or less, is desirable. Several different inorganic scintillators have been used in this type of system.

Although thallium-drifted sodium iodide (NaI[Tl]) has been used, the most common material is bismuth germinate ($Bi_4Ge_3O_{12}$ or BGO). Scintillators with decay times of a few nanoseconds using barium fluoride (BaF_2) and cesium fluoride (CsF) have been tried in TOF PET scanners. Their principal drawback is that their light output is only 10% and 5% of NaI(Tl) respectively.[1]

The original PET scanners performed tomographs with single slices. Slice resolutions of >2 cm full width half maximum (FWHM) were produced in the early 1960s at several research institutes using systems with a ring of 32 NaI(Tl) detectors. An initial improvement in resolution was realized with more complex machines that increased the number of detectors and added gantries, which moved the detectors and provided more uniform sampling of the imaged subject.

Second generation PET machines decreased detector size and tried BGO detectors and additional rings to allow simultaneous acquisition of multiple slices of the subject brain. Resolution improved to less than 1 cm FWHM. (A practical limit on the thickness of the slices is about one-half of the axial FWHM resolution.) Most of these systems were "home built" one-of-a-kind machines and had very complicated electronic and mechanical systems. Others were marketed as the first commercially available machines in the late 1970s. Production runs were of limited numbers.

As more detectors and photomultiplier tubes (PMTs) were added to different designs, the complexity of PET machines increased and their resolution and sensitivity were improved. Stacked rings of detectors, each surrounded by hundreds of PMTs, have been used to improve in-plane resolution to 5 mm or less FWHM and axial resolution to less than 10 mm FWHM.[1-3]

After a prototype single-slice system was developed at the University of Pennsylvania, a stationary array of six positron detectors arranged in a hexagon around a 50 cm diameter patient port was built and achieved a volume acquisition with a 10 cm axial field of view. This departure from the more common ring-of-detectors configuration requires a special iterative reconstruction algorithm to "fill in the gaps" because the data acquisition is limited by coming from only three pairs of projections. The machine is named PENN-PET after the University of Pennsylvania. The design is simple, offers good resolution of 5.5 mm FWHM, has high sensitivity, and is commercially available. It is marketed as being less complex and less expensive than systems with the ring detector designs.[4,5] Better and better computation has increased the quality of data produced by PET scans.[6-9] Increases in sensitivity may be quickly achieved by using wide detectors that are not faced by septa. These systems can capture and locate events that angle between any two opposing faces. This improvement does degrade image contrast a bit because the fraction of scatter radiation included in the reconstruction is increased.[10]

It is possible to calculate the quantity of radioisotope that is delivered to a given area of the brain by using complex schemes. Some techniques rely on rapid blood sampling to establish arterial input functions during isotope administration. Others use rapid and repetitive data acquisition from slices to establish rates of isotope gain or loss. Loss by attenuation is compensated for by transmission scanning with positron sources of a known radioactivity and is important in these calculations.[11-13] It is well beyond the scope of this chapter to detail these techniques. They remarkably increase the complexity of PET studies, demand meticulous quality control performed by highly trained technologists and scientists, and add to the expense of the tests performed.

With all the developments made in PET technology, there are only a few more than 100 centers worldwide. Some are devoted to clinical use but most remain dedicated to research, and many are one-of-a-kind or prototypes. By comparison, there are several dozen SPECT systems in New Mexico, which has a population of only 1.5 million people. All of these SPECT facilities are used primarily for clinical work.

PET RADIOPHARMACEUTICALS

The positron emitting radioisotopes all have different half-lives but the same energy as twin 511 keV annihilation photons is produced. The half-lives of the isotopes are measured in minutes (Table 5-1). This is both the good news and the bad news. Repeat measurements at close intervals are possible with the same or different PET radiopharmaceuticals. Most of the PET agents used medically start with production in a cyclotron in the same building as the patient and the scanner. They may be processed briefly in a "black box" synthetic device to prepare a specific pharma-

Table 5-1. Radionuclides for PET brain imaging

Radionuclide	T1/2 Minutes	Source	Generator T1/2
^{15}O	2	Cyclotron	N/A
^{13}N	10	Cyclotron	N/A
^{11}C	20.4	Cyclotron	N/A
^{18}F	110	Cyclotron	N/A
^{68}Ga	68	^{68}Ge	270 days
^{62}Cu	9.8	^{62}Zn	9.2 hr

ceutical and must be quickly administered to the patient for scanning.[14] Hundreds of different molecules have been labeled with positron emitters.

Some of these agents are used for perfusion images to measure blood flow to the brain, others are used to mark metabolic processes, and some are labeled with molecules that bind to specific receptors. ^{13}N ammonia in physiologic saline circulates with the blood after injection. It is extracted by the brain in a manner proportional to regional blood flow. Its disappearance from the brain is dominated by the physical T1/2 of 2 minutes since it has a biologic T1/2 of about 60 to 70 minutes in the brain. ^{15}O (oxygen) is prepared as $H_2{}^{15}O$-labeled water for measurement of cerebral blood flow (CBF) and displays a linear relationship between actual CBF and measured CBF up to 65 ml/min/100 g. Above that value, it underestimates CBF.[15] Inhaled $C^{15}O$ and $O^{15}O$ also allow the measurement of CBF.[16] ^{62}Cu (copper) pyruvaldehyde-bis-N^4-methyl-thiosemicarbazone (PTSM) is prepared from a ^{62}Zn (zinc) generator and shows promise as a CBF agent for clinics that do not have a cyclotron.[17]

^{18}F (fluorine) as fluorodeoxyglucose (FDG) is an excellent agent for studying glucose metabolism.[18] After extraction by metabolically active tissues in the brain, FDG is phosphorylated to FDG-6-phosphate but does not undergo glycolysis and remains trapped in the cell. Tumor, epileptic foci, and recurrent tumors (as opposed to postradiation necrosis) can be detected with FDG.

The publications in the field of labeled-receptor chemistry for brain PET, ranging from the dopaminergic receptor system to the opiate agonists, would fill texts larger than this book. A variety of ^{18}F- and ^{11}C-labeled receptor-binding pharmaceuticals are discussed in greater detail later in this chapter.

Some perfectly predictable results have been obtained from the use of ^{68}Ga (gallium)-labeled ethylenediaminetetraacetic acid (EDTA) in PET scanners. Like the traditional gamma camera agent ^{99m}Tc diethyleneaminepentaacetic acid (DTPA), iodinated contrast agents used with CT, or paramagnetic contrast agents used with MRI, the ^{68}Ga EDTA is excluded

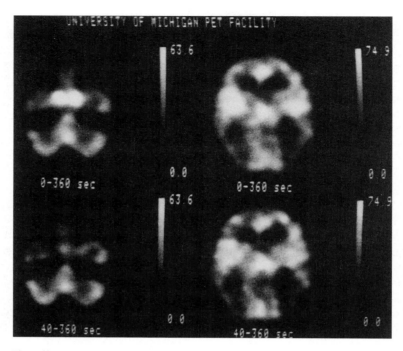

Fig. 5-1. The effect of including early data (first 40 seconds after injection) on a PET rCBF scan is to artifactually increase apparent activity in the vicinity of large arteries. The two upper images show increased activity around the internal carotid and middle and anterior cerebral arteries. The lower pair of images are from the same acquisition without the first 40 seconds of data and more accurately show the perfusion of the cortex. (From Koeppe R: J Nucl Med 28:1695-1703, 1987.)

by the intact blood-brain barrier (BBB) but will concentrate in areas where the BBB is damaged by tumor, infection, or healing infarct.[19,20]

CEREBRAL BLOOD FLOW

The most widely used PET tracer for measuring regional cerebral blood flow (rCBF) is $H_2^{15}O$. The non-invasive measurement of rCBF is valuable since it parallels the regional glucose consumption in the brain (discussed below) and changes rapidly with activation or stimulation of cortical neurons. Quantifying the absolute rCBF in units of ml/100 g/min is tricky. Some methods require rapid arterial sampling from the radial artery in order to approximate the input of the $H_2^{15}O$ in the arteries of the brain. This may be done manually or in a more precise manner by slowly bleeding the subject's radial artery through a scintillation detector. How the arterial input values should be used to establish an approximation for cerebral artery input is a mathematician's battleground.[21-32] These mathematical uncertainties make simpler static scan techniques look attractive (Fig. 5-1).

Different styles of $H_2^{15}O$ acquisition produce different measurements of rCBF. In general, the measured rCBF approximates 70 ml/100 g/min in gray matter and 20 ml/100 g/min in white matter. Obviously, one source of error when measuring these two closely

related tissues stems from the resolution of the scanner used. Different machines will be more or less accurate in the distinction of measurements made over the convoluted, millimeters thick gray/white interface. The more elegant quantitative methods require sequential, dynamic scans. Scans may be repeated rapidly using collection times of 20 seconds or more. The bolus of labeled water does not immediately equilibrate with brain tissue and might arrive at slightly different times in various parts of the brain. Early acquisitions after injection may be weighted by regional cerebral blood volume (rCBV). Some authors recommend that during sequential dynamic scans, data for the first 40 seconds after injection be omitted from rCBF calculations.

For the functional comparison of resting versus activated neurons, single static scans are attractive because they are simpler than quantitative dynamic scans. Simply measuring regional ^{15}O activity (rA) and accepting this as proportional to rCBF requires much less complex analysis.[32] The 2-minute half-life of ^{15}O limits the scanning time. Although there is not much time to gather data, sequential injections can be performed with little or no need to correct for residual radioactivity from previous injections. The resulting images will have optimal signal-to-noise ratios if acquisitions between 90 and 120 seconds long are

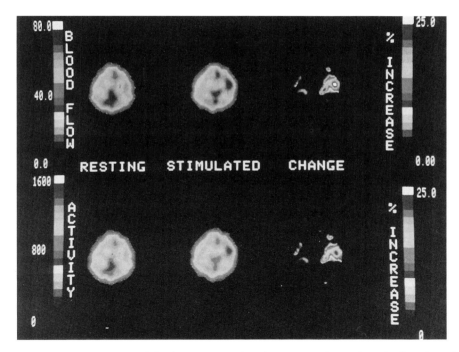

Fig. 5-2. Blood flow maps of the brain at two levels were performed at the baseline (*left*) and during left hand vibration (*center*). The effects of sensory stimulation are more obvious when the resting perfusion image is subtracted from the stimulated scan to show the increased perfusion in the stimulated sensory cortex. (Reproduced in full color in color insert.) (From Fox PT: J Nucl Med 30[2]: 141-149, 1989.)

used.[33] Unlike the quantitative dynamic schemes, the immediate postinjection period is helpful in static scans for establishing the differences between resting and stimulated brain states.[34] Keeping the subject stationary in the scanner for a few minutes after a baseline (resting) scan allows a second, stimulated-state scan to be performed after a second bolus of $H_2^{15}O$ is injected. A difference image is then made by subtracting the baseline scan from the stimulated-state scan. Activated portions of the brain should show increased perfusion (Fig. 5-2).

A wide variety of stimulated states have been investigated. Stimulation of primary somatosensory, visual, and auditory cortexes can be easily done. Testing association cortex related to these primary areas simply requires the use of any of several psychologic test paradigms. Motor cortex activity has been studied and localized during voluntary movement of the extremities by the subject. This information can be used for basic research into brain function (and its cortical location) and in preoperative planning when neurosurgical procedures must be conducted near critical areas of the cortex. Accuracy of this PET application can be extended by comparing scans of a subject in the stimulated state with averaged images from multiple subjects in the unstimulated state. Scans analyzed in this fashion must be geometrically transformed into a standardized stereotactic coordinate

system. This transformation complicates the simple subtraction or change-distribution techniques used for imaging the resting and stimulated states. To increase objectivity of the analysis, an algorithm can be used to remove observer bias.[35-49]

Alternate PET agents for rCBF measurements are available. Inhaled ^{15}O, $C^{15}O$, $C^{15}O_2$, ^{77}Kr, and (^{18}F) fluoromethane, as well as injected (^{11}C) butanol, (^{15}O) butanol, and ^{11}C-labeled chlorphentermine derivatives, can be used. The possibility of a generator-produced ^{62}Cu-PTSM rCBF agent has yet to be exploited. These agents do not enjoy the widespread use and in-depth scientific characterization of $H_2^{15}O$ rCBF measurements.[17,19,50-55]

REGIONAL CEREBRAL METABOLIC RATES OF GLUCOSE

Since the brain preferentially uses glucose as a metabolic substrate, there is ample reason to study its glucose consumption. This can be done directly in animal models with ^{14}C-labeled glucose (GLC). There appears to be a good correlation between the metabolism of GLC and [^{18}F]2-fluoro-2-deoxyglucose (FDG) in most areas of the brain. Exceptions to this relationship between FDG and GLC are found in the hippocampus, thalamus, and cerebellum, where activated cortex shows FDG uptake to be higher than CLG uptake.[56-59] The extremely long half-life of beta-

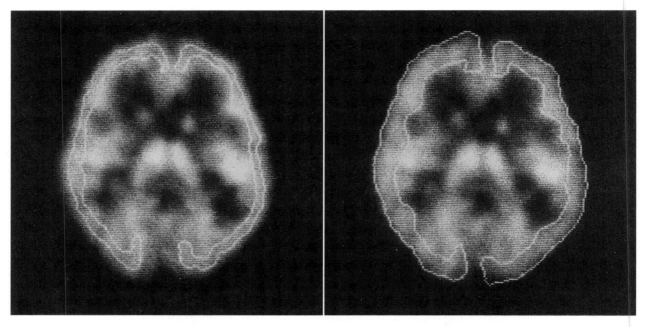

Fig. 5-3. With thin and thick outline regions of interest, differences in measurement of rCMRglc are not a surprise. From one machine to the next, marked differences in resolution of the convoluted cortical surface produce bigger variations in rCMRglc estimates. (From Jagust W: J Nucl Med 27:1358-1361, 1986.)

emitting [14]C (5730 years) and the relatively short half-life of [11]C (20.4 minutes) make these isotopes impractical to use. FDG is the best GLC approximation available for PET. With the advantage of a 2-hour half-life, a number of different synthetic methods are available to make FDG.[60-64]

The measurement of regional cerebral metabolic rates for glucose (rCMRglc) with FDG reminds me of enchilada recipes. Every dish is cooked differently, with a range of dishes produced that are both similar and unique. The cooks argue the merits of their techniques but they all call their creation enchiladas. There are many variations in the recipes for rCMRglc estimations. Many different quantitative results are expressed in units of mg/100 g/min or μmol/100 g/min.

The resolution of the PET scanner, geometric and anatomic effects of the convoluted gray matter cortex, and marked differences in data collection and analysis have produced 20% to 30% variations in rCMRglc estimates in the same brain region[65-73] (Fig. 5-3).

Measurement of rCMRglc requires rapid sampling of the arterialized 5 to 10 mCi (185 to 370 MBq) venous bolus. A classic model in FDG PET named for its author, Sokoloff, relates four rate constants and three compartments to the metabolic fate of FDG.[74] The first, k1, describes the transfer of FDG from capillary vessels to the extracellular space. Transfer back to the bloodstream is measured by k2. An independent standardization of the k1 and k2 rates was accomplished by the use of ^{11}C-labeled methyl-D-glucose, which is not taken into the cell but shares the GLC transport into and out of capillaries. The uptake of FDG from the extracellular space to the cell is measured by k3. The FDG is then phosphorylated to FDG-6-phosphate by hexokinase. It does not undergo further glycolysis and is trapped in the cell. The rate of transfer from the cell back to the extracellular space, k4, is negligible and customarily ignored in measurements made within 1 hour of injection. The relationship between GLC and FDG metabolism is established with the use of a "lumped constant," which corrects for essential differences between the two metabolisms. Normal resting values depend on the area of brain and the laboratory in question. These values range from 20 to 60 μmol/100 g/min in gray matter and 10 to 20 μmol/100 g/min in white matter.

Given the variations in PET scanners, data acquisitions, and mathematical assumptions used, standardization within a PET center is critical to the validity of any experimental studies performed. Studies of reproducibility and measurements of normal inter- and intrasubject variability show a range of 10% to 15%[75] (Fig. 5-4). Optimal experimental design frequently requires a patient to serve as his own control. Comparisons of subjects studied with sequential (on different days) FDG scans requires a computer-assisted image registration program.[76] Studies performed while the subject remains motionless in the scanner (difficult even for healthy subjects) require correction for residual FDG present when the second

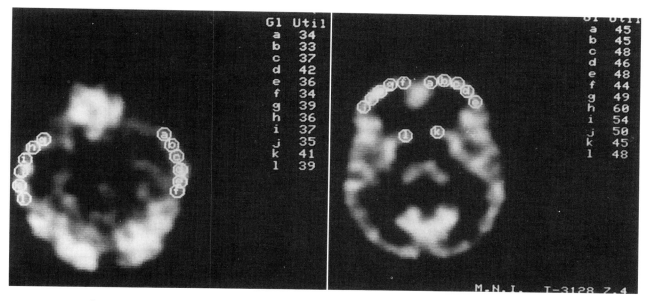

Gl	Util
a	34
b	33
c	37
d	42
e	36
f	34
g	39
h	36
i	37
j	35
k	41
l	39

Gl	Util
a	45
b	45
c	48
d	46
e	48
f	44
g	49
h	60
i	54
j	50
k	45
l	48

Fig. 5-4. Side-to-side comparison of rCMRglc calculations in one set of normal patients shows small but significant increase in left mid and posterior temporal area and caudate nucleus relative to comparison areas on the right. This further complicates the use of a normal data base which must take into account each hemisphere. (From Tyler JL: J Nucl Med 29:631-642, 1988.)

injection is performed[77,78] (Figs. 5-5 and 5-6). Accurate comparisons of studies done on different PET scanners may be impossible. "Absolute" measurements of rCMRglc from different scanners are probably correlated but may range from 30% to 120% different when older PET scanners are compared with new machines. One partial solution is to compare the rCMRglc measurements as values indexed to their respective whole brain or lobar uptake.[79] This may reduce PET results to the semiquantitative status enjoyed by SPECT results.

ISCHEMIA AND STROKE

Using combinations of PET techniques, an understanding of the acutely infarcted brain has been gained. The normal brain shows "tight coupling" between rCBF and metabolic rates described as rCMRglc and/or regional cerebral metabolic rate for oxygen (rCMRO$_2$). In some patients, immediately after a stroke the regional oxygen extraction fraction (rOEF) increases while rCBF falls greatly and rCMRglc falls slightly. This "uncoupling" of flow and metabolism indicates a compensatory metabolic shift after decreased perfusion, which is referred to as *misery perfusion*. After a week, the infarcted brain tends to increase rCBF while rCMRglc remains depressed. This phenomenon is referred to as *luxury perfusion*. After a month, rCBF and rCMRglc are at a level lower than the normal contralateral brain (and presumably lower than before the infarct) but are, again, tightly coupled.[80-90]

There is a question about the recovery of severely ischemic brain or at least the "penumbra" of viable tissue around the (irreversibly) infarcted core. PET techniques have suggested that *misery perfusion* areas peripheral to infarcts may be salvaged if adequate rCBF can be restored. Those areas that have *luxury perfusion* would not be expected to improve with intervention to increase rCBF. A stroke's end point occurs when rCBF and rCMRglc/rCMRO$_2$ are recoupled at lower than baseline rates. Interventions designed to increase rCMR at that point will not recover neuron function. In a totally expected fashion, the metabolic rates and rCBF of remote areas dependent on afferent input from the infarcted area will decrease after stroke (Fig. 5-7). A motor cortex stroke will interrupt the cerebropontocerebellar pathways and cause a drop in flow and metabolism in the contralateral cerebellar hemisphere and is referred to as *crossed cerebellar diaschisis*.

In the case where collateral circulation keeps an area of brain alive after occlusion of a primary artery, the drop in perfusion pressure is partly compensated by an increase in regional cerebral blood volume (rCBV). Dilated arterioles decrease the resistance to flow so that rCBF, rCMRglc, and rCMRO$_2$ can be maintained at normal levels. The increased rCBV indicates that the brain involved in this phenomenon has already used one compensatory mechanism to preserve perfusion (Fig. 5-8). The most sensitive PET measurement of this phenomenon is a ratio image of

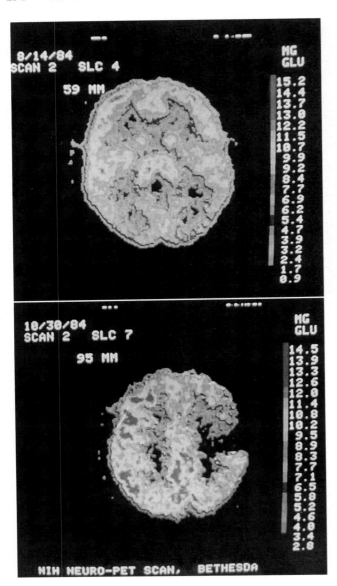

8/14/84
SCAN 2   SLC 4
59 MM
MG GLU
15.2
14.4
13.7
13.0
12.2
11.5
10.7
9.9
9.2
8.4
7.7
6.9
6.2
5.4
4.7
3.9
3.2
2.4
1.7
0.9

10/30/84
SCAN 2   SLC 7
95 MM
MG GLU
14.5
13.9
13.3
12.6
12.0
11.4
10.8
10.2
9.5
8.9
8.3
7.7
7.1
6.5
5.8
5.2
4.6
4.0
3.4
2.8

NIH NEURO-PET SCAN,   BETHESDA

Fig. 5-5. FDG image from a normal subject (*above*) and one with a brain tumor (*below*) show precisely mapped regional glucose metabolic rate measurements. With repeated scans, these values are within 5% to 10% of their respective second measurements. (Reproduced in full color in color insert.) (From Brooks R: J Nucl Med 28[1]:53-59, 1987.)

rCBF/rCBV that quantifies *perfusion reserve*. The areas with little perfusion reserve have already dilated their vessels and will have to fall back on increased rOEF if there is any additional decrease in rCBF. These measurements would seem to predict the future risk of infarction. However, there is not agreement in the literature as to the utility of rCBF/rCBV measurements in the operative management (carotid endarterectomy and extracranial-intracranial bypass) of these patients. There is a role for the use of PET in monitoring the efficacy of medical management of stroke with drugs such as nimodipine.[91,92] As medical and surgical

prevention and therapy for stroke are pursued by various researchers, PET will provide physiologic measurements to help explain clinical outcomes.[93]

PET ASSESSMENT OF DEMENTIA

Dementia includes a broad category of diagnoses that result in the loss of higher cortical functions of intellectual ability. Dementia may be completely, partly, or not at all reversible. Some dementias are associated with drug and alcohol abuse and are best treated by cessation of the abuse. Others are related to hypothyroid states, infections, and systemic illnesses such as systemic lupus erythematosus and may be medically corrected. Ischemic injury after profound shock, drowning, and carbon monoxide poisoning may also produce a dementia. Intracranial lesions such as subdural hematoma, normal pressure hydrocephalus, and primary and metastatic brain tumors may result in dementia and may or may not be correctable. Diseases that directly affect neurons include Alzheimer's, Pick's, Huntington's, Wilson's, and Parkinson's diseases, multiple sclerosis, multi-infarct dementia, and infections such as AIDS dementia and Jakob-Creutzfeldt disease. At present, little can be done to correct the dementias in these categories. "Pseudodementia" or depression in the elderly is readily treatable but can be clinically confused with dementias that do not have associated motor disorders or systemic diseases.[94]

Alzheimer's disease affects millions of elderly Americans and has been the focus of considerable PET investigation. There is a general pattern of decreased rCBF, rCMRglc, and rCMRO$_2$ that start bilaterally in the superior parietal cortex. As the disease progresses, this area of decreased flow and metabolism extends contiguously into the inferior parietal, superior temporal, and prefrontal cortex. The extent of the defects correlates with the severity of the disease. Longitudinal studies have shown that the early biparietal defects are detectable by PET at least 1 year before the clinical diagnosis can be made. The decreased flow and metabolism of the affected areas indicate intact autoregulation responding to reduced demand in the areas of histopathologically established decreased synaptic density[95-115] (Fig. 5-9). The findings of cortical atrophy by MRI and CT scan in suspected Alzheimer's disease are very nonspecific and not useful in making the diagnosis.[116-117] The pattern of cortical defects in Alzheimer's disease is not pathognomonic, and accuracy of diagnosis depends on the experience of the observer. There are patterns of hypometabolism in a small percentage of patients with Parkinson's disease and dementia that are identical to those of patients with Alzheimer's disease. Nondemented Parkinson's disease patients do not show this pattern. Either the two diseases may have a common effect on the brain

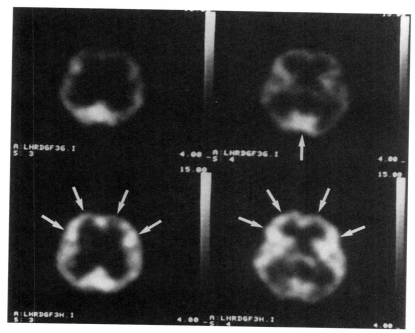

Fig. 5-6. The upper pair of PET FDG images shows preferential FDG uptake in the occipital cortex (*single arrow*) during performance of a picture preference task. In the lower images marked FDG uptake occurs in the frontal lobes (*quad arrows*) during a word fluency test. (From Chang JY: J Nucl Med 28:852-860, 1987.)

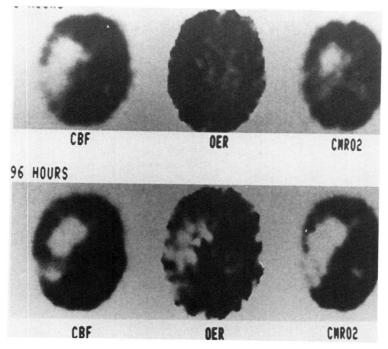

Fig. 5-7. *Upper row,* Eight hours after a stroke decreased cerebral blood flow (*CBF*) is seen in the right middle cerebral distribution. The oxygen extraction ratio (*OER*) is slightly increased and the cerebral metabolic rate for oxygen (*CmRO₂*) is slightly decreased in the same area. Flow and oxygen metabolism are uncoupled. After 96 hours (*bottom row*), a smaller area of decreased CBF and a matching reduction in OER and CmRO₂ are seen. This combination of findings at 96 hours indicates recoupling of flow and oxygen consumption at a lower than normal level. (From Boich C: Sem Nucl Med 22[4]: 224-232, 1992.)

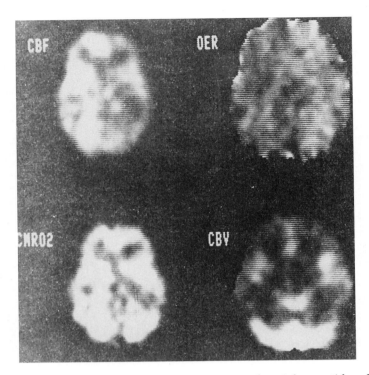

Fig. 5-8. This patient has diminished perfusion reserve after right carotid occlusion. The CBF study shows decreased flow on the right (images displayed with the right brain in the reader's right). The OER image shows higher oxygen extraction in the low-flow hemisphere. The CmRO$_2$ image shows similar side-to-side oxygen consumption. The CBU image shows an increased blood volume in the affected hemisphere. Compensatory vasodilation and increased oxygen extraction manage to preserve the brain's perfusion despite arterial insufficiency. (From Frackowiak RST: Neurol Clin 1[1]: 183-200, 1983.)

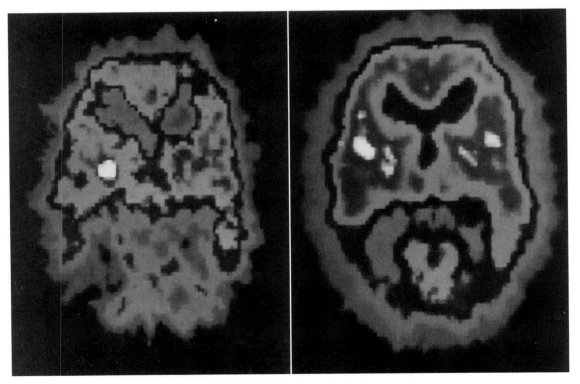

Fig. 5-9. Blood flow (*left*) and FDG uptake (*right*) maps at the level of the basal ganglia in a typical Alzheimer's disease patient. Occipital blood flow and glucose metabolism are severely decreased. (From Volkow N: J Nucl Med 28:524-527, 1987.)

or the Parkinson's disease patients may also have Alzheimer's disease.[118,119] Computer algorithms may eventually be helpful in classifying PET scan patterns.[120] The need to assess a patient with PET outside the experimental setting awaits further development of a therapy that would be too expensive or too dangerous to try empirically in a patient with clinically suspected Alzheimer's disease.

The dementia of Pick's disease is uncommon. The PET scan pattern in Pick's disease appears to be the "reverse" of that in Alzheimer's disease. Symmetric frontal and anterior temporal reduction in metabolism parallels the CT and MR findings as neuron loss progresses.[121,122] The condition of progressive supranuclear palsy produces a similar hypometabolic pattern in the superior frontal and temporal lobes on PET scans but is easily distinguished by characteristic physical findings of bradykinesia, gaze palsies, and truncal rigidity.[123,124]

While CT and MR imaging may be helpful in making the diagnosis of multi-infarct dementia by showing multiple areas of infarct that vary in size and symmetry, the PET equivalent patterns of reduced rCBF and rCMRglc must be recognized in order to differentiate them from other dementias. Crossed cerebellar diaschisis is much more common in multi-infarct dementia than in Alzheimer's disease.[96,101,125]

Huntington's and Wilson's disease affect a very small number of dementia patients, but they are of particular research interest because they are genetically determined conditions. The specific area affected in the first is the caudate nucleus, where hypometabolic changes can be seen with PET years before the onset of symptoms.[126-131] In the latter, very limited PET experience in patients with this diagnosis shows hypometabolism in the frontal and parietal white matter and cortex as well as in the caudate and lenticular nuclei.[132] Another genetically determined disorder of the nervous system is adrenoleukodystrophy, which includes adrenal insufficiency and demyelination of the cerebral white matter. PET has shown decreased rCBF and rCMRglc in the white and overlying gray matter of the temporal and occipital lobes in one case with multiple clinical findings, including memory and visual loss.[133]

One viral brain infection associated with dementia is Jakob-Creutzfeldt disease, which produces pancortical hypometabolism.[134] The dementia produced by the AIDS virus may produce a pattern very similar to that of progressive supranuclear palsy with hypometabolic areas in white matter and subcortical gray matter. The AIDS virus is probably carried across the blood-brain barrier by infected macrophages. It predominantly infects glial cells. Regional or generalized decrease in rCMRglc may precede the dysfunctional brain, which results in a characteristic clinical pattern of concentration and memory defects. The frontal regions are the most significantly affected. Favorable response to treatment of AIDS with AZT is paralleled by improved rCMRglc.[135,136]

DOPAMINE RECEPTOR PET

Dopaminergic receptors come in two varieties. The D1 receptor is inhibited by the D2 receptor. Amphetamine stimulates and neuroleptics block dopaminergic activity. One of the areas of extensive research in PET receptor imaging has come with the introduction of 6-[^{18}F]fluoro-L-dihydroxyphenylalanine (6-[^{18}F]-DOPA), which has several published syntheses.[137-143] This agent acts as an adrenergic false transmitter. It localizes in proportion to the density of dopaminergic receptors.[144] The uptake of 6-[^{18}F]-DOPA depends first on transport across the blood-brain barrier by the large neutral amino acid (LNAA) transport system and is a result of presynaptic synthesis and storage of 6-[F^{18}]-dopamine.

The accumulation of 6[^{18}F]-dopamine and its metabolites 6- [^{18}F]-3,4-dihyroxy-phenylacetic acid (^{18}F-DO-PAC) and 6-[^{18}F]- homovanillic acid (^{18}F-HVA) is responsible for its preferential localization in the striatum, which is comprised of the caudate and putamen. There is a peripheral conversion of 6-[^{18}F]-dopamine to the metabolite, O-methy-6-[^{18}F]-dopamine (^{18}F-30M- DOPA), which can decrease the striatum to background ratio as it enters the brain tissues uniformly.[145] Uptake of 6-[^{18}F]-DOPA is decreased in patients with Parkinson's disease and in those who have been exposed to 1-methyl-4-phenyl-1,2,3,6- tetrahydropyridine (MPTP), a drug that causes parkinsonism in humans.[146]

The small size of the striatum relative to the FWHM of most PET scanners makes it difficult to accurately quantify the uptake of 6-[^{18}F]-DOPA. Uncertainty about the boundaries of the striatum makes the placement of regions of interest (ROIs) difficult even when guided by MR imaging.[147-151] When severe parkinsonism is encountered, the striatum to background ratio may be <2.0. This increases errors when outlining ROIs around this structure. Various schemes to increase the striatum to background ratio of 6-[^{18}F]-DOPA have been tried. One method uses catechol-O-methyl transferase inhibitors to prevent the peripheral formation of ^{18}F-30M-DOPA.[152-153] Another strategy calls for pretreatment with a peripheral decarboxylase inhibitor, carbidopa, to increase availability of 6-[^{18}F]-DOPA in a manner similar to the clinical dependence on carbidopa to increase L-DOPA levels.[154] A third technique adds a continuous infusion of gram doses of phenylalanine started 15 to 70 or 80 minutes after the 6[^{18}F]-DOPA administration.[145,155] This saturates the BBB/LNAA transport system so that any ^{18}F-30M-DOPA present

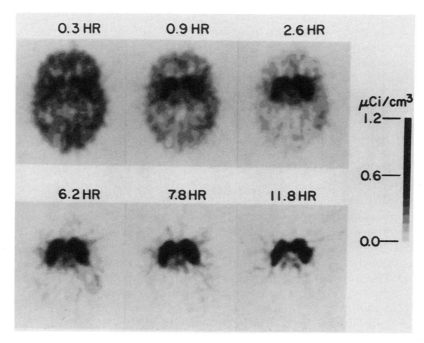

Fig. 5-10. The initial distribution of NMS is widespread. As time elapses, the caudate and putamen D-2 receptors strongly retain NMS. Standardization of acquisition time is critical to avoid false positive D-2 maps. (From Arnett CD: J Nucl Med 27: 1878-1882, 1986.)

will be displaced by mass action. This technique may double the striatum to background ratio.

An interesting side note in the study of Parkinson's disease is the ^{11}C-labeling of MPTP for PET studies in laboratory animals. This drug is sold as a street drug in combination with a meperidine analog MPPP that produces severe neuropathies. In monkeys it produces Parkinson-like symptoms and degeneration of the substantia nigra in mice. Selective arterial injections of MPTP can destroy the striatum on one side of the basal ganglia in test animals.[156]

Dopamine receptor agents studied also include ^{18}F and [11]C N- methylspiroperidol (NMS) and related butyrophenone neuroleptics such as [^{18}F]haloperidol, [^{11}C]raclopride, and [[76]Br]bromospirone. NMS binds to serotonin (S2) as well as dopaminergic receptors. Raclopride has a relatively low binding affinity for dopaminergic receptors and can be competitively displaced by increases in endogenous dopamine. Very high affinity D2 agents such as [11]C- labeled n[(2RS, 3RS)-1-benzyl-2-methyl-3-pyrrolidinyl]-5-chloro-2-methoxy-4-methylaminobenzamide (YM-09151-2) are under investigation as well[157-161] (Fig. 5-10).

Alterations in dopaminergic transmission in the brain have been related to schizophrenia. Antipsychotic drugs tend to block the dopamine receptor.[162,163] These same drugs can produce extrapyramidal side effects that are similar to the motion disorders of Parkinson's disease. Tyrosine is the amino acid precursor of noradrenaline and dopamine synthesis. A small group of schizophrenics (not taking any neuroleptic medication) have been shown by PET to have reduced transport of L-[1-^{11}C] tyrosine into the brain.[164] Where this fits in the etiology of schizophrenia is not clear. The direct, in vivo study of drugs that alter interaction with D2 receptors in schizophrenics is possible when these drugs can be labeled with PET isotopes.

There are also metabolic changes in schizophrenics that are linked to different receptors. Using measures of rCMRglc has helped delineate a subgroup of schizophrenics who tend to have chronic disease, negative symptoms, and decreased FDG uptake in the frontal lobes. Failure to increase rCMRglc in the frontal lobes during cognitive activation tasks has been linked to decreased dopamine function in these lobes. Metabolic activity in the basal ganglia has been reported as both increased and decreased in schizophrenia. Given the interconnections between the basal ganglia and the frontal lobes, it is tempting to pick one or the other as the cause or the effect of a problem. Some investigators report elevated FDG localization in the left temporal cortex of schizophrenics, but this has not been well corroborated.[165]

Studies of proposed drugs designed to have antipsychotic effects may be enhanced if they can be labeled and studied by PET. Their receptor interaction

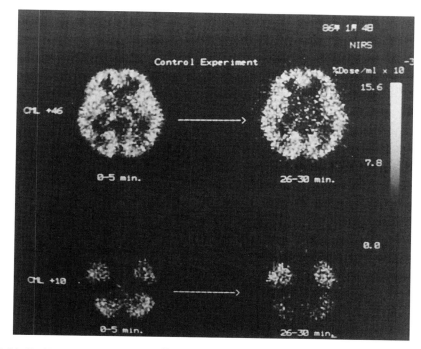

Fig. 5-11. Ro15-1788 labeled with ^{11}C distributes according to rCBF during the first 5 minutes after injection (*left*). After 25 minutes (*right*) this agent is localized in cerebral cortex in proportion to benzodiazepine receptor distribution. (From Shinotoh H: J Nucl Med 27:1593-1599, 1986.)

characteristics and gross distribution in the brain can be directly measured in humans. An excellent example of this approach is ^{18}F-labeled BMY 14802, which has gained interest as a drug with minimal D2 interaction and the ability to prevent the effects of amphetamine.[166]

OTHER RECEPTOR STUDIES IN PET PSYCHIATRIC EVALUATIONS

Benzodiazepine receptor agonists labeled with ^{11}C, such as Ro15-1788, allow the study of therapeutic effects of the benzodiazepine drugs used for treatment of anxiety and convulsive disorders. Benzodiazepine receptor levels may change during stress or seizure. Normal distribution of [^{11}C]Ro15-1788 shows high activity in the cortical brain, less in the subcortical gray matter, and low levels in the brainstem that parallel the known distribution of benzodiazepine receptors (Fig. 5-11). Presumably, the development of a good PET agent for this receptor would allow further pathophysiologic characterization.[167]

Another avenue of PET research in psychiatric disorders is fabrication of ^{11}C-labeled blockers of the serotonin (5-hydroxytryptamine; 5-HT) such as [11]C McN-5652Z. Antidepressant drugs specifically bind to and block 5-HT uptake sites. There is interest in studying 5-HT blocking drugs of abuse such as 3,4-methylenedioxymethamphetamine ("speed") and

therapeutic agents such as fenfluramine (used to treat obesity).[168]

PET STUDIES OF OTHER RECEPTORS

Central histamine receptors of the H1 subtype are found most concentrated in the frontal and temporal cortex with low H1 values in the cerebellum and brainstem. The H1 receptors are involved with arousal, locomotor activity, appetite, cardiovascular regulation, and thermoregulation. They can be imaged and saturated with ^{11}C-pyrilamine, which is displaced competitively with diphenhydramine.[169]

The muscarinic cholinergic receptors (mAChR) of the normal brain are abundant and play a role in cognition and memory. There are decreased mAChR sites in Alzheimer's, Huntington's, and Parkinson's diseases. Various PET mAChR agents including [18]F- and ^{11}C-labeled scopolamine and ^{11}C benztropine have been proposed along with ^{11}C-labeled (+)2 alpha-tropanyl benzylate, which may be easier to synthesize and has a higher uptake than scopolamine at the same receptor site.[170]

Initial work has been done to label fluoroprednisone with ^{18}F as a glucocorticoid representative of the steroid family. This offers a potential for understanding the steroid's effects on the central nervous system.[171]

A common biologic scheme uses receptors on the

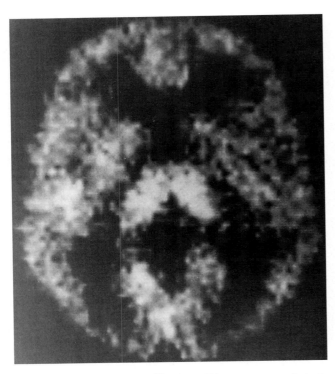

Fig. 5-12. A PET scan with [11C] DMPEA serves as a substrate for and maps the brain's distribution of monoamine oxidase in a normal patient. (From Shinotoh H: J Nucl Med 28:1006-1001, 1987.)

surface of a cell that trigger the signal amplifying action of a second messenger system inside the cell. In the neuron there is such a receptor-linked phosphatidylinositol (PI) turnover system. Phospholipase C is associated with the surface receptor and hydrolyses phosphatidylinositides into sn-1,2-diacylglycerol (DAG) and inositol phosphates. The PI turnover–protein kinase C (PKC) system is involved with higher cortical functions of memory and learning. Phorbol esters labeled with 11C bind with PKC and have been used to map PKC density directly.[172] Using 11C-labeled DAG the function of the PKC second messenger system can be traced as DAG is mixed into the PI turnover system, converted into polarized compounds and trapped inside the cell.[173,174]

A strategy similar to receptor PET imaging is that of providing substrates for intracellular enzymes. In the brain, monoamine oxidase concentrations are linked with aging, the degenerative brain diseases, alcoholism, suicides and psychiatric diseases. An in vivo measurement of this enzyme's levels could be had with a PET agent that was deaminated and subsequently trapped such as [11C]N,N-dimethylpenylethylamine[11C]DMPEA.[175] (Fig. 5-12).

PET IN THE ASSESSMENT OF EPILEPSY

The PET approach to understanding the pathophysiology of epilepsy exercises scanning techniques of metabolism and receptor studies. The typical interictal focus of abnormal electrical activity shows decreased rCMRglc (although the area in question may be small). On the basis of size alone, decreased FDG uptake may not be detectable by older systems with poor resolution. Cortical dysplasia leading to infantile spasms and the varied lesions of Lennox-Gastaut syndrome is identified by the presence of hypometabolic areas of cortex. When the angiomas of the surface of the brain in Sturge-Weber syndrome affect the underlying cortex, there will be decreased rCMRglc. The FDG scan is gaining some clinical utility as a marker of abnormal brain that can be removed surgically in hopes of curing these various seizure disorders. The best surgical results are seen in infants or children because there is a better chance of the still developing brain taking over any function lost by resection.[176,177] (Figs. 5-13 and 5-14).

The other PET approach in epilepsy research centers focuses on the use of radiolabeled opioids with both anticonvulsant and convulsant effects. The mu opiate receptor can be selectively studied with [11C] carfentanil. In the area of a seizure focus, there is an increase in mu opiate receptors (with a decrease in rCMRglc). The action of these receptors may be to stop seizure or reduce the spread of seizure activity to adjacent areas of brain. Specific agonists for the delta and kappa opiate receptors are not available, but [11C]-diprenorphine is a PET agent that has similar affinity for mu, delta, and kappa receptors and can be used to study the overall distribution of opiate receptors in the brain. In conjunction, these two agents have been used to show that increased mu receptors may coexist with normal or decreased delta and/or kappa receptors in the seizure focus. Considerably more work in this area remains to be done.[178]

PET IN THE STUDY OF COCAINE ABUSE

PET images of the brain distribution of [11C] cocaine have shown maximal uptake by the basal ganglia within a few minutes of intravenous administration. There is 50% washout of cocaine from these areas in 20 minutes. This abrupt rise and fall corresponds to the clinically manifested euphoria.[165] Acute doses of cocaine cause decreased brain metabolism as marked by FDG in the cortical and subcortical structures.[179] There is also widespread decreased rCBF as measured with 15O water and PET.[180] This is most noticeable in the frontal cortex and left hemisphere. During detoxification, the rCMRglc is abnormally increased in the basal ganglia and orbitofrontal cortex. This may be related to a pathway for control of repetitive behavior (repeat abuse) and the addicted patient's craving for the drug.[181] After a week of withdrawal there is decreased metabolic activity in the frontal cortex that persists for months. An interesting effect of chronic cocaine abuse

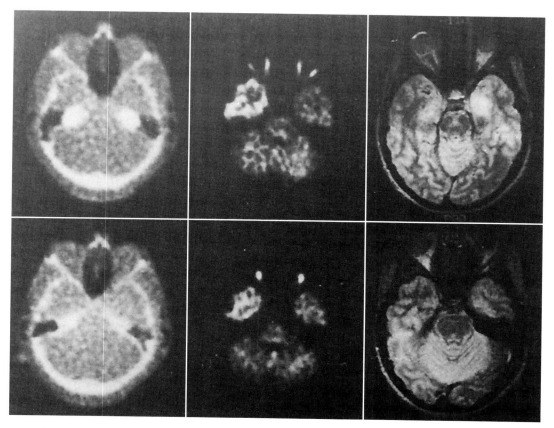

Fig. 5-13. A patient with partial complex epilepsy has a marked decrease in FDG uptake in the left temporal cortex (*reader's right, middle images*). The corresponding T2-weighted MR images (*right*) show increased signal from the medial left temporal cortex. The transmission scans (*left*) help locate anatomy on the FDG scans. (From Valk P: Radiology 1986: 55-58, 1993.)

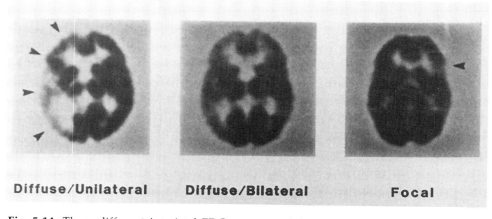

Fig. 5-14. Three different interictal FDG patterns of decreased uptake in children with Lennox-Gastaut syndrome seizures are shown. (From Chugani HT: Semin Nucl Med 22[4]: 247-253, 1992.)

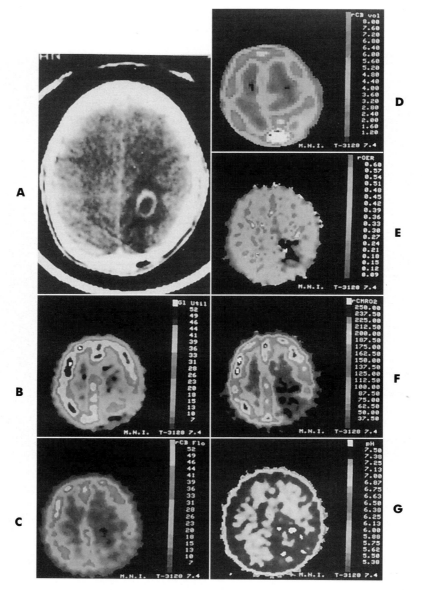

Fig. 5-15. A, Ring-enhancing lesion on CT is a grade IV glioma. **B,** Low CMRGlc, **C,** low CBF, **D,** high CBV, **E,** low OER, **F,** low CMRO$_2$, and **G,** a high pH are seen in the same area. (From Tyler JL: J Nucl Med 28[7]: 1123-1133, 1987.)

can be measured with dopamine receptor PET. NMS PET scans have shown decreased receptor availability. This probably represents compensation for dopaminergic overstimulation by the cocaine.[182,183]

BRAIN DEVELOPMENT STUDIED BY PET

The development of the brain after birth starts with regional metabolic rates that are different from those in adults. The primary sensorimotor cortex, thalamus, brainstem, and cerebellar vermis are phylogenetically old structures and control the primitive functions of the newborn. As visual functions in the second and third months develop, the rCMRglc increases in the

parietal, temporal, and visual cortex, basal ganglia, and the cerebellum. Cognitive and higher cortical functions develop during the first year, with increases in lateral and then dorsal frontal cortex. The pattern of rCMRglc appears similar to an adult at 1 year. The neonate's rCMRglc begins about 30% lower than an adult, increases to two or three times that of an adult during second through the tenth year, and then decreases to adult levels by the late teenage years. Roughly paralleling the increase and plateau of metabolic activity is rapid growth of neuron interconnections. During this phase, the brain has its maximum plasticity and recovery from injury (or surgical resec-

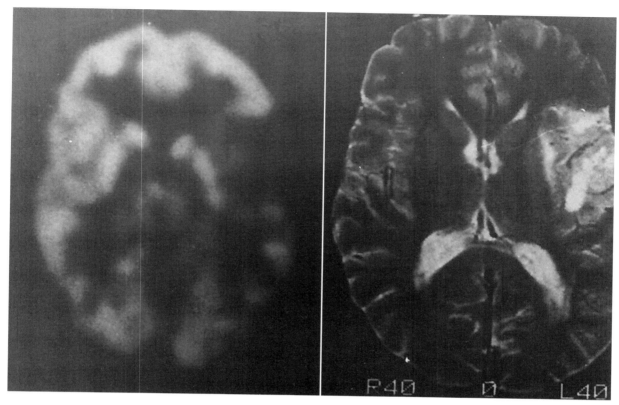

Fig. 5-16. FDG PET shows decreased left frontoparietal uptake in the same area where a T2-weighted MRI shows an increased signal after radiation. This is a characteristic of radiation necrosis. (From Coleman RE: J Nucl Med 32: 616-622, 1991.)

tion for seizure focus) is most possible. Excess connections in the brain are pruned during the teenage years. Thereafter, transfer of function after injury to other areas of the brain is less likely.[184-187] The rapidly maturing brain of an infant has a very high rate of protein synthesis. The neutral amino acid carrier mediated uptake of [^{11}C]L-methionine has been measured in infants and found to exceed adult levels by a factor of 5.[188] Measurements of rCBV, rCBF, and rCMRO$_2$ with C^{15}O, H$_2$^{15}O, and O^{15}O respectively can also be studied in the developing child.[189]

PET STUDIES IN BRAIN MALIGNANCY

A number of PET radiopharmaceuticals have been applied to the study of brain malignancies. It would be ideal to have a brain PET agent that would have a tumor uptake independent of the integrity of the blood-brain barrier and strongly dependent on the grade and biologic aggressiveness of the tumor. In addition, it should be able to differentiate viable from necrotic tumor.[190] Unfortunately, no such ideal agent exists. However, each of the metabolic agents previously discussed in the study of brain function can be applied to primary brain tumors. FDG is the most widely studied and is discussed below with labeled

amino acid and therapeutic agents. Blood-brain barrier integrity can be quantified by ^{82}Rb or ^{68}Ga-EDTA. The rCBF tends to be lower than normal gray matter in higher grade tumors. The rCBV tends to be increased. The OER and rCMRO$_2$ are generally lower. After tumor treatment with radiotherapy or chemotherapy, the rCMRglc increases for reasons that are not clear[191,192] (Figs. 5-15 and 5-16).

FDG SCANNING IN MALIGNANCY

The rapid proliferation of tumor cells is accompanied by anaerobic metabolism with energy-inefficient glycolysis, even in the presence of adequate oxygen. The standard assumptions that describe rCMRglc in normal brain may not be valid for tumors. The lumped constant that relates glucose metabolism to FDG uptake in normal brain probably does not have a constant relation to uptake in tumors. The presence of insulin stimulates the uptake of FDG in brain tumors but not in normal brain. Glucose in a recently fed patient decreases uptake of FDG in the normal brain, but probably not in a tumor. The timing of the scan is important since these tumors show increasing uptake of FDG for at least 90 minutes. These variables and others have led to

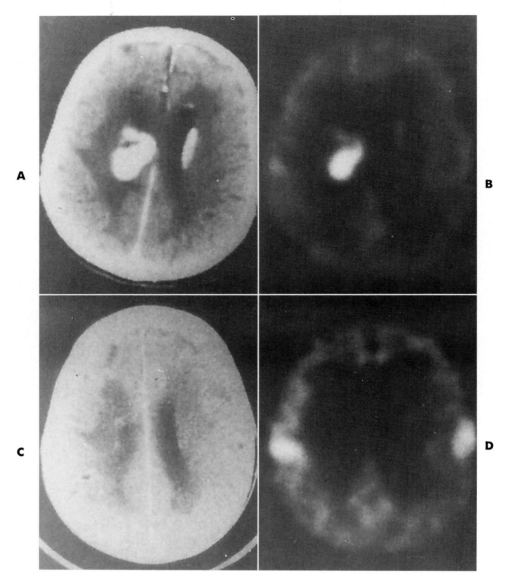

Fig. 5-17. A brightly enhancing CNS lymphoma on a CT scan (**A**) takes up FDG strongly on a PET scan (**B**) after radiotherapy. **C,** The CT scan shows a more normal appearance. **D,** The corresponding PET-FDG scan shows increased FDG localization in the motor corticals because the patient was moving her arms. The lymphoma uptake was no longer present. (From Rosenfeld S: J Nucl Med 33: 532-536, 1992.)

discordant findings. Some authors have found that FDG uptake is a good predictor of survival and histologic grade. Others find little association between tumor grade and rCMRglc.[193-200]

The FDG scan can be used to differentiate between radiation necrosis after therapy of gliomas (which does not take up the radiopharmaceutical) and recurrent tumor (which does). A blood-brain barrier scan shows uptake in both conditions. The malignant degeneration of a low-grade tumor may be signaled by an increase in FDG uptake.[201,202] Metastatic lesions in the brain are difficult to detect when they are small relative to the resolution of the PET scanner. They have been shown to have increased and decreased uptake relative to adjacent gray and white matter. As such, there is probably little use for PET in the clinical evaluation of brain metastases.[203] The FDG scan has been shown to detect central nervous system lymphoma as a lesion with abnormally high uptake, indicating aggressive biologic behavior. In AIDS patients, the differentiation of brain lymphoma from infection (usually toxoplasmosis) with decreased FDG levels has been demonstrated[204,205] (Figs. 5-17 and 5-18).

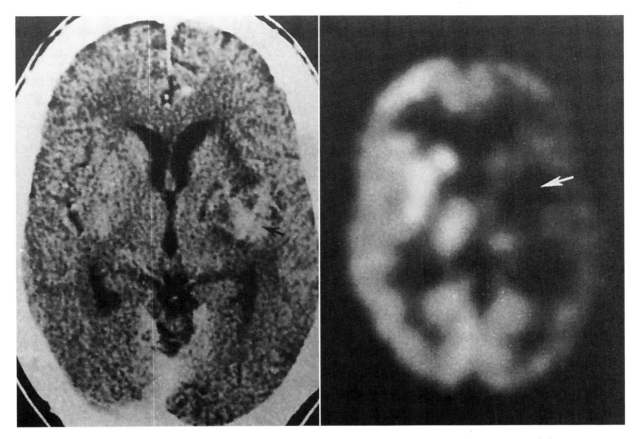

Fig. 5-18. A patient with toxoplasmosis has an area of enhancement on a CT scan (*left*), which corresponds to an area of decreased FDG uptake (*arrow*) on a PET scan (*right*). (From Hoffman J: J Nucl Med 34: 567-575, 1993.)

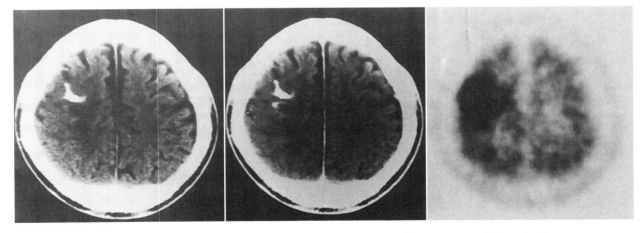

Fig. 5-19. A noncontrast CT (*left*) shows calcifications around a vague mass lesion that has an enhancing adjacent cystic component seen by intravenous contrast CT (*middle*). The methionine PET scan shows the tumor amino acid uptake and better defines the tumor, which is a grade 2 astrocytoma. (From Ogawa T: Radiology 1986: 45-53, 1993.)

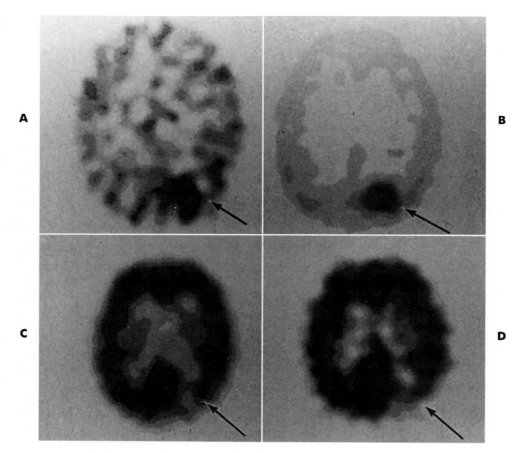

Fig. 5-20. Increasing ^{11}C putrescine uptake in a metastasis from lung carcinoma is seen at an interval of 4 months (**A,B**): corresponding glucose PET scans show a matching occipital defect (**C,D**). (From Hiesiger E: J Nucl Med 28: 1251-1261, 1987.)

PET AMINO ACIDS AND POLYAMINES

The syntheses of ^{11}C-labeled methionine, leucine, and tyrosine amino acids and ^{18}F-labeled tyrosine provide agents for studying protein metabolism in brain tumors. Methionine and tyrosine uptake levels in high-grade gliomas tend to be higher than in low-grade gliomas. Methionine PET is better at delineating the extent of tumor than CT[206-211] (Fig. 5-19).

The rapid protein metabolism of tumor cells creates an increased demand for polyamines such as putrescine, which can be labeled with ^{11}C. The uptake of putrescine by tumor is rapid and generally parallels FDG uptake. Putrescine uptake in the brain is also dependent on blood-brain barrier breakdown and is not a specific marker of malignancy. Its future PET role seems limited[212,213] (Fig. 5-20).

PET IN THE ASSESSMENT OF THERAPY FOR MALIGNANCY

Cisplatin (cis-diaminedichloroplatinum [II], DDP) has been labeled with ^{13}N and used to study the intraarterial and intravenous distribution of this radiosensitizing chemotherapeutic agent in patients with brain tumors.[214,215] Another chemotherapeutic agent used for glioma treatment is BCNU, which has been labeled with ^{11}C for similar studies.[216] The ^{18}F analog of the radiosensitizing agent misonidazole, fluoromisonidazole, specifically labels hypoxic but viable cells. Since hypoxic cells are relatively radioresistant, this PET agent would allow a rational selection of primary brain tumors for radiotherapy.[217] These and similar agents could be used clinically to guide chemotherapy and radiotherapy.

• • •

The evolution of PET techniques has been diverse and impressive from a research point of view. There are those who argue that it has a necessary clinical role. While CT and MR imaging have done much to advance the in vivo understanding of brain anatomy and pathologic anatomy in the last two decades, the PET scanner has made most of the significant advances in understanding in vivo physiology and pathophysiology of the brain. The developmental and degenerative diseases, ischemia and infarct, brain activation techniques, schizophrenia receptor physiology, malignancies, and other studies discussed here are examples of first-rate PET science advancing medicine.[218-225]

The technologic business of performing PET still has much promise. The annihilation radiation used offers "electronic" collimation with high sensitivity and a limit of resolution that is now approaching 2 mm. The ability to tag biologically interesting molecules has increased as clever chemists work out quick methods of synthesis.[8]

There is a continuing problem with the quantitation of PET data and an implied scorn for visual analysis that pervades much of the literature reviewed for this chapter. With a demand for and reliance on numerical analysis, the PET scientist has driven wedges between this technique and clinical medicine. Most of the imaging physicians in modern medicine are highly trained visual readers who use the best computer processor ever built, the human brain. A stream of precise looking but nonconvincing PET numbers costs a lot of money and time to produce and discourages most clinical radiologists and nuclear medicine physicians. The phrase "the radiologist with a ruler in hand is a radiologist in trouble" summarizes this point.[226]

This is a sensitive economic point in the world of imaging medicine. With the number of health care dollars available shrinking, it is unlikely that society will be able to afford fancy, expensive, and intellectually intriguing PET scans when less expensive, semi-quantitative SPECT techniques will suffice for clinical decision making. To install a PET scanner and cyclotron costs about $5 million. With a staff including the disciplines of physics, chemistry, and computing, in addition to technologists and physicians, the payroll of a small PET center is high in relation to the volume of clinical studies done. Operating supplies, maintenance, and other expenses add to the cost of operating a PET center; $1 million a year might cover the bill. A shift to qualitative PET, yet to be developed deliverable generator systems for metabolic PET isotopes, and production instead of engineering prototype scanners might extend PET into the clinical area. If the current model of PET scanning were expanded by an order of magnitude in the United States of America (hundreds of sites instead of tens of sites), there would still be limited access to PET and a crippling shortage of competent PET technologists, scientists, and physicians.[224,225] If clinical PET were inexpensive and widely available, it would still not survive if it did not provide answers to medical questions that would alter physicians' behavior. Few of the answers provided by PET scans of the brain have any clinical utility at this time.[227,228]

SPECT technology is cheaper than PET by an order of magnitude. A few hundred thousand dollars will put a nuclear medicine clinic into the SPECT world. Tens of thousands of dollars will provide yearly operating expenses. The throughput of examinations is also better. The cadre of trained clinical nuclear medicine practitioners is already on the job. One school of thought contends that the most important effect of clinical PET has been to stimulate and validate clinical SPECT. This is not a good answer for those who have invested their medical reputations or financial capital in pursuit of clinical PET installations. They have labored to advance PET beyond its proven research boundaries. If it turns out that clinical PET is circumvented by cheaper techniques, their efforts could be in vain and detract from the glowing record of research PET.

REFERENCES

1. Koeppe RA, Hutchins GD: Instrumentation for positron emission tomography: tomographs and data processing and display systems, Semin Nucl Med 22:162-181, 1992.
2. Ter-Pogossian MM: The origins of positron emission tomography, Semin Nucl Med 22:140-149, 1992.
3. Miller TR, Wallis JW, Grothe RA: Design and use of PET tomographs: the effect of slice spacing, J Nucl Med 31:1732-1739, 1990.
4. Muehllehner G, Karp JS: A positron camera using positron-sensitive detectors: PENN-PET, J Nucl Med 27:90-98, 1986.
5. Karp JS, Muehllehner G, Mankoff DA et al: Continuous-slice PENN-PET: a positron tomograph with volume imaging capability, J Nucl Med 31:617-627, 1990.
6. Minoshima S, Berger KL, Lee KS et al: An automated method for rotational correction and centering of three-dimensional functional brain images, J Nucl Med 33:1579-1585, 1992.
7. Minoshina S, Koeppe RA, Mintun MA et al: Automated detection of the intercommissural line for stereotactic localization of functional brain images, J Nucl Med 34:322-329, 1993.
8. Budinger TF: Editorial: advances in emission tomography: quo vadis? J Nucl Med 31:628-631, 1990.
9. Daube-Witherspoon ME, Muehllehner G: Treatment of axial data in three-dimensional PET, J Nucl Med 28:1717-1724, 1987.
10. Cherry SR, Meikle SR, Hoffman EJ: Correction and characterization of scattered events in three-dimensional PET using scanners with retractable septa, J Nucl Med 34:671-678, 1993.
11. Carson RE, Daube-Witherspoon ME, Green MV: A method for post-injection PET transmission measurements with a rotating source, J Nucl Med 29:1558-1567, 1988.
12. Ranger NT, Thompson CJ, Evans AC: The application of a masked orbiting transmission source for attenuation correction in PET, J Nucl Med 30:1056-1068, 1989.
13. Thompson CJ, Ranger N, Evans AC et al: Validation of simultaneous PET emission and transmission scans, J Nucl Med 23:154-160, 1991.
14. Saha GB, MacIntyre WJ, Go RT: Cyclotrons and positron emission tomography radiopharmaceuticals for clinical imaging, Semin Nucl Med 22:150-161, 1992.
15. Phelps ME, Hoffman EJ, Coleman RE et al: Tomographic images of blood pool and perfusion in brain and heart, J Nucl Med 17:603-612, 1976.
16. Ter-Pogossian MM, Herscovitch P: Radioactive oxygen-15 in the study of cerebral blood flow, blood volume, and oxygen metabolism, Semin Nucl Med 15:377-394, 1985.
17. Green Ma, Mathias CJ, Welch MJ et al: Copper-62-labeled pyruvaldehyde bis(N⁴-methylthiosemicarbazonato)copper(II): synthesis and evaluation as a positron emission tomography tracer for cerebral and myocardial perfusion, J Nucl Med 31:1989-1996, 1990.
18. Hamacher K, Coeen HH, Stocklin G: Efficient sterospecific synthesis of no-carrier-added 2-¹⁸F-fluoro-2-deoxy-D-glucose

using aminopolyether-supported nucleophilic substitution, J Nucl Med 27:235-284, 1986.

19. Yamamoto YL, Thompson CJ, Meyer E et al: Dynamic positron emission tomography for study of cerebral hemodynamics in cross section of the head using positron emitting ^{68}Ga-EDTA and ^{77}Kr, J Comput Assist Tomogr 1:43-56, 1977.

20. Hawkins RA, Phelps ME, Huang SC et al: A kinetic evaluation of blood-brain-barrier permeability in human brain tumors with [^{68}Ga]EDTA and positron emission tomography, J Cereb Blood Flow Metab 4:507-515, 1984.

21. Huang S-C, Carson RE, Hoffman EJ et al: Quantitative measurement of local cerebral blood flow in humans by positron emission computed tomography and ^{15}O-Water, J Cereb Blood Flow Metab 3:141-153, 1983.

22. Raichle ME, Martin WRW, Herscovitch P et al: Brain blood flow measured with intravenous H$_2$^{15}O. 2, implementation and validation, J Nucl Med 24:790-798, 1983.

23. Hutchins GD, Koeppe Ra, Hichwa RD et al: The effect of partition coefficient values for water on the estimation of lCBF and lCMRO$_2$ in PET, J Nucl Med 27:941, 1986.

24. Iida H, Kanno I, Miura S et al: Error analysis of a quantitative cerebral blood flow measurement using H$_2$^{15}O autoradiography and positron emission tomography, with respect to the dispersion of the input function, J Cereb Blood Flow Metab 6:536-545, 1986.

25. Huang S-C, Gamhbir SS, Hawkins RA et al: Investigation of Kety-Schmidt single-compartment model for O-15 water in CBF measurements using PET, J Nucl Med 27:913, 1986.

26. Koeppe RA, Hutchins GD, Rothley JM et al: Examination of assumptions for local cerebral blood flow studies in PET, J Nucl Med 28:1695-1703, 1987.

27. Kano I, Iida H, Miura S et al: A system for cerebral blood flow measurement using an O-15 H$_2$O autoradiography and positron emission tomography, J Cereb Blood Blow Metab 7:143-153, 1987.

28. Ida H, Higano S, Tomura N et al: Evaluation of regional differences of tracer appearance in cerebral tissues using [^{15}O] water and dynamic positron emission tomography, J Cereb Blood Flow Metab 8:285-288, 1988.

29. Herscovitch P, Markham J, Raichle ME: Brain blood flow measured with intravenous O-15 H$_2$O. 1. Theory and error analysis, J Nucl Med 24:782-789, 1983.

30. Dhawan V, Conti J, Mernyk M et al: Accuracy of PET rCBF measurements: effect of time shift between blood and brain radioactivity curves, Phys Med Biol 31:507-514, 1986.

31. Meyer E: Simultaneous correction for tracer arrival delay and dispersion in CBF measurements by the H$_2$^{15}O autoradiographic method and dynamic PET, J Nucl Med 30:1069-1078, 1989.

32. Fox PT, Mintun MA, Raichle ME et al: A noninvasive approach to quantitative functional brain mapping with H$_2$^{15}O and positron emission tomography, J Cereb Blood Flow Metab 4:329-333, 1984.

33. Kanno I, Iida H, Miura S et al: Optimal scan time of oxygen-15-labeled water injection method for measurement of cerebral blood flow, J Nucl Med 32:1931-1934, 1991.

34. Volkow ND, Mullani N, Gould LK et al: Sensitivity of measurements of regional brain activation with oxygen-15-water and PET to time of stimulation and period of image reconstruction, J Nucl Med 32:58-61, 1991.

35. Celesia G, Polcyn RD, Holden JE et al: Visual evoked potentials and positron emission tomographic mapping of regional cerebral blood flow and cerebral metabolism, EEG Clin Neurophysiol 54:243-256, 1982.

36. Howard BE, Ginsberg MD, Hassel WR et al: On the uniqueness of cerebral blood flow measured by the in vivo autoradiographic strategy and positron emission tomography, J Cereb Blood Flow Metab 3:432-441, 1983.

37. Fox PT, Raichle ME: Stimulus rate dependence of regional cerebral blood flow in human striate cortex, demonstrated by positron emission tomography, J Neurophysiol 51:1109-1120, 1984.

38. Mazziotta JC, Huang S-C, Phelps M et al: A noninvasive positron computed tomography technique using oxygen-15-labeled water for the evaluation of neurobehavioral task batteries, J Cereb Blood Flow Metab 5:70-78, 1985.

39. Fox PT, Fox JM, Raichle ME et al: The role of cerebral cortex in the generation of voluntary saccadic eye movements: a positron emission tomographic study, J Neurophysiol 52:348-368, 1985.

40. Fox PT, Mintun ME, Raichle ME et al: Mapping human visual cortex with positron emission computed tomography, Nature 323:806-809, 1986.

41. Roland PE, Freiberg L: Localization of cortical areas activated by thinking, J Neurophysiol 53:1219-1243, 1985.

42. Fox PT, Miezin ME, Allman JM et al: Retinotopic organization of human visual cortex mapped with positron emission tomography, J Neurosci 7:913-922, 1987.

43. Fox PT, Burton H, Raichle ME: Mapping human somatosensory cortex with positron emission tomography, J Neurosurg 67:34-43, 1987.

44. Posner MI, Petersen SE, Fox PT et al: Localization of cognitive operation in the human brain, Science 240:1627-1631, 1988.

45. Posner MI, Petersen SE, Fox PT et al: Localization of cognitive operation in the human brain, Science 240:1627-1631, 1988.

46. Petersen SE, Fox PT, Rosner ML et al: Positron emission tomographic studies of the cortical anatomy of single word processing, Nature 331:585-589, 1988.

47. Fox PT, Mintun ME, Reiman EM et al: Enhanced detection of focal brain responses using inter-subject averaging and change-distribution analysis of subtracted PET images, J Cereb Blood Flow Metab 8:642-653, 1988.

48. Conrad B, Klingelhofer J: Dynamics of regional cerebral blood flow for various visual stimuli, Exp Brain Res 77:437-441, 1989.

49. Fox PT, Mintun MA: Noninvasive functional brain mapping by change-distribution analysis of averaged PET images of H$_2$^{15}O tissue activity, J Nucl Med 30:141-149, 1989.

50. Subranamyam R, Alpert NM, Hoop B et al: A model for regional cerebral oxygen distribution during continuous inhalation of ^{15}O$_2$, C^{15}O, and C^{15}O$_2$, J Nucl Med 19:48-53, 1978.

51. Frackowiak RSJ, Lenzi G-L, Jones T et al: Quantitative measurement of regional cerebral blood flow and oxygen metabolism in man using ^{15}O and positron emission tomography: theory, procedure, and normal values, J Comput Assist Tomogr 4:727-736, 1980.

52. Holden JE, Gatley SJ, Nickles RJ et al: Regional cerebral blood flow with fluoromethane and positron emission tomography. In: Positron emission tomography of the brain, Berlin, 1983 Springer-Verlag, pp 90-94.

53. Koeppe RA, Holden JE, Polcyn RE et al: Quantitation of local cerebral blood flow and partition coefficient without arterial sampling: theory and validation, J Cereb Blood Flow Metab 5:214-224, 1985.

54. Herscovitch P, Raichle ME, Kilbourn MR et al: Measurement of cerebral blood flow and water permeability with positron emission tomography using O-15 water and C-11 butanol, J Cereb Blood Flow Metab 5(suppl 1):567-568, 1985.

55. Takahashi K, Murikami M, Hagami E et al: Radiosynthesis of ^{15}O-labeled butanol available for clinical use. In: Proceedings of the Sixth International Symposium on Radiopharmaceutical chemistry, 1986 pp 81-82.

56. Lear JL, Ackerman RF: Comparison of cerebral glucose metabolic rates measured with fluorodeoxyglucose and glucose labeled in the 1,2,3-4, and 6 positions using quantitative double labeled autoradiography, J Cereb Blood Flow Metab 8:575-585, 1988.

57. Duncan G, Pilgrim C, Stumpf W et al: High resolution autoradiographic determination of the topographic distribution of radioactivity of the hippocampal formation after injection of [1-^{14}C]-glucose or 2-deoxy [^{14}C] glucose, Neuroscience 17:99-106, 1986.

58. Ackerman RF, Lear JL: Glycolysis-induced discordance between cerebral glucose metabolic rates measured with fluorodeoxyglucose and glucose, J Cereb Blood Flow Metab 9:774-785, 1989.

59. Lear JL, Ackerman RF: Comparison of regional blood-brain transport kinetics between glucose and fluorodeoxyglucose, J Nucl Med 33:1819-1824, 1992.

60. Betz AL, Gilboe DD, Yudilevich DL et al: Kinetics of unidirectional glucose transport into the isolated drug brain, Am J Physiol 225:586-592, 1973.

61. Pardridge WM, Oldendorf WH: Kinetics of blood-brain barrier transport of hexoses, Biochim Biophys Acta 382-377-392, 1975.

62. Koster G, Muller-Platz C, Laufer P: 3-11-C-methyl-D-glucose: a potential agent for regional cerebral glucose utilization. Synthesis, chromatography, and tissue distribution in mice, J Lab Comp Radiopharm 18:855-863, 1981.

63. Vyska K, Magloire JR, Freundlieb C et al: In vivo determination of the kinetic parameters of glucose transport in the human brain using ^{11}C-methyl-D-glucose (CMG) and dynamic positron emission tomography (dPET), Eur J Nucl Med 11:97-106, 1985.

64. Feinendegen LE, Herzog H, Wieler H et al: Glucose transport and utilization in the human brain: model using carbon-11 methylglucose and positron emission tomography, J Nucl Med 27:1867-1877, 1986.

65. Hoffman EJ, Huang SC, Phelps ME et al: Quantitation in positron emission computed tomography: 1. Effect of object size, J Comput Assist Tomogr 3:299-308, 1979.

66. Huang S-C, Hoffman EJ, Phelps ME et al: Quantitation in positron emission computed tomography: 1. Effect of sampling, J Comput Assist Tomogr 3:819-826, 1980.

67. Mazziotta JC, Phelps ME, Plummer D et al: Quantitation in positron emission computed tomography: 5. Physical-anatomic effects, J Comput Assist Tomogr 5:734-743, 1981.

68. Heiss W-D, Pawlik G, Herholz K et al: Regional kinetic constants and cerebral metabolic rate for glucose in normal human volunteers determined by dynamic positron emission tomography of [^{18}F]-2-fluoro-2-deoxy-D-glucose, J Cereb Blood Flow Metab 4:212-223, 1984.

69. Jagust WJ, Budinger TF, Huesman RH et al: Methodologic factors affecting PET measurements of cerebral glucose metabolism, J Nucl Med 27:1358-1361, 1986.

70. Dhawan V, Moeller JR, Strother SC et al: Effect of selecting a fixed dephosphorylation rate on the estimation of rate constants and rCMRGlu from dynamic [^{18}F] fluorodeoxyglycose/PET data, J Nucl Med 30:1483-1488, 1989.

71. Kuwabara H, Gjedde A: Measurements of glucose phosphorylation with FDG and PET are not reduced by dephosphorylation of FDG-6-phosphate, J Nucl Med 32:692-698, 1991.

72. Kumar A, Braun A, Schapiro M et al: Cerebral glucose metabolic rates after 30 and 45 minute acquisitions: a comparative study, J Nucl Med 33:2103-2105, 1992.

73. Lucignani G, Schmidt KC, Moresco RM et al: Measurement of regional cerebral glucose utilization with fluorine-18-FDG and PET in heterogeneous tissues: theoretical considerations and practical procedure, J Nucl Med 34:360-369, 1993.

74. Sokoloff L, Reivich M, Kennedy C et al: The [^{14}C] deoxyglucose method for the measurement of local cerebral glucose metabolism: theory, procedure and normal values in the conscious and anesthetized albino rat, J Neurochem 28:897-916, 1977.

75. Tyler JL, Strother SC, Zatorre JR et al: Stability of regional cerebralglucose metabolism in the normal brain measured by positron emission tomography, J Nucl Med 29:631-642, 1988.

76. Phillips RL, London ED, Links JM et al: Program for PET image alignment: effects on calculated differences in cerebral metabolic rates for glucose, J Nucl Med 31:2052-2057, 1990.

77. Brooks RA, Di Chiro G, Zukerberg BW et al: Test-retest studies of cerebral glucose metabolism using fluorine-18 deoxyglucose: validation of method, J Nucl Med 28:53-59, 1987.

78. Chang JY, Duara R, Barker W et al: Two behavioral states studied in a single PET/FDG procedure: theory, method, and preliminary results, J Nucl Med 28:852-860, 1987.

79. Grady Cl, Berg G, Carson RE et al: Quantitative comparison of cerebral glucose metabolic rates from two positron emission tomographs, J Nucl Med 30:1386-1392, 1989.

80. Alavi A, Reivich M, Jones S et al: Functional imaging of the brain with positron emission tomography, Nucl Med Ann 10:319-372, 1982.

81. Ackerman R, Correia J, Alpert N et al: Positron imaging in ischemic stroke disease using compound labeled with oxygen-15, Arch Neurol 38:537-543, 1981.

82. Baron J, Bousser M, Comar D et al: Noninvasive tomographics study of cerebral blood flow and oxygen metabolism in vivo, Eur Neurol 20:273-284, 1981.

83. Baron J, Rougemont D, Bousser M et al: Local CBF, oxygen extraction fraction (OEF) and CMRO$_2$: prognostic value in recent supratentorial infarction in humans, J Cereb Blood Flow Metab 3:A-2 (suppl A), 1983.

84. Lenzi G, Frackowiak R, Jonres T: Cerebral oxygen metabolism and blood flow in human cerebral ischemic infarction, J Cereb Blood Flow Metab 2:321-335, 1982.

85. Kuhl D, Phelps M, Kowell A et al: Effects of stroke on local cerebral metabolism and perfusion: mapping by emission tomography of ^{18}FDG and ^{13}NH3, Ann Neurol 8:47-69, 1980.

86. Hakim A, Pokrupa R, Villanueva J et al: The effect of spontaneous reperfusion on metabolic function in early human cerebral infarcts, Ann Neurol 21:279-289, 1987.

87. Wise R, Bernardi S, Frackowiak R et al: Serial observations on the pathophysiology of acute stroke: the transition from ischaemia to infarction as reflected in regional oxygen extraction, Brain 106:197-222, 1983.

88. Baron J, Rougemont D, Bousser M et al: Local interrelationships of cerebral oxygen consumption and glucose utilization in normal subjects and in ischemic stroke patients, J Cereb Blood Flow Metab 4:140-149, 1984.

89. Baron J, Bousser M, Rey A et al: Reversal of focal "misery-perfusion syndrome" by extra-intracranial arterial bypass in hemodynamic cerebral ischemia, Stroke 12:454-459, 1981.

90. Marchal G, Evans A, Dagher A et al: The evolution of cerebral infarction with time: a PET study of the ischemia penumbra, J Cereb Blood Flow Metab 7:S99 (suppl 1), 1987.

91. Hakim A, Evans A, Berger L et al: The effect of nimodipine on the evolution of human cerebral infarction studied by PET, J Cereb Blood Flow Metab 9:523-534, 1989.

92. Heiss W, Holthoff V, Pawlik G et al: Effect of nimodipine on regional cerebral glucose metabolism in patients with acute ischemic stroke as measured by positron emission tomography, J Cereb Blood Flow Metab 10:127-132, 1990.

93. Broich K, Alavi A, Kusher M: Positron emission tomography in cerebrovascular disorders, Semin Nucl Med 22:224-232, 1992.

94. Mazziotta JC, Frackowiak RSJ, Phelps ME: The use of positron emission tomography in the clinical assessment of dementia, Semin Nucl Med 22:233-246, 1992.

95. Ferris SH, de Leon MJ, Wolf AP et al: Positron emission tomography in the study of aging and senile dementia, Neurobiol Aging 1:127-131, 1980.

96. Frackiowak R, Pozzilli C, Legg N et al: Regional cerebral oxygen supply and utilization in dementia: a clinical and physiological study with oxygen-15 and positron tomography, Brain 104:753-778, 1981.

97. Cutler NR, Haxby J, Duara R et al: Clinical history, brain

metabolism, and neurophysiological function in Alzheimer's disease, Ann Neurol 18:298-309, 1985.

98. Kuhl DE, Metter EJ, Riege WH et al: Local cerebral glucose utilization in elderly patients with depression, multiple infarct dementia and Alzheimer's disease, J Cereb Blood Flow Metab 3:s494-495 (suppl), 1983.

99. Friedland RP, Budinger TF, Ganz E et al: Regional cerebral metabolic alterations in dementia of the Alzheimer type: positron emission tomography with [18F]fluorodeoxyglucose, J Comput Assist Tomogr 7:590-598, 1983.

100. Foster NL, Chase TN, Fedio P et al: Alzheimer's disease: focal cortical changes shown by positron emission tomography, Neurology 33:961-965, 1983.

101. Benson DF, Kuhl DE, Hawkins RA et al: The fluorodeoxyglucose 18F scan in Alzheimer's disease and multi-infarct dementia, Arch Neurol 40:711-714, 1983.

102. Foster NL, Chase TN, Mansi L et al: Cortical abnormalities in Alzheimer's disease, Ann Neurol 16:649-654, 1984.

103. Friedland RP, Budlinger TF, Brant-Zawadzki M et al: The diagnosis of Alzheimer-type dementia: a preliminary comparison of positron emission tomography and proton magnetic resonance, JAMA 252:2750-2752, 1984.

104. Cutler NR, Haxby JV, Duara R et al: Brain metabolism as measured with positron emission tomography: serial assessment in a patient with familial Alzheimer's disease, Neurology 35:1556-1561, 1985.

105. Haxby JV, Duara R, Grady CL et al: Relationship between neuropsychological and cerebral metabolic asymmetries in early Alzheimer's disease, J Cereb Blood Flow Metab 5:193-200, 1985.

106. Friedland RP, Budinger TF, Koss E et al: Alzheimer's disease: anterior-posterior and lateral hemispheric alterations in cortical glucose utilization, Neurosci Lett 53:235-240, 1985.

107. Hatazawa J, Matsuzawa T, Iito M et al: Disturbance of cerebral oxidative metabolism in patients with Alzheimer's disease: a positron emission tomography study, J Cereb Blood Flow Metab 5:S129-130 (suppl 1), 1985.

108. Duara R, Grady C, Haxby J et al: Positron emission tomography in Alzheimer's disease, Neurol 36:879-887, 1986.

109. Haxby JV, Grady CL, Duara R et al: Neocortical metabolic abnormalities precede nonmemory cognitive defects in early Alzheimer's-type dementia, Arch Neurol 43:882-885, 1986.

110. Foster NL, Chase TN, Patronas NJ et al: Cerebral mapping of apraxia in Alzheimer's disease by positron emission tomography, Ann Neurol 19:139-143, 1986.

111. Lowenstein DA, Barker WW, Chang JY et al: Predominant left hemisphere metabolic dysfunction in dementia, Arch Neurol 46:146-152, 1989.

112. Jagust WJ, Friedland RP, Budinger TF et al: Longitudinal studies of regional cerebral metabolism in Alzheimer's disease, Neurology 38:909-912, 1988.

113. Haxby JV, Grady CL, Koss E et al: Heterogeneous anterior-posterior metabolic patterns in dementia of the Alzheimer type, Neurology 38:1853-1863, 1988.

114. Sherican PH, Sato S, Foster N et al: Relations of EEG alpha background to parietal lobe function in Alzheimer's disease as measured by positron emission tomography and psychometry, Neurology 38:747-750, 1988.

115. Friedland RP, Jagust WJ, Heusman RH et al: Regional cerebral glucose transport and utilization in Alzheimer's disease, Neurology 39:1427-1434, 1989.

116. Chawluk JB, Alavi A, Dann R et al: Positron emission tomography in aging and dementia: effect of cerebral atrophy, J Nucl Med 28: 431-437, 1987.

117. Fazekas F, Alavi A, Chawluk JB et al: Comparison of CT, MR, and PET in Alzheimer's dementia and normal aging, J Nucl Med 30:1607-1615, 1989.

118. Kuhl DE, Metter JM, Benson FD et al: Similarities of cerebral glucose metabolism in Alzheimer's and parkinsonian dementia, J Cereb Blood Flow Metab 5:S169-170 (suppl), 1985.

119. de la Monte SM, Wells SE, Hedley-White ET et al: Neuropathological distinction between parkinson's dementia and parkinson's plus Alzheimer's disease, Ann Neurol 26:309-320, 1989.

120. Kippenhan JS, Barker WW, Pascal S et al: Evaluation of a neuro-network classifier for PET scans of normal and Alzheimer's disease subjects, J Nucl Med 33:1459-1467, 1992.

121. Kamo H, McGeer PL, Harrop R et al: Positron emission tomography and histopathology in Pick's disease, Neurology 37:439-445, 1987.

122. Durar R, Gutterman A, Lowenstein D et al: The clinical and PET scan pattern of probable Pick's disease, Neurology 38:415 (suppl 1, abstr), 1988.

123. Foster NL, Gilman S, Berent S et al: Cerebral hypometabolism in progressive supranuclear palsy studied with positron emission tomography, Ann Neurol 24:399-406, 1988.

124. D'Antona R, Baron JC, Samson Y et al: Subcortical dementia: frontal cortex hypometabolism detected by positron tomography in patients with progressive supranuclear palsy, Brain 108:785-799, 1985.

125. Barker WW, Lowenstein DA, Chang JY et al: FDG/PET studies of crossed cerebellar hypometabolism in dementia (abstract), Neurology 38:364, 1988.

126. Kuhl DE, Phelps ME, Markham CH et al: Cerebral metabolism and atrophy in Huntington's disease determined by 18-FDG and computed tomographic scan, Ann Neurol 12:425-434, 1982.

127. Garnett ES, Firnau G, Nahmias C et al: Reduced striatal glucose consumption and prolonged reaction time are early features in HD, J Neurol Sci 65:231-237, 1984.

128. Clark CM, Hayden MR, Stoessel AJ et al. Regression model for predicting dissociations of regional cerebral glucose metabolism in individuals at risk for Huntington's disease, J Cereb Blood Flow Metab 6:756-762, 1986.

129. Hayden MR, Martin WRW, Stoessl AJ et al: Positron emission tomography in the early diagnosis of Huntington's disease, Neurology 36:888-894, 1986.

130. Hayden MR, Hewitt BS, Stoessl AJ et al: The combined use in positron emission tomography and DAN polymorphisms for preclinical detection of Huntington's disease, Neurology 37:1441-1447, 1987.

131. Mazziotta JC, Phelps ME, Pahl JJ et al: Reduced cerebral glucose metabolism in asymptomatic subjects at risk for Huntington's disease, N Engl J Med 316:357-362, 1987.

132. Hawkins RA, Mazziotta JC, Phelps ME: Wilson's disease studied with FDG and positron emission tomography, Neurology 37:1707-1711, 1987.

133. Volkow Nd, Patchell L, Kulkarni MV et al: Adrenoleukodystrophy: imaging with CT, MRI, and PET, J Nucl Med 28:524-527, 1987.

134. Benson DF, Mazziottsa JC: Positron emission tomographic scanning in the diagnosis of Jakob-Creutzfeldt disease (abstract), Ann Neurol 30:238, 1991.

135. Brunetti A, Berg G, Di Chiro G et al: Reversal of brain metabolic abnormalities following treatment of AIDS dementia complex with 3'-azido-2'3'dideoxythymidine (AZT, Zidovudine): a PET-FDG study, J Nucl Med 30:581-590, 1989.

136. Pascal S, Resnick L, Barker WW et al: Metabolic asymmetries in asymptomatic HIV-1 seropositive subjects: relationship to disease onset and MRI findings, J Nucl Med 32:1725-1729, 1991.

137. Chirakal R, Firnau G, Couse J et al: Radiofluorination with 18F-labelled acetyl hypofuorite: [18F]L-6-fluorodopa, Int J Appl Radiat Isot 35:651-653, 1984.

138. Firnau G, Chirakal R, Garnett ES: Aromatic radiofluorination with [18F] fluorine gas: 6-[18F]fluoro-L-Dopa, J Nucl Med 25:1228-1233, 1984.

139. Diksic M, Farrokhzad S: New synthesis of fluorine-18-labelled

6-fluoro-DOPA by cleaving the carbon silicon bond with fluorine, J Nucl Med 26:1314-1318, 1985.

140. Adam MJ, Ruth TJ, Grierson JR et al: Routine synthesis of L-[^{18}F]6-fluorodopa with fluorine-18 acetyl hypofluorite, J Nucl Med 27:1462-1466, 1986.

141. Chaly T, Diksic M: High yield synthesis of 6-[^{18}F]acetylhypofluorite, J Nucl Med 27:1896-1901, 1986.

142. Chirakal R, Firnau G, Garnett ES: High yield synthesis of 6-[^{18}F]fluoro-L-DOPA, J Nucl Med 27:417-421, 1986.

143. Chen J-J, Huang S-J, Finn RD et al: Quality control procedure for 6-[^{18}Ffluoro-L-DOPA: a presynaptic PET imaging ligand for brain dopamine neurons, J Nucl Med 30:1249-1256, 1989.

144. Garnett ES, Firnau G, Nahmias C: Dopamine visualizes in the basal ganglia of living man, Nature 305:137-138, 1983.

145. Doudet DJ, McLellan CA, Aigner TG et al: Delayed L-phenylalanine infusion allows for simultaneous kinetic analysis and improved evaluation of specific-to-nonspecific fluorine-18-DOPA uptake in brain, J Nucl Med 33:1383-1389, 1992.

146. Calne DB, Langstrom JW, Martin WR et al:. Positron emission tomography after MPTP: observations relating to the cause of Parkinson's disease, Nature 317:246-248, 1985.

147. Pate BD, Snow BJ, Hewitt KA et al: The reproducibility of striatal uptake data obtained with positron emission tomography and fluorine-18-L-6-flurodopa trace in non-human primates, J Nucl Med 32:1246-1251, 1991.

148. Links JM: Editorial: The influence of positioning on accuracy and precision in emission tomography, J Nucl Med 32:1252-1253, 1991.

149. Vesna S, Buckley KR, Snow BJ et al: Recovery of the human striatal signal in a slice oriented positron emission tomograph, J Nucl Med 34:481-487, 1993.

150. Yu D-C, Huang S-C, Grafton ST et al: Methods for improving quantitation of putamen uptake constant of FDOPA in PET studies, J Nucl Med 34:679-688, 1993.

151. Gjedde A, Reith J, Kuwabara H et al: Determining DOPA decarboxylase activity in the human brain in vivo: the complete fluoro-DOPA model, J Nucl Med 31:720, 1990.

152. Miletich RS, Comi G, Bankiewicz K et al: Improved 6-[^{18}F]fluoro-L-DOPA PET image contrast with combined peripheral inhibition of COMT and DOPA decarboxylase in monkeys abstract, J Cereb Blood Flow Metab 11:S154, 1991.

153. Laihinen A, Rinne JO, Rinne UK et al: PET studies on the cerebral effects of COMT inhibition with nitecapone in Parkinson's disease (abstract), J Cereb Blood Flow Metab 11:S813, 1991.

154. Hoffman JM, Melega WP, Hawk TC et al: The effects of carbidopa administration on 6-[^{18}F]fluoro-L-DOPA kinetics in positron emission tomography, J Nucl Med 33:1472-1477, 1992.

155. Doudet DJ, McLellan CA, Aigner TG et al: Postinjection L-phenylalanine increases basal ganglia contrast in PET scans of 6-^{18}F-DOPA, J Nucl Med 32:1408-1413, 1991.

156. Livini E, Spellman JP, Correia JA et al: [^{11}C]MPTP: a potential tracer for Parkinson's disease research in laboratory animals, J Nucl Med 27:1600-1603, 1986.

157. Shiue CY, Bai L-Q, Teng R-R et al: No-carrier-added N-(3-[^{18}F]fluoropropyl) spiroperidol: biodistribution in mice and tomographic studies in a baboon, J Nucl Med 28:1164-1170, 1987.

158. Arnett CD, Wolf AP, Shiue C-Y et al: Improved delineation of human dopamine receptors using [^{18}F]-N-methylspiroperidol and PET, J Nucl Med 27:1878-1882, 1986.

159. Volkow ND, Fowler JS, Wang G-J et al: Reproducibility of repeated measures of carbon-11-raclopride binding in the human brain, J Nucl Med 34:609-613, 1993.

160. Hatano K, Ishiwata K, Kawashima K et al: D2-dopamine receptor specific brain uptake of carbon-11-labeled YM-09151-2, J Nucl Med 30:515-522, 1989.

161. Zanzonico PB, Bigler RE, Schmaoo B: Neuroleptic binding sites: specific labeling in mice with [^{18}F]haloperidol, a potential tracer for positron emission tomography, J Nucl Med 24:408-416, 1983.

162. van Rossum JM: The significance of dopamine receptor blockade for the mechanism of action of neuroleptic drugs, Arch Int Pharmacodyn Ther 160:492-494, 1966.

163. Carlsson A: Antipsychotic drugs, neurotransmitters, and schizophrenia, Am J Psych 135:164-173, 1978.

164. Wiessel F-A, Blomqvist G, Halldin C et al: The transport into the human brain as determined with L-[1-^{11}C]tyrosine and PET, J Nucl Med 32:2043-2049, 1991.

165. Volkow ND, Fowler JS: Neuropsychiatric disorders: investigation of schizophrenia and substance abuse, Semin Nucl Med 22:254-267, 1992.

166. Ding Y-S, Fowler JS, Dewey SL et al: Synthesis and PET studies of fluorine-18-BMY 14802: a potential antipsychotic drug, J Nucl Med 34:246-254, 1993.

167. Shinotoh H, Yamasaki t, Inoue O et al: Visualization of specific binding sites of benzodiazepine in human brain, J Nucl Med 27:1593-1599, 1986.

168. Suehiro M, Scheffel U, Dannals RF et al: A PET radiotracer for studying serotonin uptake sites: carbon-11-McN- 5652Z, J Nucl Med 34:120-127, 1993.

169. Villemagne VL, Dannals RF, Sanchez-Roa PM et al: Imaging histamine H1 receptors in the living human brain with carbon-11-pyrilamine, J Nucl Med 23:308-311, 1991.

170. Mulholland GK, Otto CA, Jewett DM et al: Synthesis, rodent biodistribution, dosimetry, metabolism, and monkey images of carbon-11-labeled (+)-^{2}alpha-tropanyl benzilate: a central muscarinnic receptor imaging agent, J Nucl Med 33:423-430, 1992.

171. Feliu AL, Rottenberg DA: Synthesis and evaluation of fluorine-18-21 fluoroprednisone as a potential ligand for neuro-PET studies, J Nucl Med 28:998-1005, 1986.

172. Ohmori Y, Imahori Y, Ueda S et al: Protein kinase C imaging using carbon-11-labeled phorbol esters: 12-deoxyphorbol 13-isobutyrate-20-[1-^{11}C]butyrate as the potential ligand for positron emission tomography, J Nucl Med 34:431-439, 1993.

173. Imahori Y, Fujii R, Ueda S et al: Membrane trapping of carbon-11-labeled 1,2-diacylglycerols as a basic concept for assessing phosphatidylinositol turnover in neurotransmission process, J Nucl Med 33:413-422, 1992.

174. Imahori Y, Fujii R, Ueda S et al: No-carrier-added carbon-11-labeled sn-1,3-diacylglycerols by [^{11}C]propyl ketene method, J Nucl Med 32:1622-1626, 1991.

175. Shinotoh H, Inoue O, Suzuki K et al: Kinetics of ^{11}CN,N-dimethylphenylethylamine in mice and humans: potential for measurement of brain MAO-B activity, J Nucl Med 28:1006-1011, 1987.

176. Valk PE, Laxer KD, Barbaro NM et al: High-resolution (2.6-mm) PET in partial complex epilepsy associated with mesial temporal sclerosis, Radiology 186:55-58, 1993.

177. Chugani HT: The use of positron emission tomography in the clinical assessment of epilepsy, Semin Nucl Med 22:247-253, 1992.

178. Fisher RS, Frost JJ: Epilepsy, J Nucl Med 32:651-659, 1991.

179. London ED, Cascella NG, Wong DF et al: Cocaine-induced reduction of glucose utilization in human brain. A study using positron emission tomography and [fluorine-18]-fluordeoxyglucose, Arch Gen Psychiatry 47:567-574, 1990.

180. Volkow ND, Mullani N, Gould L et al:. Cerebral blood flow in chronic cocaine users, Br J Psychiatry 152:641-648, 1988.

181. Volkow ND, Fowler JS, Wolf AP et al: Changes in brain glucose metabolism in cocaine dependence and withdrawal, Am J Psych 148:621-626, 1991.

182. Dachis CA, Gould MS: New concepts in cocaine addiction: the

dopamine depletion hypothesis, Neurosci Biobehav Rev 9:469-477, 1985.

183. Volkow ND, Fowler JS, Wolf P et al: Effects of chronic cocaine abuse on postsynaptic dopamine receptors, Am J Psychiatry 147:719-724, 1990.

184. Phelps ME, Mazziotta JC: Positron emission tomography: human brain function and biochemistry, Science 228:799-809, 1985.

185. Chugani HT, Phelps ME: Maturation changes in cerebral function in infants determined by [18F]FDG positron emission tomography, Science 231:840-843, 1986.

186. Chugani HT, Phelps ME, Mazziotta JC: Positron emission tomography study of human brain functional development, Ann Neurol 22:487-497, 1987.

187. Chugani HT, Phelps ME: Editorial: Imaging human brain development with positron emission tomography, J Nucl Med 22:23-25, 1991.

188. O'Tuama LA, Phillips PC, Smith QR et al: L-methionine uptake by human cerebral cortex: maturation from infancy to old age, J Nucl Med 32:16-22, 1991.

189. Powers WJ, Stabin M, Howse et al: Radiation absorbed dose estimates for oxygen-15 radiopharmaceuticals (H$_2$^{15}O, C^{15}O, O^{15}O) in newborn infants, J Nucl Med 29:1961-1970, 1988.

190. Di Chiro G: Editorial: which PET radiopharmaceutical for brain tumors? J Nucl Med 32:1346-1348, 1991.

191. Coleman RE, Hoffman JM, Hanson MW et al: Clinical application of PET for the evaluation of brain tumors, J Nucl Med 32:616-622, 1991.

192. Tyler JL, Diksic M, Villemure J-G et al: Metabolic and hemodynamic evaluation for gliomas using positron emission tomography, J Nucl Med 28:1123-1133, 1978.

193. Patronas NJ, DiChiro G, Kufta C et al: Prediction of survival in glioma patients by means of positron emission tomography, J Neurosurg 62:816-822, 1985.

194. Di Chiro G, Hatazawa J, Katz DA et al: Glucose utilization by intracranial meningiomas as an index of tumor aggressivity and probability of recurrence: a PET study, Radiology 164:521-526, 1987.

195. Alavi JB, Alavi A, Chawluk J et al: Positron emission tomography in patients with glioma, Cancer 62:1074-1078, 1988.

196. DiChiro G, Brooks RA: PET-FDG of untreated and treated cerebral gliomas, J Nucl Med 29:421-422, 1988.

197. Herholz K, Ziffling P, Staffen W et al: Uncoupling of hexose transport and phosphorylation in human gliomas demonstrated by PET, Eur J Clin Oncol 24:1139-1150, 1988.

198. Hiesss W-D, Heindel W, Herholz K et al: Positron emission tomography of fluorine-178-deoxyglucose and image-guided phosphorus-31 magnetic resonance spectroscopy in brain tumors, J Nucl Med 31:302-310, 1990.

199. Borbely K, Fulham MJ, Brooks RA et al: PET-fluorodeoxyglucose of cranial and spinal neuromas, J Nucl Med 33:1931-1934, 1992.

200. Fischman AJ, Alpert NM: Editorial: FDG-PET in oncology: there's more to it than looking at pictures, J Nucl Med 34:6-11, 1993.

201. Patronas NJ, Di Chiro G, Brooks RA et al: Work in progress [18F]fluoro-deoxyglucose and positron emission tomography in evaluation of radiation necrosis of the brain, Radiology 144:885-889, 1982.

202. Francavilla TL, Miletich RS, Di Chiro C et al: Positron emission tomography in the detection of malignant degeneration of low-grade gliomas, Neurosurgery 24:1-5, 1989.

203. Griffeth LK, Rich KM, Dehdashti F et al: Brain metastases from non-central nervous system tumors: evaluation with PET, Radiology 186:37-44, 1993.

204. Rosenfield SS, Hoffman JM, Coleman RE et al: Studies of primary central nervous system lymphoma with fluorine-18-fluorodeoxyglucose positron emission tomography, J Nucl Med 33:532-536, 1992.

205. Hoffman JM, Waskin HA, Schifter T et al: FDG-PET in differentiating lymphoma from nonmalignant central nervous system lesions in patients with AIDS, J Nucl Med 34:567-575, 1993.

206. Langstrom B, Antoni G, Gulberg P et al: Synthesis of L- and D-[methyl-11C]methionine. J Nucl Med 28:1037-1040, 1987.

207. Mineura K, Sasajima T, Kowada M et al: Innovative approach in the diagnosis of gliomatosis cerebri using carbon-11-L-methionine positron emission tomography, J Nucl Med 32:726-728, 1991.

208. Bergstrom M, Muhr C, Lundberg PO et al: PET as a tool in the clinical evaluation of pituitary adenomas, J Nucl Med 32:610-615, 1991.

209. Ogawa T, Shishido F, Kanno I et al: Cerebral glioma: evaluation with methionine PET, Radiology 186:45-53, 1993.

210. Coenen HH, Kling P, Stocklin G: Cerebral metabolism of L-[2-18F]fluorotyrosine, a new PET tracer of protein synthesis, J Nucl Med 30:1367-1372, 1989.

211. Wienhard K, Herholz K, Coenen HH et al: Increased amino acid transport into brain tumors measured by PET of L-(2-18F)fluorotyrosine, J Nucl Med 32:1338-1346, 1991.

212. Hiesiger E. Fowler JS, Wolf AP et al: Serial PET studies in human cerebral malignancy with[1-11C]putrescine and [1-11C] 2- deoxy-D-glucose, J Nucl Med 28:1251-1261, 1987.

213. Hiesiger EM, Fowler JS, Logan J et al: Is [1^{11}C]putrescine useful as a brain tumor marker? J Nucl Med 33:192-199, 1992.

214. De Spiegeleer B, Slegers G, Vandecasteele C et al: Microscale synthesis of nitrogen-13-labeled cisplatin, J Nucl Med 27:399-403, 1986.

215. Binos JZ, Cooper AJL, Dhawan V et al: [13N]cisplatin PET to assess pharmacokinetics of intra-arterial versus intravenous chemotherapy for malignant brain tumors, J Nucl Med 28:1844-1852, 1987.

216. Tyler JL, Yamamoto YL, Diksic M et al: Pharmacokinetics of superselective intra-arterial and intravenous [11C]BCNU evaluated by PET, J Nucl Med 27:775-780, 1986.

217. Valk PE, Mathis CA, Prados MD et al: Hypoxia in human gliomas: demonstration by PET with fluorine-18-fluoromisonidazole, J Nucl Med 33:2133-2137, 1992.

218. Wagner HN: Positron emission tomography at the turn of the century: a perspective, Semin Nucl Med 22:285-288, 1992.

219. Wagner HN: Images of the brain: past as prologue, J Nucl Med 27:1929-1937, 1986.

220. Wagner HN: SPECT and PET advances herald new era in human biochemistry, J Nucl Med 27:1227-1238, 1986.

221. Wagner HN: SNM highlights—1989: "Why not?" J Nucl Med 30:1283-1295, 1989.

222. Wagner HN: Scientific highlights 1990: the universe within, J Nucl Med 31:17A-26A, 1990.

223. Wagner HN: Annual meeting highlights: molecules with messages, J Nucl Med 33, 10N-27N, 1992.

224. McGivney WT: Hurdles to technology diffusion: what are expectations for PET? J Nucl Med 32:660-664, 1991.

225. Positron emission tomography: clinical status in the United States in 1987, J Nucl Med 29:1136-1143, 1988.

226. Di Chiro G, Brooks RA: Editorial: PET quantitation: blessing and curse, J Nucl Med 29:1603-1604, 1988.

227. Jolles PR, Chapman PR, Alavi A: PET, CT, and MRI in the evaluation of neuropsychiatric disorders: current applications, J Nucl Med 30:1589-1606, 1989.

228. Dobkin JA, Mintun MA: Clinical PET: Aesop's tortoise? Radiology 186:13-15, 1993.

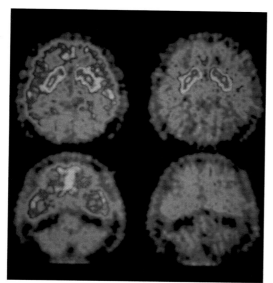

Fig. 2-10. Positron emission tomography images (sectioned through caudate and putamen) of dopamine receptors in the human brain. Leftmost images show D1 receptors, rightmost images show D2 receptors. (From Roland PE: Brain activation, New York, 1993, Wiley-Liss.)

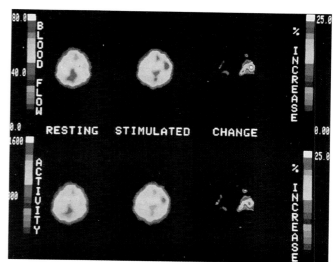

Fig. 5-2. Blood flow maps of the brain at two levels were performed at the baseline *(left)* and during left hand vibration *(center)*. The effects of sensory stimulation are more obvious when the resting perfusion image is subtracted from the stimulated scan to show the increased perfusion in the stimulated sensory cortex. (From Fox PT: J Nucl Med 30[2]: 141-149, 1989.)

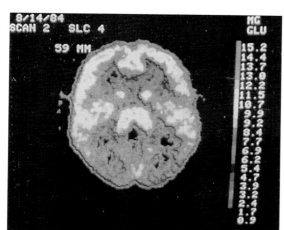

Fig. 5-5. FDG image from a normal subject *(above)* and one with a brain tumor *(below)* show precisely mapped regional glucose metabolic rate measurements. Repeated scans showed these values to be within 5% to 10% of their respective sound measurements. (From Brooks R: J Nucl Med 28[1]: 53-59, 1987.)

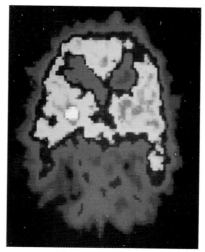

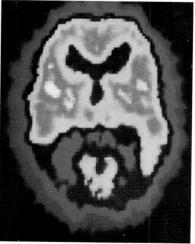

Fig. 5-9. Blood flow *(left)* and FDG uptake *(right)* maps at the level of the basal ganglia in a typical Alzheimer's disease patient. Occipital blood flow and glucose metabolism are severely decreased. (From Volkow N: J Nucl Med 28: 524-527, 1987.)

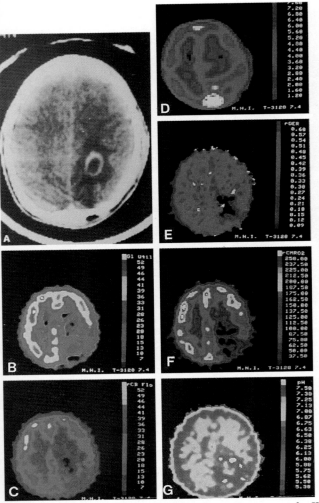

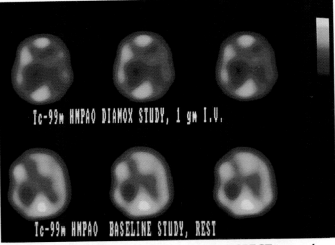

Fig. 6-14. Acetazolamide challenge HMPAP SPECT, normalized, matched axial slices are obtained without *(left)* and with *(right)* the influence of acetazolamide (Diamox). The patient was a middle-aged man with a history of CT-documented left middle cerebral artery bleeding (from an undiscovered pathologic cause) and headaches. The left middle cerebral distribution appears abnormal during the acetazolamide study because it cannot dilate further under the influence of acetazolamide. A subsequent SPECT RBC scan (not shown) showed an increased blood volume in this area at rest. These findings indicate that there is decreased flow reserve compensation for decreased blood flow distal to a partly obstructed artery caused by local vasodilation (and hence increased blood volume) in the affected area.

Fig. 5-15. A, Ring-enhancing lesion on CT is a grade IV glioma. **B,** Low CMRG1c. **C,** Low CBF. **D,** High CBV. **E,** Low OER. **F,** Low $CMRO_2$ and a high pH are seen in the same area. (From Tyler JL: J Nucl Med 28[7]: 1123-1133, 1987.)

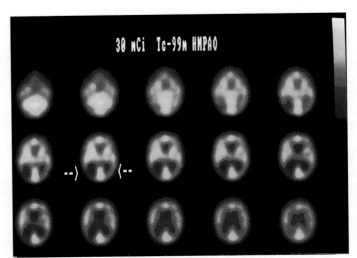

Fig. 6-15. Binswanger's disease (compare cortical HMPAO uptake with the images of Fig. 6-6, done on the same system). There is a generalized decrease in cortical labeling compared with cerebellum and calcarine cortex. Additionally, small marked focal defects are seen in the cortex *(arrowheads)*.

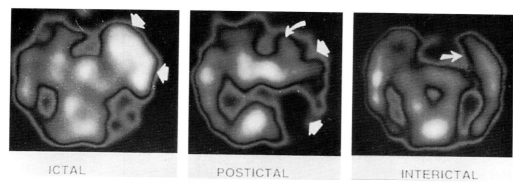

ICTAL   POSTICTAL   INTERICTAL

Fig. 6-18. HMPAO scans from a patient with left temporal lobe seizures. Hypermetabolism in the left temporal lobe is seen in the ictal scan. Injection and scan during the immediate postictal period show mild hyperfusion in the left mesial temporal region *(short curved arrow)* and generalized decreased perfusion in the rest of the temporal lobe. In the interictal scan there is a mild hypoperfusion at the mesial temporal region.

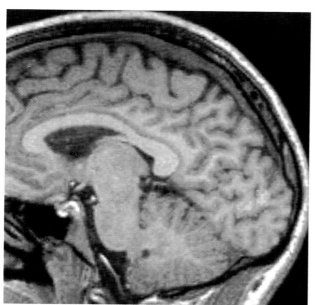

Fig. 7-2. FMRI results obtained on a clinical instrument without contrast agent injection. Location of detected activation above the calcarine fissure is expected from the applied lower visual field stimulation and is consistent with corresponding MEG localizations obtained from the same subject. The MEG source is indicated as a green square.

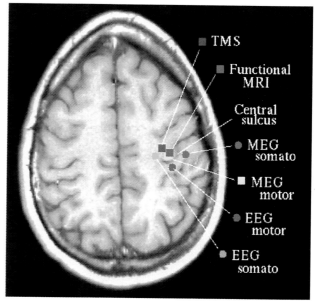

Fig. 7-101. Correlation of FMRI motor function localization with that of MEG and transcranial magnetic stimulation (TMS) in a normal volunteer.

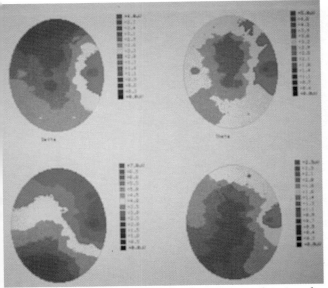

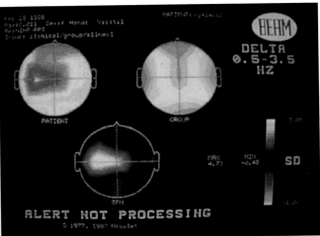

Fig. 8-42. Brain electrical activity map (BEAM) showing the spatial topography of spectral power for a schizophrenic patient. Note differences in the topography in the various frequency bands.

Fig. 8-44. BEAM and significance probability maps (SPM) for a premature neonate (30 weeks) studied 42 weeks postgestation. The infant had suffered a grade II intraventricular hemorrhage involving the left hemisphere. The BEAM map for delta activity is highly asymmetric relative to the average map for the control group. The SPM data show a statistically significant level of increased delta activity over the left hemisphere. (From Duffy FH: Issues facing the clinical use of the brain electrical activity mapping. In Pfurtscheller G, Lopes da Silva, editors: Functional brain imaging, Toronto, 1988, Han Huber Publishers.)

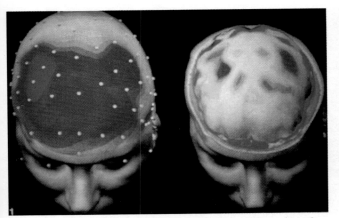

Fig. 8-45. Spatial deblurring of scalp data collected with a high-density electrode array provides increased spatial resolution of EEG data. Displayed data were collected in response to movements of one finger of each hand. In the scalp map, little detail is seen, but the deblurred image, projected just above the cortical space, shows clear bilateral activity in the vicinity of the central sulcus. (From Gevins A: Diag Imaging, Nov 1993, p 77.)

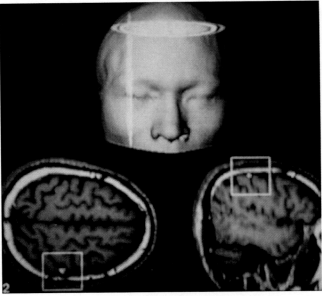

Fig. 8-46. Integration of EEG and MRI data provides for mapping of somatosensory cortex in individual subjects. EEG data collected during stimulation of the left index finger were analyzed with an equivalent dipole model. (From Gevins A: Diag Imaging, Nov 1993, p 78.)

6

Single Photon Emission Computed Tomography

Michael F. Hartshorne

The development of single photon emission computed tomography (SPECT) put a powerful physiologic imaging technology in the hands of physicians and researchers. SPECT is neither as expensive nor as complex as positron emission tomography (PET) and can be used for many of the same purposes. Most clinical centers can afford SPECT. Few can indulge in PET. Some researchers suggest that the principal function of PET technology is to expand SPECT technology. Whether or not that is true, to understand SPECT's current role in functional brain imaging it is necessary to be familiar with its technical and radiopharmaceutical aspects. Then it is possible to discuss the clinical applications of SPECT and the directions future research with this technique may take.

HISTORY OF INSTRUMENTATION

Some nuclear medicine techniques for producing noncomputed tomographs have been developed. These systems use focused imaging with gamma camera motion to blur objects that are not in the plane of focus. The tomographic systems pertinent to this discussion use computers create digital tomographs by back-projecting data from images obtained at multiple known angles. The theories that underlie tomographic imaging have existed since 1917, when the German mathematician Radon published his work dealing with reconstruction from image projections. Extension of this work by Cormack in the early 1960s and its practical application in x-ray computed tomography by Hounsfield in the early 1970s paralleled the development of nuclear tomographic techniques by Kuhl, Patton, and others.[1-4] An interesting development for nuclear medicine tomography came with Muehllehner's rotating, slant-hole collimator in the early 1970s. In this system the camera head remains stationary and the slanted collimator is turned to obtain angular projections for mathematical back-projection. However, the volume available for tomographic imaging is too limited for brain imaging.

Multiple pinhole collimators and coded-aperture tomographic systems also have restricted fields of view, images with sparse statistical information, and have not been found applicable to brain tomography.

Many of the problems of nuclear medicine tomography have been solved by the rotating gamma camera SPECT system. Work reported by Keyes in 1977 on the "Humongotron" proved the basics of this technique for tomographic brain imaging.[5] In this technique multiple angular projections are accumulated as the camera turns in an orbit around the subject's head. (The mathematically equivalent technique of holding a gamma camera head steady while rotating a patient in a chair in front of the camera has been tried successfully but has not caught on commercially.)

Two types of gamma cameras are used to create SPECT images of the brain. The most common is an orbiting gamma camera. This instrument is favored by most clinical nuclear medicine centers because it can perform a wide variety of other, nonneurologic nuclear medicine imaging procedures. The less widely used systems are those dedicated to the performance of brain images.[6]

During the last 10 years, the static planar-gamma camera has evolved to include rotating gamma camera technology. Initial problems with system alignment, orbital irregularities, and spatial distortions in the detector itself have been minimized. Because minor irregularities in the camera orbit and nonuniformities in detector sensitivity can cause artifacts and image degradation in SPECT images, mechanically precise and sturdy systems are required. These allow the detector to turn about the patient without sagging and swaying. The actual center of rotation is measured frequently by acquisitions from line or point sources. Detector nonuniformities are mapped with high-count extrinsic flood phantoms. Quality control steps like these mean residual imperfections can be compensated for by software adjustments.[7-10]

SPECT systems that use a rotating gamma camera are limited in their ability to image at long distances from the brain. The 360-degree orbit of the camera must clear the patient's shoulders. Image resolution, expressed as full width half maximum (FWHM) of point source, is as poor as 23 mm when low-energy, all-purpose collimation is used at these distances. Long-bore collimators that increase resolution can compensate for imaging at these unfavorably long distances (orbits with radii of 30 cm or more) between brain and detector. FWHM for these collimators is in the range of 11 to 17 mm. These collimators trade radiation sensitivity for improved resolution and also increase the acquisition time required to obtain sufficient image counts for reconstruction. Some systems have specially configured detector heads with a "cut-out" side that allows a closer approach to the shoulders, thereby reducing the radius of the orbit.[11] Another solution to this problem is to use a fixed 30-degree-slant collimator mounted on a camera tilted at a complementary 30 degrees. This allows acquisitions perpendicular to the axis of the orbit to be obtained closer to the patient's head, while still allowing the camera to clear the patient's shoulders.[12] Resolution from this type of collimator is much better than that from a standard collimator on the same system. Both the fixed 30-degree-slant collimator and the "cut-out" detectors show about a 30% improvement in FWHM for any collimator used for neuro-SPECT imaging (Fig. 6-1).

Cone beam or neurofocal collimation is the most advanced collimator adaptation of the rotating gamma camera to neuro-SPECT. With a two-axis converging collimator rotating about the patient's head, the sensitivity to radiation can be two to four times that of parallel or slant collimators. Resolution approaches 10 mm FWHM. However, spatial distortion in the data acquired by these systems requires special reconstruction algorithms[13] (Fig. 6-2).

Some systems dedicated to neuro-SPECT use thin rings of individual detectors just large enough to admit a patient's head. The advantages of these systems are increased resolution because of the reduced imaging distance (nearly 8 mm FWHM) and dramatically increased sensitivity because there are multiple detectors (four times the sensitivity of a gamma camera acquiring the same slice)[14-15] (Fig. 6-3). These systems can make images a single slice at a time or they may be "stacked" to produce multiple slices simultaneously. Using several gamma camera heads (two, three, or four identical detectors) rotating on a single gantry is another way to increase sensitivity.[16-18] Several commercial systems of both types are available. Experimental work with a hemispherical array of 20 small gamma cameras that acquire data independently and simultaneously has also been done[19] (Fig. 6-4).

A difficult problem in SPECT imaging is correcting for scatter. The energy window used for photon discrimination includes some off-axis, Comptom-scattered radiation that is back-projected as noise into the reconstructed image along with legitimate, on-axis photons. The deeper inside any scattering material the target image is, the worse the effect is on image resolution. Several schemes are used to compensate for this effect. A simple solution for ^{99m}Tc radiopharmaceuticals is the use of an asymmetric energy window shifted up to a photopeak of 140 to 154 keV instead of the usual centered window of 126 to 154 keV. This is a quick method that relies on the fact that most Compton-scattered radiations entering the window will be below the photopeak. It reduces the count rate of the camera and may cause nonuniform count

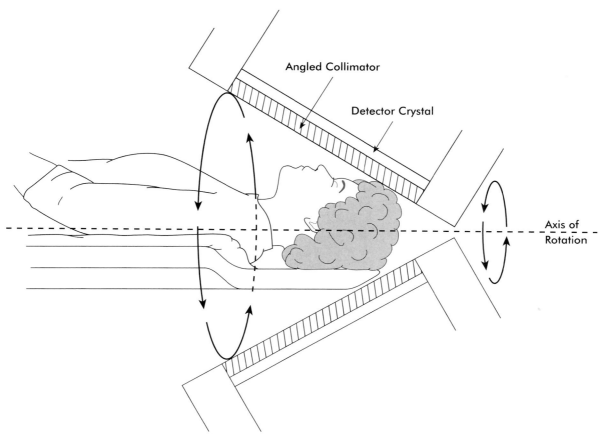

Fig. 6-1. The angle of the collimator's septations is offset by tilting the camera. The radius of rotation about the head is reduced. (See also Fig. 6-9, *B* and *C*.)

rates in different areas of the detector face. An alternative approach to ^{99m}Tc scatter correction involves simultaneous acquisition through a low energy window (92 to 125 keV), just below the symmetric window of 126 to 154 keV. Subtracting the lower window data from the primary ^{99m}Tc photopeak can improve image resolution. Scatter correction software is not currently available.[20-24]

Images are reconstructed using a variety of commercially available computers and different algorithms. Most use some form of filtered back-projection, but Fourier transformation and iterative techniques are also available. The problem of attenuation still persists. For example, generally speaking, ^{99m}Tc photons at 140 keV have a 35% attenuation when imaged at 8 cm from a patient's skull. However, variations in skull thickness around the circumference of a slice image can vary attenuation. In x-ray computed tomography (CT), the attenuation of a beam of x-rays is directly measured. In PET, the data from the patient are corrected by comparison with an attenuation image made from a transmission scan. These techniques are not applicable to SPECT imaging, and it would require the entire space allotted for this text to discuss adequately the ways to correct for attenuation in SPECT. Suffice it to say that much work remains to be done to bring a reliable attenuation correction scheme to the ordinary clinic.[25-29]

Without reliable methods for scatter and attenuation correction, SPECT techniques remain semiquantitative at best. Attempts to quantitate these studies rely on side-to-side comparison of regions of interest or comparison to benchmark regions such as the calcarine cortex or the cerebellum.[30-32]

RADIOPHARMACEUTICALS

There are several Food and Drug Administration (FDA) approved radiopharmaceuticals, several pending approval, and numerous investigational agents used for SPECT. The old standards for brain scans rely on tracer uptake in areas of blood-brain barrier (BBB) defect. ^{99m}Tc pertechnetate (with simultaneous administration of potassium perchlorate to block choroid plexus uptake), ^{99m}Tc DTPA, and ^{99m}Tc glucoheptonate (both with rapid decrease in background activity because of renal excretion) are used infrequently for SPECT imaging. SPECT regional cerebral blood volume (rCBV) measurements require a radiopharmaceu-

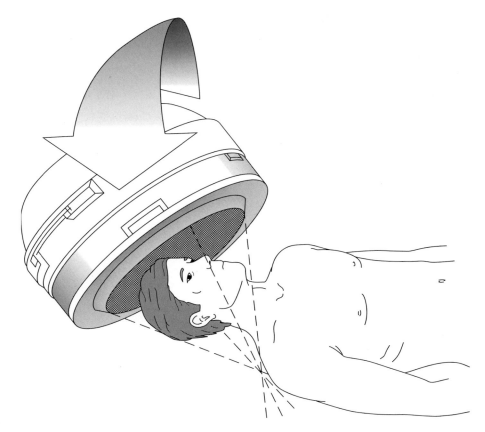

Fig. 6-2. The maximum use of the detector face involves a converging collimator rotating at an angle to the long axis of the patient's body.

tical that will stay within the vascular compartment during acquisition. ^{99m}Tc red blood cells (RBCs) are the most readily prepared. ^{99m}Tc-labeled albumin and ^{111}In or ^{113m}In-labeled transferrin have also been used.[33]

The large number of cerebral blood flow agents includes several approved by the FDA. An ideal agent would reproduce the gold standard measurement of blood flow provided by radiolabeled microspheres. The traditional regional cerebral blood flow (rCBF) standard is ^{133}Xe gas. SPECT technology replaced multiprobe imaging systems more than 10 years ago, but the technique for administration remains the same. After a brief period of ^{133}Xe inhalation, blood flow rates are mapped using sequential, rapid tomographic scans. In gray matter blood flow, rates are about 75 ml/100 g/min and in white matter about 25 ml/100 g/min. The relatively poor spatial resolution of the system (16 mm FWHM) requires imaging regions of at least 3 cm in diameter for rCBF measurement. Considering this limitation, the accuracy is surprisingly good when compared with that obtained using injected microspheres[34-38] (Fig. 6-5).

^{123}I-labeled amines include ^{123}I-N,N,N',-trimethyl-N'-[2-hydroxyl-3-methyl-5-iodo-benzyl]-1,3-propane diamine (HIPDM) and ^{123}I-n-isopropyl-p-iodoam-phetamine (IMP).[33,39-49] Brain uptake of these intravenously injected, lipophilic agents is proportional to rCBF, although HIPDM reaches peak concentrations in the brain at 10 to 15 minutes, while maximum IMP brain activity occurs 20 to 30 minutes after injection. It is believed that distribution of IMP in the brain is controlled by the presence of high-capacity, nonspecific binding sites for amines. The actual distribution of these agents is proportional to regional blood flow (Fig. 6-6). Initial retention in the lung, followed by slow release of the radiopharmaceutical into the general circulation, causes some of the variation in the brain activity detected. There is an equilibrium period of brain activity during which SPECT can be performed and washout from the brain seen. After 1 hour, the labeled amines redistribute. This process is poorly understood, and some investigators contend that areas of initial poor uptake and subsequent filling-in are ischemic, in a manner analogous to myocardial ischemia identified by ^{201}T1 studies.

IMP is FDA approved and available throughout the United States by overnight air delivery. A limited dose of 3 to 6 mCi of ^{123}I provides a marginally acceptable photon flux. If the ^{124}Xe(p,2n)^{123}Cs-> ^{123}Xe-> ^{123}I re-

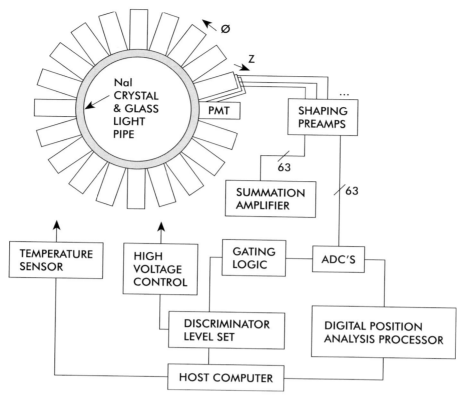

Fig. 6-3. Diagram of a ring SPECT detector, which uses an annular NaI crystal backed by a ring of photomultiplier tubes.

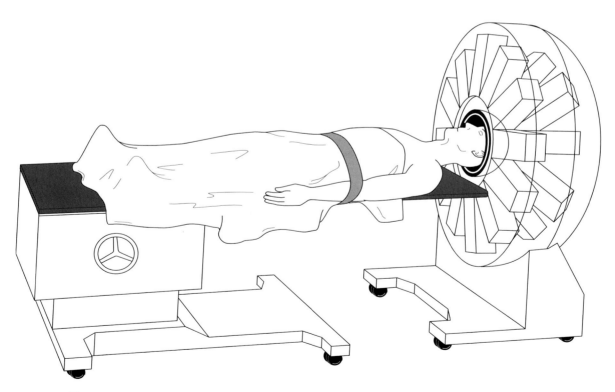

Fig. 6-4. The closest fit of detector and brain is shown with 20 stationary detectors in a hemispherical array around the head.

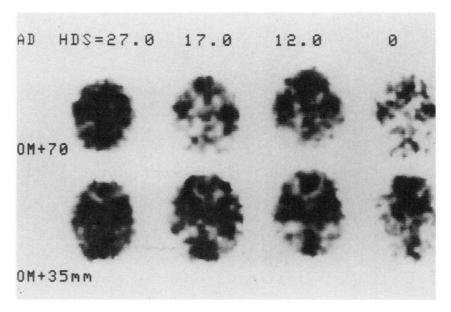

Fig. 6-5. Resolution of 15 mm FWHM in SPECT imaging of regional cerebral blood flow (rCBF) with inhaled ^{133}Xe shows symmetric, diminished perfusion in the parietal and posterior temporal lobes. The patient has Alzheimer's disease.

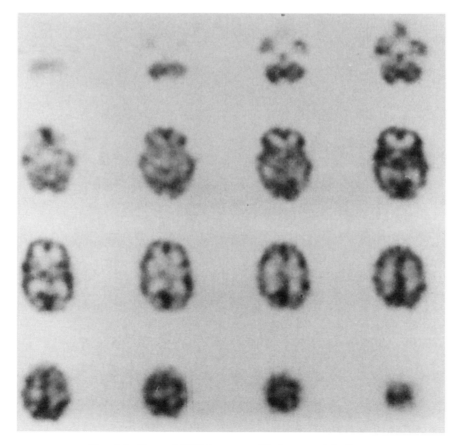

Fig. 6-6. Normal IMP images with 8 mm axial slices.

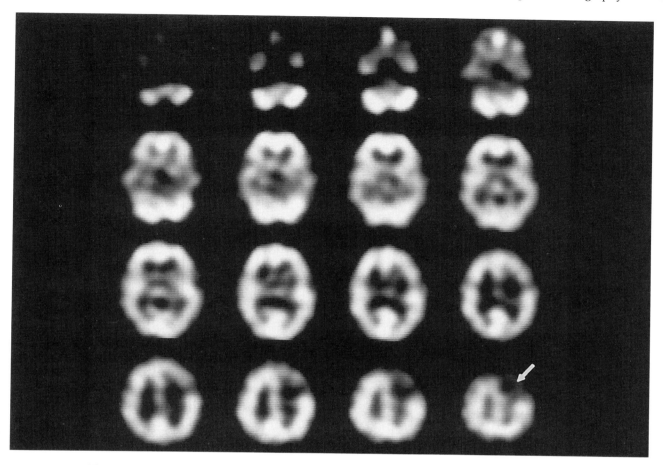

Fig. 6-7. HMPAO axial slices starting from the cerebellum show preferential uptake in gray matter. A defect in the left frontal lobe (*arrow*) corresponds to the site of a glial tumor resection.

action is used to prepare this agent, the result is relatively pure [123]I. Other reactions may be used, but [124]I contaminants degrade images and ^{125}I contaminants increase the biologic dose.

FDA approved and widely available, lipid soluble ^{99m}Tc-hexamethylpropyleneamineoxime (HMPAO) provides an excellent photon flux for SPECT imaging. It is an intravenous brain perfusion agent that almost reproduces the theoretical microsphere. The d,l isomer of HMPAO is not stable after its kit is prepared and should be injected within 30 minutes of preparation. This agent distributes according to regional blood flow and is believed to react rapidly with intracellular glutathione (GSH), converting it to a meso-isomer that is trapped inside the brain (Fig. 6-7). There is a minor initial back-diffusion from the brain to the blood that is more prominent in high blood flow regions; it explains why HMPAO tends to slightly underestimate higher rCBF.[50-57] Allowing for differences in resolution and convenience of handling, SPECT studies with ^{133}Xe, IMP and HMPAO studies correlate well in the detection of decreased rCBF.[58]

An investigational agent, ^{99m}Tc-L,L-ethyl cyteinate dimer (ECD), performs in a manner very similar to HMPAO. Uptake in the brain is rapid and final concentrations are reached within minutes (Fig. 6-8). It is probable that a polar metabolite formed in the brain cell is incapable of diffusing back into the bloodstream and is rapidly cleared by the kidneys. The reduction of blood pool activity produces an image that is "easier to read" than one obtained with HMPAO. ECD is not yet an FDA-approved new drug. Unlike the ^{123}I-labeled amines, neither ECD nor HMPAO redistributes in the brain.[59-62]

Other lipophilic ^{99m}Tc compounds such as Chloro[bis{2,3-butanedionedioxime(1-)-O}{2,3 butane-dionedioximato (2-)-N,N',N'',N''',N''''} (2-methyl-propyl borato (2-)[^{99m}Tc] (^{99m}Tc-DMG-2MP), ^{99m}Tc-O(N-2[1H pyrolylmethyl])N'-(4-pentene-3-one-2) ethane-1,2-diamine) (MRP20), and ^{99m}Tc-N1-2(mercapto-2-methylpropyl)-N2-(2-propargylthio-2-methylpropyl)-1,2-benzenediamine (T691) are impossible to spell and have no significant advantages over HMPAO or ECD.[63-65] [201]T1 diethyldithiocarba-

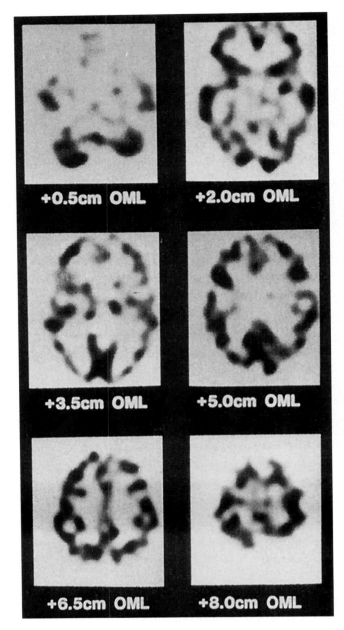

Fig. 6-8. Distribution of ECD in a normal brain at intervals above the orbital meatal line (OML).

mate (DDC) is an investigational perfusion agent that has little redistribution. The 73-hour half-life of ^{201}T1 makes imaging possible long after this agent is injected. DDC has the same poor imaging characteristics of ^{201}T1 and has largely been abandoned.[66] A host of other agents has been investigated in the search to produce the perfect "chemical microsphere" for the measurement and preferably absolute quantitation of rCBF.[67-69] Unless brain imaging is substantially improved by these radiopharmaceuticals, the millions of dollars and years of efforts required to bring them to market ensure that they

will not replace the SPECT agents currently approved by the FDA.

Investigational ^{123}I-labeled receptor antagonists are being developed for SPECT imaging. A specific D1 dopamine receptor antagonist ^{123}I[(+)-7-chloro-8-hydroxyl-1-(3'-iodophenyl) 3-methyl-2,3,4,5-tetra-hydro-1H-3 benzazepine], known as TISH, localizes in receptors in the prefrontal cortex, the hippocampus, and the amygdala.[70] ^{123}I-labeled (S-(-)-N-[(1-ethyl-2-pyrrolidinyl)methyl]-2-hydroxy-3-iodo-6-methoxy-benzamide) (IBZM) is a specific D2 receptor agonist that shows high uptake in the striatum. It can be displaced by haloperidol, which is a high-affinity D2 receptor agent.[71,72] There are other ^{125}I- and ^{123}I-labeled benzamides such as[^{123}I]-ethyl-5,6,-dihydro-7-iodo-5-methyl-6-oxo-4H-imidazo[1,5a][1,4]benzo-diazepine-3-carboxylate (conveniently referred to as Ro 16-0154) and ergolenes (such as [^{123}I]iodolisuride) that offer in vivo pharmacokinetic studies of agonists and antagonists to dopamine receptors[73-75] (Fig. 6-9). These radiopharmaceuticals are all inspired by PET investigational D1 and D2 receptor agents. The research implications include the study of the pathogenesis and therapy for Parkinson's disease, supranuclear palsy, and schizophrenia.

An experimental muscarinic acetylcholine receptor ligand ^{123}I (R)-3-quinuclidinyl-4-iodo-benzilate (IQNB) distributes on SPECT images as expected from postmortem studies of this receptor. IQNB may allow in vivo study of changes in the density of muscarinic acetylcholine receptors during the progression of Huntington's chorea and Alzheimer's disease.[76]

Another line of SPECT radiopharmacy research involves the use of ^{123}I L-3-iodo-alpha-methyl tyrosine (IMT) to characterize brain tumors. In parallel with established PET techniques for ^{11}C amino acid studies, greater uptake of IMT implies a higher grade (grades II, III, and IV) glioma. Competitive loads of nonlabeled amino acids have shown that the uptake of IMT requires the operation of a carrier system in the intact BBB (Fig. 6-10). Presumably, tumors without astrocytes (such as meningiomas and metastases) are not capable of producing the BBB that modulates IMT transport and controls glucose and other small molecule transport in a very selective fashion. Without a BBB these tumors do not selectively take up IMT.[77-82]

Exploration of possible SPECT glucose analogs has been stimulated by PET researchers' experiences with ^{18}F-fluorodeoxyglucose (FDG). ^{99m}Tc glucarate has been used as a marker of ischemic brain injury for SPECT imaging. It does not, however, appear to be transported by the sugar-carrying mechanism responsible for the uptake of FDG. It may turn out to be an expensive BBB defect agent.[83,84]

A final class of SPECT radiopharmaceuticals being studied for brain investigations relies on monoclonal

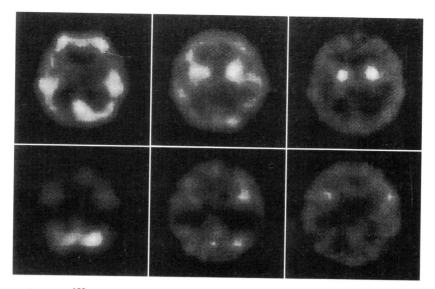

Fig. 6-9. SPECT [^{123}I]iodolisuride (ILIS) images of a schizophrenic patient treated with haloperidol (*left*) shows little or no D2 uptake in the striatum. Middle images show an intermediate D2 uptake in the basal ganglia in a patient with progressive supranuclear palsy. On the right there is intense, preferential ILIS-D2 uptake in the striatum.

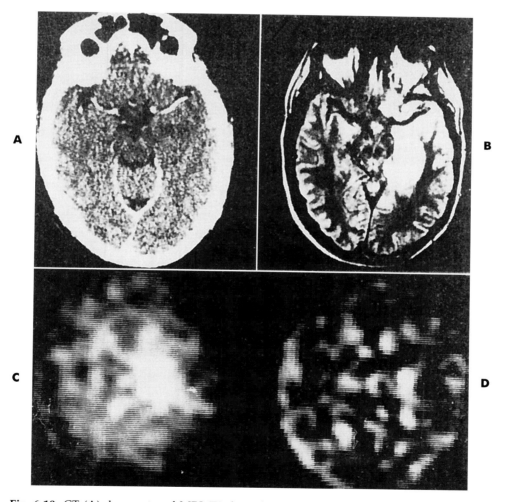

Fig. 6-10. CT (**A**) does not and MRI (**B**) does show a grade II astrocytoma. When IMT is given during fasting (**C**), the SPECT images show intense tumor uptake of the amino acid. With an infusion of amino acids (**D**), the IMT is not well taken up by tumor and normal brain.

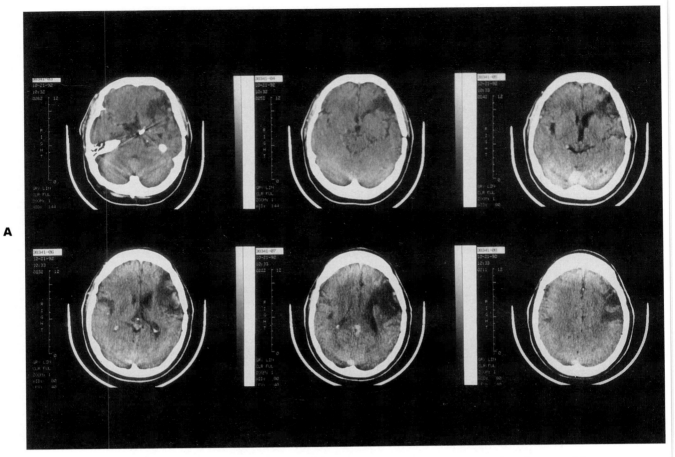

Fig. 6-11. A, Cerebral infarction CT shows an extensive infarct associated with a carotid cavernous fistula with low-density areas in the anterior portions of the left middle cerebral distribution 5 weeks after a stroke.

antibodies labeled with ^{123}I or [99m]Tc. A ^{99m}Tc murine monoclonal antibody targeted to beta/A4 amyloid has been described in postmortem brain tissue studies and is proposed for use in in vivo detection of amyloid angiopathy in Alzheimer's disease.[85] ^{123}I-labeled antibodies against epidermal growth factor receptor (EFR) and against placental alkaline phosphatase (PLAP) have been used to detect gliomas.[86] Another ^{123}I murine monoclonal antibody, 81C6, has been reported to react with an epitope of tenascin that is located in the extracellular matrix of glioma cells.[87]

Radiotherapeutic treatment by intravenous or intracarotid injections of ^{131}I-labeled EFR and PLAP antibodies of a few patients showed some transitory improvement.[86] Antibody preparations have the disadvantage of nonspecific labeling that may mean high uptake in the liver, spleen, and other organs. More tumor-specific antibodies and better beta emitters such as [90]Yt hold an elusive promise for glioma treatment.

CEREBRAL INFARCTION

Normal rCBF is strongly associated with the metabolism of oxygen. Autoregulation with vasodilata-tion adjusts rCBF when metabolic demands change. SPECT of rCBF agents map these changes. Cerebral infarction represents one end of this spectrum. Stroke is usually simple to diagnose. CT is used only to detect a hemorrhagic lesion. Imaging with rCBF agents immediately locates all but small (i.e., lacunar) infarcts but is not clinically needed to establish the diagnosis (Fig. 6-11). It might gain a role if it proves useful for early evaluation of stroke patients. SPECT studies done within 24 hours of clinical stroke show that lesion size correlates well with clinical outcome, although many studies done of patients in the subacute period have resulted in confusing conclusions about prognosis. Studies done with HMPAO or [133]Xe 10 to 14 days after a stroke may show luxury perfusion. Also, the size of the infarct may be underestimated or the infarct may not even be seen during this period. However, IMP scans at the same time as HMPAO studies continue to show the infarct. Later, in the subacute period of recovery, differences in the size of a lesion seen on CT scans compared with a lesion seen on SPECT predicts the patient's recovery potential. The larger the lesion as seen on SPECT rather than CT, the

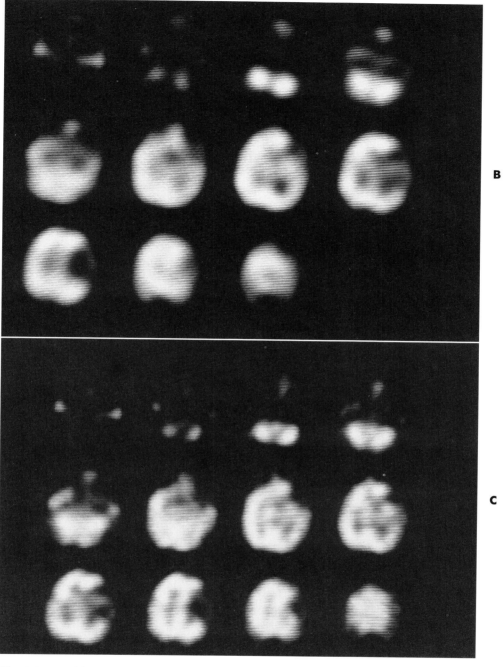

B

C

Fig. 6-11, cont'd. B, The HMPAO SPECT brain scan done with a single head camera and parallel collimation shows an area of marked decrease in perfusion, which was judged to extend more posteriorly than the CT abnormality. This probably represents an ischemic penumbra that is viable but dysfunctional. **C,** An immediate repeat SPECT study with a 30-degree slant collimator (see Fig. 6-1) shows a modest improvement in image resolution. Note decreased blurring of the cortical details and improved resolution of the basal ganglia.

better the prognosis. The discrepancy between the two images probably represents viable but dysfunctional tissue that has potential for improved function if it is reperfused.[88-93]

Neurologic activity in one area of the brain that is influencing the activity in another area may confuse the unwary imaging physician. Brainstem infarcts may be too small to detect with SPECT, yet they may produce major reductions in rCBF in the cortex. Basal ganglia infarcts can cause areas of decreased ipsilateral cortical rCBF. Crossed cerebellar diaschisis or hypoperfusion is seen after contralateral cortical infarcts or metabolic depression of cortical brain decreases flow to cerebellar neuronal activity.[94]

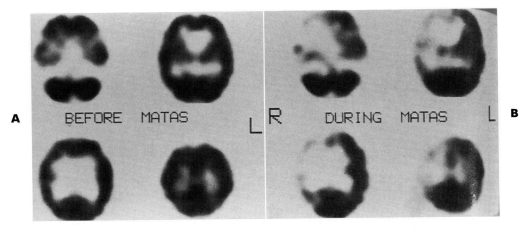

Fig. 6-12. A, Baseline SPECT study (*left*) shows symmetric cerebral labeling with HMPAO. **B,** A second HMPAO injection during manual compression of the right common carotid provides SPECT images, which show little perfusion to the right, middle, and anterior cerebral artery distributions. Sacrifce of the right carotid would risk massive infarction since collaterial flow through the circle of Willis was not shown.

CEREBRAL ISCHEMIA

Simple methods to convert SPECT data for the FDA-approved brain agents into absolute rCBF (in units of ml/100 g/min) have not been developed. Rapid, dynamic images that require a dedicated ring detector have been used in a scheme to quantify rCBF with IMP.[95] Arterial-input-curve measurement using HMPAO is a cumbersome technique done in conjunction with single-acquisition SPECT to make the same measurement.[96,97] Both methods are equipment-specific and difficult enough to preclude their routine clinical use. A few centers equipped to do ^{133}Xe SPECT may achieve routine, absolute rCBF measurements. Semiquantitative techniques express rCBF as a ratio of a lesion to similar normal brain (L/N). As established by ^{133}Xe SPECT studies, the rCBF threshold for CNS symptoms of ischemia is in the range of 33 to 36 ml/100 g/min. The threshold for irreversible damage is 19 to 23 ml/100 g/min. The corresponding IMP L/N ratios have been established at 65% to 72% and 39% to 49%, respectively. An obvious limitation to the widely used L/N ratio is the assumption that one side is normal.[98]

An additional limitation of IMP, HMPAO, and ECD measurements of rCBF is seen by the comparison of these agents with ^{133}Xe SPECT. IMP slightly underestimates the rCBF. (The IMP contrast between normal and reduced CBF areas is slightly less than that of [133]Xe.) The contrast between normal and reduced CBF, as measured with either HMPAO or ECD, is even less. However, the actual differences are small and more than offset by the advantages of the ^{99m}Tc agents.[47,99]

Subjective interpretation of HMPAO scans can be useful in detecting vasospasm-induced ischemia.[100] HMPAO corticocerebellar ratios (carefully established to avoid measuring the cerebellar hemisphere af-

fected) can be used to determine whether angioplasty has improved a patient's rCBF after vasospasm induced by subarachnoid hemorrhage. A study of 10 patients reports an improvement from an average corticocerebellar vasospasm ratio of 80% to a postangioplasty value of 90%.[101] Subjective assessment of HMPAO SPECT and analysis of IMP SPECT with a modification of the "bull's-eye" program are used to detect improvement and degradation in cerebral perfusion after carotid endarterectomy.[102,103] External-to-internal carotid artery bypass results can also be evaluated with this technique.[104]

HMPAO SPECT also can be used to detect areas of hypoperfusion of the contused brain after closed head injury.[105,106] One report describes the serendipitous detection of subdural hematoma with HMPAO.[107] Corticocerebellar ratios with HMPAO and ^{133}Xe SPECT techniques are used to demonstrate reductions in the rCBF of the cerebrum compressed by the hematoma and improvements in rCBF after surgical evacuation of the hematomas. It is possible that SPECT may become a useful tool for evaluation of nonspecific neurologic symptoms seen in patients with closed head injuries.[108,109] One report suggests that mild, reversible ischemia can be detected by HMPAO SPECT when the small amount of blood-bound HMPAO and minor back-leak of HMPAO from normal brain cause 4-hour fill-in of defects found on 30-minute scans.[110]

The Matas test involves trial occlusion of the carotid artery before surgery that might require sacrifice of that vessel. The test can be done with manual compression of a carotid artery or during angiography by using temporary balloon occlusion to test the adequacy of collateral circulation (Figs. 6-12 and 6-13). This procedure is ideally suited for SPECT with

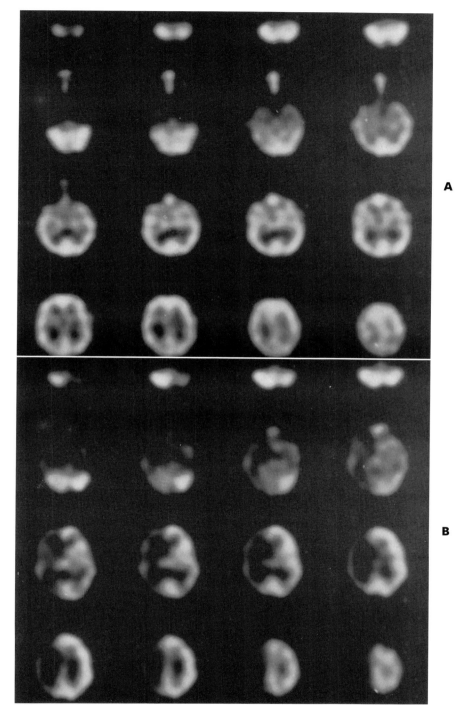

Fig. 6-13. A, Angiographic Matas test. The baseline SPECT HMPAO study is normal in this patient, who is being evaluated prior to surgery to treat a meningioma and in whom sacrifice of the right internal carotid may be necessary. **B,** With an angioplasty balloon temporarily inflated in the right internal carotid artery, a second injection of HMPAO allows delayed, postangiography SPECT images. These show a massive area of diminished perfusion in the right cerebral hemisphere. This forced an alternate surgical approach to the meningioma resection.

HMPAO injected intravenously during the occlusion. The SPECT imaging is done after the angiography is completed. Symmetric cerebral perfusion despite carotid artery occlusion predicts that the patient can tolerate sacrifice of the carotid. Decreased ipsilateral perfusion dictates an alternate surgical approach to avoid pre- or postoperative infarct.[111-114]

The Wada test relies on intracarotid amobarbital sodium injection to predict postoperative memory function in patients being considered for temporal lobectomy or hemispherectomy to treat tumors or control seizures. If the amobarbital distributes to and anesthetizes the mesial temporal lobe on the side of injection, then memory function can be tested with the patient using only the contralateral temporal lobe. HMPAO injected along with the amobarbital can be used to complement the angiographic estimation of amobarbital distribution.[115,116]

VASODILATORY RESERVE

Carbon dioxide (CO_2) is the most potent cerebral vasodilator. For obvious reasons, increasing arterial CO_2 is not used in clinical medicine, and data on CO_2 are largely from animal experiments.[112-115] In patients with normal CT scans and a history of transient ischemic attack (TIA), rCBF studies can be improved with an acetazolamide challenge. This carbonic anhydrase inhibitor is given intravenously in gram quantities. It causes a uniform increase in rCBF of as much as 70% that peaks at 20 to 30 minutes. Abnormal arteries cannot dilate. SPECT-rCBF scans, with and without acetazolamide, are compared in a fashion somewhat analogous to dipyridamole-challenge myocardial perfusion scans. Separate day scans done with the same radiopharmaceutical, rapid sequence ^{133}Xe and IMP or HMPAO, and very carefully windowed IMP and HMPAO scans done simultaneously are used to evaluate transient ischemic attack, stroke, arteriovenous malformation, and other vascular pathologies. The value of the simultaneously acquired HMPAO baseline and IMP acetazolamide SPECT studies is that the image registration for the two studies is superb.[120-127]

HMPAO acetazolamide-challenge studies can be interpreted either using complex mathematics and technically difficult measurements of rCBF or by eye. A common pattern is seen in those patients who have major cerebral vessel occlusive disease. A baseline study that shows a defect that becomes larger and/or

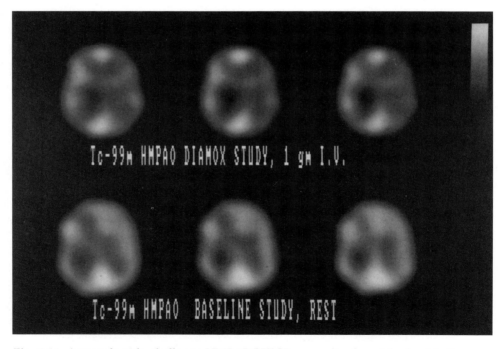

Fig. 6-14. Acetazolamide challenge HMPAP SPECT, normalized, matched axial slices are obtained without (*left*) and with (*right*) the influence of acetazolamide (Diamox). The patient was a middle-aged man with a history of CT-*documented* left middle cerebral artery bleeding (from an undiscovered pathologic cause) and headaches. The left middle cerebral distribution appears abnormal during the acetazolamide study because it cannot dilate further under the influence of acetazolamide. A subsequent SPECT RBC scan (not shown) showed an increased blood volume in this area at rest. These findings indicate that there is decreased flow reserve compensation for decreased blood flow distal to a partly obstructed artery caused by local vasodilation (and hence increased blood volume) in the affected area.

less well perfused after acetazolamide indicates a decrease in flow reserve (in the ischemic area). A decreased perfusion pressure distal to arterial obstruction has already caused compensatory vasodilation and increased rCBV in the affected area. Little additional dilation can occur in the ischemic area, which has already done all it can to keep tissues alive. The areas elsewhere in the brain with normal blood supply do not vasodilate until forced to do so by the acetazolamide (Fig. 6-14).

Another pattern seen is an initial area of decreased rCBF, which improves after acetazolamide. This ability to increase blood flow indicates preserved perfusion reserve and may imply a good collateral supply to the ischemic area. An alternative explanation is that the baseline hypoperfused area has already lost neurons or afferent input and so has a decreased metabolic rate compared with normal brain. In either case, these patients may not be good candidates for vascular reconstructive surgery.[128-132]

Cerebral circulatory reserve can also be evaluated using SPECT to compare rCBF with rCBV. This is conveniently accomplished by doing SPECT image with both an rCBF agent and [99mTc] RBCs. These studies are performed sequentially using two agents having different energies ([133Xe] and [99mTc] RBCs). This combination requires that the initial acquisition be with rCBFs, followed immediately by infusion of tagged RBCs for a second acquisition. A frame-by-frame subtraction of the first acquisition from the second produces a third data set, reflecting the rCBV.

The resulting SPECT-based index of cerebral circulatory reserve is an extension of established PET techniques.[133-136]

BRAIN DEATH

HMPAO can be used to perform conventional radionuclide angiography studies in cases of suspected brain death. The planar or SPECT images obtained can assist in the evaluation of posterior fossa perfusion. The quality of the bolus is immaterial. Absence of brain uptake with HMPAO is a strong confirmation of brain death, whereas brain perfusion of the HMPAO-labeled agent indicates potential recovery.[138-141]

DEMENTIA

Relatively specific patterns of cerebral perfusion are seen in rCBF SPECT examinations or patients with different dementias. The classic example, Alzheimer's disease, appears to have bilateral posterior temporal defects that subsequently extend into the parietal cortices as the disease progresses. These were first identified with PET, [133Xe], and IMP (Figs. 6-5 and 6-15). With the classic pattern, the likelihood that the patient has Alzheimer's disease by National Institute of Neurologic Disease and Stroke/Alzheimer's Disease and Related Disorders Association criteria (NINDS/ADRDA) exceeds 80%. On the other hand, if the patient is demented and has a normal scan, there is still a 20% chance that he or she has the disease (perhaps in an early phase). Early cases studied with HMPAO

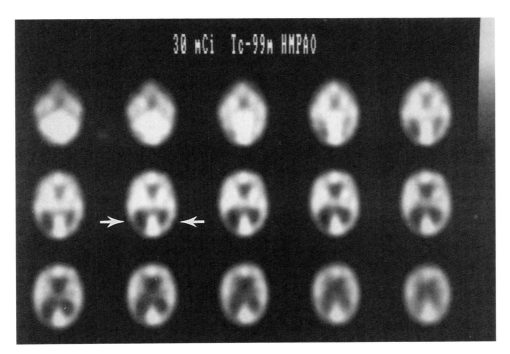

Fig. 6-15. The [99mTc] HMPAO distribution in a patient with Alzheimer's disease shows a marked symmetric decrease uptake in the posterior temporal and parietal lobes.

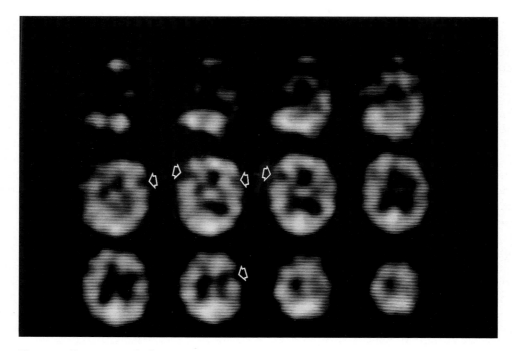

Fig. 6-16. Binswanger's disease (compare cortical HMPAO uptake with the images of Fig. 6-6 done on the same system). There is a generalized decrease in cortical labeling compared with cerebellum and calcarine cortex. Additionally, small marked focal defects are seen in the cortex (arrow heads).

corticocerebellar ratios show a generalized decrease in the perfusion of the whole cerebrum, particularly in the frontal, temporal, and parietal cortex. A large study with quantitative histologic examination, as opposed to clinical diagnosis, of the recently scanned brain has yet to be done. Such a study would help refine the relationships between the clinical, scan, and histologic features of this form of dementia.[142-150]

A somewhat different pattern is seen in Binswanger's disease. This is a subcortical atherosclerotic encephalopathy caused by atherosclerosis of penetrating cerebral arteries. Decreases in cerebral perfusion seen in generalized areas are evaluated by using corticocerebellar ratios. The most profoundly affected area is the thalamus, unlike the preferential parietal decreased rCBF seen in the Alzheimer's patient. Multiinfarct dementia involves larger vascular distributions[144-147] (Fig. 6-16). Preferential, frontal lobe–decreased rCBF is characteristic of Pick's disease but can also be seen in progressive supranuclear palsy (progressive dementia with motor neuron disease) and after trauma. Some, but not all, schizophrenics show decreased frontal rCBF by different SPECT techniques. There is enough overlap in the SPECT rCBF patterns that they cannot always be differentiated. Some utility for SPECT remains for the diagnosis of the clinically depressed, but not demented, elderly patient, who will have a normal rCBF pattern.[148-151]

Acquired immunodeficiency syndrome dementia complex (ADC) has also received attention from researchers employing rCBF SPECT. The HIV infection can directly cause ADC, and matters are made more complex by concomitant opportunistic CNS infection. Cortical and particularly subcortical (basal ganglia) rCBF asymmetries are seen in HIV-seropositive patients with and without symptoms. Early abnormalities are seen in the frontal cortex. Severe involvement with ADC has been reported to involve the white matter as well as the gray.[152-156]

Cocaine abusers show very similar patterns. The mechanism of injury may involve drug-induced vasospasm. Multiple infarcts resulting from vascular diseases and these dementias cannot be differentiated by SPECT appearances. Recent work with HMPAO SPECT shows that the brain perfusion defects of cocaine users are partly reversible with abstinence.[159-161]

EPILEPSY

Detection of seizure foci is important for presurgical planning. SPECT rCBF studies with ^{133}Xe show interictal hypoperfusion in only about 50% of cases. The better spatial resolution of HMPAO SPECT allows the detection of hypoperfused seizure foci in many cases (about 75%), which is similar to PET results (Figs. 6-17 and 6-18). False-positive results have been reported when images were interpreted

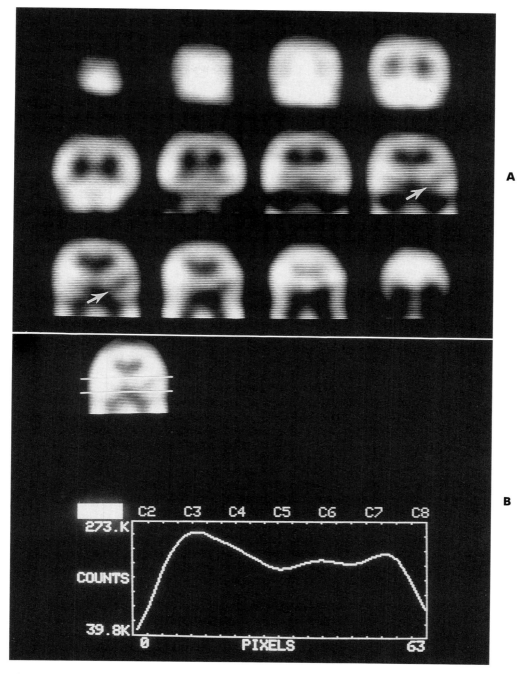

Fig. 6-17. A, Interictal HMPAO SPECT in a patient with left temporal lobe seizures. An area of decreased temporal lobe perfusion is seen in the coronal sections (*arrows*). **B,** The line-profile region of interest technique shows graphically the reduced temporal lobe labeling.

visually. Various authors report different accuracies depending on the radiopharmaceutical, SPECT system, and criteria for comparison (i.e., EEG versus surgical corticography). Additional preoperative studies may be unnecessary if EEG and SPECT rCBF determinations are concordant for detection of the seizure focus.[164-168]

The elusive solution to the problem of seizure foci detection is ictal scanning. The hyperperfusion that accompanies activation of a seizure focus is particularly easy to find on SPECT images. Although locating a seizure focus in an ictal scan made using a [123]I rCBF agent can be very accurate (93% in one series), this procedure may mean waiting for hours until a seizure

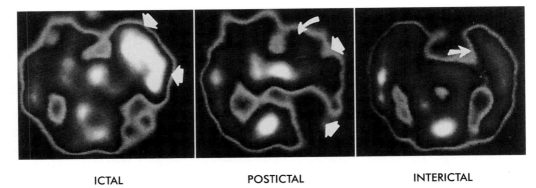

ICTAL   POSTICTAL   INTERICTAL

Fig. 6-18. HMPAO scans from a patient with left temporal lobe seizures. Hypermetabolism in the left temporal lobe is seen in the ictal scan. Injection and scan during the immediate postictal period shows mild hyperfusion in the left mesial temporal region (*short curved arrow*) and generalized decreased perfusion in the rest of the temporal lobe. In the interictal scan there is mild hypoperfusion at the mesial temporal region.

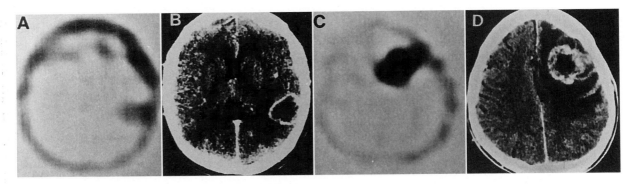

Fig. 6-19. Thallium uptake in astrocytomas. Two cases of high-grade astrocytoma (Grade IV: **A,B**; Grade III: **C,D**) with thallium localization are shown in SPECT images **A** and **C**. These correspond to rim-enhancing lesions on CT scans **B** and **D**. The apparent intensity of thallium uptake can be reduced by volume averaging of a large necrotic center (as in **A** and **B**).

occurs so that the agent can be injected during or immediately after it. HMPAO would work as well if a seizure occurred within the 30-minute window available after kit reconstitution.[164-168]

PSYCHIATRIC APPLICATIONS

Inconsistent results from studies on the changes in cerebral perfusion and metabolism in psychiatric patients before and after treatment make it difficult to draw conclusions about a clinical role for SPECT imaging.[169,170] Some researchers associate depression and decreased rCBF in the lateral prefrontal cortex.[171-173] Others have used PET to demonstrate an association with increased regional cerebral glucose metabolism (rCGM).[171] It is not unreasonable to speculate that SPECT might find rCBF abnormalities in the same area. Discrepancies between rCBF and SPECT results may in part be related to variations in populations, diagnoses, medications, and duration of disease.[174,175] Temporal lobe rCBF abnormalities have also been reported in schizophrenics.[176] A tendency for decreased rCBF in the left cerebral hemisphere that is measurable by PET and SPECT has been reported.[172,177-179]

INCREASED rCBF

There are physiologic conditions in which both metabolism and blood flow are increased. HMPAO SPECT detected increased rCBF in visual cortex stimulated by strobe lights as the agent was injected. IMP patients, however, do not show changes in visual cortex rCBF if strobe light stimulation is applied during the redistribution phase (165 minutes after injection).[177,176] Activation of motor cortex increases HMPAO uptake when the radiopharmaceutical is administered during rhythmic hand exercise.[182]

Pathologic conditions that increase rCBF as a result of inflammation include encephalomyelitis, which

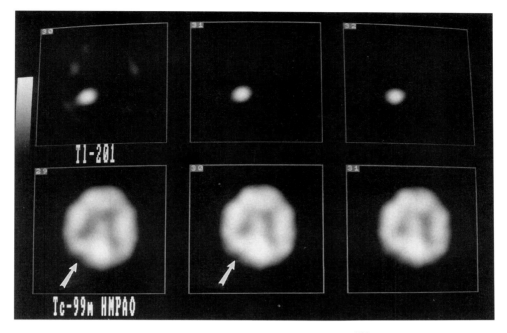

Fig. 6-20. Brain metastasis from adenocarcinoma of the lung. [201]Tl SPECT axial images (*upper row*) show a focus of intense ^{201}Tl uptake. The matched HMPAO images (*bottom row*) have a focal defect (*arrows*) at the location of the metastasis.

showed areas of increased rCBF when imaged with HMPAO,[183,184] and brain abscess,[185] when imaged with ^{201}Tl SPECT. Increased IMP localization in primary and secondary auditory areas of the brain has been reported in a case of a patient with auditory hallucination.[186]

PEDIATRIC APPLICATIONS

SPECT rCBF agents can be used in neonates. Continued maturation of the brain after birth is demonstrated by increasing rCBF values. Cortical rCBFs measured by ^{133}Xe at birth are lower than adult values. At 5 to 6 years of age these increase to levels higher than those seen in adults and then decrease to adult levels by the late teens. IMP SPECT shows greater thalamic perfusion than cortical perfusion until the end of the second month of life. Parietal and occipital areas are well seen at birth, and their visibility rises thereafter. Frontal perfusion seems absent at birth but quickly becomes apparent after the second month of life.[187-189]

Areas of decreased brain perfusion are detectable after extracorporeal membrane oxygenation that temporarily or permanently sacrifices the right carotid artery.[190] Neonatal and childhood SPECT rCBF measurements may gain a role in defining areas of anoxic damage resulting in cerebral palsy. Future longitudinal studies are needed to assess the predictive value of SPECT-identified rCBF lesions.[191] Some cases of con-

genital dysphagia have been associated with perfusion defects of language areas in the brain.[192,193]

BRAIN TUMORS

Using rCBF agents to evaluate meningiomas is of marginal utility. Standard static SPECT imaging of these tumors shows lesion-to-normal (L/N) tissue ratios of less than 1. Dynamic SPECT systems using early acquisitions, done at 2-minute intervals, show increased presence of IMP but not of HMPAO. The early IMP uptake appears proportional to the vascularity of the meningioma. Angioblastic tumors have L/N ratio measurements three times normal, while fibrotic meningiomas have a L/N ratio less-than or equal to 1. This is not surprising, considering the data from contrast-enhanced computed tomography, magnetic resonance imaging, and angiography.[194,195]

Some data support the theory that GSH plays a role in trapping HMPAO inside the brain cell by showing that primary tumors of the brain take up HMPAO in proportion to their GSH content, which is variable within classes of tumors and within different areas of the same tumor. Consequently, HMPAO uptake measurements might gain some importance. A link between tumor resistance to cytoreductive chemotherapy and tumor GSH levels has been suggested. If this proves to be the case, then HMPAO SPECT studies might allow us to discrimi-

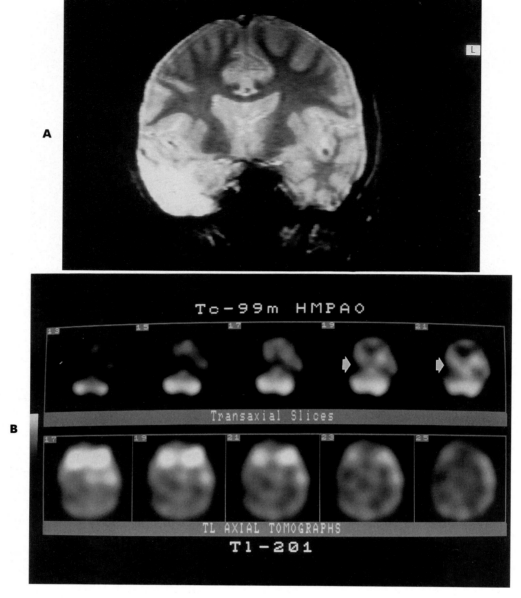

Fig. 6-21. A, Exclusion of recurrence after surgical resection and radiation therapy of a right temporal lobe primary brain tumor. The coronal MR image shows postsurgical changes in the right temporal lobe. **B,** Arrowheads mark decreased HMPAO uptake in the right temporal lobe on transaxial images. Matched ^{201}Tl slices show no uptake in this area.

nate between gliomas that will and will not respond to treatment.[196-198]

The use of ^{201}Tl SPECT to image brain primary and secondary tumors has been explored (Figs. 6-19 to 6-21, **A** and **B**). Cationic ^{201}Tl, like the iodinated CT contrast agents and the Gd-labeled MRI contrast agents, will not cross the intact BBB. Disruption of the BBB is not enough to localize ^{201}Tl, however. Viable tumor cells with an intact Na+/K+ ATP-ase pump are required. The vascular supply, disruption of the BBB, and the

metabolic rate of the tumor cell each play a part in the localization of ^{201}Tl. Higher grade malignancies and recurrent tumors after radiotherapy are readily detectable[199,200] (Fig. 6-21, **C**). Neurotoxicity from chemotherapy, like necrosis after radiotherapy, has been suggested to show no uptake on ^{201}Tl SPECT scans.[201] Preliminary work with ^{99m}Tc (2-methoxyisobutylisonitrile technetium [I]), which is used as a ^{99m}Tc-labeled myocardial perfusion agent under the trade name Cardiolite (Dupont, N. Billerica, MA), suggests

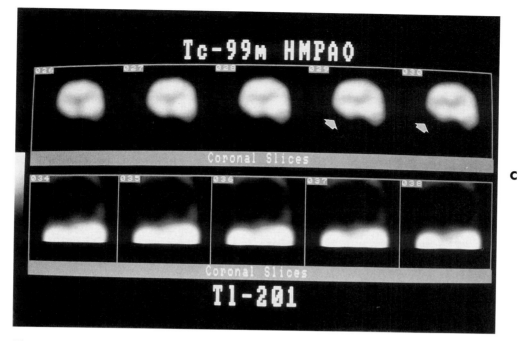

Fig. 6-21, cont'd. C, Matched HMPAO (*upper row*) and [201]Tl (*lower row*) coronal images show absence of HMPAO uptake in the temporal lobe (*arrowheads*) without a corresponding ^{201}Tl uptake.

that this agent may behave in a fashion similar to ^{201}Tl and thus could be useful for evaluating CNS tumors.[202]

• • •

Avenues are open for the application of brain SPECT imaging. The evaluation of dementia with rCBF agents awaits a clearer therapeutic strategy that includes better differentiation of the dementias. If a particularly expensive or risky treatment would work on Alzheimer's patients but not on multiinfarct patients, then it would be of value to do brain rCBF SPECT first.[203] If prospective tumor therapy requires pretreatment differentiation between high-grade and low-grade lesions, then the use of ^{201}Tl SPECT is in order. If a decision depends on differentiation between recurrent tumor and radiation necrosis, again ^{201}Tl is useful. Unfortunately, however, because neither of these conditions can be treated effectively in most cases, this technique is not currently of much value.

Subtypes of schizophrenia might be better delineated for selective therapy with rCBF measurements. Confusion now reigns in the discussion of the various rCBF findings in schizophrenic patients, which may indicate the complexity of the psychiatric diagnoses.

Functional measurements with stimulated and baseline rCBF SPECT may have investigational applications, particularly when these are done as "fusion" images with SPECT data painted on top of MRI or CT coregistered images.[204] The use of Diamox and baseline rCBF SPECT is slowly gaining a role in the understanding of cerebral perfusion dynamics.

Labeled-antibody SPECT (with implications for beta and gamma emitter therapy in some cases) is a wide-open field limited only by the nonspecific binding of some antibody preparations. With continuing investigation, more specific agents may become available. Labeled receptor agonists and antagonists are another avenue of research that should keep radiochemists busy for decades. As some of these clinical, basic science, and chemistry problems are solved, the clinical SPECT camera will be waiting and widely available.

REFERENCES

1. Croft BY: History and coordinate system in single-photon emission computed tomography, Chicago, 1986, Year Book.
2. Kuhl DE, Edwards RQ: Image separation radioisotope scanning, Radiology 80:653-662, 1963.
3. Kuhl DE, Edwards RQ: Cylindrical and section radioisotope scanning of the liver and brain, Radiology 83:926-936, 1964.
4. Patton JA, Brill AB, Erickson JJ et al: A new approach to the mapping of thee-dimensional radionuclide distributions, J Nucl Med 10:363, 1969.
5. Keyes, JW et al: The Humongotron—a scintillation-camera transaxial tomograph, J Nucl Med 18:381-387, 1977.

6. Heller SL, Goodwin PN: SPECT instrumentation: performance, lesion detection, and recent innovations, Semin Nucl Med 18:184-199, 1987.

7. Goodwin PN: Recent developments in instrumentation for emission computed tomography, Semin Nucl Med 10:322-334, 1980.

8. Esser PD: Improvements in SPECT technology for cerebral imaging, Semin Nucl Med 15:335-346, 1985.

9. Cerqueira MD, Matsuoka D, Ritchie JL, Harp GD: The influence of collimators on SPECT center of rotation measurements: artifact generation and acceptance testing, J Nucl Med 29:1393-1397, 1988.

10. Croft BY: Instrumentation and computers for brain single photon emission computed tomography, Clin Nucl Med 20:281-289, 1990.

11. Larsson SS, Bergstrand G, Befgstedt H: A specially designed cut-off gamma camera for high spatial resolution SPECT of the head, J Nucl Med 25:1023-1030, 1984.

12. Polak JF, Holman BL, Moretti JL et al: I-123 HIPDM brain imaging with a rotating gamma camera and slant-hole collimators, J Nucl Med 25:495-498, 1984.

13. Jaszczak RJ, Greer KL, Coleman RE: SPECT using a specially designed cone beam collimator, J Nucl Med 29:1398-1405, 1988.

14. Genna S, Smith AP: The development of ASPECT, an annular single crystal brain camera for high efficiency SPECT, IEEE Trans Nucl Sci NS-35:654-658, 1988.

15. Holman BL, Carvalho PA, Zimmerman RE et al: Brain perfusion SPECT using an annular single crystal camera: initial clinical experience, J Nucl Med 31:1456-1461, 1990.

16. Jaszczak RJ, Chang LT, Stein NA et al: Whole-body single photon emission computed tomography using dual, large-field-of-view scintillaton cameras, Phys Med Biol 24:1184-1191, 1986.

17. Lim Y, Gottschalk S, Walker R et al: Triangular SPECT system for 3-D total organ volume imaging: design concept and preliminary results, IEEE Trans Nucl Sci NS-32:741-747, 1985.

18. Kimura K, Hawhikawa K, Etani H et al: A new apparatus for brain imaging: four-head rotating gamma camera single-photon emission computed tomograph, J Nucl Med 31:603-609, 1990.

19. Rowe RK, Aarsvold JN, Barrett HH et al: A stationary hemispherical SPECT imager for three-dimensional brain imaging, J Nucl Med 34:474-480, 1993.

20. Jaszczak RJ, Gloyd CE, Coleman RE: Scatter compensation techniques for SPECT, IEEE Trans Nucl Sci NS-32:786-793, 1985.

21. Oppenheim BE: Scatter correction for SPECT, J Nucl Med 25:928-929, 1984.

22. Koral KF, Wang X, Rogers WL et al: SPECT Compton-scattering correction by analysis of energy spectra, J Nucl Med 29:195-202, 1988.

23. Koral KF, Swailem FM, Buchbinder S et al: SPECT dual-energy-window Compton correction: scatter multiplier required for quantification, J Nucl Med 31:90-98, 1990.

24. Macey DJ, DeNardo GL, Denardo SJ: Comparison of three boundary detection methods for SPECT using Compton scattered photons, J Nucl Med 29:203-207, 1988.

25. Kemp BJ, Prato FS, Dean GW et al: Correction for attenuation in technetium-99m-HMPAO SPECT brain imaging, J Nucl Med 33:1875-1880, 1992.

26. Kim HJ, Zeeberg BR, Fahey FH et al: Three-dimensional SPECT simulations of a complex three-dimensional mathematical brain model and measurements of three-dimensional physical brain phantom, J Nucl Med 32:1923-1930, 1991.

27. Kim HJ, Zeeberg BR, Reba RC: Compensation for three-dimensional detector response, attenuation and scatter in SPECT grey matter imaging using an interative reconstruction algorithm which incorporates a high-resolution anatomical image, J Nucl Med 33:1225-1234, 1992.

28. Moore SC, Kijewski MF, Muller SP, Holman BL: SPECT image noise power: effects of nonstationary projection noise and attenuation compensation, J Nucl Med 29:1704-1709, 1988.

29. Parker JA: Quantitative SPECT: basic theoretical considerations, Semin Nucl Med 19:3-12, 1989.

30. Junck L, Moen JG, Hutchins GD et al: Correlation methods for centering, rotation, and alignment of functional brain images, J Nucl Med 31:1220-1276, 1990.

31. Hooper HR, Alexander JM, Lentle BC et al: Interactive three-dimensional region of interest analysis of HMPAO SPECT brain studies, J Nucl Med 31:2046-2051, 1990.

32. Honda N, Machida K, Mamiya T et al: Value of three-dimensional surface display of brain perfusion imaging: comparison with tomographic imaging, Clin Nucl Med 17:106-109, 1992.

33. Ell PJ, Jarritt PH, Costa DC et al. Functional imaging of the brain, Semin Nucl Med 17:214-229, 1987.

34. Conn HL: Measurement of organ blood flow without blood sampling, J Clin Invest 34:916-917, 1955.

35. Mallett BL, Veall N: The measurement of regional cerebral clearance rates in man using xenon-133 inhalation of extra-cranial recording, Clin Sci 29:179-191, 1965.

36. Obrist WD, Thompson HK, King CD et al: Determination of regional cerebral blood flow by inhalation of xenon-133, Circ Res 20:124-135, 1967.

37. Obrist WD, Thompson HK, Wang HS et al: Regional cerebral blood flow estimated by xenon-133 inhalation, Stroke 6:245-256, 1975.

38. Rezai K, Kirchner PT, Armstrong C et al: Validation studies for brain blood flow assessment by radioxenon tomography, J Nucl Med 29:348-355, 1988.

39. Hill TC, Holman L, Lovett R et al: Initial experience with SPECT (single photon emission computerized tomography) of the brain using N-isopropyl-(I-123)-p-iodoamphetamine: concise communication, J Nucl Med 23:191-195, 1982.

40. Hill TC, Magistretti PL, Holman BL et al: Assessment of regional blood flow (rCBF) in stroke using SPECT and N-isopropyl-(I-123)-p-iodoamphetamine (IMP), Stroke 15:40-45, 1984.

41. Magistretti PL, Uren RF, Royal HD et al: N-isopropyl-^{123}I-p-iodoamphetamine imaging in epilepsy. In Magistretti PL: Functional radionuclide imaging of the brain. New York, 1983, Raven Press, pp 247-251.

42. Gemell HG, Sharp PF, Besson JAO et al: Single photon emission tomography with ^{123}I-isopropyl-amphetamine in Alzheimer's disease and multi-infarct dementia, Lancet ii:1348, 1984.

43. Kuhl DE, Bariio JR, Huang SC et al: Quantifying local cerebral blood flow by N-isopropyl-p-^{123}I-iodoamphetamine (IMP) tomography, J Nucl Med 23:196-203, 1982.

44. Lassen NA, Henriksen L, Holm S et al: Cerebral blood-flow tomography: xenon-133 compared with isopropyl-amphet-amine-iodine-123: concise communication, J Nucl Med 24:17-21, 1983.

45. Winchell HS, Horst WD, Braun L et al: N-isopropyl-^{123}I-p-iodoamphetamine: single-pass brain uptake and washout; binding to brain synaptosomes; and location in dog and monkey brain, J Nucl Med 21:947-952, 1980.

46. Lear JL, Ackermann RF, Kameyama M et al: Evaluation of [123]isopropyliodoamphetamine as a tracer of local cerebral blood flow using direct autoradiographic comparison, J Cerebr Blood Flow Metab 2:179-185, 1982.

47. Nishizawa S, Tanada S, Yonekura Y et al: Regional dynamics of N-isopropyl-(^{123}I)p-iodo-amphetamine in human brain, J Nucl Med 30:150-156, 1989.

48. Greenburg JH, Kusher M, Rango M et al: Validation studies of

iodine-123-iodoamphetamine as a cerebral blood flow tracer using emission tomography, J Nucl Med 31:1364-1369, 1990.

49. Yonekura Y, Fujita T, Nishizawa S et al: Temporal changes in accumulation of N-isopropyl-p-iodoamphetamine in human brain: relation to lung clearance, J Nucl Med 30:1977-1981, 1989.

50. Lear JL: Quantitative local cerebral blood flow measurements with technetium-99m HM-PAO: evaluation using multiple radionuclide digital quantitative autoradiography, J Nucl Med 29:1387-1392, 1988.

51. Hung JC, Corlija M, Volkert WA, Holmes RA: Kinetic analysis of technetium-99m d,l-HM-PAO decomposition in aqueous media, J Nucl Med 29:1568-1576, 1988.

52. Fienstein-Jaffe I, Boazi M, Tor Y: Assessment of the purity of d,l HM-PAO from diastereomeric mixtures using NMR techniques, J Nucl Med 30:106-109, 1989.

53. Ballinger JR, Reid RH, Gulenchyn KY: Technetium-99m HM-PAO stereoisomers: differences in interactions with glutathione, J Nucl Med 29:1988-2000, 1988.

54. Gemmell HG, Evans NTS, Besson JAO et al: Regional cerebral blood flow imaging: a quantitative comparison of technetium-99m-HMPAO SPECT with $C^{15}O_2$ PET, J Nucl Med 31:1595-1600, 1990.

55. Ballinger JR, Gulenchyn KY, Reid RH: Radiopharmaceutical factors in the variable quality of [^{99m}]HM-PAO images of the brain, J Nucl Med 31:118-122, 1990.

56. Villanueva-Meyer J, Thompson D, Mena I, Marcus CS: Lacrimal gland dosimetry for the brain imaging agent technetium-99m-HMPAO, J Nucl Med 31:1237-1239, 1990.

57. Tubergen K, Corlija M, Volkert WA, Holmes BL: Sensitivity of technetium-99m-d,l-HMPAO to radiolysis in aqueous solutions, J Nucl Med 32:111-115, 1991.

58. Nakano S, Kinoshita K, Jinnouchi S, Hoshi H: Comparative study of regional cerebral blood flow images by SPECT using xenon-133, iodine-123 IMP, and technetium-99m HM-PAO, J Nucl Med 30:157-164, 1989.

59. Holman BL, Hellman RS, Goldsmith SJ et al: Biodistribution, dosimetry, and clinical evaluation of technetium-99m ethyl cyteinate dimer in normal subjects and in patients with chronic cerebral infarction, J Nucl Med 30:1018-1024, 1989.

60. Walovitch RC, Hill TC, Garrity ST et al: Characterization of technetium-99m-L,L-ECD for brain perfusion imaging, Part 1: Pharmacology of technetium-99m ECD in nonhuman primates, J Nucl Med 30:1892-1901, 1989.

61. Leveille J, Demonceau G, De Roo M et al: Characterization of technetium-99m-L,L-ECD for brain perfusion imaging, Part 2: Biodistribution and brain imaging in humans, J Nucl Med 30:1902-1910, 1989.

62. Leveille J, Demonceau G, Walovitch RC: Intrasubject comparison between technetium-99m-ECD and technetium-99m-HMPAO in healthy human subjects, J Nucl Med 33:480-484, 1992.

63. Narra RK, Nunn AD, Kuczynski BL et al: A neutral lipophylic technetium-99m complex for regional cerebral blood flow imaging, J Nucl Med 31:1370-1377, 1990.

64. Bossuyt A, Morgan GF, Deblaton M et al: Technetium-99m-MRP20, a potential brain perfusion agent: in vivo biodistribution and SPECT studies in normal male volunteers, J Nucl Med 32:399-403, 1991.

65. Taylor SF, Frey KA, Baldwin RM et al: Technetium-99m-N1-(2-mercapto-2-methylpropyl0-N2-(2-propargylthio-2-methylpropyl)-1,2-benzenediamine (T691): preclinical studies of a potential new tracer of regional cerebral perfusion, J Nucl Med 33:1836-1842, 1992.

66. Bruine JF, van Royen EA, Vyth A et al: Thallium-201 diethyldithocarbamate: an alternative to iodine-123 N-isopropyl-p-iodoamphetamine, J Nucl Med 26:925-930, 1985.

67. Di Rocco RJ, Silva DA, Kuczynski BL et al: The single-pass cerebral extraction and capillary permeability-surface area product of several putative cerebral blood flow imaging agents, J Nucl Med 34:641-648, 1993.

68. Ell PJ: Editorial: mapping cerebral blood flow, J Nucl Med 33:1843-1845, 1992.

69. Kung HF, Ohmomo Y, Kung MP: Current and future radiopharmaceuticals for brain imaging with single photon emission computed tomography, Semin Nucl Med 20:290-302, 1990.

70. Mozley PD, Zhu X, Kung HF et al: The dosimetry of iodine-123-labeled TISCH: a SPECT imaging agent for the D1 dopamine receptor, J Nucl Med 34:208-213, 1993.

71. Kessler RM, Ansari MS, de Paulis T et al: High affinity dopamine D2 receptor radioligands. 1. Regional rat brain distribution of iodinated benzamides, J Nucl Med 32:1593-1600, 1991.

72. Seibyl JP, Woods SW, Zoghbi SS et al: Dynamic SPECT imaging of dopamine D2 receptors in human subjects with iodine-123-IBZM, J Nucl Med 33:1964-1971, 1992.

73. Beer HF, Blauenstein PA, Hasler PH et al: In vitro and in vivo evaluation of iodine-123-Ro 16-0154: a new imaging agent for SPECT investigations of benzodiazepine receptors, J Nucl Med 31:1007-1014, 1990.

74. Innis RB, Al-Tikriti MS, Zoghbi SS et al: SPECT imaging of the benzodiazepine receptor: feasibility of in vivo potency measurements from stepwise displacement curves, J Nucl Med 32:1754-1761, 1991.

75. Chabriat H, Levasseur M, Vidailhet M et al: In-vivo SPECT imaging of D2 receptor with iodine-iodolisuride: results in supranuclear palsy, J Nucl Med 33:1481-1485, 1992.

76. Eckelman WC, Reba RC, Rzeszotarski WJ et al: External imaging of cerebral muscarinic acetylcholine receptors, Science 223:291-293, 1984.

77. Biersack HJ, Coenen HH, Stocklin G et al: Imaging of brain tumors with L-3-[^{123}I]iodo-alpha-methyl tyrosine and SPECT, J Nucl Med 30:110-112, 1989.

78. Langen KJ, Coenen HH, Roosen N et al: SPECT studies of brain tumors with L-3-[^{123}I] iodo-alpha-methyl tyrosine: comparison with PET, ^{124}IMT and first clinical results, J Nucl Med 31:281-286, 1990.

79. Kawai K, Fujibayashi Y, Saji H et al: A strategy for the study of cerebral amino acid transport using iodine-123-labeled amino acid radiopharmaceutical: 3-iodo-alpha-methyl-L-tyrosine, J Nucl Med 32:819-824, 1991.

80. Langen KJ, Roosen N, Coenen HH et al: Brain and brain tumor uptake of L-3-[^{123}I]iodo-alpha-methyl tyrosine: competition with natural L-amino acids, J Nucl Med 32:1225-1228, 1991.

81. Oldendorf WH: Saturation of amino acid uptake by human brain tumor demonstrated by SPECT (editorial), J Nucl Med 32:1229-1230, 1991.

82. Ell PJ: Brain tumor uptake of iodo-alpha-methyl-tyrosine (letter to the editor), J Nucl Med 32:2193, 1991.

83. TenKate CI, Fischman AJ, Wilkinson RA et al: ^{99m}Tc-glucaric acid: a glucose analog, Eur J Nucl Med 31:451, 1990.

84. Yaoita H, Uehara T, Brownell AL et al: Localization of technetium-99m-glucarage in zones of acute cerebral injury, J Nucl Med 32:272-278, 1991.

85. Majocha RE, Reno JM, Friedland RP et al: Development of a monoclonal antibody specific for beta/A4 amyloid in Alzheimer's disease brain for application to in vivo imaging of amyloid angiopathy, J Nucl Med 33:2184-2189, 1992.

86. Kalofonos HP, Pawlikowska TR, Hemingway A et al: Antibody guided diagnosis and therapy of brain gliomas using radiolabeled monoclonal antibodies against epidermal growth factor receptor and placental alkaline phosphatase, J Nucl Med 30:1636-1645, 1989.

87. Schold SC, Zalutsky MR, Coleman RE et al: Distribution and dosimetry of I-123-labeled monoclonal antibody 81C6 in patients with anaplastic glioma, Invest Radiol 28:488-496, 1993.

88. Oshima M, Tadokoro M, Sakuma S: Comparison of ^{99m}Tc HMPAO fast SPECT with ^{99m}Tc HMPAO conventional SPECT in patients with acute stroke, Clin Nucl Med 17:18-22, 1992.

89. Helman RS, Tikofsky RS: An overview of the contribution of regional cerebral blood flow studies in cerebrovascular disease: is there a role for single photon emission computed tomography? Semin Nucl Med 20:303-324, 1990.

90. Mountz JM, Modell JG, Foster NL et al: Prognostication of recovery following stroke using the comparison of CT and technetium-99m HM-PAO SPECT, J Nucl Med 31:61-66, 1990.

91. Limburg M, van Royen EA, Hijdra A, Verbeeten B: rCBF-SPECT in brain infarction: when does it predict outcome? J Nucl Med 32:382-387, 1991.

92. Oshima M, Tadokoro R, Makino N, Sakuma S: Role of fast data acquisition method with ^{99m}Tc HMPAO brain SPECT in patients with acute stroke, Clin Nucl Med 15:172-174, 1990.

93. Isaka Y, Iiji O, Ashida K et al: Cerebral blood flow and magnetic resonance imaging in locked-in syndrome, J Nucl Med 34:291-293, 1993.

94. Yamauchi H, Fukuyama H, Yamaguchi S et al: Crossed cerebellar hypoperfusion in unilateral major cerebral artery occlusive disorders, J Nucl Med 33:1632-1636, 1992.

95. Takeshita G, Maeda H, Nakane K et al: Quantitative measurement of regional cerebral blood flow using N-isopropyl-(iodine-123-p-iodoamphetamine and single-photon emission computed tomography, J Nucl Med 33:1741-1749, 1992.

96. Pupi A, De Cristofaro MTR, Bacciottini L et al: An analysis of the arterial input curve for technetium-99m-HMPAO: quantification of rCBF using single-photon emission computed tomography, J Nucl Med 32:1501-1506, 1991.

97. Rattner Z, Smith EO, Woods S et al: Toward absolute quantitation of cerebral blood flow using technetium-99m-HMPAO and a single scan (editorial), J Nucl Med 32:1506-1507, 1991.

98. Nakano S, Kinoshita K, Jinnouchi S et al: Critical cerebral blood flow thresholds studied by SPECT using xenon-133 and iodine-123 iodoamphetamine, J Nucl Med 30:337-342, 1989.

99. Devous MD, Payne JK, Lowe JL, Leroy RF: Comparison of technetium-99m-ECD to xenon-133 SPECT in normal controls and in patients with mild to moderate regional cerebral blood flow abnormalities, J Nucl Med 34:754-761, 1993.

100. Soucy JP, McNamara D, Mohr G et al: Evaluation of vasospasm secondary to subarachnoid hemorrhage with technetium-99m-hexamethyl-propyleneamine oxime (HM-PAO) tomoscintigraphy, J Nucl Med 31:972-977, 1990.

101. Lewis DH, Eskridge JM, Newell DW et al: Brain SPECT and the effect of cerebral angioplasty in delayed ischemia due to vasospasm, J Nucl Med 33:1789-1796, 1992.

102. Ramasy SC, Yeats MG, Lord RS et al: Use of technetium-HMPAO to demonstrate changes in cerebral blood flow reserve following carotid endarterectomy, J Nucl Med 32:1382-1386, 1991.

103. Maurer AH, Siegel JA, Comerota AJ et al: SPECT quantification of cerebral ischemia before and after carotid endarterectomy, J Nucl Med 31:1412-1420, 1990.

104. Ohashhi K, Fernancez-Ulloa M, Hall LC: SPECT, magnetic resonance and angiographic features in a moyamoya patient before and after external-to-internal carotid artery bypass, J Nucl Med 33:1692-1695, 1992.

105. Abdel-Dayem HM, Sadek SA, Kouris K et al: Changes in cerebral perfusion after acute head injury: comparison of CT with ^{99m}Tc-HM-PAO SPECT, Radiology 165:221-226, 1987.

106. Roper SN, Mena I, King WA et al: An analysis of cerebral blood flow in acute closed-head injury using technetium-99m-HMPAO SPECT and computed tomography, J Nucl Med 32:1684-1687, 1991.

107. Coupland D, Lentle B: Bilateral subdural hematomas diagnosed with technetium-99m-HMPAO brain SPECT, J Nucl Med 32:1915-1917, 1991.

108. Isaka Y, Imaizumi M, Itoi Y et al: Cerebral blood flow imaging with technetium-99m-HMPAO SPECT in a patient with chronic subdural hematoma: relationship with neuropsychological test, J Nucl Med 33:246-248, 1992.

109. Provenzale J: The current role of SPECT in imaging subdural hematoma (editorial), J Nucl Med 33:248-250, 1992.

110. Hayashida K, Nishimura T, Imakita S, Uehara T: Filling out phenomenon with technetium-99m HMPAO brain SPECT at the site of mild cerebral ischemia, J Nucl Med 30:591-598, 1989.

111. Matsuda H, Higashi S, Asli IN et al: Evaluation of cerebral collateral circulation by technetium-99m HM-PAO brain SPECT during Matas test: report of three cases, J Nucl Med 29:1724-1729, 1988.

112. Palestro CJ, Sen C, Muzinic M et al: Assessing collateral cerebral perfusion with technetium-99m-HMPAO SPECT during temporary internal carotid artery occlusion, J Nucl Med 34:1235-1238, 1993.

113. Mathews D, Walker BS, Purdy PD et al: Brain blood flow SPECT in temporary balloon occlusion of CAROTID and intracerebral arteries, J Nucl Med 34:1239-1243, 1993.

114. Askienazy S, Lebtachi R, Meder JF: SPECT HMPAO and balloon test occlusion: interest in predicting tolerance prior to permanent cerebral artery occlusion (editorial), J Nucl Med 34:1243-1245, 1993.

115. Jeffery PJ, Monsein LH, Szabo Z et al: Mapping the distribution of amobarbital sodium in the intracarotid Wada test by use of ^{99m}Tc HMPAO with SPECT, Radiology 178:847-850, 1991.

116. Friedman D: Mapping distribution of amobarbital sodium in the intracarotid Wada test with use of ^{99m}Tc HMPAO with SPECT, Radiology 181:605, 1991.

117. Waltz AG: Effect of PaCO2 on blood flow and micro vasculature of ischemic and nonischemic cerebral cortex stroke, Stroke 1:27-37, 1970.

118. Eklof B, Lassen NA, Nilsson L et al: Blood flow and metabolic rate of oxygen in the cerebral cortex of the rat, Acta Physiol Scand 88:587-589, 1973.

119. Kontos HA, Wei EP: Oxygen-dependent mechanisms in cerebral autoregulation, Ann Biomed Eng 13:329-334, 1985.

120. Karatzas ND, Sfakianakis GN, Pappas D et al: Experimental increase in brain HIPDM uptake by hypercapnia, J Nucl Med 29:1675-1682, 1988.

121. Chollet F, Celsis P, Clanet M et al: SPECT study of cerebral blood flow reactivity after acetazolamide in patients with transient ischemic attacks, Stroke 20:458-464, 1989.

122. Vorstrup S, Boysen G, Brun B, Engell HC: Evaluation of the regional cerebral vasodilatory capacity before carotid endarterectomy by the acetazolamide test, Neurol Res 9:10-18, 1987.

123. Tikorsky RS, Hellman RS: Brain single photon emission computed tomography: new activation and intervention studies, Semin Nucl Med 21:40-57, 1991.

124. Bonte FJ, Devous MD, Reisch JS: The effect of acetazolamide on regional cerebral blood flow in normal human subjects as measured by single photon emission computed tomography, Invest Radiol 23:564-568, 1988.

125. Devous MD, Gassaway SK: Simultaneous SPECT imaging of ^{99m}Tc and I-123-labeled brain agents in patients using the PRISM™ scanner, J Nucl Med 31:877, 1990.

126. Devous MD, Payne JK, Lowe JL: Dual-isotope brain SPECT imaging with technetium-99m and iodine-123: clinical validation using xenon-133 SPECT, J Nucl Med 33:1919-1924, 1992.

127. Devous MD, Lowe JL, Payne JK: Dual-isotope brain SPECT imaging with technetium and iodine-123: validation by phantom studies, J Nucl Med 33:2030-2035, 1992.

128. Gibbs JM, Wise RJS, Leenders KL, Jones T: Evaluation of cerebral perfusion reserve in patients with carotid-artery occlusion, Lancet 8372:310-314, 1984.

129. Higano S, Uemura K, Inugamia et al: Studies on cerebral blood flow and oxygen metabolism in patients with chronically obstructive carotid disease, using positron emission tomography (PET)–in consideration of the indication for EC/IC bypass surgery, Jpn J Nucl Med 24:809-815, 1987.

130. Burt R, Rdddy R, Mock B et al: Acetazolamide enhancement of HIPDM brain blood flow distribution imaging, J Nucl Med 27:1627, 1986.

131. Burt RW, Witt RM, Cikrit D, Carter J: Increased brain retention of ^{99m}Tc HMPAO following acetazolamide administration, Clin Nucl Med 16:568-571, 1991.

132. Matsuda H, Higashi S, Kinuya K et al: SPECT evaluation of brain perfusion reserve by the acetazolamide test using ^{99m}Tc HMPAO, Clin Nucl Med 16:572-579, 1991.

133. Knapp WH, Kummer R, Kubler W: Imaging of cerebral blood flow-to-volume distribution using SPECT, J Nucl Med 27:465-470, 1986.

134. Buell U, Stirner H, Braun H et al: SPECT with ^{99m}Tc-HMPAO and ^{99m}Tc-pertechnetate to assess regional cerebral blood flow (rCBF) and blood volume (rCBV): preliminary results in cerebrovascular disease and interictal epilepsy, J Nucl Med Commun 8:519-524, 1987.

135. Kanno I, Lassen NA: Two methods for calculating regional cerebral blood flow from emission computed tomography of inert gas concentrations, J Comput Assist Tomogr 3:71-76, 1967.

136. Toyama H, Takeshita G, Takeuchi A et al: Cerebral hemodynamics in patients with chronic obstructive carotid disease by rCBF, rCBV, and rCBV/rCBF ratio using SPECT, J Nucl Med 31:55-60, 1990.

137. Reid RH, Gulenchyn KT, Ballinger JR: Clinical use of technetium-99m HM-PAO for determination of brain death, J Nucl Med 30:1621-1626, 1989.

138. Laurin NR, Driedger AA, Hurwitz GA et al: Cerebral perfusion imaging with technetium-99m HM-PAO in brain death and severe central nervous system injury, J Nucl Med 30:1627-1635, 1989.

139. Larar GN, Nagel JS: Technetium-99m-HMPAO cerebral perfusion scintigraphy: considerations for timely brain death declaration, J Nucl Med 33:2209-2213, 1992.

140. Hoch DB: Brain death: a diagnostic dilemma (editorial), J Nucl Med 33:2211-2213, 1992.

141. Wieler H, Marohl K, Kaiser KP et al: ^{99m}Tc HMPAO cerebral scintigraphy: a reliable, noninvasive method for determination of brain death, Clin Nucl Med 18:104-109, 1993.

142. Bonte FJ, Ross ED, Chehabi HH et al: SPECT study of regional cerebral blood flow in Alzheimer disease, J Comput Assist Tomogr 10:579-583, 1986.

143. Sharp P, Gemell H, Cherryman G et al: Application of iodine-123-labeled isopropylamphetamine imaging to the study of dementia, J Nucl Med 27:761-768, 1986.

144. Johnson KA, Mueller ST, Walshe TM et al: Cerebral perfusion imaging in Alzheimer's disease: use of SPECT and I-123 IMP, Arch Neurol 44:165-168, 1987.

145. Perani D, Di Piero V, Vallar G et al: Technetium-99m HM-PAO-SPECT study of regional cerebral perfusion in early Alzheimer's disease, J Nucl Med 29:1507-1514, 1988.

146. Komatani A, Yamaguchi K, Sugai Y et al: Assessment of demented patients by dynamic SPECT of inhaled xenon-133, J Nucl Med 29:1621-1626, 1988.

147. Bonte FJ, Horm J, Tintner R, Weiner MF: Single photon tomography in Alzheimer's disease and the dementias, Semin Nucl Med 20:342-352, 1990.

148. Holman BL, Johnson KA, Gerada B et al: The scintigraphic appearance of Alzheimer's disease: a prospective study using technetium-99m-HMPAO SPECT, J Nucl Med 33:181-185, 1992.

149. Bonte FJ, Tintner R, Weiner MF et al: Brain blood flow in the dementias: SPECT with histopathologic correlation, Radiology 186:361-365, 1993.

150. Kawabata K, Tachibana H, Sugita M et al: A comparative I-123 SPECT study in Binswanger's disease and Alzheimer's disease, Clin Nucl Med 18:329-336, 1993.

151. Ohnishi T, Hoshhi H, Jinnouchi S et al: The utility of cerebral blood flow imaging in patients with the unique syndrome of progressive dementia with motor neuron disease, J Nucl Med 30:688-691, 1990.

152. Johnson KA, Sperling RA, Holman BL et al: Cerebral perfusion in progressive supranuclear palsy, J Nucl Med 33:704-709, 1992.

153. Dierckx RA, Saerens J, De Deyn PP et al: Evolution of techetium-99m-HMPAO SPECT and brain mapping in a patient presenting with echolalia and palilalia, J Nucl Med 32:1619-1621, 1991.

154. Cohen MB, Lake RR, Graham LS et al: Quantitative iodine-123 IMP imaging of brain perfusion in schizophrenia, J Nucl Med 30:1616-1620, 1989.

155. Pohl P, Vogl G, Fill H et al: Single-photon emission computed tomography in AIDS dementia complex, J Nucl Med 29:1382-1386, 1988.

156. Kramer EL, Sanger JJ: Brain imaging in acquired immunodeficiency syndrome dementia complex, Semin Nucl Med 20:353-363, 1990.

157. Dinh YRT, Mamo H, Cervoni J et al: Disturbances in the cerebral perfusion of human immune deficiency virus-1 seropositive asymptomatic subjects: a quantitative tomography study of 18 cases, J Nucl Med 30:1601-1607, 1990.

158. Masdeu JC, Yudd A, Van Heertum RL et al: Single-photon emission computed tomography in human immunodeficiency virus encephalopathy: a preliminary report, J Nucl Med 32:1471-1475, 1991.

159. Holman BL, Garada B, Johnson KA et al: A comparison of brain perfusion SPECT in cocaine abuse and AIDS dementia complex, J Nucl Med 33:1312-1315, 1992.

160. Holman BL, Carvalho PA, Mendelson J et al: Brain perfusion is abnormal in cocaine-dependent polydrug users: a study using technetium-99m-HMPAO and ASPECT, J Nucl Med 32:1206-1210, 1991.

161. Holman BL, Mendelson J, Garada B et al: Regional cerebral blood flow improves with treatment in chronic cocaine polydrug users, J Nucl Med 34:723-727, 1993.

162. Devous MD, Leroy RF, Horman RW: Single photon emission computed tomography in epilepsy, Semin Nucl Med 20:325-341, 1990.

163. Rowe CC, Berkovic SF, Austin MC et al: Visual and quantitative analysis of interictal SPECT with technetium-99m-HMPAO in temporal lobe epilepsy, J Nucl Med 32:1688-1694, 1991.

164. Grunwald F, Durwen HF, Bockisch A et al: Technetium-99m-HMPAO brain SPECT in medically intractable temporal lobe epilepsy: a postoperative evaluation, J Nucl Med 32:388-394, 1991.

165. Ramsay SC, McLaughlin AF, Greenough R et al: Comparison of independent aura, ictal and interictal cerebral perfusion, J Nucl Med 33:438-440, 1992.

166. Shen W, Lee BI, Park HM et al: HIPDM-SPECT brain imaging in presurgical evaluation of patients with intractable seizures, J Nucl Med 31:1280-1284, 1990.

167. Newton MR, Austin MC, Chan JG et al: Ictal SPECT using technetium-99m-HMPAO: methods for rapid preparation and optimal deployment of tracer during spontaneous seizures, J Nucl Med 34:666-670, 1993.

168. Gzesh D, Goldstein S, Sperling MR: Complex partial epilepsy: the role of neuroimaging in localizing a seizure focus for surgical intervention, J Nucl Med 31:1839-1843, 1990.

169. Devous MD, Rush AJ, Schlesser MA et al: Single-photon tomographic determination of regional cerebral blood flow in psychiatric disorders, J Nucl Med 25:P57, 1984.

170. O'Connell RA, Van Heertum RL, Billick SB et al: Single photon emission computed tomography (SPECT) with ^{123}I IMP in the differential diagnosis of psychiatric disorders, J Neuropsychiatry 1:145-153, 1989.

171. Baxter LR: PET studies in cerebral function in major depression and obsessive-compulsive disorder: the emerging prefrontal cortex consensus, Ann Clin Psychiatry 3:103-109, 1991.

172. Devous MD: Imaging brain function by single-photon emission computed tomography. In Andreasen N, ed: Brain imaging applications in psychiatry, Washington, DC, 1988 American Psychiatric Press, pp 147-234.

173. Paulman RG, Devous MD, Gregory RR et al: Hypofrontality and cognitive impairment in schizophrenia: dynamic single-photon tomography and neuropsychological assessment of schizophrenic brain function, Biol Psychiatry 27:377-399, 1990.

174. Bajc M, Medved V, Basic M et al: Cerebral perfusion inhomogeneities in schizophrenia demonstrated with single-photon emission computed tomography and ^{99m}Tc-hexamethylpropyleneamine-oxime, Acta Psychiat Scand 80:427-433, 1989.

175. Geraud G, Arne-Bes MC, Guell A, Bes A: Reversibility of hemodynamic hypofrontality in schizophrenia, J Cereb Blood Flow Metab 7:9-12, 1987.

176. Devous MD, Paulman RG, Herman J et al: Single-photon tomography studies with schizophrenic patients, J Clin Exp Neuropsychol 10:321-322, 1988.

177. Alavi A, Hirsch LJ: Studies of the central nervous system disorders with single-photon emission computed tomography and positron emission tomography: evolution over the past two decades, Semin Nucl Med 21:58-81, 1992.

178. Van Heertum RL, O'Conell RA: Functional brain imaging in the evaluation of psychiatric illness, Semin Nucl Med 21:24-39, 1991.

179. Gur RE, Resnick SM, Gur RC: Laterality and frontality of cerebral blood flow and metabolism in schizophrenia: relationship to symptom specificity, Psychiatry Res 27:325-334, 1989.

180. Woods SW, Hegeman IM, Zubal IG et al: Visual stimulation increases technetium-99m-HMPAO distribution in human visual cortex, J Nucl Med 32:210-215, 1991.

181. Weber DA, Cabahug C, Klieger P et al: Effects of visual stimulation on the redistribution of iodine-123-IMP in the brain using SPECT imaging, J Nucl Med 32:1866-1872, 1991.

182. Ebmeier KP, Murray CL, Dougall NJ et al: Unilateral voluntary hand movement and regional cerebral uptake of technetium-99m-exametazime in human control subjects, J Nucl Med 33:1637-1641, 1992.

183. Meyer MA: Focal high uptake of HM-PAO in brain perfusion studies: a clue in the diagnosis of encephalitis, J Nucl Med 31:1094-1098, 1990.

184. Broich K, Horwich D, Alavi A: HMPAO-SPECT and MRI in acute disseminated encephalomyelitis, J Nucl Med 32:1897-1900, 1991.

185. Krishna L, Slizofski WJ, Katsetos CD et al: Abnormal intracerebral thallium localization in bacterial brain abscess, J Nucl Med 33:2017-2019, 1992.

186. Matsuda H, Gyobu T, Ii M, Hisada K: Iodine-123 iodoamphetamine brain scan in a patient with auditory hallucination, J Nucl Med 29:558-560, 1988.

187. Denays R, Van Pachterbeke T, Tondeur M et al: Brain single photon emission computed tomography in neonates, J Nucl Med 30:1337-1341, 1989.

188. Rubenstein M, Denays R, Ham HR et al: Functional imaging of brain maturation in humans using iodine-123 iodoamphetamine and SPECT, J Nucl Med 30:1982-1985, 1989.

189. Chiron C, Raynaud C, Maziere B et al: Changes in regional cerebral blood flow during brain maturation in children and adolescents, J Nucl Med 33:696-703, 1992.

190. Park CH, Spitzer AR, Desai HJ et al: Brain SPECT in neonates following extracorporeal membrane oxygenation: evaluation of technique and preliminary results, J Nucl Med 33:1943-1948, 1992.

191. Denays R, Tondeur M, Toppet V et al: Cerebral palsy: initial experience with ^{99m}Tc HMPAO SPECT of the brain, Radiology 175:111-116, 1990.

192. Denays R, Tondeur M, Foulon M et al: Regional brain blood flow in congenital dysphasia: studies with technetium-99m HM-PAO SPECT, J Nucl Med 30:1825-1829, 1989.

193. O'Tuama LA, Urion DK, Janicek MJ et al: Regional cerebral perfusion in Landau-Kleffner syndrome and related childhood aphasias, J Nucl Med 33:1758-1765, 1992.

194. Nakano S, Kinoshita K, Jinnouchi S et al: Dynamic SPECT with iodine-123 IMP in meningiomas, J Nucl Med 29:1627-1632, 1988.

195. Nakano S, Kinoshita K, Jinnouchi S et al: Dynamic SPECT with technetium-99m HM-PAO in meningiomas—a comparison with iodine-123 IMP, J Nucl Med 30:1101-1105, 1989.

196. Suess E, Malessa S, Ungersbock K et al: Technetium-99m-d,l-hexamethylpropyleneamine oxime (HMPAO) uptake and glutathione content in brain tumors, J Nucl Med 32:1675-1681, 1991.

197. Babich JW: Technetium-99m-HMPAO retention and the role of glutathione: the debate continues (editorial), J Nucl Med 32:1681-1683, 1991.

198. Cleto EM, Holmes RA, Singh A et al: Radiographic and neuro-SPECT imaging in an immature third ventricle teratoma: case report, J Nucl Med 33:435-437, 1992.

199. Carvalho PA, Schwartz RB, Alexander III E et al: Extracranial metastatic glioblastoma: appearance on thallium-201-chloride/technetium-99m-HMPAO SPECT images, J Nucl Med 32:322-324, 1991.

200. Kim KT, Black KL, Marciano D et al: Thallium-201 SPECT imaging of brain tumors: methods and results, J Nucl Med 31:965-969, 1990.

201. Even-Sapir E, Barnes DC, Llewellyn CG, Langley GR: Methotrexate-induced neurotoxicity: appearance on indium-111 white blood cells, gallium-67-citrate and thallium-201-chloride scintigraphy, J Nucl Med 34:1377-1381, 1993.

202. O'Tauma LA, Packard AB, Treves ST: SPECT imaging of pediatric brain tumor with hexakis (methoxyisobutylisonitrile) technetium (I), J Nucl Med 31:2040-2041, 1990.

203. Holman BL, Devous MD: Functional brain SPECT: the emergence of a powerful clinical method, J Nucl Med 33:1888-1904, 1992.

204. Holman BL, Zimmerman RE, Johnson KA et al: Computer-assisted superimposition of magnetic resonance and high-resolution technetium-99m-HMPAO and thallium-201 SPECT of the brain, J Nucl Med 32:1478-1484, 1991.

Functional Magnetic Resonance Imaging

John A. Sanders
William W. Orrison, Jr.

While MR imaging of anatomic structures has long been widely appreciated, the emergence of functional magnetic resonance imaging (FMRI) methods for localizing brain activity has significantly expanded the potential clinical role of MRI. Correspondingly, interactions between both clinical and research neuroscientists have also expanded. This new MRI technique produces images of activated brain regions by detecting the indirect effects of neural activity on local blood volume, flow, and oxygen saturation, and it is a promising new tool for furthering the understanding of the relationships among brain structure, function, and pathology. The noninvasive nature of this technology and the potentially easy integration of it into existing clinical practice make it an appealing technique for neuroradiologists, neurologists, and neurosurgeons.

Structural imaging techniques alone are not adequate for defining functional neuroanatomy. For example, a study by Sobel et al[1] found a large amount of observer variability in identifying the central sulcus from serial MR images of normal subjects. This identification becomes even more difficult when intracranial lesions are present, where mass effects and functional reorganizations occur. Techniques that can localize functional activity can provide clinically relevant information in cases of distorted or uncertain brain anatomy.

Functional imaging is also valuable in the surgical treatment of brain lesions. In many cases, the precise localization of essential functional cortex is required to minimize postoperative neurologic deficit, yet allow maximum removal of diseased or dysfunctional tissue. The preoperative identification of essential functional regions allows evaluation of both surgical feasibility and approach. The resulting clinical benefits include improved identification of candidates for successful surgery, improved outcome of those surgeries undertaken, and reduced overall treatment cost.

Presurgical localization of critical functional regions is an area where FMRI can be immediately clinically useful. FMRI offers the possibility of performing these localizations routinely and on existing rather than expensive new instrumentation. Image acquisition and processing times are similar to those for structural MRI examinations and allow the ready integration of FMRI into existing radiology practice. However, there are many other potential clinical applications of this technology, in areas ranging from characterizing particular pathologic conditions to furthering the understanding and treatment of more subtle psychologic or cognitive disorders.

An example of an FMRI image of right hand motor activation obtained using a standard clinical MR scanner is seen in Fig. 7-1. FMRI can directly identify functional regions at high resolution and directly provide an anatomic basis to these localizations since there is a natural correspondence of FMRI data with MRI structural images. FMRI can also readily identify multiple diffuse regions of activation without the modeling or registration complications of other functional imaging techniques. The noninvasive nature of this modality allows repeated examinations of the same patient so that it can also provide information on the posttreatment neural reorganization and recovery of function. While the initial reports have stimulated a great deal of activity in neuroscience research, the possibility of performing these measurements on routine clinical instrumentation offers a tremendous potential for clinical applications of noninvasive func-

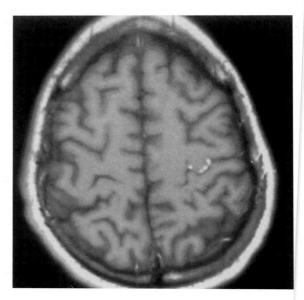

Fig. 7-1. Sample FMRI image of right-hand motor activation obtained on a standard clinical MRI instrument.

tional localization. Furthermore, this capability would come at little or no additional capital cost to medical centers already having a clinical MRI unit.

While FMRI is a promising technology, it is by no means an established technique. An exact understanding of the mechanisms involved, robust examination procedures, and application limitations have yet to be firmly established. Another significant question is whether the encouraging results obtained in normal persons can be routinely obtained in patients who have pathologic conditions or who are subject to the influence of pharmacologic interventions, which may alter the local blood flow and blood oxygenation responses that underlie the imaging contrast mechanism of current FMRI techniques. Also, there are still important instrumentation questions that will determine the extent of clinical availability and utility of FMRI. However, considering the large and increasing number of successful studies, none of these remaining problems appears to have the potential to severely disrupt the beneficial application of FMRI technology.

FMRI is a technique based on hemodynamic responses and is thus likely to overlap in application with alternative modalities such as SPECT or PET. Given its higher spatial and temporal resolution, lack of ionizing radiation, and lower cost, FMRI may become more widely used than these technologies for clinical functional brain mapping based on hemodynamic responses to neural activation. While FMRI applications may overlap with those of MEG and EEG, these modalities are based on very different mechanisms and have largely complementary temporal and localization characteristics. It is likely that as these functional imaging techniques mature, clinical circumstance will determine the use of one or more of these modalities.

HISTORY

Over the past few years, techniques have been developed that allow the formation of MR images that localize changes in tissue blood volume or deoxyhemoglobin levels. These changes have been directly correlated with evoked brain activity. These FMRI results are formed from the differences between acquisitions obtained during both stimulated and nonstimulated states. Although the initial reports employed consecutive bolus injections of paramagnetic contrast agents and utilized prototype imaging systems, more recent efforts have shown that it is possible to successfully obtain FMRI results using readily available clinical hardware and without contrast agents (Fig. 7-2).

As with any scientific advance, current progress rests on a base of previous work. In the case of FMRI, the base is particularly wide as a result of the many contributions from physics, chemistry, physiology, and radiology that were required to demonstrate that brain activation changes could be identified and localized by MR imaging techniques. While FMRI reflects the most recent in the continuing series of medical NMR advances, the fundamental concepts of NMR signal loss by proton diffusion in the presence of magnetic field gradients date from the late 1940s, and tissue flow and volume measurements using indicator dilution techniques were first described over 100 years ago.

One interpretation of the history of work that led to FMRI is that two related streams of work came together to provide MR functional images—namely, the development of NMR indicator dilution methods and the characterization of observations regarding image contrast changes with blood oxygenation. Progress in both of these areas was heavily dependent on advances in imaging hardware and sequence design and on the production and characterization of MRI contrast agents that were safe and effective for use in humans.

PET studies and, more recently, MR studies have shown that changes in neuronal activity are accompanied by local changes in cerebral blood flow (CBF),[2] cerebral blood volume (CBV),[3,4] and blood oxygenation.[3,5,6] FMRI techniques are based on imaging sequences sensitive to these changes.

Extending kinetic tracer techniques to MR through the use of bolus administrations of Gd-DTPA, Belliveau, Rosen, and coworkers[4,7,8] demonstrated that changes in regional CBV resulting from functional (i.e., visual) activation could be localized. This work relied on the ability to link MR image appearance and paramagnetic contrast agent concentration. This linkage was provided by the efforts of several groups

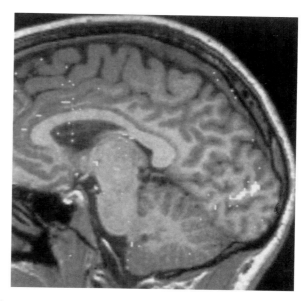

Fig. 7-2. FMRI results obtained on a clinical instrument without contrast agent injection. Location of detected activation above the calcarine fissure is expected from the applied lower visual field stimulation and is consistent with corresponding MEG localizations obtained from the same subject. The MEG source location is indicated as a green square in Fig. 7-101 in the color insert (p. 212). (Reproduced in full color in color insert.)

studying the characteristics of paramagnetic contrast agents and of water in tissue. Investigators discovered that a first-pass transit curve can be fitted to the intensities of a series of images taken during contrast agent injection, allowing estimation of contrast-accessible blood volume. Differences in computed CBV images obtained using bolus applications made during activated and nonactivated states provide an image that identifies the location of volume changes resulting from functional activity. The newly developed specialty echo planar imaging (EPI) systems were well suited to these bolus Gd-DTPA techniques because they could produce images at rates (40 to 100 msec each) adequate to precisely map the time course of the first pass of the injected contrast agent.

Unlike its clinical tissue T1 relaxation mechanism, the effect of Gd-DTPA exploited by these studies is the associated local changes in magnetic susceptibility, which lead to signal loss in microscopic regions of susceptibility-induced magnetic field inhomogeneity. It has been established in solution studies[9,10] that local susceptibility changes also result from the intrinsic paramagnetism of deoxyhemoglobin. Ogawa and Lee et al[11,12] showed that in high-field, high-resolution imaging, image contrast around vessels was related to the level of blood oxygenation. They further suggested that this effect could be used to monitor regional changes in oxygenation. Even though susceptibility effects are reduced at clinical imaging field strengths compared to effects seen with high-field, small-bore or

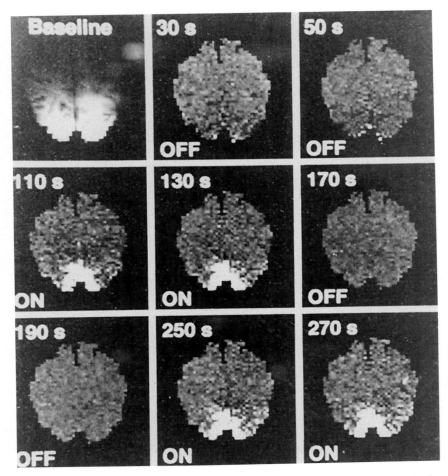

Fig. 7-3. Landmark demonstration of intrinsic deoxyhemoglobin contrast signal changes with photic stimulation. (From Kwong KK et al: Proc Natl Acad USA 89:5675, 1992.)

prototype whole body systems, procedures have been developed based on changes in the capillary and venous concentration of deoxyhemoglobin that enable the localization of function without exogenous contrast agents.

The effect of deoxyhemoglobin is also a local T2* effect that is modulated by local blood volume.[11-14] As hemoglobin becomes deoxygenated, it becomes paramagnetic and creates a magnetically inhomogeneous environment, leading to a local signal decrease. These inhomogeneous regions extend two (or more) times the radius beyond the confines of the vessel. Therefore the venous blood oxygenation will influence the signal of significantly more tissue than the approximately 2% to 4% content of the microvasculature.

Oxygen delivery, CBF, and CBV all increase with activation; however, because blood oxygen extraction increases only slightly,[3,4] the venous blood oxygenation increases and the concentration of deoxyhemoglobin decreases. The decrease in the tissue-blood susceptibility difference causes less intravoxel dephasing to occur, which in turn leads to more signal

observable on T2*- or T2-weighted images (Fig. 7-3).

Detection of these small signal changes (probably no more than 5% at 1.5 T)[9,14-16] associated with brain functional activity is technically demanding and had been thought to require specialized instrumentation, such as high-field or echo planar systems. However, several groups have demonstrated that MR functional images can be successfully obtained on clinical MR instruments without the need for the administration of contrast agents.

The administered contrast-based (Gd-DTPA) techniques continue to be developed and provide increasingly quantitative estimates of tissue perfusion. Dynamic imaging of bolus Gd administration is being extended to other areas, for example, assessing membrane permeabilities, determination of tissue structure (compartmentalization), and classification of tissue based on dynamic responses. The completely noninvasive oxygenation contrast methods are evolving rapidly and have an even greater potential to make brain functional mapping a part of routine radiologic practice.

The initial period of demonstration of basic FMRI capabilities has given way to more careful and applied studies. Functional responses to a wide range of mechanical and cognitive stimuli, previously examined by other modalities such as PET, have been demonstrated, and FMRI studies are now being focused toward fully characterizing the underlying mechanisms and addressing specific clinical and research questions.

Since FMRI is based on the combination of several technologies and since the mechanisms of image contrast changes with activation are still being determined, it is appropriate to review a range of relevant basic concepts before addressing the specifics of FMRI image formation and application.

BASIC PRINCIPLES

The order in which the following basic principles are presented somewhat reflects the historical development of the technology. The fundamental areas of indicator dilution methods and image appearance dependence on blood oxygenation, along with the basics of tissue blood flow and exchange, will be reviewed in the course of explaining how NMR measurements can be employed to detect changes in local blood volume, blood flow, blood oxygenation, and, ultimately, changes in brain activity.

This extensive background is necessary for two reasons:

1. The appearance of MR images reflects a complex relationship between the MR sequence design and the detailed physical, chemical, and physiologic nature of the tissue. This is particularly true for MR images representing functional activation.
2. The details characterizing this relationship for this relatively new technique are still under study, and several aspects of the information encoding have yet to be fully validated.

FMRI images are formed from the signal differences between activated and nonactivated image acquisitions. The basic mechanism for these signal differences is most often attributed to the diffusion of water in local inhomogeneous magnetic fields caused by susceptibility differences between tissues. These local inhomogeneous fields can be caused by either introduced (Gd-DTPA) or intrinsic (deoxyhemoglobin) contrast agents. These processes will be discussed in more detail.

Magnetic Susceptibility

The magnetic properties of materials can be classified into three categories: paramagnetic, diamagnetic, and ferromagnetic (or superparamagnetic). Paramagnetic and ferromagnetic materials have molecules with permanent magnetic dipole moments. These electronic magnetic moments are much larger (on the order of 700 times) than the nuclear magnetic moments that are the basis of NMR signals.

In paramagnetism, the individual magnetic moments do not interact strongly with one another and are normally randomly oriented, giving no net bulk magnetization. In the presence of an external magnetic field, the dipoles become partially aligned in the direction of the field and act to increase the magnetic field. However, for ordinary external field strengths, and like the weaker *nuclear* magnetic properties, only a very small fraction of the magnetic moments will be aligned with the field. Because thermal motion tends to randomize their orientation, the resulting contribution from these magnetic moments to the total magnetic field is very small. Elements having unpaired electrons, such as iron (Fe^{+2}), gadolinium (Gd^{+3}), and dysprosium (Dy^{+3}), show these paramagnetic characteristics, and their induced magnetization will tend to align with the external field.

Ferromagnetism is a much more complicated phenomenon. Because neighboring magnetic dipoles in a crystal structure ("domains") synergistically interact with each other, a high degree of alignment can result from even weak external magnetic fields. The aligned magnetic moments make a significant contribution to the total resulting field. When there is no external magnetic field, the intrinsic mutual alignment of the magnetic dipoles can lead to the ferromagnetic material having a bulk magnetic moment, as seen in the case of permanent magnets. If the size and nature of the domains are such that thermal motions disrupt this intrinsic alignment (in the absence of a magnetic field), the material is referred to as being superparamagnetic.

Diamagnetic materials have no permanent magnetic dipole moment. However, when an external magnetic field is applied, a magnetic moment is induced in the material and is oriented opposite the direction of the external field. This effect occurs in all materials but is small enough to be masked by any paramagnetic or ferromagnetic effects.

The direction of the induced magnetic field of the material is in the direction of the external magnetic field for paramagnetic and ferromagnetic materials, and it is oriented in the opposite direction for diamagnetic materials (Fig. 7-4). For paramagnetic and diamagnetic materials the amount of induced magnetization, M, is directly proportional to the intensity of the magnetic field, B, that it experiences, $M = \chi B$. The proportionality constant, χ, relating the applied magnetic field and the resulting magnetization is called the magnetic "susceptibility" of the material. Since M and B have the same dimensions, the susceptibility constant is dimensionless and will be positive for paramagnetic materials and negative for diamagnetic materials.

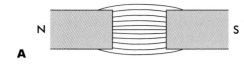

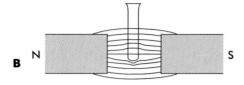

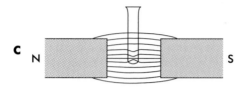

Fig. 7-4. Lines of force in **A**, vacuum; **B**, a diamagnetic substance; **C**, a paramagnetic substance.

As shown in Table 7-1, χ is typically much less than 1. Susceptibility is related to the magnetic permeability of the material, μ, by $\mu = (1 + \chi)\mu_o$. Because the susceptibility values are so small (compared to 1), the magnetic permeability of paramagnetic and diamagnetic materials is very close to that of free space, μ_o.

From the molecular point of view, χ is made up of two contributions: the inherent magnetic polarizability of the material and the alignment in the field of any molecules present having permanent magnetic moments. The alignment of permanent molecular moments is opposed by the randomizing effect of thermal vibration and motion.

Diffusion

Diffusion is central to many aspects of NMR and FMRI. In particular, the mechanism of NMR signal changes observable after brain activation is primarily considered to be the result of diffusion. There are several different ways to examine the diffusion of molecules, reflecting the general importance of this process. We will emphasize the so-called stochastic model of diffusion, in which the spatial drift of molecules is due to their kinetic motions, which are driven by ambient thermal energy.

The physical model of diffusion is one of successive small, random steps (Fig. 7-5). It is termed random since the size and direction of each step are unrelated to those of the preceding ones. Since any direction is equivalent, after a large number of individual steps there will, on average, be no net displacement of a molecule from its starting location. However, there will

Table 7-1. Magnetic susceptibility of some common substances

Substance	$\chi_m \times 10^{-8}*$ (per Kg at 18°C)
Ethanol	−1.00
Water	−0.91
Sulfur	−0.62
Gold	−0.19
Copper	−0.11
Tin	+0.03
Tungsten	+0.35
Aluminum	+0.81

From Beall PT, Amtey SR, Kasturi SR, editors: The NMR handbook for biomedical applications, New York, 1984, Pergamon Press.

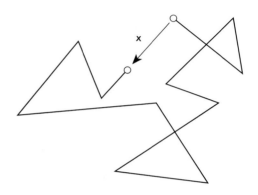

Fig. 7-5. Random walk pattern of diffusive movements.

be a region around the starting location in which the molecule can be expected at any one time (Fig. 7-6). After a large number of steps, the mean-squared (expected) displacement from the starting location, $\overline{\Delta x^2}$, is directly related to the mean-squared displacement, $\overline{d^2}$, of each step and the number of steps taken, N_s:

$$\overline{\Delta x^2} = N_s \, \overline{d^2} \qquad (7\text{-}1)$$

If τ is the average time between steps, then N_s is equal to the total diffusion time, t, divided by the step time, τ. Equation 7-1 can be rewritten as

$$\overline{\Delta x^2} = \left(\frac{\overline{d^2}}{\tau}\right) t = 2Dt \qquad (7\text{-}2)$$

This equation indicates that the mean-squared displacement of the molecule from its starting point is directly proportional to the length of diffusion time. The constant of proportionality, $D\ (= \overline{d^2}/2\tau)$, is termed the "free diffusion coefficient." This equation applies to the interdiffusion of molecules of a single type and can be measured experimentally by the use of NMR excitation or radioactive isotope labeling. A molecule will, as a result of its random movement, find itself

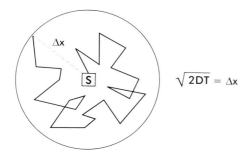

Fig. 7-6. On average, there will be no *net* displacement from the starting location but, over time, there will be an increasingly large region in which the molecule can be expected at any one time.

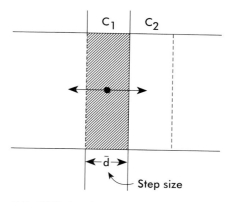

Fig. 7-7. Diffusion in a concentration gradient.

some distance, x, from its starting point after an elapsed amount of time, t. Because this is not a direct velocity but rather a molecular drift, x increases only as $\sqrt{t}$.

Diffusion in a concentration gradient. In order to understand how diffusion can also lead to net displacements, consider the one-dimensional situation illustrated in Fig. 7-7, where a gradient of concentration exists along a tube. During the time interval, τ, during which each molecule is expected to take a step of average size $\bar{d}$, one half of the molecules are expected to move left and one half will move right. This occurs for each location along the tube. This means that half of the number of molecules within a step-sized distance to an arbitrary plane (of area S) will cross the plane from left to right. That number of molecules is the volume times the concentration, C_1 (number per volume), and will be $\frac{1}{2}\bar{d}SC_1$. Similarly, the number crossing the same plane from right to left will be $\frac{1}{2}\bar{d}SC_2$. The net flux, J, or net movement across the plane (of area S) per time τ is the difference between these numbers.

$$J = \frac{\bar{d}}{2\tau} S (C_1 - C_2) \qquad (7\text{-}3)$$

The concentrations of the two regions located a distance $\bar{d}$ apart (in the x direction) can be related in terms of the concentration gradient, dC/dx, along the tube in that direction. For $C_1 > C_2$,

$$C_2 = C_1 - \left(\frac{dC}{dx}\right)\bar{d} \qquad (7\text{-}4)$$

Substituting this expression for the concentration C_2 into equation 7-3,

$$J = -S \left(\frac{\bar{d}^2}{2\tau}\right)\left(\frac{dC}{dx}\right) \qquad (7\text{-}5)$$

Noting that the diffusion coefficient, D, defined above

is equal to the first term in this equation, we can rewrite this equation to be:

$$J = -SD \frac{dC}{dx} \qquad (7\text{-}6)$$

This result is known as Fick's first law of diffusion and describes the fundamental phenomenon that diffusion acts to even out concentrations. Unless some opposing force is applied, a net flux or drift of molecules will result, moving molecules from the more concentrated to the more dilute solution. Even though it is typically the solvent (not solute), this process applies to water as well, and there will be an "osmotic" force moving water to lower concentrations (i.e., toward a more concentrated solute solution).

It also means that the concentration gradient represents (chemical) potential energy and provides the driving force for this process of net diffusive movement. By considering the concentration gradient as a thermodynamic force, one can derive the Stokes-Einstein equation:

$$D = \frac{RT}{N_{av}6\pi\eta a} \qquad (7\text{-}7)$$

relating D (diffusibility) to the molecular size, a, and the fluid viscosity, η. R is the ideal gas constant, N_{av} is Avogadro's number (6.022×10^{23}), and T is the temperature in degrees Kelvin.

Barriers to diffusion/permeability. Since diffusion acts to eliminate any concentration differences, there needs to be a mechanism by which living systems can maintain unequal chemical solutions. This is possible through the use of membrane barriers surrounding individual compartments (e.g., cells or organelles). If the membrane has a structure that inhibits free movement of molecules, then diffusion across the membrane is physically restricted.

Fick's first law describes the flux across some arbitrary plane at one instant in time. His second law of diffusion describes the situation of two solutions of different concentrations separated by a membrane of thickness Δx and surface area S, as shown in Fig. 7-8. In this case the flux across the membrane may be described by:

$$J = D_m S \frac{(C_1 - C_2)}{\Delta x} \quad (7\text{-}8)$$

where D_m is the membrane diffusion coefficient. In general, the value for D_m decreases with increasing molecular size. Since the thickness of the membrane may not be known, the membrane "permeability" is defined as:

$$P = \frac{D_m}{\Delta x} \quad (7\text{-}9)$$

Often the surface area of the membrane is not known or is difficult to determine. In these cases the combined PS product may be easier to measure experimentally.

Most biologic membranes are considered to be semipermeable membranes, meaning that they allow relatively free movement of water and small solute molecules but rapidly become completely impermeable to larger molecules or charged ions. This behavior is often characterized by the presence of a large number of small holes or pores in the membrane (Fig. 7-9). While the pores are larger than water molecules and allow them relatively free movement, they are too small for larger molecules to pass through.

Cerebral Circulation

The cerebral circulation has many specialized characteristics that differ from other organs. In particular, the blood-brain barrier helps to isolate and protect the brain from ionic changes and other stimuli. Larger arteries account for a relatively greater portion of vascular resistance in the brain than in other vascular beds, and cerebral vessels are very responsive to changes in arterial pressure, implying tight autoregulatory processes.[17] Cerebral vessels are also unusually responsive to chemical stimuli, and hypercapnic acidosis and hypoxia produce pronounced vasodilation.

Tissue structure. The structure at the tissue level can be represented by the basic model shown in Fig. 7-10, with the interstitial fluid (ISF) being the fluid external to the cells of the tissue. This space comprises from 4% to 12% of the tissue volume.[19] It can be argued that the rest of the circulatory system functions as plumbing necessary to provide oxygenated blood to, and remove waste from, the tissue capillary bed. Furthermore, the flow of plasma allows the maintenance of concentration gradients between the tissue compartments. The endothelial cells lining the capillary do more than just contain the blood; they regulate the transmembrane motions of all molecules and account for 95% of all transport exchange across the membrane.

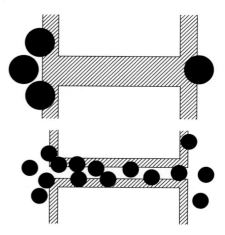

Fig. 7-9. Pore theory considers semipermeable membrane characteristics to be the result of physical obstruction of larger molecules. (From Curry Fitz-Roy E: Handbook of physiology, vol IV, Bethesda, MD, 1983, American Physiological Society, p 346.)

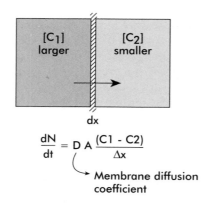

$$\frac{dN}{dt} = D\, A\, \frac{(C1 - C2)}{\Delta x}$$

Membrane diffusion coefficient

Fig. 7-8. Diffusion across a finite membrane separating two solutions of different concentrations.

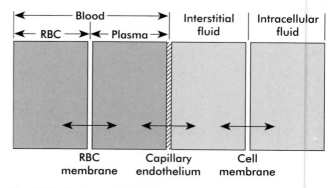

Fig. 7-10. Basic model of tissue organization. Exchange of substances occurs between compartments.

This membrane is often characterized as a molecular sieve — a porous structure generally with junctions between endothelial cells (Fig. 7-11). This structure allows the transmembrane movement of water and small solutes (up to approximately 68 kD) but is essentially impermeable to large molecules. In the absence of capillary flow (and when there is sufficient time for exchange across the BBB) the ISF will have approximately the same concentration of small solutes as plasma.

Vascular structure. As shown in Figs. 2-94, 2-95, and 2-98, there is a complex system of blood vessels supplying the needs of the brain. The brain is supplied primarily by two carotid and two vertebral arteries, with the internal carotid artery being the main source of cerebral blood flow (CBF) to the brain in humans. However, this is not necessarily the case in animal models that may be studied. The major arteries communicate with one another through the anastomoses that form the circle of Willis, but, under normal conditions, there is little mixing of blood flow from the major arteries.[17] The complex vascular supply to the brain can make it difficult to accurately measure CBF at this level since it may be difficult to separate blood flow to extracranial and intracranial compartments.

The brain is drained by two systems of veins. Blood from the cerebral cortex flows through veins on the surface of the brain, collecting into the venous sinuses. Blood from the basal areas collects into the deep sinus system, including the large vein of Galen and the straight sinus. Venous blood leaves the skull through the internal jugular and other veins, where there is some potential for mixing with veins draining extracranial areas.[17]

Fig. 7-12 depicts the variation in size and wall thickness of the various vascular components. Table 7-2 summarizes the physical characteristics of the different types of vessels. The elastic walls of the arterial system serve to smooth out the pulsatility of cardiac output to the point where, at the capillaries,

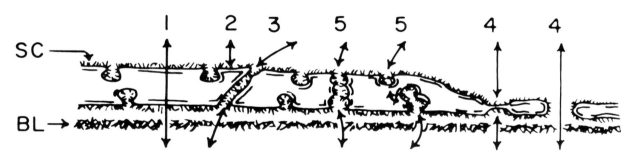

Fig. 7-11. Transport pathways in capillary endothelium. *1*, Endothelial cell pathway; *2*, lateral membrane diffusion pathway; *3*, intercellular junctions; *4*, endothelial cell fenestrae; *5*, endothelial cell vesicles. *BL*, Basal lamina; *SC*, cell surface coat. (Modified from Renkin[121]; in Curry Fitz-Roy E: Handbook of physiology, vol IV, Bethesda, MD, 1983, American Physiological Society, p 370.)

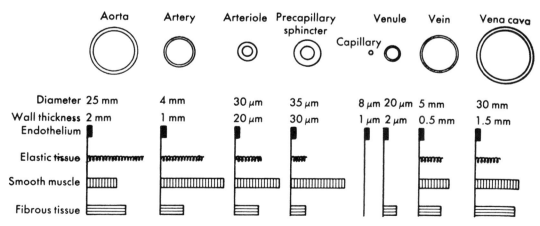

Fig. 7-12. Comparison of vessel size and construction. Figure is not drawn to scale because of the huge range in sizes between the aorta and the capillary vessels. (From Berne RM: Physiology, St Louis, 1983, Mosby.)

Table 7-2. Physical characteristics of the different vascular components

Type of vessel	Diameter (mm)	Number	Total cross-sectional area (mm²)	Length (mm)	Fraction of total volume (%)	Intravascular pressure (mm Hg)	Pressure gradient ΔP length (mm Hg/mm)
Aorta	10	1	0.8×10^2	4×10^2	2.0	100	0.0075
Large arteries	3	40	3×10^2	2×10^2	4.0	97	0.0215
Main artery branches	1	600	5×10^2	10^2	3.4	92.7	0.129
Terminal branches	0.6	1800	5×10^2	10	1.7	79.8	0.330
Small arteries	0.019	4×10^7	1.1×10^4	3.5	2.7	76.5	5.97
Arterioles	0.007	4×10^8	1.5×10^4	0.9	1.0	55.6	32.1
Capillaries	0.0037	1.8×10^9	1.8×10^4	0.2	0.3	25.1	89.6
Postcapillary venules	0.0073	5.8×10^9	2.5×10^5	0.2	3.6	4.5	1.90
Venules	0.021	1.2×10^9	3.7×10^5	0.1	25.6	4.1	0.3
Small veins	0.037	8×10^7	8×10^4	3.4	18.6	3.8	0.5
Main venous branches	2.4	600	2.7×10^3	10^2	18.6	2.1	0.004
Large veins	6.0	40	1.1×10^3	2×10^2	15.2	1.7	0.002
Vena cava	12.5	1	1.2×10^2	4×10^2	3.4	1.3	0.003

Data from Schmid-Schonbein (2).
From Johnson P: Peripheral circulation, New York, 1978, Wiley, p. 3.

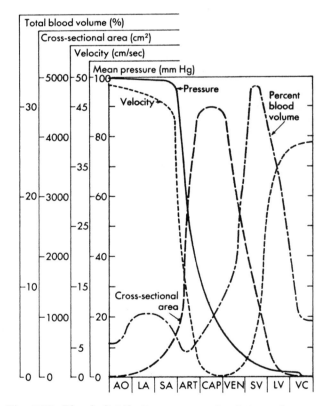

Fig. 7-13. Blood distribution among circulatory elements. *AO*, Aorta; *LA*, large arteries; *SA*, small arteries; *ART*, arterioles; *CAP*, capillaries; *VEN*, venules; *SV*, small veins; *LV*, large veins; *VC*, venae cavae. (From Berne RM: Physiology, St Louis, 1983, Mosby.)

the blood flow is relatively steady. The smaller arteries and arterioles serve as the resistance vessels of the system. Their cross- sectional diameter dynamically varies in order to regulate flow and pressure in the face of varying local demands. The capillaries are the exchange vessels, where the thin walls and large combined surface area allow ready exchange of substances with the tissue. Postcapillary venules and small veins have distensible walls and serve to contain the body blood reservoir. As diagramed in Fig. 7-13, most of the blood volume in the body at any one time is contained within the venous system distributed throughout the peripheral circulation.

Microvasculature. As shown schematically in Fig. 7-14, successive branching to the capillary level leads to a tremendous increase in surface area for tissue exchange. The diameter of the precapillary arteriole segments controls the blood flow through the capillaries, and these segments are the principal points of resistance supporting the blood pressure. The venous blood is maintained at relatively low pressures of 6 to 15 mm Hg.

The structure of the microcirculation in a tissue is distinctively characteristic of that tissue and varies among regions having specialized functionality. There can be flow heterogeneity within tissues, reflecting local metabolic demands or patterns of growth.[18] Intercapillary distances correlate with the metabolic activity of the tissue and vary from the dimensions of a single cell up to that of 10 cells. The fraction of blood in tissue provides an approximate estimate of the capillary density and, to some extent, the metabolic rate.[19] Given the variability and complexity of microvascular structure (Fig. 7-15), it is less surprising that morphologic descriptions and dimensions are generally provided only in approximate terms. Thus parameters used in FMRI modeling studies should be considered as being very approximate.

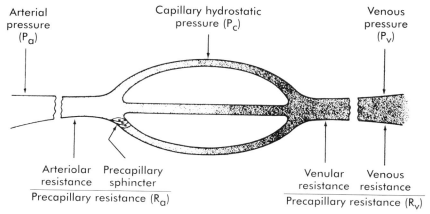

Fig. 7-14. Schematic model of the microvasculature. (From Berne RM: Physiology, St Louis, 1983, Mosby.)

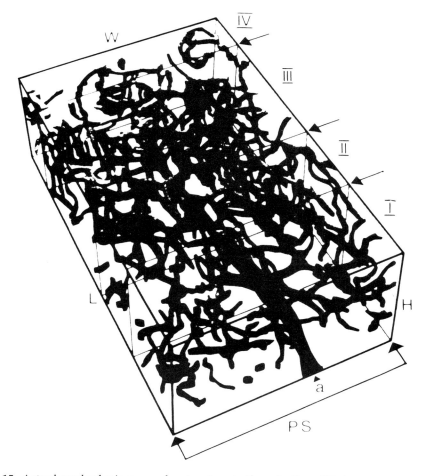

Fig. 7-15. Actual cerebral microvascular structure in the cat. (From Wiedeman MP: Handbook of physiology, vol IV, Bethesda, MD, 1983, American Physiological Society, p 311.)

The results reported by Pawlik et al[20] on microscopy of the cat cerebral cortex serve as a standard reference for information as to capillary morphology. The mean capillary diameter of 5.1 ± 0.84 μm is notably smaller than the average size of the red blood cells (RBCs) (Fig. 7-16), implying that they must deform for passage through the capillaries. In contrast to the parallel, evenly spaced capillaries often seen in heart and skeletal muscle beds, cerebral capillaries are short (with segment lengths ranging from 12 to 302 μm), tortuous, and intertwined with no evidence of a parallel arrangement. This supports the common modelling assumption of a random distribution of capillary orientation. The median intercapillary distance (24.2 μm) and the volume fraction of capillaries (2.1% ± 0.51%) vary among different regions in the brain. As a drawing of their observations suggests (Fig. 7-17), the actual brain capillary structure is quite different from the classic (Krogh) cylinder model.

Another standard reference,[21] using fluorescent (plasma) markers in quick-frozen and sectioned rat brain, determined an average capillary diameter of 6.1 ± 1.05 μm and capillary volume fractions that

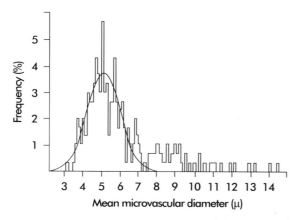

Fig. 7-16. Frequency distribution of microvascular mean diameters measured in cat cerebral cortex. Solid curve represents the maximum likelihood of normal distribution of intracortical capillary mean diameters. (From Pawlik G, Rackl A, Bing RJ: Brain Res 208:42, 1981.)

varied regionally from 4.2% to 7.8%. The relatively large number of capillaries within the volume of an imaging voxel (5700/mm^3) allows them to be considered on a statistical basis.

These studies are typical in that they assess microcirculatory morphology by anatomic dimensions and fractions rather than by effective or functional values.

Blood. Blood consists of a cellular component and a plasma component. The cellular component of blood contains erythrocytes (red blood cells or RBCs), various leukocytes (white blood cells), and platelets. RBCs contain hemoglobin (Hb) with bound oxygen or deoxyhemoglobin (dHb) without oxygen. RBCs are transported to tissues via the circulatory system and provide oxygen for tissue metabolism. The percentage of RBCs in blood is known as the hematocrit and is approximately 48% of blood in men and 42% of blood in women. RBCs are shaped like biconcave disks, having a diameter of 7 to 8 μm, a thickness of 2 μm, and a volume of approximately 85 μm^3. This, combined with deformation during transit through the smaller capillaries, indicates that spherical RBC models are only very approximate.

In the normal human adult, plasma makes up approximately 55% to 60% of blood. Plasma contains a huge number of dissolved substances including molecular oxygen (O_2), carbon dioxide (CO_2), nitrogen and nitrogen breakdown products, electrolytes, proteins, lipids, carbohydrates (e.g., glucose), amino acids, vitamins, and hormones. Plasma consists of approxi-

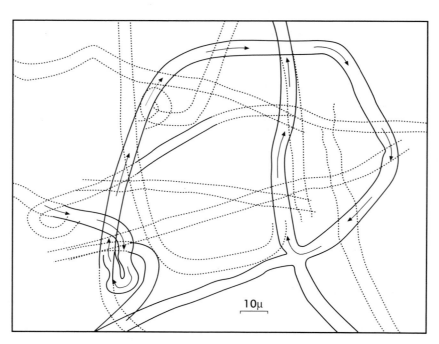

Fig. 7-17. Drawing of local capillary structure in the cat brain. (From Pawlik G, Rackl A, Bing RJ: Brain Res 208:42, 1981.)

mately 91% water and 7% protein, the bulk of which is primarily albumin, globulins, and fibrinogen.[22] In blood of normal hematocrit, the water content is approximately 80%,[23] with extracellular water (protons) being almost twice the intracellular content.[24]

Blood-brain barrier. The blood-brain barrier (BBB) is characterized by relatively tight junctions between the endothelial cells lining the microvasculature and minimal transmembrane transport by pinocytotic vesicles (temporary pores).[25-27] Therefore, there is virtually a continuous layer of cells separating the blood from brain parenchyma, and all solutes must cross the endothelial membrane. This effectively limits the transport of protein and polar substances out of blood and into the cerebral extravascular fluid, reducing any corresponding movement of water. However, specialized active transport mechanisms exist for the effective uptake of sugars, amino acids, and other metabolites. The BBB is absent in several areas of the brain, including area postrema, choroid plexus, pituitary gland, pituitary stalk, pineal gland, and some parts of the hypothalamus.

The transmembrane movement of water can occur by either diffusion (down concentration gradients) or by convection (bulk flow driven by hydrostatic pressure). In most tissue, the primary pathway of water movement between the plasma and the interstitium is through the cellular junctions or clefts. However, in brain, these junctions are not available and bulk water flow cannot readily occur. The presence of an intact blood-brain barrier results in a slow exchange of water between the extracellular and plasma spaces relative to that in other tissues.[19] In the occurrence of changes in hydrostatic pressure, the slowed transmembrane exchange causes the brain to shrink or swell more slowly than other tissues.

Intravascular water does not freely equilibrate with tissue water at normal perfusion flow rates. The exchange is also slow with respect to NMR measurement times.[28,29] Because the capillary space exchanges water with tissue so slowly (exchange times are ~500 ms),[28,29] the vascular water can be considered to be isolated from the tissue volume during a typical TE (≤ 100 msec).

Even though the exchange of water between the intravascular compartment and tissue is slow in the brain, the RBC intracellular/extracellular water exchange appears to be relatively fast, on the order of 8 msec. In addition, extracellular water rapidly exchanges with neuronal intracellular water.[23] This implies that cell membranes impose only minor restrictions on water movement[30] and that the water in both compartments separated by the BBB is well mixed.

A number of perturbations are known to elevate

BBB permeability. Among those that irreversibly open the endothelial structure are wounds, freeze lesions, irradiation, some tumors, and heavy metal poisoning. Reversible increases in BBB permeability can be produced by osmotic imbalances, hypertension, seizures, ischemia, and hypercapnia.[31] The resulting increase in transmembrane water permeability typically leads to water transfer from intravascular to extravascular spaces, and cerebral edema results.

Hemodynamics

The brain consists of a large number of specialized regions, with an extensive range of primary functional activities including local neuronal activity, afferent and efferent connections, neurotransmitter production and processing, endocrine activity, and glucose uptake and utilization. It is to be expected that such diversity will be similarly reflected in the characteristics of the local blood flow in these regions. Detailed analysis of local flow patterns in a rat model[32] revealed that the local blood flow varies 18-fold between different brain regions and was particularly high in neuroendocrine structures. Marked differences were found even within some structures.

Local cerebral blood flow measured in animals is on the order of 1 ml/g/min. The most commonly accepted explanation for regional variations in blood flow is dissimilarities in the number of capillaries in the tissue, rather than differences in capillary flow velocities.[31] The capillary density in brain is relatively high, especially in gray matter, and the ratio of capillary density in gray and white matter is approximately 2 : 1 to 3 : 1.[33] This may also be reflected in the difference between gray (81.9%) and white (71.6%) matter water content.[34] However, from functional measurements, the CBF gray:white ratio is 4 : 1, almost twice that of the CBV ratio of 2 : 1, indicating that white matter transit times are longer than those of gray matter.[35]

Flow rates within capillaries are on the order of 0.5 to 3.0 mm/sec[20] (Fig. 7-18). The mean transit times of blood through the parenchymal microvessels is approximately 0.3 to 0.6 sec for gray matter and 0.6 to 0.9 sec for white matter,[36] which is much longer than the times required for RBC/plasma exchange. However, there seems to be some ambiguity whether flow in individual capillaries is continuous (although slowed during rest) or intermittent. Several reports using intravital preparations indicate that flow stops periodically as a consequence of the vasomotor activity of the arterioles.[21,37,38] However, with invasive preparations there may be inflammatory reactions and some degree of vasodilatory effect. Other microscopic studies suggest that slow, continuous flow in capillaries is the more typical behavior,[39] with fluctuating[40] or periodic on/off patterns seen less frequently.[20] The intermittent flow duty cycle and/or the continuous

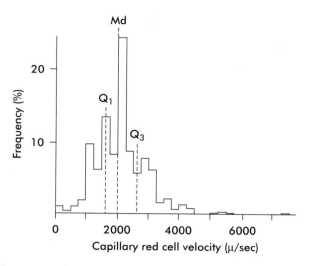

Fig. 7-18. Relative frequency of red cell velocities in cat intracortical capillaries (mean length 188 μm, mean diameter 5.7 μm), recorded in periods of 2.5 msec for 2 seconds. Median (*Md*) and first and third quartile (*Q1* and *Q3*, respectively) are indicated by broken lines. Mean velocity is 2103 ± 770 μm/sec. (From Pawlik G, Rackl A, Bing RJ: Brain Res 208:42, 1981.)

flow rates are generally considered to vary in accordance with metabolic demands and metabolite levels in the local vicinity of the capillary. The primary mechanism for blood flow change appears to be altered vessel flow velocity rather than vessel density (recruitment).[23] This implies that the mean transit time decreases with conditions that lead to increased blood flow.

The hematocrit within parenchymal microvessels is generally 45% to 75% of the arterial hematocrit, suggesting that RBCs move more rapidly through the brain microvessels than do plasma and its dissolved substances.[31] In addition, at capillary branching points, the branch with a faster stream will receive most of the RBCs.[40] This helps to explain the nonuniformity of hematocrit distribution in the capillaries.

Flow Regulation and Neural Control

The brain requires a constant delivery of flow regardless of the demands imposed by the rest of the body.[41] The circulation of blood carries out a variety of functions, including delivery of nutrients to the tissue, removal of waste products, and maintenance of tissue fluid volume. In keeping with this range of activities, the blood flow in some organs is much greater than that required to meet local nutritional needs. Thus it seems inappropriate to assume that blood flow regulatory mechanisms are geared entirely to satisfying tissue nutritional requirements.[39]

The arteries on the brain surface and larger arterioles inside the brain tissue are supplied by a network of sympathetic and parasympathetic nerve fibers.

Maximal stimulation of sympathetic nerves reduces CBF by 5% to 10%,[41-43] and a similar level of vasodilator response to parasympathetic stimulation has also been shown.[41,44] These results indicate that nervous control of cerebral blood flow is much less than for most other tissues. It appears that sympathetic nerves counteract the autoregulatory CBF response (for increased flow) to significantly lowered blood pressure. Sympathetic regulation mechanisms may also play a significant protective role during acute increases in blood pressure.[17] No physiologic role has been generally assigned to the parasympathetic innervation.[39] The low level of nervous regulation also allows the cerebral neurotransmitters to function without interference from released cholinergic and adrenergic compounds.

The moment-to-moment regulation of vascular tone in the brain is largely carried out by local control mechanisms that are not neural in nature.[39,41] These mechanisms are active in response to changes in local conditions including blood flow, intravascular pressure, or tissue metabolism. In the brain, blood flow and pressure are tightly regulated, and constant flow is maintained with arterial pressure kept within the range of 80 to 160 mm Hg. The same mechanisms that maintain capillary pressure also provide adequate nutrient flow.

Neuronal activity is associated with an increase in metabolic activity and blood flow. Functional hyperemia describes this increase in blood flow accompanying an increase in tissue activity. While it seems intuitively obvious that there must be some linkage between tissue metabolism and blood flow and between oxygen supply and oxygen demand, the details of the mechanism are not known.

Johnson[39] describes three possible mechanisms for this control. In the first mechanism, the link between blood flow and metabolism may be through a vasodilator substance that is continuously produced by normal metabolic processes. As metabolism increases or blood flow falls, the vasodilator metabolite concentration would rise, leading to a compensatory increase in flow. A substance that would fit into this category is carbon dioxide, CO_2. CO_2 is a normal product of metabolism in all tissues, and its concentration can be shown to vary with blood flow. Increased CO_2 levels in arterial blood have been shown to produce vasodilation in the brain,[45] although in the brain the direct effect of CO_2 is apparently secondary to a corresponding increase in H^+ ion concentration.[46] The weakness of CO_2 being central to this proposed mechanism is that the rate of CO_2 production depends on the availability of oxygen. If oxygen delivery falls because of a drop in arterial O_2 content, CO_2 production will also fall. A general increase in tissue osmolality has also been suggested for this mechanism.

A second proposed mechanism envisions the linkage involving the production of a vasodilator metabolite, which is not ordinarily present, when the blood supply falls below metabolic needs. A substance such as lactic acid fits this second category: it is produced when flow and oxygen delivery are insufficient to meet metabolic demand. However, the functional importance of lactate appears to be limited. The sensitivity of the blood vessels to introduced lactate is not great, with the associated pH changes causing more significant responses. Lactate levels may come into play only when tissue intravascular oxygen tension, pO_2, falls to very low levels and anaerobic metabolism becomes dominant. Another substance that may fit into this second category is adenosine. Decreases in blood flow or pO_2 or increases in metabolism increase adenosine levels, and they have been found to have strong vasodilator effects.[47,48]

In Johnson's third mechanism, arterial blood may contain a vasoconstrictor substance that is utilized by the tissue at a rate dependent on the tissue metabolism. This substance then would be a vasoconstrictor material carried by the bloodstream and consumed in proportion to tissue metabolism. It is logical to consider that oxygen may act in this manner. Reduction of oxygen in arterial blood leads to peripheral vasodilation in the brain, and microvascular tone and flow are strongly influenced by oxygen levels. However, significant questions remain as to how oxygen levels could be sensed and regulated at this level of the microvasculature. There is little evidence that a direct effect of oxygen is important in local regulation.

The substance or substances responsible for linking tissue activity and blood flow are still under investigation. At this time, there is evidence that implicates carbon dioxide, H^+ ion (pH), K^+ ion, tissue osmolality, and adenosine.[17,39] In the brain, the end products of tissue metabolism may play a key role in functional hyperemia and the release of potassium may also contribute to vasodilation during increased cerebral activity. These metabolic products as well as other regional regulators may exert their effect through local arteriolar endothelial dependent vasoactive substances such as nitric oxide. A problem with theories based on regulation by metabolic products, and a subject of active research, is how influences are propagated to regulatory (i.e., vascular smooth muscle) regions upstream of exchange sites.

There appears to be little or no local control in the postcapillary venules. The control of venous vessels appears to be largely under nervous regulation. This probably indicates that the local blood volume of the tissue is less important than the local blood flow supplying nutrients to the tissue. With functional activation the postcapillary blood volume can be expected to increase. Under resting conditions, the veins are partially contracted by a normal level of sympathetic stimulation. It is estimated that in the absence of sympathetic tone, the blood volume would increase by approximately 20% and would decrease by 30% during maximal sympathetic tone.[39]

With the development of methods able to make localized measurements of CBF, the previously held concepts regarding steady continuous flow to the brain under all conditions have been revised to reflect a local coupling of metabolism and blood flow. Even though there is a tight autoregulation of cerebral blood pressure and blood flow, work using chronically implanted oxygen electrodes has shown that local brain pO_2 levels fluctuate and the periodic oscillations correspond to local blood flow changes.[49] The direct association between increased neuronal activation (metabolism) and local blood flow is supported by the results of electroencephalography (EEG),[17,50-52] radioisotope,[53] and PET[5,58] studies.

The resting distribution pattern of blood flow is rapidly and readily altered by changes in activity of different portions of the hemisphere[17] (Fig. 7-19). Specific motor or sensory stimulation causes focal increases in flow to the corresponding functional centers of the brain. More complex mental activity causes more widespread changes in blood flow, presumably because more extensive areas of the hemisphere are activated. Interestingly, *total* CBF and oxygen consumption are little changed between sleeping (rapid eye movement) and waking states.[54]

Motor (i.e., hand) activation causes a corresponding 50% to 100% increase in local CBF in cortical sensorimotor regions.[55] It has also been shown that this local CBF change is associated with increased oxygen uptake[56] and a slight increase in pO_2.[41,57] Since the percentage rise in CBF (and oxygen delivery) exceeds the rise of local oxygen uptake, oxygen itself is not likely to be the primary local control mediator.

PET studies have also shown than the oxygen delivery to the tissue in response to activation exceeds local metabolic demands[58] (Fig. 7-20). Using ^{15}O-labeled water and oxygen, this study found that during somatosensory stimulation, CBF increases by 29%, oxygen utilization increases by 5%, and oxygen extraction fraction decreases by 19%, demonstrating a local uncoupling between blood flow and oxygen demand. The decrease in oxygen extraction corresponds to an increase in local pO_2 and hemoglobin oxygen saturation.

During an epileptic seizure, oxygen uptake and blood flow increase,[17,41,59,60] which indicates that local physiologic control mechanisms continue to be intact in these cases. A commensurate decrease in oxygen uptake and blood flow occurs in cases of depressed neuronal activity, such as during surgical

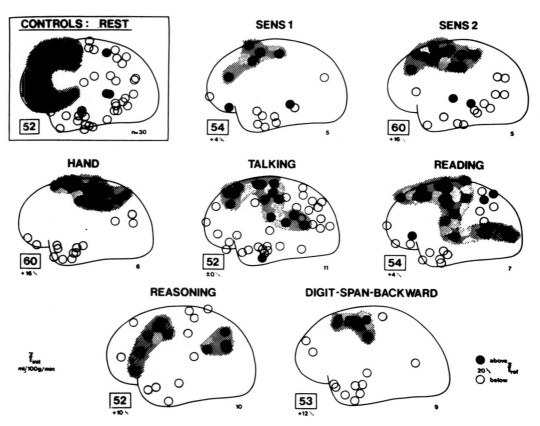

Fig. 7-19. Resting and activated distribution of CBF as measured by ^{133}Xe tracer kinetic studies. (From Ingvar DH: Brain Res, 107:181, 1976.)

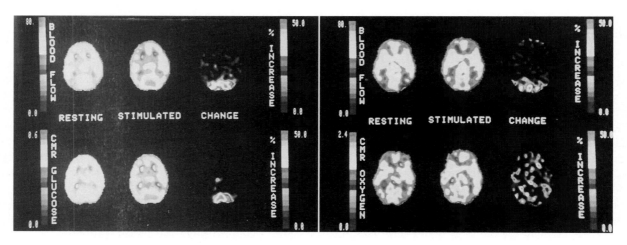

Fig. 7-20. Landmark PET results demonstrating that oxygen uptake (5%) during visual activation does not increase as much as blood flow (49%) or glucose utilization (50%). (From Fox PT: Science 241:463, 1988.)

anesthesia.[61] However, deeper anesthesia interferes with activation-induced responses.[62]

Depriving brain cells of oxygen or both oxygen and glucose leads to a large variety of cellular changes.[63] In particular, cells tend to acquire NaCl along with water, which leads to swelling and the consequent reduction in the volume fraction of the extracellular space.

Ischemia causes cell injury by reducing CBF to well below 50% of normal flow.

Respiratory challenges, such as anoxia and hypercapnia, cause rapid adjustments of blood flow and blood volume to maintain cerebral aerobic metabolism. Anoxia produces changes in blood oxygen content, as well as in blood volume and blood flow.[64] Hypercapnia causes greater blood flow with a constant oxygen consumption rate, producing a decrease in arteriovenous oxygen difference and therefore an increase in the oxygen content of venous blood.[65]

All of these processes should be observable with FMRI techniques.

Diffusion in Magnetic Field Gradients

Diffusion of excited spins in an inhomogeneous magnetic field leads to reduced NMR echo signal intensity. This effect was first noted by Hahn[66] early in the development of NMR. The random movement of spins from one field value to another changes their precessional frequency and, over time, their accumulated phase relative to completely stationary spins. Since the motion is random, the acquired phase is also random and the cancellation among the random distribution of phases reduces the echo amplitude.

Carr and Purcell[67] examined the case of diffusion in a constant linear gradient, G, using a sequence as shown in Fig. 7-21. They showed that the additional signal decay of a single echo caused by diffusion at time TE is by a factor of

$$S = S_0 \exp\left[\frac{-\gamma^2 G^2 D\, TE^3}{12}\right] \qquad (7\text{-}10)$$

where S_0 is the signal, S, without diffusion gradients, γ is the proton gyromagnetic ratio, and D is the diffusion coefficient. This decay factor can be very large for long echo times because the TE^3 factor increases rapidly. In the case of a multiecho experiment where a repeated train of 180-degree pulses causes echo signals to form at intervals of TE (Fig. 7-22), the diffusion time is split into a series of shorter diffusion times equal to the TE used. The refocussing by the 180-degree pulse causes the diffusion effects to be less, and after N echoes the decay factor becomes

$$S = S_0 \exp\left[\frac{-\gamma^2 G^2 D\, TE^3}{12N^2}\right] \qquad (7\text{-}11)$$

The decay factor is now a function of the selected 180-degree pulse spacing. Note that if it were possible to pulse fast enough (with short TE) to form a large number of echoes, N, the effects of diffusion could be made negligible.

On the other hand, these signal effects can be used to measure the diffusion coefficient, and NMR methods provide an effective way of doing so. In a previous chapter the same multiple spin echo sequence without the constant gradient was used to measure the T2 decay properties of the material. A value for the diffusion coefficient can be obtained by making two measurements, one with and one without the constant

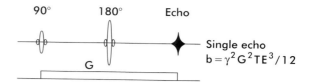

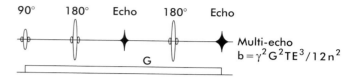

Fig. 7-21. Constant gradient sequence for measurement of diffusion.

Fig. 7-22. Multiecho sequence with a constant gradient.

gradient, in order to identify the additional decay by diffusion in the gradient. In practice the applied gradient, G, must be made substantially larger than the inhomogeneity in the static magnetic field. Since this gradient is on during the collection of echo, the echo's duration will be shorter, the sampling is required to be faster, the corresponding bandwidth will be wider, and the associated extra noise will lower the signal-to-noise ratio.

Stejskal and Tanner[68] avoided these problems by using short gradient pulses to sensitize the sequence to diffusion while avoiding having a gradient on during data collection or RF pulsing. As shown in Fig. 7-23, the gradient pulses are applied for a duration δ and are spaced apart by a time Δ. The resulting signal decay factor is then

$$S = S_0 \exp\left[\gamma^2 G^2 D\delta^2 \left(\Delta - \frac{\delta}{3}\right)\right] \qquad (7\text{-}12)$$

A similar expression can be obtained for a multiecho sequence. The areas of the gradient pulses, the product of the amplitude and duration, are carefully kept equal so that stationary spins experience no net phase encoding from these large pulses.

The effects of a constant background gradient, as seen in Fig. 7-21 and equation 7-10, can be considered by combining this decay factor with the one for the pulsed gradients. This case arises when modeling the effects of diffusion in inhomogeneous magnetic fields.

The preceding expressions for the diffusion decay factor have all been of the form, $exp[-bD]$, where the "b factor" is characteristic of and determined by the details of the pulse sequence.

MR imaging sequences can be similarly modified for diffusion sensitivity, and most diffusion-weighted MRI sequences have been extensions of the Stejskal-Tanner spin echo paired gradient sequences. In these

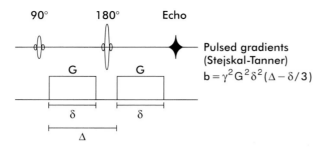

Fig. 7-23. Stejskal-Tanner pulsed gradient diffusion measurement sequence.

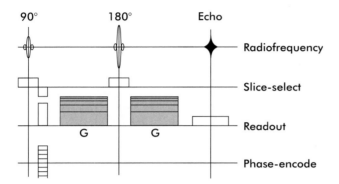

Fig. 7-24. Diffusion imaging sequence incorporating large pulsed gradients.

sequences (Fig. 7-24), the additional sensitizing gradients are made large enough that the effects of diffusion in the rest of the imaging gradients are negligible.[69] For quantitative purposes, diffusion in the gradients used for imaging must also be considered, and the more complicated b factor is usually computed numerically. The change in the phase-encoding gradient amplitude with each projection complicates a complete analytic analysis of the b factor for imaging sequences.

To create diffusion images, two (or more) separate acquisitions are obtained, each using a different diffusion gradient and thus having a different b factor. Since this is the only change between the sequences, taking the ratio of the images, S_1 and S_2, will result in the cancellation of all effects other than the diffusion in the gradients used. The sequence of gradient events is reflected in the corresponding b factors, b_1 and b_2:

$$\frac{S_1}{S_2} = \frac{\exp{[-b_1 D]}}{\exp{[-b_2 D]}} = \exp{[(b_2 - b_1)D]} \quad (7\text{-}13)$$

Taking the logarithm of the ratio image and dividing each point by the (known) quantity $b_2 - b_1$ produces an image of the diffusion coefficient.

The diffusion coefficients measured for water in vivo are rarely as high as those measured for in vitro water samples and, as indicated in Table 7-3, are on the

Table 7-3. Diffusion coefficients ($\times 10^{-5}$ mm^2/sec) in vivo in the human brain and in vitro at 37° C

	In vitro (free diffusion)	In vivo
Water	2.97	2.94 CSF 0.78 (gray matter) 0.22 (corpus callosum) 0.43 (white matter, perpendicular to fibers) 1.03 (white matter, parallel to fibers)

From Functional MRI of the brain: a workshop presented by the Society of Magnetic Resonance in Medicine and the Society for Magnetic Resonance Imaging. June 17-19, 1993 (Table 1, p. 26).

order of 10^{-5} cm^2/sec for soft tissue and body fluid specimens. Most models of water in tissue lead to the supposition that a substantial fraction (20% to 40%) of the cell water is hydration water, or that the diffusion coefficient of the cytoplasmic water is reduced substantially from the free water value.[70]

The large diffusion gradients in these imaging sequences make the images very sensitive to other types of motion as well, particularly patient motion and blood flow. They also make these images sensitive to system RF and gradient instability, eddy currents induced by the large diffusion gradient pulses, and internal susceptibility variations. Furthermore, diffusion is quite temperature sensitive (2.4%/°C), and local variations may influence the measured coefficients.[71] In consideration of these contributions to the measured value of D, the results from this type of MR experiment are more correctly referred to as the "apparent diffusion coefficient" (ADC).[72]

Restricted diffusion. Diffusion pulse sequences can be used to measure restricted diffusion in systems where partitions (e.g., membranes) limit the freedom of molecular motion. This was recognized in the original NMR literature,[68,73,74] and the principles have been subsequently extended for use in imaging sequences.[30,75-77]

In these experiments, the time over which the diffusion is measured must be accurately known. In Stejskal-Tanner sequences, the time during which the random motion of the spins lead to dephasing, which acts to reduce the measured signal, is set primarily by the time, $\Delta - \delta/3$, between gradient pulses. This factor can be considered to be the interpulse period Δ if the pulse width δ is relatively short. If Δ is short, the diffusing molecules will only infrequently reach, and be impeded by, the tissue partitions, and the signal characteristics will be similar to those diffusing in a free environment. As Δ becomes longer, the molecules bounce off the partitions and will be limited in the

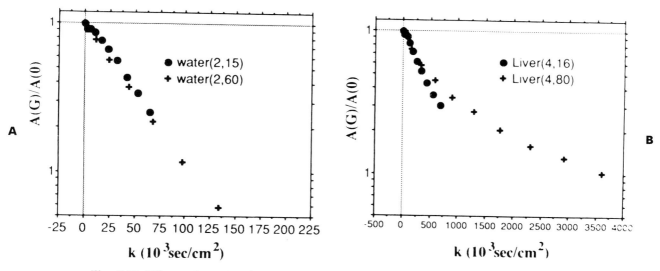

Fig. 7-25. Effects of restricted diffusion can be seen in liver (**B**) but not in water (**A**). Increasing values of k represents measurement by sequences with increasing diffusion sensitivity. (From Zhong J, Gore JC: Magn Reson Med 19:276, 1991.)

amount of dephasing they accumulate. This effect reduces the measured diffusion coefficient. In a spin echo sequence, the loss of signal from intrinsic T2 processes limits the amount of potential sequence diffusion time. An alternative approach is to vary the diffusion sensitizing gradient while keeping Δ constant[77] (Fig. 7-25). It is also possible to incorporate diffusion encoding into other types of sequences that are less sensitive to this T2 decay.[78,79]

For small values of Δ, D will have a constant value. As Δ is increased, D will be decreased and will have a value dependent on the particular Δ used. Knowing the diffusion coefficient for short Δs and the value of Δ when D becomes time independent, one can estimate the average separation between partitions[74] (Fig. 7-26). The average distance traveled by the molecules during the time Δ is $\sqrt{2D\Delta}$, and this will be approximately the measured spacing between partitions. The Δs in MRI diffusion experiments are in general sufficiently long that the potential restriction of water diffusion by cellular (e.g., membrane) and intracellular (e.g., macromolecules) obstructions needs to be considered.

The models that have been proposed to explain the observed reduction in tissue diffusion coefficient, as compared to the free diffusion coefficient, focus on two general mechanisms.[70] The tissue water may diffuse at the same rate as free water, but continual collisions with obstructions, cellular or intracellular, slow travel and lead to the measurement of a lower D. Alternatively, the diffusion of water is not free, and the bulk diffusive motions (and measured D) are reduced by slowing caused either globally or locally by hydration and/or ordering at macromolecular surfaces. It appears that a combination of both processes is

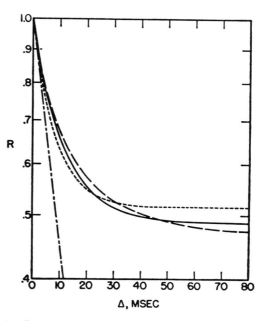

Fig. 7-26. Restricted diffusion results in the signal attenuation becoming independent of the diffusion time. R is the theoretical attentuation, Δ is the diffusion time. (From Tanner JE, Stejskal EO: J Chem Phys 49[4]:1768, 1968.)

responsible for reducing measured diffusion. While membrane and macromolecular obstructions do contribute to this reduction, the overall diffusive motion of water in cells appears to be reduced from that of free water.[80]

Anisotropic diffusion. Up to this point we have considered the process of diffusion to be isotropic, or identical in all directions. This is not required by any fundamental limitation of NMR measurements since

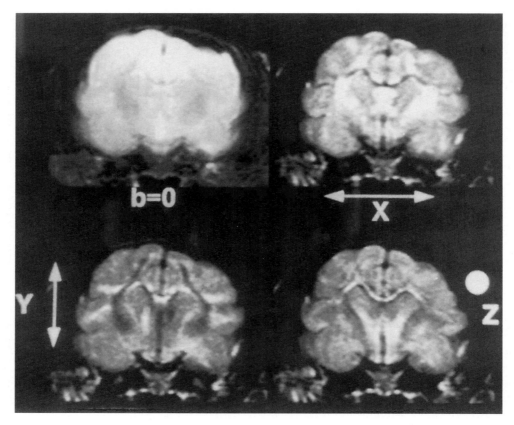

Fig. 7-27. Diffusion anisotropy can be identified by changing the direction of the diffusion-encoding gradient and repeating the diffusion imaging measurement. (From Moseley ME et al: Magn Reson Med 19:321, 1991.)

the direction of the diffusion sensitizing gradient pulses can be controlled and the ADC can be measured in any arbitrary direction (Fig. 7-27). Full characterization of diffusion anisotropy requires measurement of the diffusion tensor, which is the (scalar) diffusion rate as a function of direction.

The presence of nonrandom intracellular obstructions or irregular cellular dimensions will cause proton diffusion to be anisotropic, resulting in a lower ADC for protons along a more hindered direction compared to that in a direction in which the protons can move more freely. Departures from isotropy reflect the underlying structure of tissue and can be considered to be another tissue microstructural parameter measurable by MRI.[75,81]

Perfusion Measurement

There are three general approaches taken toward the measurement of tissue perfusion with MRI. The first approach uses long-established principles of indicator dilution analysis of the measured time course of injected paramagnetic indicator substances as they pass through the tissue capillary bed. Detection of changes in measurable tissue parameters using these methods was the first FMRI method

demonstrated; such methods will be discussed in more detail shortly. Despite sensitivity limitations, the second approach for measuring perfusion, using specific MRI sequences designed to be sensitive to perfusion- (and diffusion-) induced phase shifts, may eventually be extended to detect cerebral perfusion changes with functional activation. The third approach, that of detecting tissue signal changes as a result of perfusive movement into the imaging region, is also limited in sensitivity but is likely to accompany signal changes observed during non-Gd-DTPA FMRI procedures.

Phase-sensitive methods. With in vivo measurements, diffusion-weighted sequences will also be sensitive to blood flow in the capillary bed of the tissue. Since the capillaries are approximately randomly oriented, this perfusive microcirculatory flow can be considered as a pseudodiffusive process on the measurement scale of the image voxel size. The combination of diffusion and perfusion is often referred to as "intravoxel incoherent motions" (IVIM), and procedures have been proposed to separate out their individual contributions.[69,72,82] As shown in Fig. 7-28, IVIM images, even without separating perfusion

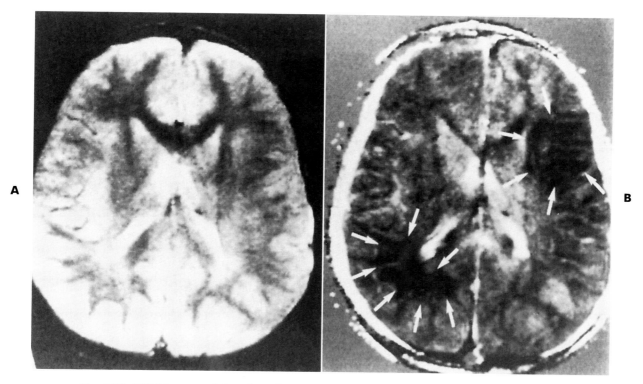

Fig. 7-28. IVIM images of the adrenal cortex, without isolation of perfusion and diffusion components, may identify lesions not distinguished by normal MRI contrast mechanisms. **A**, T2-weighted image; **B**, IVIM image. (From Le Bihan D et al: Radiology 168:497, 1988.)

and diffusion contributions, may also provide additional clinical diagnostic information.

If the direction of the perfusive flow in the capillaries changes often during the time of the measurement sequence, the flow can be modeled as a diffusive process (Fig. 7-29). The pseudodiffusion coefficient, D^*, associated with perfusive flow depends on the capillary geometry and blood velocity and is estimated to be approximately 10 times larger than the diffusion coefficient of water.[72,82] The microcirculatory perfusion contribution to the signal decay is similar in form to regular diffusion, $exp[-bD^*]$ but will only apply to the volume fraction, f, of flowing blood in the tissue. This fraction will additionally experience attenuation by diffusion while the remaining $(1 - f)$ nonperfusing fraction of the tissue is attenuated only by diffusion.

Most methods for separating the perfusion and diffusion contributions to the signal attenuation use multiple acquisitions, each with identical RF and gradient timing but having different motional sensitivities (diffusion gradient amplitudes). The model and procedure proposed by LeBihan[72] use three images, with large, medium, and small amounts of velocity encoding (Fig. 7-30). The signal attenuation resulting from both perfusion and diffusion is given by

$$S_b = S_0 e^{-bD}[(1 - f) + Ff] \qquad (7\text{-}14)$$

where F is the additional attenuation factor (i.e., $exp[-bD^*]$) for the moving blood. The gradient b factors used in these acquisitions are assumed to be large enough that the remaining signal contribution of flowing spins is insignificant for both medium and large encoding images $(F \sim 0)$. The signal loss by perfusing spins is assumed to be negligible $(F \sim 1)$ in the small encoding images having small gradients and b factors. It can be shown[72] that since the tissue fraction of capillaries is small

$$ln\left(\frac{S_0}{S_b}\right) = f + Db \qquad (7\text{-}15)$$

Therefore the slope and intercept of a plot of $ln(S_0/S_b)$ (the logarithm of the ratio images without, S_0, and with, S_b, encoding gradients) as a function of the b factor used correspond to the diffusion constant, D, and the capillary volume fraction, f, respectively (Fig. 7-31). Acquiring data with multiple gradient (b) values increases the accuracy of these measurements.[83] While this measurement may not measure actual tissue perfusion—that is, it does not distinguish between blood flow to a tissue and blood flow through the tissue[84] (unless assumptions are made regarding vascular structure[85])—it does provide an estimate of diffusion, which can be used for tissue discrimination, and vascular volume fraction, which is an important physiologic parameter.

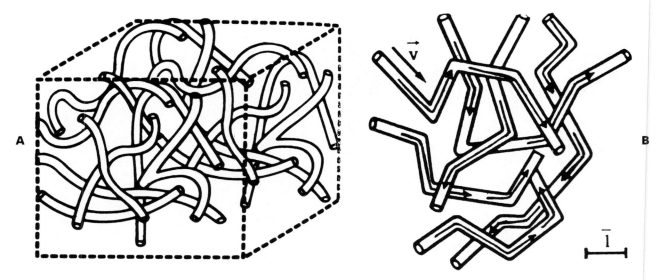

Fig. 7-29. Perfusive motion of blood can lead to signal attenuations similar to diffusion. **A,** Tissue structure within a voxel can be modeled as a large number of randomly oriented capillary segments. **B,** If the segment lengths are shorter than the distance spins move during the sequence, the signal dephasing will be similar to that from diffusion. (From Le Bihan D et al: Radiology 168:497, 1988.)

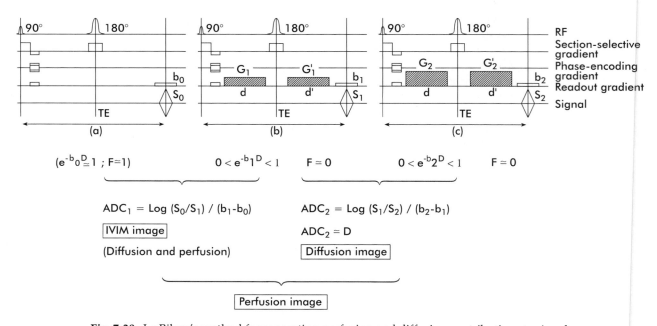

Fig. 7-30. Le Bihan's method for separating perfusion and diffusion contributions to signal decay analyzes the results from three sequences having different motion sensitivities. (From Le Bihan D et al: Radiology 168:497, 1988.)

An alternative approach to perfusion measurement[86] assumes that the intravoxel distribution of capillary orientation is, in fact, nonuniform. The small net directionality ("intravoxel coherent motion") and associated phase shift can be observed using images with sufficiently sensitive velocity-encoding gradients oriented in that direction.

A limitation in using most direct perfusion measurement methods for MR functional imaging is that only on the order of 2% of a typical tissue consists of (flowing) capillaries. This means that there will be only a 2% perfusion contribution to the signal arising from the volume. The use of a long TE will somewhat increase the sensitivity by weighting the signal in

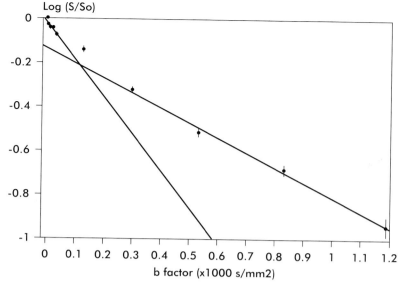

Fig. 7-31. Sample IVIM results from cat brain cortex showing the plot of logarithm of signal attenuation versus sequence b factor. Primarily diffusion effects are seen at larger b values while small b factors additionally show perfusion effects. The value at the intercept gives an estimation of the vascular volume fraction. (From Le Bihan D, Turner R: Magn Reson Med 19:221, 1991.)

favor of blood (with a long T2) with respect to brain parenchyma (with a shorter T2),[87] but SNR is also reduced at long echo times. Given that perfusion changes with brain activation are less than 100%, the available SNR limits the ability to detect small activation changes. As mentioned previously, diffusion (perfusion) imaging requires very large gradient pulses for encoding, which makes it subject to a number of potential sources of error, any of which would act to obscure small activation changes.[88,89]

T1/inflow methods.   Saturation or inversion of blood T1-weighted signal can be used to quantify perfusion. In the method of Detre and coworkers,[90,91] two images are made with and without saturating upstream sources of flow. This approach is based on (1) the delivery of water to a tissue being proportional to the rate of perfusion and (2) the fact that changes in the NMR properties of tissue water are significantly affected by perfusion. The water spins outside of the ROI are either saturated or inverted. These spins then perfuse into the ROI and exchange with tissue water. As these spins lose their label, the tissue magnetization changes at a rate dependent on the apparent T1 value and the rate of perfusive delivery of spins to the region. Given sufficient time for the flow of the saturated spins to perfuse the tissue, a difference image between the two acquisitions shows a signal proportional to the amount of perfusion through the image slice. Since the label can exchange out of the vascular compartment, the potential signal changes are not limited by the volume fraction of the vasculature.

This relationship between T1 and regional blood flow can be described[90,92] by

$$\frac{1}{T1_{app}} = \frac{1}{T1} + \frac{f}{\lambda} \qquad (7\text{-}16)$$

where $T1_{app}$ is the observed (apparent) longitudinal relaxation time with flow effects included, $T1$ is the true tissue longitudinal relaxation time in the absence of flow, f is the flow in ml/g/unit time, and λ is the brain- blood partition coefficient of water (approximately 0.95 ml/g[93]). Kwong et al[13] further expanded upon this model, measuring T1 changes associated with blood flow changes. Assuming that tissue T1 remains constant with neural activation, a change in blood flow Δf will lead to a change in the observed $T1_{app}$:

$$\Delta\left(\frac{1}{T1_{app}}\right) = \Delta\left(\frac{f}{\lambda}\right) \qquad (7\text{-}17)$$

In this way, the MR signal change can be used to estimate the change in blood flow. For an inversion recovery sequence with TI ~ T1 and assuming constant proton density, a 2% change in MR signal intensity implies a change in flow of ~50 ml/100 g/min. This is in good agreement with previous PET results with visual stimulation.[2,94,153,154]

Contrast Agents

Gd-DTPA is the only MRI contrast agent currently approved for routine human use in the United States.

The common use of this agent is the result of its demonstrated ability to enhance the conspicuity of lesions associated with a compromised BBB (Fig. 4-34). More details regarding its clinical applications are available elsewhere.[95-97] A typical injection dose is approximately 0.1 mM/kg body weight, although relaxation effects can be observed at significantly lower concentrations.[98]

Another lanthanide paramagnetic compound used in experimental studies is dysprosium (Dy). This agent does not have as much of a direct relaxivity effect as Gd-DTPA[99,100] (Fig. 7-32) and is more likely to be toxic. Additionally, the relaxation characteristics of superparamagnetic iron particles have been studied,[101] and these results have particular clinical relevance when considering and modeling the effects of iron in hemorrhage.

The presence of paramagnetic compounds can induce shifts in nuclear spin resonance frequencies or increase nuclear spin relaxation rate constants, or, usually, both. In the former capacity such compounds are often called "shift agents" and in the latter, "relaxation agents." In MRI, paramagnetic compounds are typically used as image "contrast agents" that, for routine clinical work, rely on their capacities as relaxation agents.[102] These paramagnetic contrast agents affect the image appearance through two primary mechanisms: dipolar relaxivity and local susceptibility effects.

The relaxivity effects result from a direct dipolar interaction between the unpaired electrons of the paramagnetic compound and nearby proton nuclear spins. This results in the enhancement of both T1 and T2 relaxation rates. Because T1 rates are intrinsically slower than T2 rates in most tissues, relaxation time changes on a percentage basis are much greater for T1 than T2. For this reason, Gd-DTPA, whose main clinical mechanism of action is this dipole-dipole relaxation enhancement, is often considered to be a "T1 agent," reflecting the dominant effect of shortening T1 relaxation times.[76,103-105] The effect on T1 is generally linear with Gd-DTPA concentration and results in increased signal intensity on MR images from sequences designed to be sensitive to T1 relaxation differences.

The second mechanism of image contrast is due to the localized variation in tissue magnetic fields produced when there is a nonuniform distribution of these high-susceptibility paramagnetic substances (Fig. 7-33). This process can affect T2-weighted images as direct dipolar relaxivity affects T1-weighted images.[99] This mechanism becomes significant in clinical imaging and FMRI because the distribution of administered Gd-DTPA is nonuniform in brain tissue. Gd-DTPA is not able to pass through the normal intact BBB, does not enter the erythrocytes, is not bound to plasma protein,[24,96,106] and is therefore limited in access to the plasma space of the blood. The amount of inhomogeneity depends on the difference in susceptibility between materials and the size and geometry of the structures. Small objects, like capillaries or RBCs, can lead to very large field gradients even if the susceptibility differences are not large.[99] These high-susceptibility plasma regions are much closer along the capillary length than between adjacent capillaries. The overlap in gradients along the length of the

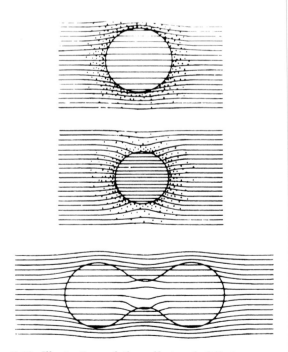

Fig. 7-33. Illustration of the effects of differing magnetic susceptibilities on the local magnetic field patterns for various particle geometries. *Top,* $\chi_{in} < \chi_{out}$; *middle,* $\chi_{out} < \chi_{in}$; *bottom,* lines of flux in the erythrocyte. (From Brindel KM et al: Biochem J, 180:37, 1979.)

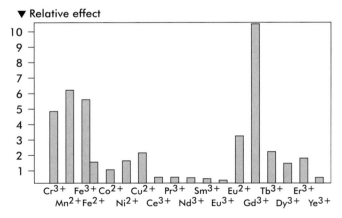

Fig. 7-32. Influence of a variety of paramagnetic ions on proton spin-lattice relaxation times. (From Weinman HJ et al: AJR 142:619, 1984.)

capillary yields field patterns that, to the tissue, look more like those for cylinders than for the spheres that are often considered in analytic or experimental models.[107-109]

The change in magnetic susceptibility of a compartment containing Gd-DTPA chelates is due to the partial alignment of the magnetic moments of the paramagnetic molecules by the magnetic field.[102] This shift depends not only on the susceptibility of the compartment occupied by the host molecule but also on the shape of the compartment and its orientation in the magnetic field. The magnetic susceptibility difference affects local resonance frequencies by modifying the local magnetic fields experienced by the water protons. This can affect the signal from a particular voxel in three ways:

1. If the field distribution within the voxel is nonuniform as a result of the susceptibility differences, the signals from tissue water will occur over a range of frequencies and the net signal intensity will be decreased because of phase cancellation. This will be a T2* effect similar to that observed when there is inhomogeneity in the static magnetic field. Sequences that do not refocus inhomogeneity dephasing, such as gradient echo sequences, will be particularly sensitive to these effects.

2. For sequences that refocus inhomogeneity effects, such as spin-echo sequences, the presence of intravoxel field gradients will indirectly lead to signal reduction by diffusion in these gradients during the imaging time. This appears as a T2 effect that increases with increasing diffusion times (i.e., TE). As mentioned previously, these effects can be distinguished from intrinsic spin-spin relaxation through the use of relatively diffusion-insensitive sequences such as a Carr-Purcell-Meiboom-Gill (CPMG) multiecho sequence with short echo times.

3. The spatial extent of the susceptibility differences may be large enough and the voxel sizes may be small enough that the field distribution within the voxel is still relatively uniform but is shifted by a net field and frequency offset. This shift in resonance frequency will lead to signal phase shifts observable in phase-sensitive images, and these effects will increase with increasing TE.[76]

Diffusion Near Local Inhomogeneities

The influences of paramagnetic compounds on signals were recognized early in the development of NMR, and a basic theoretical framework for their direct relaxivity effects was established by the early work of Soloman and Bloembergen.[110-112] Supporting the thorough study of the characteristics of paramag-

netic contrast agents for routine clinical use, a number of theoretical models have been proposed to more fully address the additional mechanism of signal loss in the inhomogeneous fields near the paramagnetic particles.

There are three basic categories of models to explain how diffusion in these regions of susceptibility differences influences the measured signal.[113] The first class of "fast exchange" models[114] assumes that there is rapid movement of the water through the regions of inhomogeneous fields and is similar to models used in relaxation theory. This model assumes that all tissue water molecules have direct and ready access to coordination sites of the paramagnetic ion in time frames that are short compared with the measurement and relaxation times.[76] More specifically, the rate of diffusion past a dipole (source of inhomogeneity) is greater than the variation in frequency (field) caused by the dipole. These models have provided analytic expressions predicting measured T2 relaxation rates. The motional assumptions underlying these models are appropriate in cases where the size of the high-susceptibility regions is small (such as near ferritin deposits within a hemorrhage) or where water diffusion rates are high. However, relevance of this model to the brain may be limited by the presence of an intact blood-brain barrier that will inhibit the free diffusion of tissue water and access to paramagnetic sites in the plasma compartment.

The second class of models[115] considers the opposite situation, where the water spins are assumed to experience only a small region of the inhomogeneous magnetic field during the echo time. In this "slow exchange" model, the magnetic field inhomogeneity experienced by the diffusing spins can be approximated as a linear field gradient. By modeling the distribution of such linear gradients in space, expressions for the attenuation of the transverse magnetization can be derived. The assumptions of this model are likely to be satisfied in cases where the regions of inhomogeneous magnetic field are large or when the diffusion coefficient of water is small.

The "intermediate exchange" models,[107,116,117] as may be expected, consider the water exchange to be neither fast nor slow. In these models, analytic expressions for relaxation behavior become difficult to derive because the inhomogeneous field patterns and signal influences are not simplified by assumptions of exchange speed. Numerical simulation techniques are often employed to compute the effects on the echo signal phase as a spin moves along random paths through the inhomogeneous fields. This approach has been used to predict field strength distributions[116] and to predict the signal loss by diffusion.[107,116] This more complicated situation may more realistically represent the conditions present with tissue perfusion with Gd-

DTPA,[76,107,113,118] and the results from this model will be described shortly.

BOLUS INJECTION PRINCIPLES
Indicator Dilution Methods

Indicator dilution methods have been used for measurement of tissue parameters for many years in physiology, and there is a large body of experience and literature to draw upon.[119,120] The "functional" parameters that can be measured by these techniques, using either single or multiple simultaneous indicators, include tissue blood volume, tissue blood flow (perfusion), tissue compartmentalization, and membrane permeability.

The choice of using a particular indicator dilution or tracer kinetic method is determined by whether the indicator substance is diffusible or nondiffusible. Diffusible substances are those that are membrane permeable to some extent. A great deal of previous work in this discipline has been primarily concerned with the use of diffusible agents, whose exchange properties between the vasculature and the tissue can be exploited to assess membrane characteristics and analyze tissue compartmentalization. The use of diffusible markers has been extended to NMR, for example, in studies using deuterium or fluorine substituted compounds. Methods utilizing nuclei other than protons are described in Chapter 10 on MR spectroscopic methods. The current discussion will be limited to nondiffusible indicator substances. The methods used in FMRI are based on the use of bolus injections, which characterize the tissue response to an abrupt introduction of a marker, or indicator, substance. In FMRI, Gd-DTPA is used as the intravascular indicator substance. These nonequilibrium indicator dilution methods are related to the steady state constant infusion techniques first described over 100 years ago[121] and were mathematically characterized using the principles of conservation of mass 35 years later.[122] Constant infusion methods are more difficult to apply when using Gd-DTPA because of its rapid transit and recirculation times (since it remains completely intravascular) combined with its relatively slow clearance from blood.

Previous CT work[123,124] with nondiffusible contrast agents has laid the groundwork for subsequent MR imaging studies. Gd-DTPA is considered to be nondiffusible since it is completely confined to the cerebral intravascular space (if there is an intact BBB) and the amount of (cerebral) extravascular leakage is negligible. Additionally, Gd-DTPA fulfills the requirement that the indicator be neither retained nor metabolized within the tissue.

In most indicator methods, including x-ray and CT applications, there has been a direct relation between the measurement (e.g., CT or Hounsfield number) and the amount or concentration of the indicator (contrast) material in the sample. Therefore, it is possible to identify the concentration of the indicator in the measurement sample. In MRI with Gd-DTPA, this critical relationship is less direct. This will be discussed in more detail when the extension of these methods to MRI is described. A primary feature of these experiments is that measurements are made over time at a particular tissue or vascular location.

The nonflowing stationary case is straightforward; if a known amount (mass, M) of indicator is added to a volume, the volume after complete mixing can be readily determined by measuring the concentration, C, in a single sample.

$$V = \frac{M}{C} \qquad (7\text{-}18)$$

Outflow detection. The case of flow into and out of the (tissue) volume is somewhat more complicated, since the rate of material entering and leaving the central mixing volume must be considered. However, simple mass conservation indicates that the amount of material accumulated in the tissue is equal to the amount of material delivered to the tissue by the flow minus the amount of material removed by drainage during the same time.

In a closed system, such as the vasculature, recirculation of flow complicates the situation and limits the type of measurements that can be done. In particular, techniques using a constant infusion of indicator material are made more difficult by the repeated recirculation of the added material back through the tissue before equilibrium infusion and measurement conditions are established.

A simple flowing model to consider is the single mixing compartment model depicted in Fig. 7-34, which assumes that no recirculation occurs. As illustrated, the indicator material is injected upstream and is sampled downstream of a mixing volume, which represents the tissue blood volume. The flow represents the blood supply to the tissue. Given the additional assumptions that the contrast agent completely mixes throughout the volume of the tissue volume and that all of the injected material is eventually washed out of the volume, we can determine the flow between the injection and collection sites. An additional assumption required for nondiffusible indicators is that the indicator behaves like, and moves at the same speed as, the rest of the flow.

In practical consideration of the rapid recirculation times in the cerebral vasculature, a rapid "bolus" injection of material is used to administer the contrast agent and a set of measurements is obtained without the contrast agent ever reaching its equilibrium concentration throughout the blood volume. After the

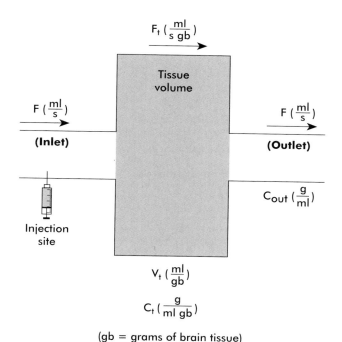

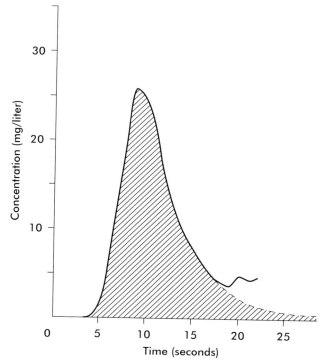

Fig. 7-34. A basic tissue mixing model for indicator dilution measurements.

Fig. 7-35. Example concentration-time curve showing effects of recirculation. (Redrawn from Axel L: Radiology 137:679, 1980.)

bolus injection, the concentration at the measurement site will, after a delay, increase to a maximum value and then decay toward zero. In practice, recirculation occurs before complete washout of the indicator is finished (Fig. 7-35).

Since we are assuming that all of the injected material (of mass, M) leaves the system, we can continuously sample the outflow concentration until all of the material has washed out. Ideally, one collects and measures the concentration of all of the outflowing mixture, but in actuality only samples are obtained from the output stream for each time interval Δt. The amount of material leaving the system during the sample time will be the sample volume times the sample concentration, C_{out} (amount per volume). The sample volume will be equal to the flow rate, F (volume per time), multiplied by the sample collection time, Δt. The summation over all of these samples, which becomes an integral as the sample time Δt becomes small, gives the total outflowing indicator mass.

After complete washout, this measured mass will be equal to the injected mass, M:

$$M = \int_0^\infty F(t)C_{out}(t)dt \qquad (7\text{-}19)$$

The repeated measurements provide a record of sample concentration per time, and the initial injected mass (M) is known, so the total flow (F) to and from the

mixing volume can be calculated. If the flow is not constant (i.e., is pulsatile) an average flow will be determined, allowing the constant (not time-dependent) value of F to be taken out of the integral and the equation to be rewritten so as to solve for the flow:

$$F = \frac{M}{\int_0^\infty C_{out}(t)dt} \qquad (7\text{-}20)$$

While the time limits of this integral are theoretically from zero to infinity, complete washout of the contrast agent is finished, or recirculation of contrast occurs, after some finite length of measuring time. Recirculation will distort the measurements if the flow is slow and the washout is not complete by the time that mass previously washed out (and measured) cycles back through the system to be remeasured. The denominator of this equation is the measured sample concentration per time (Fig. 7-35) and is known as the "concentration-time curve." The integral over these measurements is essentially the area under the measurement curve.

Recirculation correction. The recirculation of indicator can be compensated for if the concentration-time curve for an equivalent tissue bed is available, whose arterial supply does not receive the initial bolus injection. The mixed blood recirculating back through will contain the indicator, and the measured time course can be used as a correction for the measured curve. However, such tissue selectivity is not often feasible, particularly for the venous injections used in most in vivo studies.

In the case of washout from a single mixing compartment, the shape of the descending tail of the concentration-time curve will follow a monoexponential decay of the form[119,123]

$$C_{out}(t') = C_0 e^{\frac{-t'}{T_w}} \qquad (7\text{-}21)$$

where C_0 is the concentration at some time point, defining $t' = 0$, early on the steepest slope part of the tail of the washout curve and T_W is the exponential time constant. The presence of recirculation effects can therefore be recognized as a deviation from linearity on a semilogarithmic plot, ln (concentration) versus time (Fig. 7-36). The exponential decay property of the concentration-time curve can be used to extrapolate the curve past the time where recirculating contrast starts to interfere with the measurements. In practice, the measured $C_{out}(t)$ curve is numerically integrated up to time t' (prior to recirculation), and the fitted exponential curve, which is the estimated washout curve in the absence of recirculation, is integrated analytically. Even though the measurements may have been limited in time, the extrapolation and area calculation should be extended out to the limit of infinite washout time.[119] The time constant, T_W, of this decay is given by V_t/F_t, and identification of this decay constant can also provide another estimate of the tissue flow per volume.

The tail of the washout curve is not purely monoexponential, but the difference in most cases is small.[125] Another procedure to eliminate recirculation without the requirement of arbitrarily choosing starting points on the washout curve is to fit the data curve with a gamma-variate function with a recirculation cutoff.[124,126,127] The gamma-variate function is of the form

$$S = [f(t - t_0)]^r e^{-\frac{t - t_0}{b}} \qquad (7\text{-}22)$$

where f, r, and b are fit parameters chosen to match the collected data (Fig. 7-37). The time parameter t_0 is the time where the injected material first appears in the measurements and the exponent r controls the steepness of the fitted curve on the rising part of the concentration-time curve.

Central volume principle. The direct application of this approach (and equation 7-20) is limited for several reasons, particularly the difficulty in determining the actual mass, M_t, of indicator delivered to the tissue from a remote injection site. In order to measure the

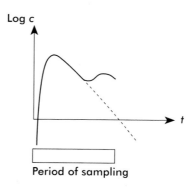

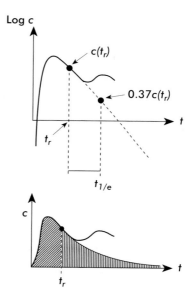

Fig. 7-36 *Top,* Recirculation of indicator can be identified by the deviation of the measured ln(C) from linearity. *Middle,* Using the choice of a time point, t_r, early on the descending part of the curve, the contribution from recirculation can be removed. *Bottom,* The area under the curve can be obtained numerically up to time t_r, and analytically thereafter. (From Lassen NA, Perl W: Tracer kinetic methods in medical physiology, New York, Raven Press, p 28, 1979.)

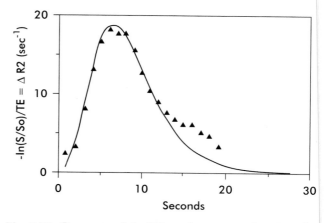

Fig. 7-37. Gamma-variate fitting of concentration-time data is also used to eliminate the effects of inductor recirculation. (From Belliveau JW: Magn Reson Med 14:538, 1990.)

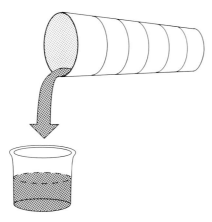

If 1 ml leaves per second and the transit time ($\bar{t}$) is 6 seconds, then with the plug flow (*F*), the entire tube volume Vd has been displaced into the collecting bucket in 6 seconds;

that is $Vd = F \times \bar{t}$
$= 1 \times 6$
$= 6$ ml

$\bar{t} = $ *turnover time*

Fig. 7-38. The simplest possible flow model consisting of plug flow in a tube. The transit time is equal to the volume to flow rate ratio. (From Lassen NA, Perl W: Tracer kinetic methods in medical physiology, New York, 1979, Raven Press, p 28.)

tissue parameters of interest (i.e., flow and volume), an alternative approach must be taken. The most common approach utilizes the concept of the "mean transit time" (MTT) for the tissue system. As shown in Fig. 7-38 for the simplest tissue model case of steady plug flow in a tube, the value of the MTT characterizes the volume to flow ratio

$$MTT = \frac{V_t}{F_t} \qquad (7\text{-}23)$$

of the system. This parameter characterizes the amount of time for the injected material to enter the system, become mixed, and leave the tissue. For assessment of tissue perfusion, it is often of more interest to determine the ratio of blood flow per unit indicator-accessible tissue volume

$$\frac{1}{MTT} = \frac{F_t}{V_t} \qquad (7\text{-}24)$$

In either form, this relationship is known as the "central volume principle."

The MTT is the average time it takes any given particle of contrast agent to pass through the tissue following an ideal instantaneous injection. In the case of a tissue mixing volume, the concentration-time curve measured at the venous outflow provides a record of the distribution of transit times through the tissue. As indicated in Fig. 7-35, the curve is not sharp and is extended over time. For an ideal injection bolus, where all of the injected indicator is delivered to the tissue in a time shorter than the shortest transit time through the tissue, the MTT corresponds to the time of the center-of-gravity (first moment) of the concentration-time curve:

$$MTT = \frac{\int_0^\infty t C_{out}(t)dt}{\int_0^\infty C_{out}(t)dt} = \frac{V_t}{F_t} \qquad (7\text{-}25)$$

which does not necessarily correspond to the time of the curve peak. The MTT is referenced using a time zero as the start of the injected material entering the tissue volume. The flow through the tissue volume can therefore be calculated from the estimated value of the mean transit time, where the flow F_t has units of ml/min per measured amount (g or ml) of tissue and V_t is the volume of distribution of agent within the tissue.[119,123,128] For a completely intravascular material such as Gd-DTPA, this volume is the tissue blood volume and is expressed in milliliters per measured amount of tissue.

In this simple tissue model, the first moment of the outlet concentration-time curve can be used to estimate the MTT, and from a known value of the injected mass and using equation 7-20 to estimate the tissue flow F_t, the tissue blood volume can be determined. The parameters obtained from this type of outlet detection characterize the entire upstream tissue system; no information is available regarding regional variations within the tissue.

The central volume principle is difficult to directly apply because of the practical difficulties encountered in performing these studies. This relation assumes that the injected material is completely mixed within the tissue volume; errors in the estimation of the MTT will occur if this is not the case (the measured concentration curve will be distorted). If the marker compound is not completely intravascular, the exchange of the substance between tissue compartments and associated transit delays must also be modeled. In practice, the delivery of indicator to the tissue as an ideal bolus is very difficult to implement. Fortunately, with additional measurements, it may be possible to correct for the effects of nonideal input injection profiles.

Mean injection time/arterial input function. Gd-DTPA does not exchange out of the blood plasma space, but the administered mass cannot be considered to arrive at the tissue as an instantaneous pulse. This is particularly the case when venous injection is used and the injection pulse is broadened during circulation through the pulmonary system and the heart prior to delivery to the tissue of interest (Fig. 7-39). Like the mean transit time, a mean injection time, MIT, can be defined as the center of gravity of another concentration-time curve obtained at a measurement site immediately before the tissue volume. The real nature of the input profile can be considered to be the result of an ideal input pulse to an imaginary input volume located ahead of, and in series with, the actual tissue system. The observed mean transit time measurement, MTT_{obs}, is therefore[120,123,125]

$$MTT_{obs} = MIT + MTT \qquad (7\text{-}26)$$

The sum of the mean transit times of each of the two systems in series gives the mean transit time for the total system. If the time course of the injection can be accurately determined, then the flow per unit volume can be determined.

With a noninstantaneous injection time course, the measured concentration time curve, $C(t)_{obs}$, will be a convolution of the input time course, $I(t)$, and the actual tissue response, $C(t)$[76,119,123]:

$$C(t)_{obs} = I(t) * C(t) \qquad (7\text{-}27)$$

This can be recognized by considering each subdelivery of indicator to the tissue over the time of the injection profile as being an ideal input pulse with an individual $C_i(t)$ curve. The detector measures the summation of current values over these individual curves as they simultaneously play out over time. In order to deconvolve the measured curve to find the actual concentration-time curve and accurately estimate the MTT, the input time course must be measured. This input function is often referred to as the "arterial input function," reflecting that it represents the time course of the injection at the level of the arterial vessels immediately supplying the tissue. Note that this deconvolution is conveniently performed using the multiplication property of the Fourier transform (FT). The FT of the tissue curve divided by the FT of the arterial curve, followed by an inverse FT, performs this operation.

This arterial input function can be obtained by direct blood sampling, as is often done in animal and radioisotope experiments. Given sufficient MRI, temporal, spatial, and contrast resolution, $I(t)$ can be determined from additional imaging measurements of the arterial indicator concentration in vessels directly supplying the tissue. In order to adequately characterize both $I(t)$ and $C(t)$ curves, frequent and high-resolution image measurements must be obtained, requiring short imaging times.

In summary, the concentration-time curve measured at the venous outflow after an ideal bolus injection has several features[130]:

1. There is a delay before the indicator appears at the exit. Thus it takes time for the indicator molecules to travel through the tissue volume.
2. The measured curve rises and falls without necessarily having a very sharp peak. This indicates that not all indicator molecules traverse the tissue volume in the same amount of time.
3. The first moment of the measured curve provides an estimate of the mean transit time for an indicator particle, and this time is equal to the ratio of the accessible tissue volume to the tissue blood flow.

Residue Detection

In MRI, the signals in the tissue (as opposed to the signals at the venous outflow) are typically what is being measured over time following the administration of the contrast agent. A signal time course curve can be measured, and the processing and analysis can be performed for each pixel of a temporal series of coregistered images. This measurement observes the concentration of the agent remaining within the system (tissue blood volume) rather than the concentration measured at the venous outlet. Furthermore, the value from each voxel generally measures a subregion of the tissue volume supplied by an upstream injection of indicator. In these experiments, the measured concentration-time curve (for each voxel) actually measures the amount or "residue" (amount of indicator per amount of measured tissue) of indicator remaining within the tissue (within each voxel), so these procedures are often referred to as being residue or external detection measurements.

Residue detection avoids complications associated with multiple possible outlets (measurement sites) from the mixing volume. This approach also accommo-

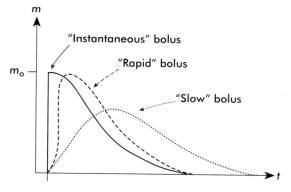

Fig. 7-39. Experimental bolus injection procedures typically do not deliver an ideal pulse of indicator to the tissue. (From Lassen NA, Perl W: Tracer kinetic methods in medical physiology, New York, Raven Press, p 28, 1979.)

dates multiple (arterial) inputs to the tissue volume and does not require that all inlets have the same arterial input curve (i.e., all act as one inlet). With residue detection, all that is required is that the fraction of indicator delivered by an inlet is directly proportional to the fraction of the total flow it receives and that all of the indicator bolus is delivered to the tissue before an appreciable amount has left the tissue.[119]

The tissue residual measurements can be related to the concentrations that would be measured at the venous outlet in order to see how the previously discussed concepts of MTT and flow or volume estimates apply. Before this relationship can be described, the situation for measurements made at the tissue outlet must be further characterized. As long as the entire outlet flow of indicator is adequately resolved and sampled, it does not matter if these outlet measurements are made using an imaging method or by some other method. Since it is possible to correct for nonideal bolus injections, we can proceed under the assumption that the indicator input to the tissue is an ideal pulse.

The amount of indicator leaving the tissue system during some small time interval, t to $t+dt$, is the concentration of indicator at the outlet, $C_{out}(t)$, multiplied by the volume of fluid leaving the system during this time interval, $F\,dt$,

$$M_{out}(t) = FC_{out}(t)dt \qquad (7\text{-}28)$$

where the subscripts serve to reemphasize that these measurements are made at the venous outlet of the tissue. The flow, F, is flow rate at the arterial injection and venous outlet sites. Since all of the injected indicator eventually leaves the tissue system and passes the outlet detector, the total sum over each individual amount leaving the system must equal the total amount of indicator that was supplied to the tissue, M_{inj}:

$$M_{inj} = \int_0^\infty M_{out}(t)dt = F\int_0^\infty C_{out}(t)dt \qquad (7\text{-}29)$$

This equation, as we have seen before (equation 7-20), can be rearranged to solve for the steady flow if the amount of injected mass supplied to the tissue is known.

From equation 7-28, it can be seen that the *fraction* of the total injected indicator leaving the system during the time interval t and $t+dt$, $h(t)$, is simply the amount leaving divided by the total injected amount of indicator

$$h(t) = \frac{FC_{out}(t)}{M_{inj}} = \frac{C_{out}(t)}{\int_0^\infty C_{out}(t)dt} \qquad (7\text{-}30)$$

where the rightmost term is obtained by replacing F using equation 7-29 (or equation 7-20).

From this expression, it can be seen that $h(t)$ is directly proportional to, and has the same shape as, the $C_{out}(t)$ curve measured at the outlet of the tissue. Assuming an ideal bolus introduction of the indicator to the tissue volume, the function $h(t)$ describes the distribution of transit times through the system, which is characteristic of the structure of the tissue.[129] In other words, $h(t)$ represents the relative proportions of indicator particles taking paths of different duration through the tissue and thus characterizes the relative amount of indicator particles that will arrive at the outlet to be measured at any time after the injection. As a physical example, if the tissue blood volume were composed of individual capillaries having equal diameters, $h(t)$ would represent the distribution of capillary lengths spanning from the inlet to the outlet (Fig. 7-40).

Each different path through the tissue has an associated volume determined by the tissue flow rate, F_t, and the time, t, it takes for a particle (and/or fluid) to traverse its length (see Fig. 7-38). $h(t)$ describes the fraction of all path lengths that have a transit time of t, so the fraction of the total tissue volume, dV_t, contributed by all paths having transit time t will be

$$dV_t = F_t t h(t) \qquad (7\text{-}31)$$

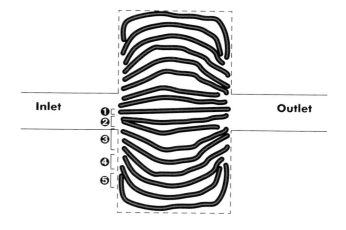

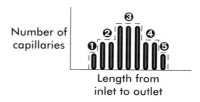

Fig. 7-40. If the tissue blood volume were composed of individual capillaries having equal diameters (*top*), then (as illustrated at the *bottom*), $h(t)$ would represent the distribution of capillary lengths spanning from inlet to outlet.

The total tissue blood volume is the sum over all the volumes contributed by paths of different lengths:

$$V_t = F_t \int_0^\infty t h(t) dt \qquad (7\text{-}32)$$

Using the expression for $h(t)$ from equation 7-30 and comparing with the definition of MTT (equation 7-25), we again obtain a statement of the central volume principle:

$$V_t = F_t \int_0^\infty t h(t) dt = F_t \, MTT \qquad (7\text{-}33)$$

This equation reiterates that the tissue volume to flow ratio can be determined by calculating the MTT from the first moment of the concentration-time curve measured at the *outlet* of the tissue.

Tomographic measurement. Tomographic imaging techniques generally measure the amount of residual indicator in the tissue. Furthermore, the measured signal curve for each voxel only measures the amount of indicator from the tissue subregion within that voxel (Fig. 7-41). At this point each voxel and each tissue segment can be considered separately. If $h(t)$ is the indicator fraction that leaves the tissue at time t, the fraction of indicator remaining in the tissue, $R(t)$, to be measured by residue detection

is 1 minus all of the fractions that have left since the injection and up to time t, $H(t)$:

$$R(t) = 1 - \int_0^t h(\tau) d\tau = 1 - H(t) \qquad (7\text{-}34)$$

This equation describes the relationship between a concentration measured at the tissue outlet and a concentration measured in the tissue. In the case of a bolus injection, the concentration measured at the draining veins will be proportional to the time derivative of the residual tissue concentration, $dR/dt = -h(t)$.[123,130,131] This can be seen by taking the time derivative of both sides of equation 7-34.

If the amount of indicator delivered to the voxel-sized region of tissue is M_0, the amount remaining in the tissue at time t will be $M_0 R(t)$. The measured tissue signal from a voxel, $S(t)$, is assumed to be proportional to the tissue concentration of indicator. As the delivered amount of indicator, M_0, is specified in terms of a weight per amount of measured (voxel) tissue, it will actually represent a measured bulk tissue concentration, and the signal measured at time t can be expressed as

$$S(t) = k M_0 R(t) \qquad (7\text{-}35)$$

where the proportionality constant, k, has units of amount measured tissue per indicator weight in order

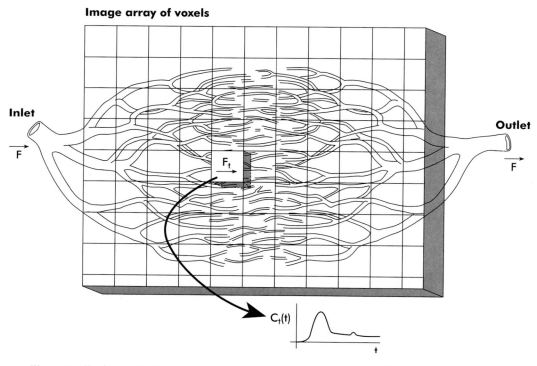

Image array of voxels

Inlet

Outlet

F

F_t

F

$C_t(t)$

t

Fig. 7-41. Each voxel of an imaging measurement measures the signal characteristics of only that voxel-sized region of tissue.

for the signal to be dimensionless. Therefore, the total measured tissue residue signal over time will be

$$\int_0^\infty S(t)dt = kM_0 \int_0^\infty R(t)dt \qquad (7\text{-}36)$$

Since $dR/dt = -h(t)$, this equation can be rewritten as

$$\int_0^\infty S(t)dt = kM_0 \int_0^\infty th(t)dt \qquad (7\text{-}37)$$

Incorporating the definition of MTT from equation 7-33, we end up with

$$\int_0^\infty S(t)dt = kM_0\, MTT = kM_0 \frac{V_t}{F_t} \qquad (7\text{-}38)$$

After all of this painful development, the significance of residual measurements made by tomographic imaging methods can be evaluated. First, equation 7-38 indicates that the area under the measured signal curve, $S(t)$, can be used to determine the tissue volume to flow ratio only if the amount of indicator actually delivered to the tissue in the voxel, from a total injected quantity of M_{inj}, is known. In general, the amount reaching the measurement voxel, M_0, from an upstream injection site will be unknown but may be considered to be in proportion to the fraction of the total flow at the indicator injection site, F, that actually supplies the tissue within the measurement voxel, F_t. In that case, equation 7-38 can be rewritten as

$$\int_0^\infty S(t)dt = kM_{inj}\frac{F_t}{F}\frac{V_t}{F_t} = kM_{inj}\frac{V_t}{F} \qquad (7\text{-}39)$$

Thus the collected signal curve for a completely intravascular indicator only provides information as to the local tissue blood volume.[132] Absolute volume measurements are possible if additional measurements are made (e.g., using equation 7-20) to determine the flow at the injection site. Relative tissue volume measurements can be made if the tissues to be compared are both supplied with blood from the same injection flow, which is likely to be the case for repeated measurements (i.e., stimulated/nonstimulated) at the same tissue site. These relative volume measurements do not depend on the detailed structure of the tissue at the comparison sites.

Flow measurements. Equation 7-39 provides no information about the tissue blood flow, F_t. For measurements made at the tissue *outlet*, tissue flow information is available from the *MTT* $(= V_t/F_t)$ obtained by computing the first moment of the measured concentration-time curve. However, as shown by

Weisskoff et al[131] and the above equations, the first moment of the measured curve does not provide the value of the MTT when using tissue residue detection. Equation 7-37 indicates that the zero moment (area) of the measured residue signal curve is proportional to the first moment (center of mass) of the outlet-detected concentration-time curve. (This can be more clearly seen by replacing $h[t]$ using equation 7-30.) Computing the first moment of the tissue residue signal curve will actually be related to the *second* moment of the outlet concentration-time curve, which is not simply related to the MTT and tissue volume or flow. While the first moment of the residue signal curve is related to the tissue volume to flow ratio, it additionally depends on the variance of transit times and on the detailed microvascular pathway structure within the voxel. Even though the details of this relationship may be complex, a center of mass calculation using the residue curve does provide information about tissue blood flow, whereas none is available from the area calculation (equation 7-39). Based on both analytic and simulation analysis, Weisskoff et al[131] concluded that absolute tissue flow measurements were reliable only in the rare circumstance where the detailed structure of the tissue vasculature had been adequately modeled. However, relative (ratio) tissue blood flow measurements are feasible if the microvascular topology is similar. Microvascular changes that may be expected to occur with functional activation, such as recruitment of additional vessels or dilation of a fixed number of vessels, will not severely affect relative flow measurements as long as the distribution of capillary path lengths does not change markedly.

In summary, for each resolution volume (voxel), the measured residue signal is the concentration of indicator in the total tissue volume within the voxel. The area under the recorded residue concentration-time curve is proportional to the local blood volume, and an image of this area calculation provides a map of the local plasma volumes. For MRI measurements of the residual concentration remaining in the tissue, the first moment of the residue concentration-time curve is not simply related to the MTT and the tissue volume to flow ratio. Unless an exact model of the vasculature is available, absolute tissue perfusion cannot be obtained from the first moment; however, this value can be used to obtain relative measurements of flow without specifying detailed models.

Volume measurements. Measuring the size of the various possible tissue compartments is generally difficult, requiring washout studies with different diffusible indicators having different exchange properties. However, determination of the accessible tissue blood volume is relatively straightforward with a purely intravascular indicator substance. Equation

7-39 specified that the area under the measured residual signal curve is proportional to the injected mass, M_{inj}, the injection and outlet flow rate, F, and the tissue blood (plasma) volume. If the injected mass is known, the tissue volume can be estimated if the flow rate can be determined.

If the injected mass is unknown, it is still possible to estimate the tissue volume if an arterial input time course, $I(t)$, is obtained from a location where all of the flow (and fraction of injected mass) is directed toward the tissue site of the residual measurement. The relationship of equation 7-20 can be employed for both the pretissue (arterial input) and posttissue (outlet) time courses. At the appropriate measurement location, the flow F_t values in both equation 7-38 (for the residual measurement) and equation 7-20 (which holds for the arterial input measurement) are equal and the equivalent delivered indicator mass divides out when rearranging to solve for the tissue volume

$$V_t = \frac{\int_0^\infty S(t)dt}{\int_0^\infty I(t)dt} \qquad (7\text{-}40)$$

The measurement of integrated area requires less temporal resolution than does the accurate determination of the center of mass (first moment),[76] so blood volume determinations by MRI are more likely to be successful than an estimation of tissue perfusion.

Vascular volume fraction. Many of the tissue parameters of interest are specified in relation to the amount of total tissue being measured. For example, tissue perfusion is typically specified in terms of flow rate per 100 g of tissue. The volume of tissue within a measurement voxel can usually be determined from the pulse sequence design, and this assessment of measurement volume may in fact be more accurate than that of other noninvasive external methods (e.g., volume of effective radioisotope counting). However, conversion to tissue weight requires an assumption regarding the density of the measured tissue.

The vascular space, particularly the microvasculature of interest in tissue exchange, is some fraction of the tissue volume, $f = V_t/V_{tot}$, and this parameter is often of interest. Note that this vascular volume is composed primarily of capillaries and small veins. Having an estimate of tissue blood volume, V_t, measured in a voxel by MRI, the blood volume fraction can be estimated using the size of the voxel as specified by the pulse sequence.

The volume fraction can also be estimated by concentration-time measurements made in both the tissue and the arterial blood using the relation[123]

$$f = \frac{\int_0^\infty C_t(t)dt}{\int_0^\infty C_a(t)dt} \qquad (7\text{-}41)$$

To obtain the information for the upper part of this equation, the tissue signal is measured with the image positioned to avoid major vessels. The information for the lower part can be obtained by measuring the concentration in a larger vessel. In practice, the arteries are difficult to use to get accurate measurement of concentration. The small size and limited imaging resolution lead to volume averaging with nearby parenchyma. Alternatively, the arterial levels can be obtained by direct, invasive arterial sampling.

Another possible method[133] estimates the fractional volume by making a tissue measurement after equilibrium of the indicator throughout the blood volume (assuming slow renal clearance) and obtaining a blood sample to get the arterial concentration.

MR Signal Strength Versus Gd Concentration

Indicator dilution analysis of measured concentration-time curves can provide estimates of both tissue flow and volume. The most important component necessary to be able to apply these concepts to MRI is the relationship between the measured signal characteristics and the local concentration of the injected paramagnetic contrast agent. To define the link between image intensity and contrast agent concentration, characterization of the mechanism, exchange kinetics, and compartmentalization of the compound are required. This relationship allows the measured signal intensity versus time curves to be converted into concentration versus time curves.

Bulk properties. The pharmacology of Gd-DTPA and the relaxation effects of Gd-DTPA in bulk solution are well established,[98,134-136] with both T1 and T2 rates showing a linear relationship with concentration (Fig. 7-42). At a field strength of 0.5 T, these relationships are reported[98] to be

$$\begin{aligned} T1^{-1} &= 0.39 + 4.52C \\ T2^{-1} &= 0.50 + 5.66C \end{aligned} \qquad (7\text{-}42)$$

where C is the concentration in mM/liter and 1/T1 and 1/T2 are in units of $\sec^{-1}$. However, the compartmentalization of the contrast agent to the vascular space leads to inhomogeneous distribution of the paramagnetic material and the formation of susceptibility-induced magnetic field gradients that further reduce the observed T2 of the tissue.

A number of experimental studies indicate a

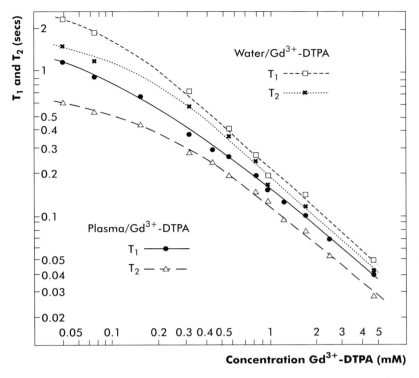

Fig. 7-42. Experimental results showing that relaxation is a function of Gd-DTPA concentration at 20 MHz. (From Gadian DG et al: J Comput Assist Tomogr 9[2]:242, 1985.)

linear relationship between Gd-DTPA concentration and T1 relaxation rate in other organs[136] and blood.[24] In general, these data were obtained under equilibrium conditions where the intravascular and extracellular concentrations have equalized. Most MRI flow/volume studies are nonequilibrium experiments with measurements obtained after a bolus injection of contrast agent in order to avoid recirculation and renal clearance effects.

In tissues other than the brain (with its blood-brain barrier), Gd-DTPA leaks out of the vasculature and causes a decrease in the signal of T1-weighted images. For a given tissue, the relationship is of the form

$$\Delta\left(\frac{1}{T1_{bulk}}\right) = \Delta R1_{bulk} = k_1 C_t \qquad (7\text{-}43)$$

where $\Delta R1_{bulk}$ is the difference between T1 rates with and without the presence of contrast agent, k_1 is a tissue and field strength specific constant, and C_t is the tissue concentration of the agent.[76,113] Recalling the exponential nature of relaxation rates, a linear rate change corresponds to a change in the monoexponential (measured) signal decay time course. This equation assumes a fast-exchange model where tissue water has ready access to relaxation sites on the paramagnetic ion (Gd^{3+}). In most tissues, the exchange across the endothelial membrane is relatively fast. In brain, the reduction in exchange rates by the BBB will not support a fast exchange model, and a medium exchange model may be more appropriate.

For dynamic observation of bolus injections, the effects on tissue signal may be lessened since there is less time for exchange. This is particularly true in the brain with an intact BBB where only small T1 effects on the tissue signal are observed.[99] These small effects can perhaps be attributed to the small volume fraction of the vascular blood where intravascular water has ready access to the paramagnetic species. In direct measurements of arterial signals (e.g., to obtain arterial input concentrations), the direct paramagnetic relaxation of the vascular water should be considered. While the tissue water is restricted in access to Gd-DTPA sites by the BBB, vascular water is not and the T1 shortening can be more significant than T2* effects at short TE. However, in vessels large enough for practical imaging measurements, there is usually sufficient inflow of relatively unsaturated spins to replace saturated spins and to minimize the signal increases resulting from direct T1 shortening.[137]

The work by Villringer et al[138] indicated that the degree of signal loss parallels the relative strengths of the magnetic moments (susceptibility) of a variety of injected agents and was not correlated with longitudinal relaxivities of the ions. This study used Dy-DTPA rather than Gd-DTPA since the former does not show any correlation between molar susceptibility and T1 relaxation. This allows a more clear evaluation of the susceptibility-induced signal effects. Since the signal loss occurs in T2- but not T1-weighted images, it can be concluded that the direct dipolar relaxation mechanism is not significant.

Susceptibility effects. The limited T1 relaxation rate effects of Gd-DTPA in the brain allows the signal effects from susceptibility differences to be more readily observed. The previously described medium exchange model of diffusion in inhomogeneous fields indicates that there will be an approximately linear relationship between Gd-DTPA concentration (tissue susceptibility difference) and signal relaxation rate.[8] The theoretical fast and slow exchange models of diffusion near paramagnetic particles predict that there will be a second-power relationship between T2 relaxation rate changes and contrast agent concentration. However, empirical data[76] support the results from the medium exchange simulations,[107,116] indicating that the relationship is closer to linear. The three models show more agreement (as to a nonlinear relationship) for isolated spheres, but cylindrical shapes represent a more realistic vascular model for agents confined to the plasma compartment.

Villringer et al[99] experimentally verified that the relationship between signal change, T2 relaxation rate change ($\Delta R2$), and brain tissue concentration can be approximated by a single exponential of the form

$$S = S_0\, e^{[-TE(\Delta R2)]} \qquad (7\text{-}44)$$

In this equation, S_0 is the signal, S, in the absence of contrast agent. This equation can be rearranged

$$-\frac{ln\left(\dfrac{S_0}{S}\right)}{TE} = \Delta R2 = k_2 C_t \qquad (7\text{-}45)$$

to show a linear relationship between the T2 rate change, $\Delta R2$, and the tissue concentration, C_t (Fig. 7-43). The constant of proportionality, k_2, is specific to the particular tissue, field strength, and pulse sequence.[113] The tissue specificity of k_2 can be further ascribed to variations in the underlying microvascular size, spacing, and orientation with respect to the static magnetic field.[139] These parameters can be expected to change with tissue type and pathologic conditions. The linearity of the relationship between relaxation rate and Gd-DTPA concentration may not hold for high amounts of contrast agent.

Changes in cerebral blood volume may be due to changes in the size of the vessels (distention) or to changes in the vessel density (recruitment) or both. Assuming that there is no overlap in field inhomogeneities from capillary to capillary, results from the numerically computed intermediate exchange models indicate that relaxation rate changes ($\Delta[1/T2]$ for SE

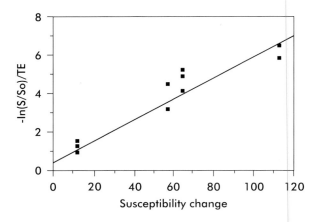

Fig. 7-43. Experimental results showing the linear relationship between T2 rate change and susceptibility (which is proportional to the concentration of contrast agent). (From Rosen BR, Belliveau JW, Chein D: Magn Reson Q 5[4]:263, 1989.)

sequences and $\Delta1/T2^*$ for GRE sequences) will increase monotonically with the microvascular volume fraction.[107] However, if the volume changes are due to distention, the rate changes will vary nonlinearly with volume fraction.[107] For volume fractions significantly higher than those typically found in tissue, the increases in relaxation rate should change to decreases with further volume fraction increases.

The susceptibility-induced signal changes affect the signal from significantly more tissue than just the intravascular volume of the tissue. The magnetic field gradients resulting from the susceptibility differences occur in the tissue immediately surrounding the vessel. The resonance frequency shift in the capillary is a few parts per million, and the shift decreases with the square of the distance from the capillary[99] (Fig. 7-44). Because the capillaries are so small (approximately 5 μm in diameter), a susceptibility difference of 1 ppm can induce an average field gradient in the tissue near the capillary of approximately 60 G/cm.[99] Using the simple model shown in Fig. 7-44, Villringer[99] estimated that diffusion would cause 62% of the protons in the tissue to experience these field gradients and become dephased by the echo time. This is relative to the approximately 4% vascular content of the tissue.

White and co-workers[140] noted that under equilibrium intravascular contrast agent conditions (using an iron-dextran compound) in animal studies, the apparent image signal intensity increased after cessation of blood flow. They proposed an extension to the contrast agent T2* signal decay mechanism to account for microvascular plasma motion. The large size of the RBCs relative to capillary dimensions leads to a model such as that shown in Fig. 7-45, whereby contrast agent confined to the plasma space alternates with RBCs. The motion of this periodic arrangement of

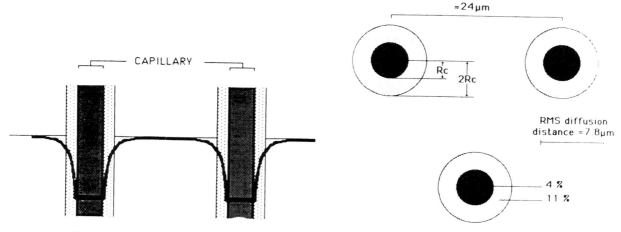

Fig. 7-44. Amplification of signal changes beyond the tissue microvascular content occurs from the susceptibility effects on the signal of surrounding tissue. (From Villringer A et al: Magn Reson Med 6:164, 1988.)

contrast agent is similar to the situation of diffusion in a periodic arrangement of gradients, the theory of which has been previously analyzed.[141,142] This motional model describes additional local field inhomogeneities that may contribute to the observed signal changes.

With the presence of pathology that alters the permeability of the BBB to Gd-DTPA, the relationship between relaxation rate changes and concentration will be altered. This is the result of two processes[35]: (1) the exchange of the contrast agent into the interstitial space will lead to a more uniform susceptibility distribution and a decrease in the amount of local signal-reducing field gradients and (2) the tissue water will have a more ready access to the paramagnetic ions and will experience direct dipolar relaxations leading to increased contrast on T1 images. These T1 effects can be assessed by observing the increasing signal intensity (accumulation) over time and can be reduced by lowering the T1 weighting (reduce TR and/or flip angle) of the imaging sequence.

Albert et al[143,144] have described and demonstrated the use of bolus injections of saline after a constant infusion of contrast agent. This interesting approach represents the converse situation to the bolus agent injections more commonly employed and should produce even larger susceptibility differences between tissue and vasculature.

MRI Volume/Flow Measurement

The potential for using measurements of relative blood volume changes for observing brain functional activity was recognized early in the development of MR susceptibility-contrast indicator methods.[4] The rapid development of these methods made them ready for application to stimulus conditions that produce an altered local CBV or CBF. A firm base from

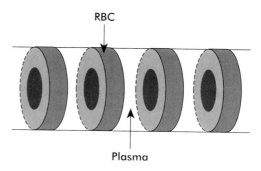

Fig. 7-45. Simple model for the extra signal decay resulting from motion of paramagnetic plasma regions.

previous PET,[145-147] CT,[148,149] and other work[150-151] supported these extensions. This previous work not only characterized the currently accepted FMRI mechanism—that cortical activation leads to increases in cerebral metabolism as well as blood flow—but also provided experience in areas of stimulus paradigm design, appropriate analysis procedures, and identification of expected anatomic locations of activation. While these administered contrast (Gd-DTPA) methods relied on previous PET and CT reports, the subsequent development of FMRI methods using only intrinsic deoxyhemoglobin as a contrast agent rapidly extended these concepts.

With the linkage between (signal) relaxation rate change and tissue concentration established, indicator dilution analysis for nondiffusible indicators can be applied to the measured first-pass intensity curves. To identify local CBV/CBF changes, two bolus doses are required, one during resting state and one during an activated state. With the renal clearance of Gd-DTPA, circulating levels of agent are low enough to allow the administration to be repeated within a half hour. Indicator methods that record flow at the venous outflow from an organ cannot assess regional flow variations within the organ. For this, direct external monitoring of the indicator concentration in the tissue is required. A linear system is preferred, so that a doubling of the flow causes a doubling of the indicator delivery to the tissue and a doubling of the detected response. The relationship between signal relaxation rate change and tissue concentration of Gd-DTPA has been shown to be approximately linear.

In MRI, susceptibility-based methods have a distinct advantage over methods that directly measure the signal characteristics of moving blood—namely, that the signal changes arise from significantly more tissue than just the small tissue volume fraction consisting of flowing vessels. As we have seen, the susceptibility-induced gradients extend beyond the boundaries of the capillaries and influence the signals arising from nearby extravascular tissue. An advantage of MRI methods over previous mapping technologies is in the reduced CBV measurement sensitivity to larger vessels, which can cause problems with radioisotope methods. Radionuclide CBV maps are dominated by macro- rather than microvasculature, while FMRI is more sensitive to microvascular changes.

Accurate measurements of the postinjection concentration-time curves can be obtained using the high temporal resolution offered by EPI instruments. The first pass transit time of the contrast agent bolus through the tissue is rapid, requiring fast imaging measurements to adequately record the accompanying intensity variations. In normal brain, cerebral circulation time (artery to vein) is on the order of 3.4 seconds[152] and with venous injection of a bolus, the delivery of contrast to the brain occurs after approximately 30 to 40 seconds. In the absence of ultrafast imaging capabilities, an alternative method for obtaining measurements of the transit curve with high temporal resolution is to image in only a single dimension, selecting a column passing through the desired region of interest.

Acquisition of relative CBV images using indicator dilution methods is easier than obtaining the data necessary for forming relative CBF images. This is because an accurate measurement of the arterial input function is required to deconvolve the measured concentration-time curve to obtain an accurate estimate of the MTT and thus, using the central volume principle, the relative flow image. Relative CBV measurements, with respect to some imposed stress or change, can be made without determination of the proportionality constant, k_2, relating signal relaxation rate and concentration. Quantitatively characterizing k_2 can prove to be difficult, requiring rapid (multiple) measurements of relaxation rate rather than single measurements of intensity.[133]

The arterial input information is potentially obtainable using MRI by measuring the time course of signal change in an imaging slice positioned through the cerebral arteries supplying the tissue of interest. This approach has been validated in animal experiments where direct arterial blood sampling confirmed the MRI results[4] (Fig. 7-46). The orientation of the artery of the measurement must be noted since arteries parallel to the field will show little susceptibility effect on surrounding tissue. Perman et al[137] demonstrated the use of a modified FLASH sequence designed to simultaneously make images from the brain and the internal carotid arteries in order to obtain the arterial input function (Fig. 7-47).

General findings. The limited number of studies reporting on this technique reflects more the excitement generated by subsequent developments in non-contrast FMRI methods rather than any lack of effectiveness of Gd-DTPA methods. The results using this technique focused on in vivo validations of the measured CBV changes using interventions with known CBV responses. The results using visual stimulation have been shown[8] to agree with those of previous PET studies.[2,153,154]

Belliveau et al[4] demonstrated that visual stimulation produces measured CBV changes of 32% ± 10% within the primary visual cortex[8] (Fig. 7-48). This and subsequent reports indicate that bolus injections of 0.1 mM/Kg Gd-DTPA result in peak signal losses on the order of 20% to 80% at 1.5 T[155] and 20% to 40% at 1.0 T,[156] reflecting a good measurement dynamic range (Fig. 7-49). Synthetic CBV maps in this region of the calcarine cortex have an image SNR of 30 or 40 : 1, which implies the ability to see changes on the order of 3%. This sensitivity may result in Gd-DTPA methods being preferred over intrinsic-contrast FMRI methods for investigation of more subtle stimuli and responses.

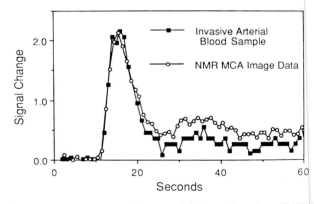

Fig. 7-46. Experimental data validating the use of NMR measurements of arterial input function. (From Rosen BR et al: Magn Reson Med 19, 285, 1991.)

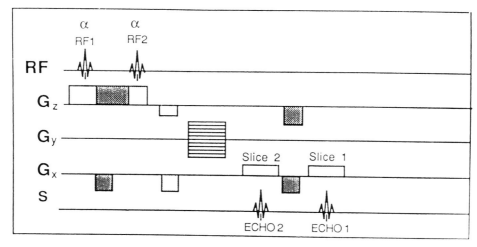

Fig. 7-47. Modified FLASH sequence that simultaneously obtains data from an additional input slice location. (From Perman WH et al: Magn Reson Med 8:74, 1992.)

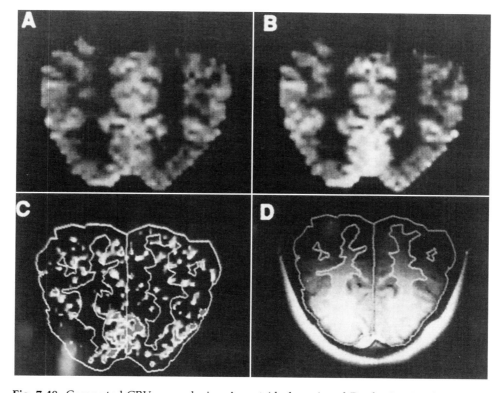

Fig. 7-48. Computed CBV maps during **A**, rest (darkness) and **B**, photic stimulation. The difference image (**C**) is superimposed on an anatomic image (**D**) to show activated regions of the primary visual cortex. (From Belliveau JW et al: Science 254:716, 1991.)

Equilibrium studies. Volume calculations using equilibrium (i.e., not first pass) T1 relaxation measurements have been shown in animals using Gd-DTPA bound to the plasma protein albumin.[157-159] Values of absolute CBV (volume/volume%) can be calculated from normalized signal intensities of post-contrast-enhanced minus pre-contrast-enhanced tissues over those arising solely from blood protons (such as those

measured in the slow flowing sagittal sinus) in the region of interest. The large size and slow clearance of this indicator substance allow equilibrium measurements to be made of both the tissue and the arterial concentrations of indicator. These equilibrium estimates of CBV did not require dynamic imaging or an estimate of MTT. In using Gd-DTPA for human studies, the relatively fast renal clearance of contrast agent formulations complicates this type of equilibrium analysis.

Applications. Measurement of CBV with MRI techniques has a number of diagnostic applications. CBV maps appear to be closely correlated with tumor grade, with low-grade lesions showing low CBV and more aggressive lesions demonstrating elevations of CBV at or above that of normal brain.[8] This is similar to previous PET reports.[160,161] MRI CBV maps can identify regional variations within tumors, with the focal

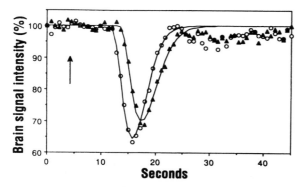

Fig. 7-49. Measured first-pass signal intensity curves obtained during rest and visual stimulation. These results show a 32% ± 10% increase in CBV with activation. (From Belliveau JW et al: Science 254:716, 1991.)

increases in CBV corresponding to local regions of elevated PET ^{18}F-deoxy-glucose uptake (Fig. 7-50). Another potential application is in aiding the currently difficult differential diagnosis (from MRI findings) of radiation necrosis or recurrent tumor. A decreased local CBV is consistent with postradiation changes.

Validation. A number of experimental studies have supported the validity of CBV and CBF measurements using MRI of injected Gd-DTPA. These have shown that MR signal changes and CBV/CBF measurements are consistent with changes expected in previously characterized systems. For example, by varying the arterial pCO_2, which is known to correlate with blood volume and flow, the relationship between susceptibility-induced signal change and brain blood volume was determined in a dog model[4] (Fig. 7-51). These changes, as well as the resting blood volume ratio of gray and white matter ($\sim 2:1$, Fig. 7-52), showed good agreement with the results obtained by other methods.

Although there is no single method to measure CBF that is clearly accepted as valid and to which other methods can be compared with complete confidence,[17] several alternative methods are available to corroborate the MRI findings. An accurate method, but one that is inappropriate for human studies, is the use of microspheres or "molecular microspheres" such as

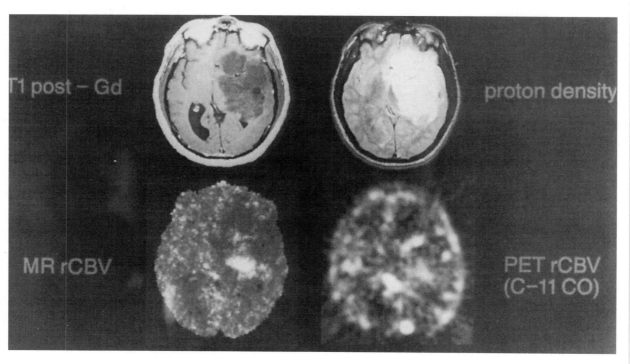

Fig. 7-50. MRI CBV maps can demonstrate regional variations within tumors, and these results are consistent with PET findings obtained on the same subject. (From Rosen BR et al: Magn Reson Med 19:285, 1991.)

lipid-soluble ligands that bind to receptors.[19] The microspheres are fully extracted from the flow and are deposited within the tissue. Measurement of local tissue concentration and comparison with a reference arterial sample can provide estimates of absolute flow to the tissue. Other CBF methods include SPECT imaging of pharmacologic agents with high first pass extraction (e.g., HMPAO), PET imaging of diffusible tracers such as $H_2^{15}O$, and x-ray CT imaging of both diffusible (^{131}Xe) and nondiffusible (iodinated chelates) agents.

Assessment of BBB permeability. Paramagnetic relaxation agents have long been used for nonimaging measurements of cellular permeability and water exchange times.[113,161,162] In normal brain the BBB prevents the contrast agent from leaving the plasma compartment of tissue and exchanging into the interstitial spaces. When the BBB is impaired by pathologic processes, the contrast agent does leak into the extravascular (but still extracellular) space and acts to reduce signal intensity. The time course of this leakage provides information as to the severity of BBB disruption. With the availability of very fast imaging methods, it is possible to extend observational studies toward quantitative analysis of BBB permeability.[106,164]

The dynamic imaging of the time course of tissue uptake measures the temporal characteristics of tissue, and this can be used as another tissue parameter for

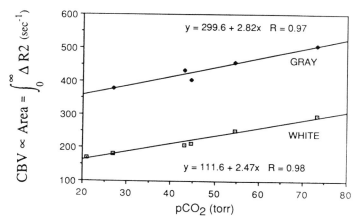

Fig. 7-51. Data showing cerebral blood volume changes with pCO_2 changes in a dog model. (From Belliveau JW et al: Magn Reson Med 14:538, 1990.)

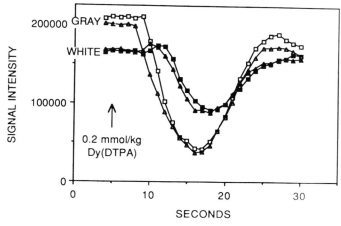

Fig. 7-52. Concentration-time data obtained using a dog model show a resting gray/white matter blood volume ratio of approximately 2 : 1. (From Belliveau JW et al: Magn Reson Med 14:538, 1990.)

discriminating between different tumor or tissue types. Using the imaging speed of EPI and other fast imaging techniques, the time after an inversion preparation pulse can be interactively adjusted to set tumor intensity to low values, thus increasing the sensitivity to changes from an injected Gd-DTPA bolus.[165]

A qualitative assessment of BBB permeability (or disruption of such) can be had by repeated measurement of postinjection signal change. The slope of the intensity measurements versus time indicates the exchange of the contrast agent into the interstitial space. This simple modeling can be extended using diffusible indicator methods[164] where a compartmental model is used to relate the observed signal characteristics to the tissue concentration. It is also possible to measure the permeability-surface product, PS, using brain uptake and arterial concentrations. This may prove to be useful in the characterization of tumors and their response to treatment.

DEOXYHEMOGLOBIN PRINCIPLES
Blood Oxygenation

A small amount of the blood oxygen at microvascular oxygen tensions is in the form of directly dissolved paramagnetic ^{17}O, but this contributes only a negligible amount (~ 0.02 sec^{-1}) to the relaxation rate of blood.[10] The remainder of blood oxygen is bound to hemoglobin, with up to four oxygen molecules per hemoglobin molecule.

Hemoglobin. Hemoglobin (Hb), with a molecular weight of 64,500, is the predominant macromolecule in blood.[10] The net concentration of hemoglobin in blood is approximately 15 g/100 ml, with intracellular concentrations of approximately 38 g/100 ml or 5.5 to 6.0 mM. Hemoglobin consists of two pairs of polypeptide chains (jointly called globin), each of which is attached to a heme group, which is a complex of iron and

protoporphyrin (Fig. 7-53). The attachment of oxygen is dependent on the local partial pressure of oxygen (also known as oxygen tension or pO_2), allowing oxygen to be released at the tissues when local metabolic activity causes local oxygen depletion. The hemoglobin oxygen dissociation curve displays a sigmoidal profile (Fig. 7-54). This profile means that oxygen binding (or affinity) is stronger when one or two oxygen molecules are already bound to the molecule. The converse is also true, in that when oxygen tension is reduced, dissociation will occur more readily after one oxygen has been released from the fully oxygenated hemoglobin.

The paramagnetic nature of deoxygenated hemoglobin and its influences on the NMR signal were recognized long before the development of clinical MRI.[22,166] In deoxygenated hemoglobin, dHb, the heme iron is in a high-spin ferrous (Fe^{2+}) state characterized by four of its six outer electrons being unpaired. The unpaired electron spins have a very large magnetic moment, and the associated paramagnetic properties make it behave in a manner similar to exogenous paramagnetic contrast agents. With oxygenated hemoglobin (Hb), one of the electrons is transferred to the oxygen molecule, and the heme iron changes to a low-spin state and has no magnetic moment or paramagnetic effects.[167]

T1 effects. The bulk relaxation of whole blood is similar to relaxation of Hb solutions, so the effects of the RBC cell membrane and of the presence of plasma protein appear to be limited.[10] However, paramagnetic dHb is relatively inefficient in causing direct T1 relaxation of solutions.[168] Thus direct paramagnetic

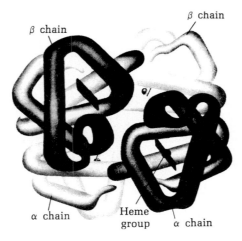

Fig. 7-53. Hemoglobin molecular structure. (From Berne RM, Levy MN [eds]: Physiology, St Louis, 1983, Mosby.)

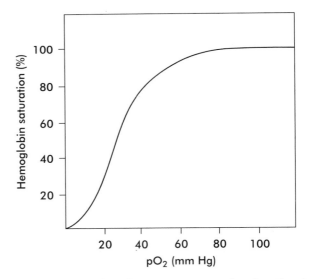

Fig. 7-54. Hemoglobin dissociation curve showing the sigmoidal relationship between hemoglobin oxygen saturation and local pO_2. (From Berne RM, Levy MN [eds]: Physiology, St Louis, 1983, Mosby.)

relaxation of water protons is generally considered to be negligible because the four unpaired electrons of the iron are well sequestered within the dHb molecule.[10] This is not the case with methemoglobin, which is formed during blood breakdown. In this case the access of water protons to the (now) five unpaired electron sites on the paramagnetic ion is improved and direct relaxation effects will come into play.[10,169,170]

Bulk T2/susceptibility effects. As opposed to administered contrast agents, which are restricted to the plasma compartment, paramagnetic dHb is confined to the intracellular space of the RBCs. The applied magnetic field causes the paramagnetic ion to align with the field with its large characteristic susceptibility producing a relatively large local field. The confinement of the dHb in the RBCs causes them to have different susceptibility than that of the surrounding tissue and plasma, leading to a inhomogeneous local magnetic environment (Fig. 7-55). Field inhomogeneity does not affect longitudinal (T1) relaxation rates since there is no motional component at frequencies near the Larmor frequency to promote energy trans-

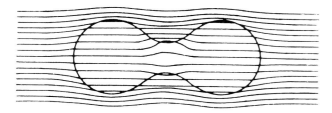

Fig. 7-55. Alteration of local lines of magnetic field near a red blood cell. (From Brindle KM et al: Biochem J 180:37, 1979.)

fer. Transverse relaxation is affected by the motion of protons in the inhomogeneous fields, which causes them to experience different field strengths, to precess at different frequencies, and to lose phase coherence.

Fully deoxygenated RBCs have a susceptibility 0.2 ppm greater than fully oxygenated blood.[9,10,171] The magnetic field mapping results from Weisskoff et al[171] demonstrate a linear relationship between susceptibility and blood oxygenation at 1.5 T (Fig. 7-56). The relative susceptibility difference between paramagnetic dHb inside RBCs and the surroundings leads to local regions of inhomogeneous magnetic field. As described previously, there are several possible theoretical models to describe the effects of diffusion on the signal from inhomogeneous field environments. These models are characterized by assumptions as to the spin exchange between the different local field environments. In the case of dHb sequestered within RBCs, the relative contributions of water diffusion through intracellular, extracellular, or transmembrane field gradients toward the observed reduction in T2 relaxation time are of additional interest.[172]

The exchange time of water between blood intracellular and extracellular environments is rapid, with an intracellular residence time of approximately 6 to 8 ms.[10,162] Several studies have estimated a diffusion time constant from data of measured T2 relaxation versus sequence echo time in order to see how it compares with the cellular exchange time. In addition, shifts in blood proton resonance frequency upon deoxygenation have been recorded, indicating a field difference between compartments. The results have been varied, attributing the primary source of signal loss to extracellular gradients,[173] intracellular gradi-

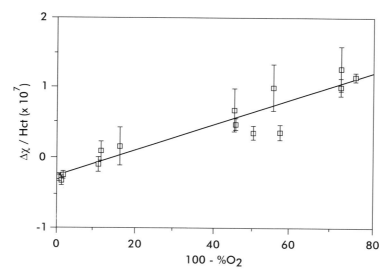

Fig. 7-56. MRI susceptometry results showing a linear relationship between blood oxygenation and susceptibility. (Susceptibility is normalized to hemoatocrit.) (From Weiskoff RM, Kiihne S: Magn Reson Med 24:375, 1992.)

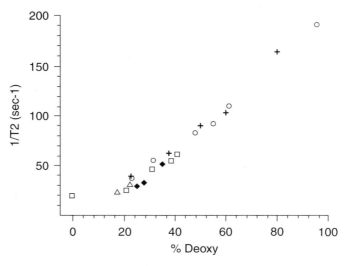

Fig. 7-57. The dependence of the blood water T2 relaxation rate on the level blood oxygenation at 7 T. The various symbols represent the different measurement samples. (From Ogawa S, Lee TM, Barrere B: Magn Reson Med 29:205, 1993.)

ents,[114] transmembrane exchange,[168,174] combination of intracellular and extracellular factors,[9] and equal but isolated contributions.[172]

Blood T2 oxygenation dependence. The T2 relaxation rate of blood solutions can be directly related to the level of oxygen saturation of Hb. Results from a high field (7 T) study[10] are shown in Fig. 7-57, indicating that a linear relationship exists between percent oxygen saturation and measured T2 values. These relationships can be utilized in human imaging studies where, in regions of uniform distribution of dHb (e.g., in the sagittal sinus when it is oriented parallel to the static magnetic field), the pO_2 in venous blood can be estimated by measuring the T2 and comparing to an in vitro calibration curve.[10,175] Wright et al[175] demonstrated that accurate estimates of blood oxygenation could be measured in this way using conventional imaging systems, even in the presence of steady blood flow.

Blood T2 field dependence. The susceptibility-induced frequency difference between the RBC and the surroundings depends on the strength of the applied magnetic field. Therefore, the inhomogeneity contribution to the signal decay will also be some function of the magnetic field strength. The T2 for whole blood was measured by Thulborn et al[9] at frequencies from 80 to 469 MHz. They examined the amount of diffusion in the inhomogeneous fields by comparing CPMG measurements of oxygenated and deoxygenated blood. Subsequently, similar measurements were made by Gomori et al[174] at frequencies closer to those used for MRI (8 to 60 MHz) but with longer TEs for more diffusion weighting. The results of

both of these studies indicate that T2 relaxation rate of blood increases approximately quadratically with field strength (Fig. 7-58). Brooks and DiChiro[10] imaged samples of blood of varying oxygenation states at both 0.5 and 1.5 T and found that the inhomogeneity effects on deoxygenated Hb images are visually striking at 1.5 T and are observed to a lesser extent at 0.5 T.

Arteriovenous oxygenation differences. Arterial blood typically contains approximately 20 ml oxygen/ 100 ml blood at a partial pressure of 100 mm Hg.[176] As the blood flows from the heart into the cerebral arterial network, it enters regions where there are radial (around the vessel) gradients favoring oxygen loss. The radial pO_2 gradient across large arteries is the arterial pO_2 (~100 mm Hg) minus tissue pO_2 (10 to 20 mm Hg). Although this gradient is large, the amount of oxygen lost from the large arteries is not great because the ratio of surface area to blood volume within these vessels is low. However, as the arteries branch successively, the surface-to-volume ratio increases and the amount of oxygen loss becomes greater. In practical terms the oxygen loss becomes significant somewhere in the small precapillary arterioles[17,176-178] (Fig. 7-59). Intravascular pO_2 has been reported to decrease from 100 mm Hg in vessels approximately 230 μm in diameter to 73 mm Hg in arterioles approximately 20 μm in diameter. Although this decrease in pO_2 represents only a small reduction in blood oxygen content, it is not correct to assume that oxygen loss occurs only within capillaries. Longitudinal (along the vessel) oxygen gradients occur as well as radial gradients, resulting in the venous blood having a different oxygenation than that of arterial blood. As oxygen consumption by the tissue increases

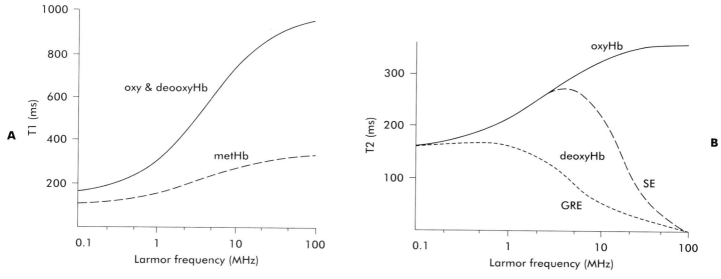

Fig. 7-58. Dependence of T1 (**A**) and T2 (**B**) on magnetic field strength for bulk blood solutions. (From Brooks RA, Di Chiro G: Med Phys 14[6]: 1987.)

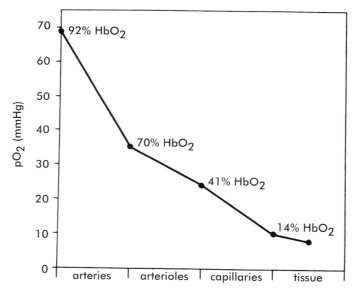

Fig. 7-59. Oxygen loss and decreased pO_2 at different levels in the vasculature. (From Intaglietta M, Johnson PC: Peripheral circulation, New York, 1978, Wiley.)

(without additional delivery), these gradients become more pronounced and exchange in precapillary vessels may become more significant.

Venous blood oxygenation levels depend on both the supply and the consumption of oxygen delivered to the tissue. Using Fick's principle, the tissue oxygen extraction, OE (ml O_2/g/min), can be related to the cerebral blood flow, CBF (ml/g/min), and the difference between the venous, O_v, and arterial, O_a, blood oxygenation (ml O_2/ml):

$$OE = CBF(O_a - O_v) \qquad (7\text{-}46)$$

During brain activation, PET measurements have determined that OE does not change much relative to the resulting increase in CBF. Therefore, the arteriovenous oxygenation difference will decrease with increased delivery, and in particular, the venous oxygenation increases to be closer to the arterial oxygenation. The venous volume will be simultaneously increasing, and it is the balance between the MR signal effects of the venous oxygenation change and the venous volume change that dictates how the image appearance is affected.

Oxygenation Image Appearance

The general image appearance resulting from paramagnetic dHb is hypointensity (or complete signal void) resulting from the signal dephasing acquired

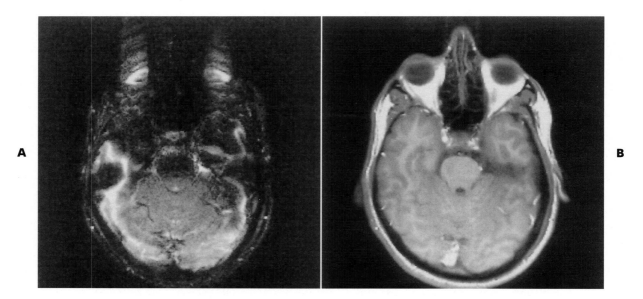

Fig. 7-60. A, Gradient echo images with very long TEs can be severely distorted at normal tissue susceptibility interfaces. **B,** Corresponding spin echo image.

during diffusion in the local inhomogeneous fields. Variations in magnetic susceptibility may also introduce effects that are similar to chemical shifts. Chemical shift image contrast has been reported,[179,180] as has direct encoding of susceptibility shifts into image phase[181,182] and frequency.[183] These methods generally use subtraction of repeated image acquisitions to remove other sources of contrast.

Tissue susceptibility differences. The image effects of intrinsic tissue susceptibility discontinuities can be observed in long TE images of normal anatomy. Even without consideration of blood oxygenation factors, susceptibility-caused image distortion at tissue interfaces, particularly air/tissue boundaries, can obscure the normal anatomy. Deep-lying structures such as the hippocampus and olfactory bulb and areas near the sinuses and petrous bone are often distorted. Gradient echo images with TEs longer than approximately 65 msec will give severely distorted images at 1.5 T (Fig. 7-60). As expected with the more pronounced frequency differences caused by susceptibility differences at 4.0 T, gradient echo images with TEs longer than 25 msec give poor image quality.[184] In cases of large inherent variations in tissue susceptibility, spin echo sequences, with their insensitivity to static inhomogeneity artifacts, may be preferred over gradient echo sequences despite the reduced susceptibility-induced signal attenuation, representing a reduced sensitivity to changes in dHb levels.

Increased spatial resolution can be used to reduce image artifacts at tissue susceptibility interfaces. However, since the susceptibility variations of interest to blood oxygenation measurements are microscopic and subvoxel, dHb sensitivity is not expected to change

with increasing resolution.[185] In fact, signal responses to oxygenation changes will often increase with increasing resolution as a result of the reduction of partial volume effects obscuring focal changes. Sequences can be designed to measure susceptibility values, and Weisskoff et al[171] developed an offset spin-echo EPI technique to measure bulk susceptibility of solutions from their image appearance.

The image appearance of local susceptibility variations from dHb and metHb is of significant clinical concern in cases of hemorrhage or hematoma. After hemorrhage, oxygenated blood hemoglobin becomes deoxygenated and is converted to methemoglobin and ultimately to hemosiderin. The readily apparent image hypointensity (particularly on gradient echo sequences) caused by signal loss near the paramagnetic centers can be used for detection and characterization of these lesions.[186-189]

Vascular Oxygenation Appearance

At this point we begin to specifically consider the nature of oxygenated/deoxygenated blood in the microvasculature, as opposed to that in bulk solution. Under these conditions, dHb acts similarly to administered paramagnetic contrast agents. Both materials are completely confined to the intravascular space, although Gd-DTPA occupies the plasma space while dHb remains inside RBCs. In both cases, the tissue microvasculature appears to cylinders of different magnetic susceptibility.

Orientation dependence. At high fields and in high-resolution images, the image effects of paramagnetic blood are particularly apparent. Fig. 7-61 shows these effects for a capillary tube phantom filled with

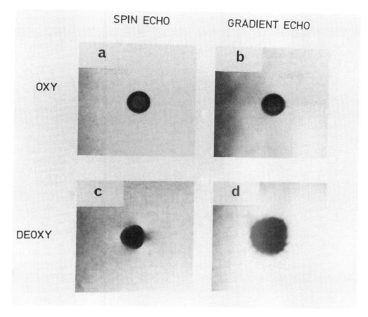

SPIN ECHO   GRADIENT ECHO

OXY   a   b

DEOXY   c   d

Fig. 7-61. Phantom results showing the image effects of susceptibility differences at high field strengths. (From Ogawa S, Lee TM, Nayak AS, Glynn P: Magn Reson Med 14:68, 1990.)

blood.[11] The decrease in signal from the material surrounding the tube is present with deoxygenated, but not oxygenated, blood samples. As expected, images from spin echo sequences are less affected by the inhomogeneity induced by dHb than those from gradient echo sequences.

In Fig. 7-61, the capillary tube was oriented perpendicular to the direction of the main magnetic field. An orientation dependence (with respect to the static field) is characteristic of susceptibility effects; orienting the capillary tube parallel to the magnetic field results in little effect on either GRE or SE images of dHb. This orientation dependence can also be seen in the images of Fig. 7-62, taken to show the inplane image susceptibility appearance.[12] When the capillary tube is oriented so that it is parallel to the static magnetic field, the magnetic field does not pass through susceptibility discontinuities in the material and there will be little field variation around the tube. When the tube is placed perpendicular to the static field, there will be regions of magnetic field inhomogeneity around the interface between the dissimilar (susceptibility-wise) materials. The variation in frequency, ω_S (i.e., magnetic field), around a long cylinder of radius a (microvessel model) at a distance r from the center ($r \geq a$) (Fig. 7-63) can be expressed[11,190] as:

$$\frac{\omega_S}{\omega_0} = 2\pi\Delta\chi\left(\frac{a}{r}\right)^2 (2\cos^2\theta - 1) \qquad (7\text{-}47)$$

where $\Delta\chi$ is the difference in susceptibilities, θ is the angle between the radial direction and the static field direction, and ω_0 is the resonance frequency far away from the interface. The value of $\Delta\chi$ is proportional to

the degree of oxygenation (and dHb). Taking $\Delta\chi$ to be 0.06×10^{-6} for 50% oxygenation, the variation in ω_S/ω_0 can be estimated[11] to be ± 0.08 ppm at a distance of one radius away from the tube ($r = 2a$). Depending on the pulse sequence details, this amount of variation is likely to cause complete dephasing and signal loss, and regions at least twice as large as the actual vessel size will have a dark image appearance. This expression also indicates that the frequency differences and image appearance will depend on the strength of the magnetic field, reflected in both ω_S and ω_0. The use of image appearance to estimate degree of tissue (as opposed to bulk) blood oxygenation is complicated by this dependence on the (unknown) microvascular size and orientation.

RBC motion. Unlike administered Gd-DTPA, which is confined to the plasma space, dHb is confined to RBCs that, for small capillaries, may act as moving point sources of magnetic field inhomogeneity. The phase of nearby proton spins may be affected by the motion of the RBC more than the diffusive motion of the proton.

Venography. Using tailored RF pulses to suppress normal tissue, Cho et al[191] demonstrated the use of susceptibility images to visualize primarily venous structures (MR venogram) based on their higher levels of dHb.

Responses to Imposed Oxygenation Changes

The signal dependence on the level of blood oxygenation provides a mechanism by which changes in oxygenation can be observed using MRI. Changes in

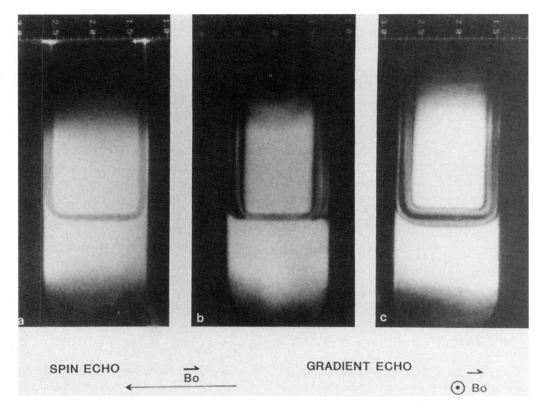

SPIN ECHO $\overrightarrow{Bo}$ **GRADIENT ECHO** $\overrightarrow{Bo}$

$\odot$ Bo

Fig. 7-62. The effect of magnetic field orientation at 7 T on images of a U-shaped capillary tube filled with deoxygenated blood in a saline bath. With the magnetic field parallel to the horizontal axis (the read gradient axis) of the image. **A,** A spin echo image. **B,** A gradient echo image with the magnetic field perpendicular to the slice plane. **C,** A gradient echo image. In all cases, the plane of the U-tube was contained in the slice plane. The capillary tube (1.5 mm o.d. and 1.0 mm i.d.) was filled with deoxygenated blood. (From Ogawa S, Lee TM: Magn Reson Med 16:9, 1990.)

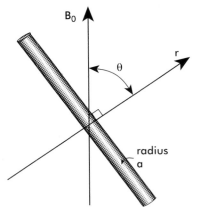

Fig. 7-63. Model for determining the effects of orientation with respect to magnetic field.

paramagnetic deoxyhemoglobin levels can be correlated with local blood flow, and thus to local brain activity. This was first recognized in extremely high-field (7 and 8.4 T) and high-resolution (65 μm) images of rodents[11] and has been termed "blood oxygen level dependent" (BOLD) contrast (Fig. 7-64). In these

studies it was shown that image contrast associated with venous blood vessels correlated well with the oxygenation of the breathing mixture and thus with the vascular oxygenation. In general, because the number of variables that contribute to the activation-induced signal change is large, it is difficult to quantitatively relate signal change, dHb levels, and neuronal activity. However, when using two acquisitions obtained under different neurologically active conditions, relative oxygenation changes can be mapped to form FMRI images.

Under normoxic conditions, BOLD contrast in the brain primarily reflects the microvasculature for venous blood.[192] Venous oxygenation levels result from the combination of oxygen extraction by the tissues and the blood flow delivery of oxygen to the tissue. The balance of these factors may be altered by changes in tissue metabolism in response to neuronal activation or by imposed changes in arterial blood oxygenation. The association of activation-induced signal effects with dHb level is supported by the lack of significant contrast changes with the introduction of carbon monoxide (carbon monoxyhemoglobin is not

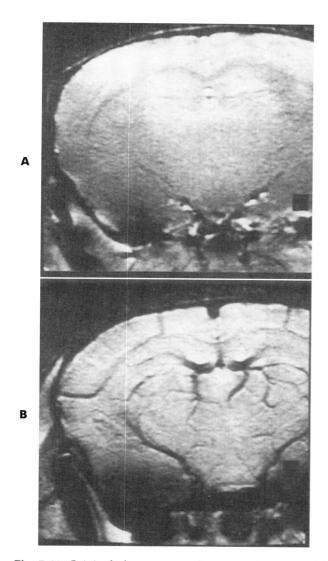

Fig. 7-64. Original observations of oxygenation contrast in rat images at 7.0 T. **A**, 100% oxygen breathing mixture (GRE image). **B**, 20% oxygen breathing mixture (GRE image). (From Ogawa S et al: Magn Reson Med 14:68, 1990.)

potential areas of application where more subtle stimuli or cognitive tasks may elicit smaller activation changes.

Bulk T2* changes between oxygenated and deoxygenated blood samples depend quadratically on the field strength.[9,10] In tissue, signal changes resulting from an activation-induced oxygenation change are also expected to increase at a nonlinear rate with increasing field strength. A number of simulation models,[107,171,193] approximating vessels as paramagnetic cylinders predict that for a constant echo time, the change in relaxation rate for a given change in blood susceptibility should vary as a power of the static field (B0) in the range of 1.6 to 2.0. At very high fields, the contribution of deoxygenated blood water to the calculated image can be neglected because of its short T2 relative to the echo time. At lower fields, the contribution of the tissue blood water to the intravoxel signal should be taken into account. The simulations identify diffusive movement through the local field gradients as being important for accurate prediction of relaxation rate, at least for vessels of capillary dimensions.

Turner et al[184] compared the results from visual stimulation at 1.5 and 4.0 T obtained under approximately equal conditions. Using a gradient echo EPI sequence, they found mean changes in signal intensity of approximately 15% at 4.0 T and approximately 4.7% at 1.5 T (Fig. 7-65). These results indicate that transverse relaxation rate change exhibits a greater than linear (1.5 to 1.8) dependence on static field strength, also consistent with susceptibility dependence being the dominant signal change mechanism.

SNR considerations. FMRI at higher field strengths can benefit from two important mechanisms. We have seen that the susceptibility-related changes in transverse relaxation rates increase nonlinearly with an increase in magnetic field strength. In addition, the image SNR generally increases with field strength, potentially allowing the detection of even smaller signal changes.

However, Jezzard et al[194] reported on a preliminary study comparing in vivo background noise at both 1.5 T and 4.0 T. These results suggest that the physiologic contribution to background variations (in gray matter) is approximately equal at both field strengths. These results showing that the image noise sources are not particularly field dependent are consistent with the dominant mechanism of image-to-image variability ("noise") as being physiologic rather than from electronic noise sources that are expected to be reduced at higher field.

In addition to improving the conspicuity of activation-induced responses, the increased signal response to oxygenation changes at high (4.0 T) fields may be applied to the use of sequences (e.g., SE) that

paramagnetic) breathing mixtures. Sequence behavior is also consistent with paramagnetic effects, in that image appearance increases with increasing TE and has an orientation dependence and the appearances are much more apparent on GRE images as compared with SE images.

Field dependence of oxygenation changes. Since BOLD contrast was first described at field strengths far above those available in whole body systems, an immediate issue arises as to the hardware requrements for effective human study—more specifically, whether systems with field strengths higher than the 1.5 T of most currently available systems are required. This is also central to questions as to the potential clinical accessibility of FMRI systems and in regard to the

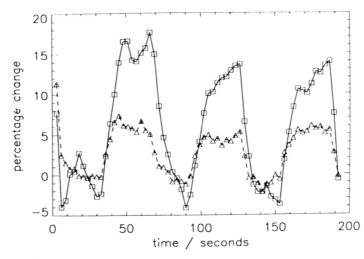

Fig. 7-65. Signal changes caused by visual stimulation for a volunteer studied at both 1.5 T and 4.0 T. (From Turner R et al: Magn Reson Med 29:277, 1993.)

are less sensitive to susceptibility changes but have other desirable characteristics. As will be discussed, spin echo and gradient echo sequences show differing sensitivities toward vessel size.

It is often difficult to directly compare SNR and BOLD characteristics between field strengths because tissue relaxation rates also increase with field strength. In addition, susceptibility artifacts increase with field strength. This primarily affects the available choice of TE at the different field strength. In the study mentioned before, Turner et al[184] selected a TE of 40 msec at 1.5 T and a TE of 25 msec at 4.0 T for their comparisons.

It is clear that FMRI at higher field strengths has advantages. However, the volume of 1.5 T work and the apparent quality of results indicate that 4.0 T may not be *required* for clinical FMRI research and application. The high field strength advantages in observing small signal changes may be lessened as 1.5 T systems become more stable, allowing smaller changes to be visible. In addition, sequence and procedural improvements continue to be developed to reduce unwanted sources of image signal change with brain activation. All MRI instrument manufacturers continue to develop improved systems with higher performance. Now that FMRI is being established, these specific requirements are being incorporated.

Signal with respect to oxygenation changes. The sensitivity to blood oxygenation depends on the extent of blood susceptibility change and the blood vessel volume fraction of the tissue within the imaging voxel. There is some indication that venous oxygen saturation dominates other factors.[193]

Ogawa and Lee[10] showed that in rats, at 7 T changes in the blood oxygenation from 0 to 100% results in a gradient echo (TE = 15 ms) signal change of 15% to 20% in regions where there are no obvious large blood vessels. Spin echo signals over the same oxygenation range showed a change of only a few percent. The tissue T1 was found to be insensitive to oxygenation.

In their landmark paper presenting photic stimulation results at 1.5 T, Kwong et al[13] estimated the amount of signal change that could be expected. Assuming that blood volume increases by 30%[4] and blood flow increases by 70%, an initial venous oxygenation of 60%, with constant oxygen consumption,[5,58] will become a final venous oxygenation of 75% during stimulation. Since the volume susceptibility difference ($\Delta\chi$) between totally deoxygenated blood and the surrounding brain is approximately 6.4×10^{-8} (cgs units),[171] visual stimulation should decrease the blood/tissue susceptibility difference from 3.8 to 1.5×10^{-8}. Modeling the cerebral vasculature as a set of randomly oriented cylinders[195] and neglecting T1 effects caused by increased flow, tissue with an initial blood volume fraction of 4% should show a 2% signal increase in GRE images at TE = 40 msec. This prediction is in good agreement with the experimental results showing primary visual cortex signal changes of 1.8% ± 0.8% with visual stimulation (Fig. 7-66).

Subsequently, work by a number of groups[184,196,197] at 1.5 to 2.0 T reported average signal changes with visual stimulation of 1% to 6% on GRE images. Groups working at 4.0 T typically report changes on the order of 5% to 20%.[184,198,199]

Simulation. A medium exchange computer model can be employed to predict the dependence of T2 or T2* relaxation rate changes on a number of parameters.[118] Physiologic parameters include diffusion co-

Photic Stimulation -- GE Images

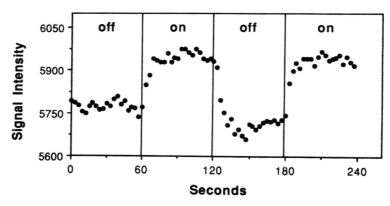

Fig. 7-66. EPI data detailing the time course of activation during visual stimulation at 1.5 T. (From Kwong KK et al: Proc Natl Acad USA 89:5675, 1992.)

efficient, blood volume fraction, vessel size, and blood oxygenation. Assuming that the susceptibility difference between fully deoxygenated blood and the surrounding tissue is approximately 7×10^{-8} cgs units[171] and that blood flow increases represent an increase in number of vessels (recruitment) rather than an increase in vessel size, the signal changes resulting from flow increases (for reasonable physiologic parameters) are as shown in Fig. 7-67. For a 70% increase in flow, approximately 1.5% changes at 1.5 T and 6% changes at 4.0 T are expected for gradient echo images. Spin echo (T2) relaxation rate changes are expected to increase more rapidly with field strength than gradient echo changes (T2*). This simulation is expected to overestimate the signal effects, while experimental results indicate that this may in fact be an underestimation.

Time course/mechanism. Using the rapid imaging times of EPI hardware and sequences, the results of FMRI studies show that signal intensity changes are observable within seconds after the onset of stimulation. The latency of the activation-induced BOLD signal change in primary cortical regions is approximately 5 to 8 seconds from stimulus onset to 90% max and is 5 to 9 seconds from stimulus cessation to 10% above baseline.[13,200,201] Often a transient undershoot after the end of stimulation is seen, and occasionally a decrease in baseline value is observed after the first activation period during cyclic activation[197] (Fig. 7-68).

The rise in signal most likely reflects a transient hyperoxemia and increased local blood volume as a result of regulatory overcompensation of blood flow to only a mild increase in tissue demand for oxygen. This is similar to the mechanisms previously proposed from PET studies. The rise times may represent the vascular transit times of the tissue.[13] The bulk of the activation-induced T2* change is not expected to be detected

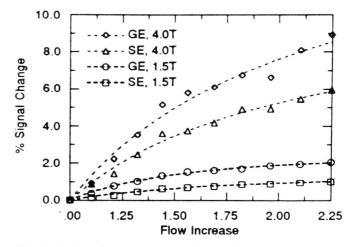

Fig. 7-67. Signal changes expected from blood flow changes at both 1.5 T and 4.0 T. These simulation results consider that the flow increases by increasing the number of vessels rather than increasing vessel size. (From Weisskoff R et al: Functional MRI of the brain: a workshop, SMRM and SMRI, June 1993, p. 103.)

until the blood has transited the capillary bed and the (relatively) oxygenated blood fills the venous capacitance vessels. The observed signal rise times (~4 seconds) are in reasonable agreement with the cerebrovascular transit times measured with ^{15}O-labeled carboxyhemoglobin.[150]

Turner et al[14] showed in animal studies that signal intensity changes were observable within seconds of lowered blood oxygenation induced by changes in breathing mixture. They also observed a similar 6-second signal rise and distinct overshoot when oxygenation was restored (Fig. 7-69). The signal profile returns to normal after 10 minutes. These authors suggest that the overshoot indicates a transient decoupling between blood flow and oxygen utilization during the first minute of restoration of oxygen. It is known that CBF is enhanced during temporary

Temporal Resolution: 3.0 s

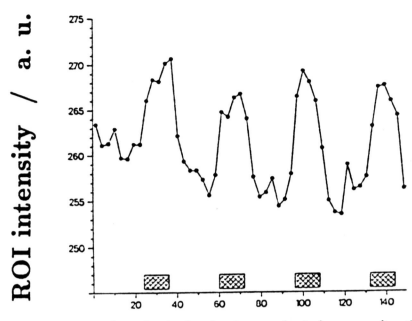

Fig. 7-68. Time course of visual activation showing overshoot of recovery after stimulation and a decreasing baseline throughout repeated cycles. (From Frahm J et al: Functional MRI of the brain: a workshop, SMRM and SMRI, June 1993, p 154.)

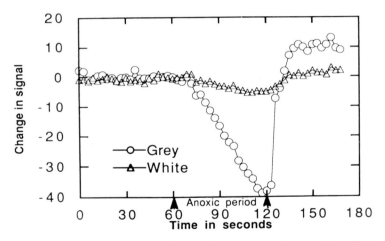

Fig. 7-69. Time course of cat anoxia experiments showing overshoot of signal intensity after restoration of oxygen. (From Turner R et al: Magn Reson Med 22:159, 1991.)

anoxia,[202] and there may be an excess oxygen delivery when normoxia is resumed. The depression of metabolism during anoxia, and hence oxygen extraction, may also persist temporarily after reoxygenation of the blood. In further correlative optical studies on cats, Turner et al[203] found that the basal level of arterial oxygen saturation is close to maximal and that the observed signal overshoot during recovery is therefore unlikely to reflect arterial dHb levels. Furthermore, the arterial oxygen saturation is only a rough measure of the oxygenation state in capillaries and venules.

Temporal resolution requirements. These studies suggest that the temporal resolution available with FMRI techniques for following brain activation is limited more by physiology than by technology. Current EPI and other fast imaging methods have a time resolution more than adequate to accurately follow the time course of the hemodynamic responses, but these occur several orders of magnitude slower than the actual neural responses observed using electrophysiologic techniques such as EEG or MEG. FMRI is appropriate for localization of sustained activations of distinct populations of activated neurons but is less appropriate for investigating the dynamics of interaction between these populations.

IMAGING PROCEDURES

The currently accepted physiologic mechanism underlying current FMRI techniques is that cortical activation leads to increases in cerebral metabolism as well as blood flow and volume. The deoxyhemoglobin (BOLD) contrast mechanism further assumes that the increase in oxygen delivery exceeds the tissue demands and consumption, so the oxygenation of the venous blood pool increases and the concentration of paramagnetic dHb decreases.

While Gd-DTPA bolus tracking methods can be effectively used to detect a number of these responses, the development of BOLD techniques for identifying activation changes (without administered contrast agents) has led to the bolus methods being largely superseded. Most current FMRI procedures localize regions of brain activation by detection of either local blood flow changes or changes in local blood susceptibility.

FMRI is based on observing signal differences between two acquisitions obtained under conditions of different neural activity, typically during stimulation and rest. In general, the sensitivity of these procedures to slight motions and misregistrations requires that these two states be imposed during the same imaging session. Relatively short stimulation and rest intervals are usually cycled repeatedly in order to reduce the possibility of response saturation while obtaining additional data for averaging and SNR improvement.

FMRI Sequences

Although FMRI applies some of the latest developments in MRI sequence design, the procedures can be discussed in terms of the two familiar classes of imaging sequences: gradient recalled echo (GRE) and spin echo (SE). In making a distinction between "fast" and "slow" imaging methods, echo planar imaging (EPI) can represent the fast techniques, with both GRE and SE variants, while the slow group is represented by FLASH (GRE) and standard SE.

Susceptibility sensitivity. The primary choice between SE and GRE sequences is whether the property of refocusing static field inhomogeneities is desired. As discussed below, the choice between these types of sequences has important implications regarding the source of signal (i.e., small versus large vessels). It is well known that spin echo (SE) sequences refocus phase accumulations as a result of static magnetic field variations such as main magnetic field inhomogeneity. However, dynamic phase accumulations such as those

from diffusional motion are not refocused by the 180-degree pulse. Gradient recalled echo sequences (GRE) only refocus phase shifts caused by the application of the gradient and do not refocus either static inhomogeneity–caused shifts or those from moving spins. Even more than FLASH imaging, GRE EPI at long echo times often has problems with artifacts from static field inhomogeneities and typically requires a global shim linewidth of better than 50 Hz. This is particularly the case at higher fields (4.0 T), where structures near air-tissue interfaces are often obscured by artifact.

Temporal resolution. Bolus injection FMRI methods place perhaps the highest temporal resolution demands on imaging sequences because the results are so dependent on obtaining a sufficient number of images during the rapid first pass through the tissue. The accuracy of CBV/CBF estimations depends directly on how precisely the concentration-time curve can be determined from the available data. The reduced temporal resolution requirements of BOLD methods potentially allow successful FMRI studies on instruments not capable of the imaging rates required by Gd-DTPA methods.

However, even in BOLD studies, EPI temporal resolution is often an advantage, particularly when response time courses are of interest or when images from extensive spatial regions are required. EPI methods utilize special gradient and data acquisition hardware to obtain a full image approximately every second with an echo time of 14 to 64 msec. Although an entire image is acquired in only 20 to 100 msec, a delay is normally imposed before the next acquisition to allow for the recovery of longitudinal magnetization. However, the availability of the specialized instrumentation required for EPI is still limited, and other imaging sequence approaches can be employed that offer comparable imaging times.

SE sequence speed. Other than by single shot techniques such as SE EPI, it can be relatively difficult to effectively speed up FMRI spin echo acquisitions. RF power deposition (by the repeated RF pulsing) considerations can limit the use of RARE and other fast spin echo sequences, particularly at fields much above 2.5 T.[204] The primary effect of field inhomogeneities (caused by dHb) on images from SE sequences is the result of spin diffusion taking place during the time prior to the echo. As seen in CPMG sequences, the rapid application of repeated 180-degree pulses in fast spin echo techniques can be expected to make the sequence relatively insensitive to both diffusion and susceptibility. However, a preliminary demonstration of FMRI using this type of sequence has been presented.[205]

GRE sequence speed. While there are several reasons for faster imaging, the temporal resolution available with conventional single-slice FLASH sequences (~3 to 10 seconds) is on the order of the temporal response times of the FMRI hemodynamic mechanisms. In order to obtain further speed increases, there are several approaches to obtaining faster gradient recalled imaging. Some of these methods have been introduced in a previous chapter on MRI principles, and additional procedures will be discussed further after the characteristics of GRE and SE have been more fully described.

Signal-to-noise ratio. Temporal resolution is not the only advantage that EPI may have over FLASH imaging. In a single shot technique like EPI, all of the equilibrium longitudinal magnetization is available for excitation and production of the encoded signals. FLASH imaging (and other multishot techniques) has an available magnetization dependent on the equilibrium established by the TR and flip angle parameters and is typically only a fraction of the total equilibrium magnetization. The repeated nature of these sequences (for acquiring all of the Fourier lines) does provide a theoretical SNR improvement, but this only goes up as the square root of the number of acquisitions. For brain imaging, an EPI image with 40 msec acquisition time has been found to have approximately the same SNR as a FLASH image (with optimized bandwidth) taking over 2 seconds to acquire. Faster FLASH images will generally have a poorer SNR than EPI.[204]

Coil/hardware choices. The current methods of obtaining FMRI localizations generally benefit from increasing magnetic field strength and from many advanced instrumentation features such as echo planar imaging and active shielded gradient coils to reduce eddy currents.[13,14,198]

As in other types of MR imaging, the choice between whole head and localized surface coils is primarily a trade-off between improved SNR for detection of small activation-induced signal changes and a limited field of view, restricting the area where the image information can be effectively obtained. Surface coils have been successfully used in measurement of visual reponses because of the relatively convenient superficial location of primary visual cortex. However, detection of additional visual areas may be limited by the rapid decrease in sensitivity away from the coil. Surface coils may also be employed to study somatomotor cortex (among other sites), but the limited FOV most likely does not allow observation of bilateral or contralateral activations.

As an alternative to the expensive implementation of whole body gradient coils and amplifiers capable of the fast switching and large currents required for EPI, small head–sized gradient coil systems are often employed. These 26 to 33 cm (ID) coils support rapid gradient switching in either all three or perhaps just one (typically the Z) orthogonal direction.[71,184,196] A potential drawback to the use of these gradient coils may be in reduced patient acceptance toward relatively long functional imaging sessions in such a confining head coil system. In addition, presentation of some types of stimulus may be made less convenient.

Sequence Sensitivity to Vessel Size

There is an increasing amount of evidence suggesting that SE signals from tissue arise primarily from capillaries while GRE signals arise from both capillaries and larger venules/veins. Evidence for this is primarily based on modeling and simulation results, but there are also experimental results indicating that FMRI activations spatially correspond to vessel locations as identified by high-resolution imaging and angiography. The simulation results indicate that vessels of less than 30 μm diameter dominate the contrast changes in spin echo images, while gradient echo images are sensitive to susceptibility changes in vessels of any diameter.[107]

Simulation. Numerical simulation models[107,206] indicate that spin echo and gradient echo images will have greatly differing sensitivities to the size scale of field inhomogeneities, which in turn reflect the size and shape of the region of differing susceptibility.

The results from computer simulation and experimental testing of relaxation rate changes with respect to the size of spherical magnetic field perturbers are shown in Fig. 7-70. From these results,[118] it can be seen that the relaxation rate depends on the size of the particle and that spin echo and gradient echo images show similar signal changes for small particles. However, unlike gradient echoes, spin echo signal relaxivities decrease with increasing particle size. The peak relaxivity occurs at a size characteristic of the peak frequency shift caused by the particles. While the general properties of these curves are fairly independent of the exact shape of the perturbers, more exact predictions do depend on the shape. Fig. 7-71 compares the relaxivity caused by spherical and cylindrical models for the same susceptibility change and volume fraction. These results[118] show that cylinders tend to produce greater relaxation at small size than comparable spheres, although somewhat smaller relaxation at larger size.

While related to medium exchange models discussed previously, a similar biophysical model incorporating diffusion is given by Ogawa et al.[193,207] In this computational model (also using Monte Carlo simu-

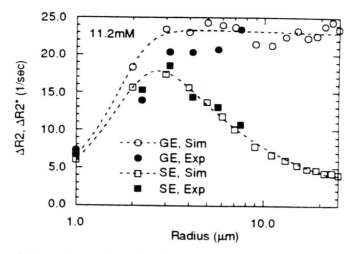

Fig. 7-70. Simulation and experimental relaxation rate results for Dy solutions and microsphere particles of different sizes. These results predict that spin echo and gradient echo images will have differing sensitivity to the size scale of the field inhomogeneities. (From Weisskoff R et al: Functional MRI of the brain: a workshop, SMRM, June 1993, p 107.)

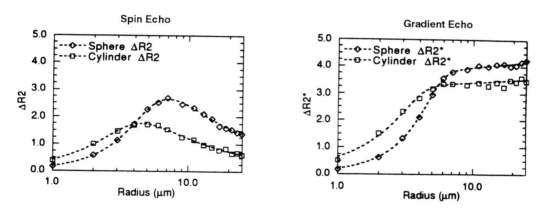

Fig. 7-71. Dependence of predicted GRE/SE size sensitivity on the shape of the magnetic field perturber. Cylindrical shapes tend to produce greater relaxation at small size than comparable spheres but somewhat smaller relaxation at larger size. (From Weisskoff R et al: Functional MRI of the brain: a workshop, SMRM, June 1993, p 103.)

lation), an image voxel is considered to be composed of a large number of small cubic compartments, each with a blood-containing cylinder running through the center. The size and number of the cubes depend on the blood volume fraction, and it is assumed that the orientation of the cylinders is uniformly distributed. Water molecules make random walks through each cube, and the accumulated signal phase caused by the local field induced by the susceptibility of the blood-containing cylinders is averaged over all cubes to give the voxel SE and GRE signals.

This model allows the signal influence of various physical parameters to be examined. For a given blood volume, blood oxygenation, field strength, and TE value, the ratio $\Delta R2/\Delta R2^*$ is dependent on the water diffusion coefficient and the vessel radius. For a given diffusion coefficient, $\Delta R2/\Delta R2^*$ decreases with increas-

ing radius (Fig. 7-72). $\Delta R2$ has a maximum at a diffusion distance approximately equal to the vessel radius, and $\Delta R2^*$ increases continuously with increasing radius. These results imply that the effect of water molecule diffusion is strong for the case of small blood capillaries, but, for larger venous blood vessels, water diffusion is not an important determinant of deoxyhemoglobin-induced signal dephasing. Given the field strength dependence of relaxation rate changes, these results further suggest that the field strength dependence of the fractional signal change on stimulation is linear for venules and larger veins but quadratic for capillaries.

Ratios/relative size contribution. The above discussion of differences in size sensitivity of spin echo and gradient echo sequences suggests that differences

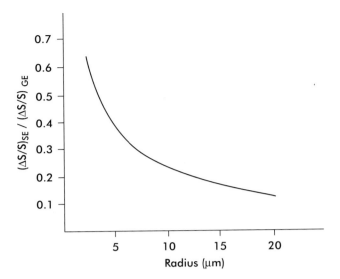

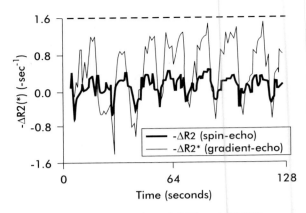

Fig. 7-74. Results from combined GRE and SE EPI sequence. As expected, GRE results are more sensitive to susceptibility changes than SE. (From Bandettini PA et al: SMRM 12th annual meeting, Vol 1, p 169, 1993.)

Fig. 7-72. Simulation results indicate that the ratio of spin echo to gradient echo signal change will decrease with increasing vessel radius giving rise to the signal. (From Ogawa S et al: Biophys J 64:803, 1993.)

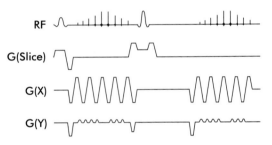

Fig. 7-73. Combined gradient echo and spin echo EPI sequence. (From Bandettini PA et al: SMRM 12th annual meeting, Vol 1, p 169, 1993.)

or ratios between the results from both sequences can be used to identify signal changes arising from larger veins. The simulation results indicate that if the ratio of the changes in SE to GRE images is small (e.g., less than 0.2), then the measured image intensity changes are probably arising from vessels greater than 20 μm. On the other hand, if the two types of images give a similar response, the observed intensity changes are more likely arising at the capillary level.[193,208] Bandettini et al[209] have shown that it is possible to obtain both SE and GRE data simultaneously using a modified EPI sequence. This type of simultaneous acquisition (Fig. 7-73) avoids the misregistration problems of sequential acquisitions. From a bilateral finger experiment, they found an average activation $\Delta R2^*/\Delta R2$ ratio of 3.57 ± 0.27. Example results from a single activated pixel are shown in Fig. 7-74.

Experimental findings. The T2* rate changes with susceptibility alterations are expected to have a de-

pendence on magnetic field that is between linear and quadratic.[184,193] Menon et al,[210] using a somewhat conservative linear extrapolation from their 4.0 T results, predict 1% to 2% changes in gray matter areas and 5% to 6% changes in larger vessels for GRE sequences. They conclude that at 1.5 to 2.0 T and at short echo times, the 5% changes reported likely correspond to larger vessels.

Lai et al[211] used high-resolution MR angiography to identify veins as the source of the largest signal changes (Fig. 7-75) and concluded that activation-induced signal changes at 1.5 T are primarily from T2* effects originating from the macroscopic venous structures on the surface of the cortex rather than from the parenchyma.

Significance of venous contribution. The significance of large vessel sensitivity is primarily in regard to the accuracy of FMRI identifications of activated cortex. If there is no size selectivity, there is a concern that large draining veins carrying hyperoxygenated blood away from activated regions will influence the MR signal from surrounding tissue. This tissue, having no functional relationship to the stimulus response, will appear from the FMRI image data as being involved. This type of concern is not new in functional imaging; PET has long been subject to emphasizing the signals from larger vessels.

While the evidence of sensitivity of GRE sequences to venous signal changes at 1.5 T is compelling, the practical significance of this finding has not been established, particularly concerning how far this artifactual activation extends from the ''actual'' site of neural activation. An example of an FMRI result apparently showing strong signal from large vessels is shown in Fig. 7-76. However, the central sulcus is correctly identified in this patient. For localized areas of activation, it seems likely that downstream venous

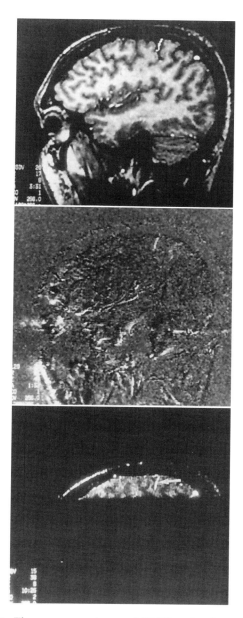

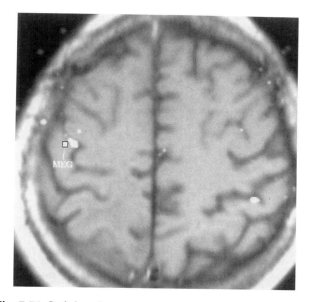

Fig. 7-76. Left-hand motor activation shows signal changes apparently corresponding to larger vessels. However, the activation correctly identifies the central sulcus and is consistent with the corresponding MEG localization in the same tumor patient.

Fig. 7-75. The correspondence of FMRI activation with the location of vascular structures identified on high-resolution MRA implicates venous vessels as being a significant site of observed activation changes. (From Lai S et al: Magn Reson Med 30:387, 1993.)

oxygenation changes will be rapidly diluted by drainage from uninvolved areas. Resolving this question is likely to be complicated by regional variations in microvascular anatomy and venous drainage patterns.

SE EPI and GRE EPI regions of signal change are similar,[204] indicating that the complication of signal contribution from larger draining veins may not be large. The scale of significance of localization errors is perhaps best referenced to the application of FMRI to presurgical planning. In this application, localization errors of over 10 mm begin to negatively affect clinical

utility. However, only with recent developments in intraoperative localization-digitization systems can measurements on the scale of 1.0 mm have clinical significance. The localization errors arising from the larger vessel sensitivity of GRE FMRI at 1.5 T are likely to fall into the intermediate range.

Sequence Sensitivity to Flow

The FMRI mechanism assumes that venous oxygenation changes are the result of changes in local cerebral blood flow. These blood flow changes can be detected using flow-sensitive sequences. Because susceptibility-induced field gradients extend into the tissue outside the vessels, signal changes from the BOLD contrast mechanism arise from significantly more tissue than just the 2% to 4% volume fraction of the microvasculature. This will not be the case with directly flow-sensitive methods. Bandettini et al[196] estimated the expected extent of signal changes with inflow of less saturated spins into the imaging volume. Given a blood T1 of 1.0 second and a steady state (EPI) TR of 2 seconds, the saturated blood in the imaging region will be at 85% of equilibrium longitudinal magnetization. If all of the tissue blood (say 4% volume fraction) is replaced during activation, the maximum flow-related signal enhancement would only be approximately 0.6% ([1 − 0.85] × 0.04).

FMRI measurements based on T1 measurements were demonstrated by Kwong et al,[13] who used a T1-weighted inversion recovery SE (IRSE) sequence (although TE = 42 msec) to observe blood flow

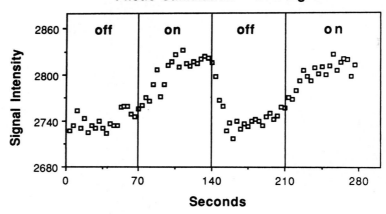

Fig. 7-77. Results obtained during visual stimulation using a SEIR sequence. (From Kwong KK et al: Proc Natl Acad USA 89:5675, 1992.)

changes in the primary visual cortex (V1); they found approximately the same extent of change (1.8%) as in GRE images. In another study, Kwong et al[212] found that the average GRE percentage signal change at V1 was 2.5% ± 0.8%, the average T2 SE signal change was 0.7% ± 0.3%, and the average T1 IRSE signal change was 1.5% ± 0.5%.

These SEIR signal changes (Fig. 7-77) result from tissue T1 changes that occur from the inflow of spins into the imaging volume, as detailed by Detre et al,[90-92] and they may influence additional signal from tissue outside of the vasculature. Kwong et al[13] estimated that the observed 2% signal changes correspond to perfusion changes of approximately 55 ml/min/100 g, which is consistent with previous PET reports.[2,153] Previous Gd-DTPA work[4] shows that local blood volume increases by approximately 30% with visual activation, which may provide additional signal change.

Inflow contribution. EPI images, with measurement times of less than 100 msec, are less influenced by blood flow and motion. However, inherent to FLASH GRE sequences is spin saturation, particularly when large flip angles are used. This results in a sensitization to inflow effects, which may be accentuated when flow-compensating gradient waveforms are used. Therefore, measured GRE signal changes from activation are likely to contain significant contributions from direct blood flow effects associated with the increased cerebral activity. Implications of this in regard to FMRI localization accuracy are similar to those discussed for vessel size dependence.

The stronger the T1 saturation of the stationary spins, the brighter the signal will be from unsaturated spins moving into the imaging region. The sensitivity of FLASH images to inflow can be reduced by using lower flip angles. The demonstration of this by Frahm et al[185] is shown in Fig. 7-78.

A number of preliminary experimental reports indicate that relaxation rate changes with functional activation are strongly influenced by direct inflow effects. Observation of FMRI responses at very low field strengths (0.15 T), below the effective field strength for the susceptibility mechanism,[213] supports the concept of a significant influence of inflow on observed signal changes. Duyn et al[214] assessed inflow using saturation bands on either side of image slice, the addition of which reduced the observed signal changes from 30% to 5% from photic stimulation. From these and other tests, they concluded that the large signal changes of other reports are caused mainly by direct inflow effects. Van Yperen et al[215] used turbo spin echo sequences to check the effect of inflow and found that the 8% responses observed after motor stimulation could be all attributed to inflow effects.

Sequence Bulk Motion Sensitivity

The appearance of motion in images is a significant problem in FMRI, producing artifactual changes that can appear to be correlated with the stimulation and confounding interpretation of FMRI results. This type of bulk motion is likely to become more of a problem with patients than with cooperative volunteers.

Since FMRI images represent the difference between activated and nonactivated acquisitions, any movement between images can give rise to artifacts on the difference images. Even motions of less than the dimensions of a single pixel can produce significant artifacts. This motion sensitivity emphasizes the importance of effective head restraint during the imaging session. Common methods employed include fitted head holders, evacuated styrofoam surgical padding, and bite-bar systems. It is possible that monitoring of external sensors or markers can be used to identify the extent of bulk motion. Even with external restraint, there will always be some degree of

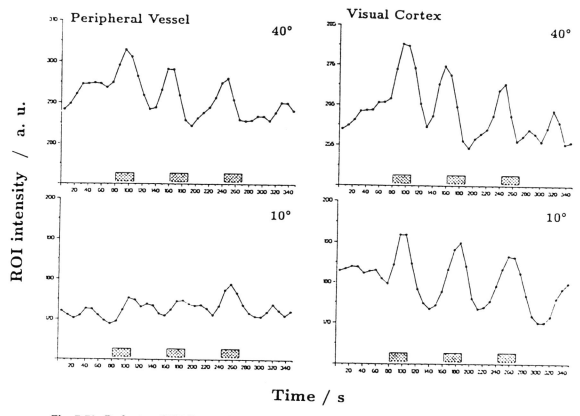

Fig. 7-78. Reducing GRE flip angle reduces inflow effects and signals arising from vessels while the susceptibility mechanism maintains signal changes from cortical regions. (From Frahm J, Merboldt KD et al: Functional MRI of the brain: a workshop, SMRM, June 1993, p 154.)

internal motion. The brain itself, not just CSF, undergoes significant bulk motion[216] throughout the cardiac cycle, although these brain motions tend to return back to original position (Fig. 7-79).

Motion-insensitive sequences can be implemented for FMRI applications, and reduction of these artifacts may allow smaller activation changes to be observed using conventional imagers. Glover et al[217] demonstrated the use of both spiral scan and projection reconstruction techniques for reducing artifacts from brain pulsatile motions. These approaches take advantage of the oversampling of low spatial frequencies that is characteristic of these methods.

Some reports have gone as far as to conclude that all activation at 1.5 T can be explained by local motion artifacts correlated to the stimulus presentation.[166] A study by Hajnal et al[218,219] analyzing small (subpixel) image-to-image displacements found that the presentation of the visual stimulus caused small flinch responses on the part of volunteers that could lead to image appearances similar to activation (Fig. 7-80). Their Doppler ultrasound measurements also indicated 20% to 30% velocity increases in the posterior cerebral artery with visual stimulation. The associated perfusion changes may result in the physical displace-

ment of venous and tissue structures and lead to artifactual enhancement on difference images. These results emphasize the importance of patient motion restraint and/or application of image registration procedures to avoid motion artifacts.

Sequence Parameters

As in normal imaging, sequence parameters such as TR, TE, and flip angle are available for tuning. In FMRI studies, the objective is not to maximize general tissue contrast but rather to maximize contrast specifically with respect to changes in susceptibility and deoxyhemoglobin levels.

Choice of TE. The longer the time spins are allowed to experience the local field distortions caused by susceptibility differences, the more dephasing and signal loss will occur. Thus susceptibility effects on image contrast will increase with increasing TE. However, the measurable signal strength simultaneously decreases with TE because of intrinsic T2 relaxation processes. The selection of sequence TE is an important choice in FMRI studies since this parameter directly influences the sequence sensitivity to susceptibility changes. In addition, the choice of TE

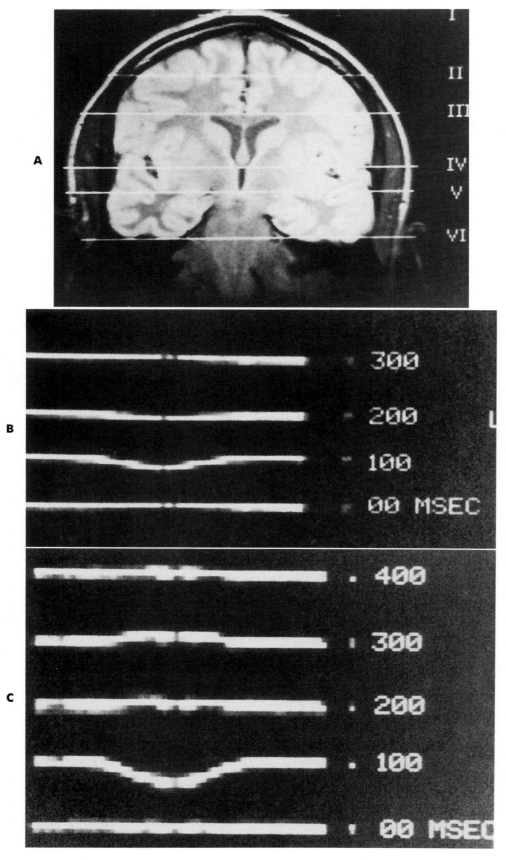

Fig. 7-79. Craniocaudal (V$_z$) velocity image results showing significant brain movement at various times after the R wave. **A** indicates the measurement locations. **B** corresponds to level IV, and **C** corresponds to level V. (From Feinberg DA, Mark AS: Radiology 163:793, 1987.)

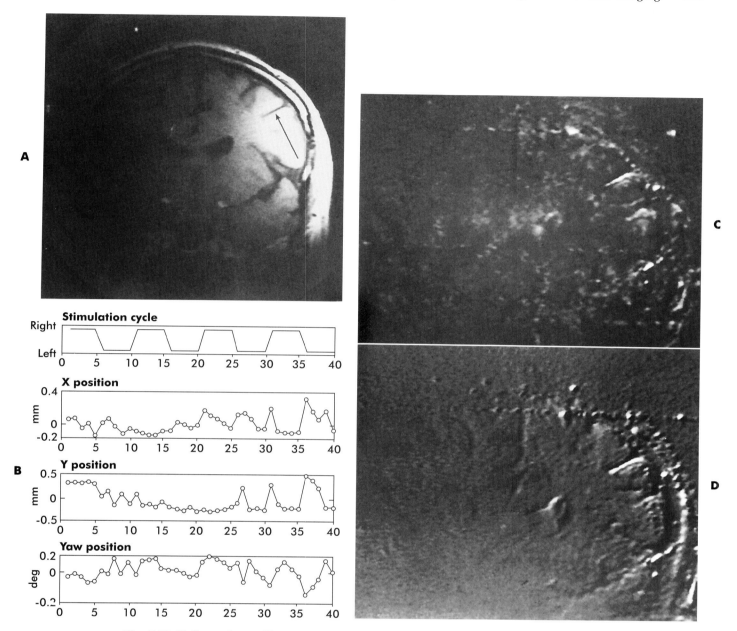

Fig. 7-80. Bulk motion artifact can give rise to image appearances similar to those from functional activation. Measured pattern of head displacement (**B**) during FMRI at location shown in (**A**) results in (**C**) an appearance that is similar to that of an FMRI activation image (**D**). (From Hajnal JV et al: Magn Reson Med 31:283, 1994.)

will often determine the amount of time required to obtain a phase encode line. Therefore, along with the desired number of spatial slices and image phase encode lines, TE will directly determine TR and the imaging speed.

The numerical simulation results of Fisel et al[107] indicate that both spin echo and gradient echo susceptibility-induced signal attenuations increase with increasing echo time (Fig. 7-81). However, the exponential signal attenuation dependence on TE:

$$A(TE) = e^{-a(TE)^b} \qquad (7\text{-}48)$$

is not predicted to be linear ($b = 1$), with b being approximately 1.2 for gradient echo sequences and 1.4 for spin echo sequences. Furthermore, the effectiveness of this equation in describing the attenuation behavior decreases with higher ($\sim$100 msec) TEs, particularly for spin echo sequences.

For GRE sequences, the use of very long TEs may be inappropriate because of the increasing amount of image artifacts at intrinsic tissue susceptibility interfaces that may obscure the desired signal changes. System instabilities also become more apparent at longer echo times. Even though susceptibility weighting is increasing at longer echo times, the measurable signal strength is simultaneously decreasing.

Menon et al[210] used a multiple gradient echo sequence to empirically examine the dependence of activation response on TE time. The use of multiple echoes allows this comparison to be more direct because images are acquired over a single, rather than repeated, FMRI functional activation. Echo times ranged from 10 to 60 msec. The results are shown in Fig. 7-82.

Frahm et al[185,220] also experimentally determined

FLASH FMRI results at a number of different echo times (at 2.0 T). They found that there was little difference between echo times in the range of 30 to 60 msec and suggest that a TE setting of 30 to 40 msec is a good compromise between susceptibility weighting and image SNR. These results (Fig. 7-83) also show that a significant T1-weighted flow response in gray matter areas remains with the use of short TEs.

The optimum TE that maximizes susceptibility weighting and image signal-to-noise (i.e., susceptibility contrast-to-noise) can be shown to be equal to the $T2^*$ of the local (i.e., gray matter) tissue of interest.[201,210,221] This $T2^*$ value can be lengthened by localized magnetic field shimming, and an improvement in $T2^*$ (with a correspondingly longer TE) from

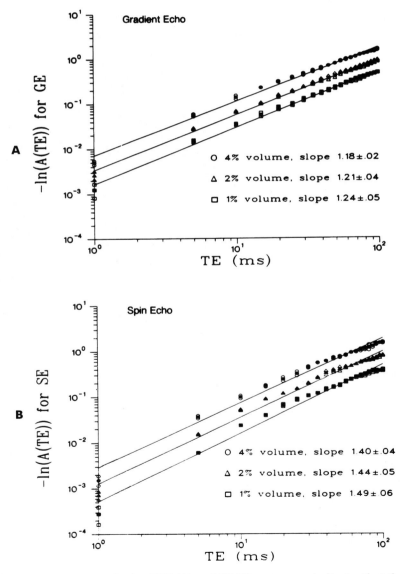

Fig. 7-81. Simulation results for GRE (**A**) and SE (**B**) sequences indicates that there should be a nearly linear increase in signal attenuation with echo time. (From Fisel CR et al: Magn Reson Med 17:336, 1991.)

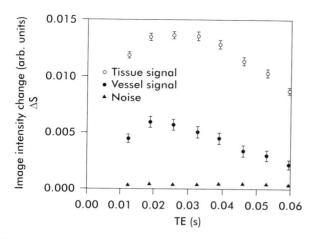

Fig. 7-82. A plot of the difference in image intensity (S) between stimulation and control states as a function of the echo time. Note that the peak for the tissue signal is found at TE = 28 msec while the peak for the venous vessels is found at TE = 20 msec, consistent with their local T2* values. (From Menon RS et al: Magn Reson Med 30:380, 1993.)

20 to 60 msec represents a significant improvement in susceptibility contrast-to-noise ratio. The local T2* can be measured by acquiring a series of GRE sequences with fixed TR and with TEs varied from 15 to 80 msec. When the local T2* value is unknown, a TE value of 40 msec is a reasonable and common compromise value.

Shimming. T2* can be increased, allowing TE to be increased for more susceptibility weighting, by shimming the magnetic field. This is done in the region where slice images are to be taken. Shimming is most easily performed if the imaging system also supports spectroscopy measurements. A slice selective free induction decay (FID) sequence can be selected to cover the region of the imaging slices. Only a few minutes of manual shimming are required to obtain local T2* values in the range of 40 to 50 msec.

Voxel size. Susceptibility effects will be affected by voxel size only when the field inhomogeneities are approximately the same size as the voxel. If field gradients are assumed to extend twice the vessel

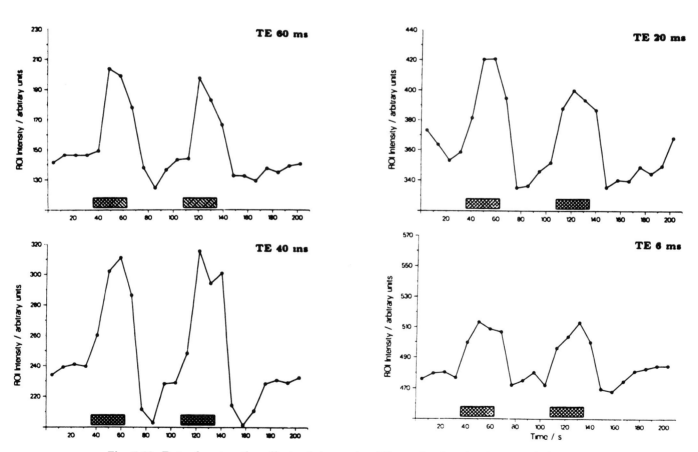

Fig. 7-83. Data showing the effects of decreasing TE on visual activation signal changes using a FLASH sequence. (FA = 40 degrees, TR = 70, 128 × 256, FOV = 250, 0.5/image). Note that significant activation is observed even at short echo times. (From Frahm J, Merboldt KD, Hanicke W: Magn Reson Med 29:139, 1993.)

radius, given a venule diameter of approximately 50 μm, the voxel sizes would have to be reduced to less than 100 μm = $(0.1 \text{ mm})^3$ before a size dependence would be expected. This is below the practical resolution limit of most whole body imaging systems, so a susceptibility dependence on voxel size is usually not seen experimentally.[196,220]

The regions of activation anticipated from previous neurophysiologic studies will be limited to only a 1 to 3 mm thick layer of cortical gray matter, with the homuncular extent varying from approximately 5 to 30 mm, depending on the type of neural response. However, the complicated and convoluted structure of the brain surface causes the anatomic region of activation to have a correspondingly complicated three-dimensional structure. MRI voxel size scales larger than 1 to 3 mm may lead to the contribution of nearby noninvolved static tissue toward the total signal from the voxel. This is a classic partial volume effect that will tend to dilute or obscure the responses from focal sources. Experimental studies comparing imaging resolutions[211,220,222] have shown that

activation-induced signal changes are often more apparent at higher resolution because of reduced partial volume effects (Fig. 7-84). The limit to voxel size reduction is determined, as usual, by the SNR and the ability to detect small activation-induced signal changes among background noise and signal drift. Conversely, high SNR image differences showing large amounts of activation changes imply that imaging resolution can be reduced and more of the available imaging time applied to other requirements, such as increasing spatial coverage or reducing imaging times.

Slice number. The number of spatial image slices required depends on a combination of desired anatomic coverage, desired temporal resolution, and any uncertainty as to the location of activity (Fig. 7-85). In the case of visual experiments, the location of the primary visual cortex along the banks of the calcarine fissure is readily identified on MR images. However, magnetoencephalography (MEG) results indicate that there are additional active sources that are superior,

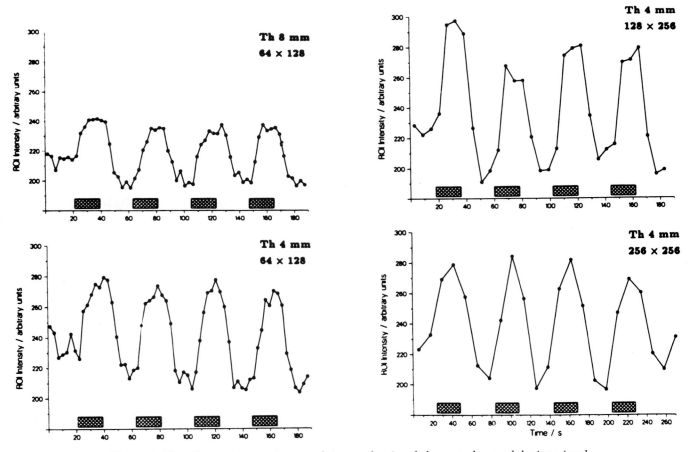

Fig. 7-84. The effects of decreasing voxel size on the signal changes observed during visual stimulation using FLASH. The increasing magnitude of observed response with smaller voxel sizes indicates the extent of partial volume effects on the measurements. (From Frahm J, Merboldt KD, Hanicke W: Magn Reson Med 29:139, 1993.)

inferior, and lateral to the primary striate source in the visual area along the calcarine fissure. Motor activation is typically more focal, but there is often more uncertainty concerning its location adjacent to the central sulcus.

While the majority of initial FMRI reports employed a single imaging slice, effective placement of a single slice often requires a priori knowledge as to the location of cortical activation. This information is what FMRI studies are often meant to provide. Slice placement becomes even more difficult with intracranial lesions where mass effects and functional reorganizations occur. Oblique slice orientations provide flexibility for minimizing the thickness and number of slices required. Given sufficiently fast acquisition and processing times and sufficiently strong evoked responses, interactive "functional scout" images (quick FMRI images to locate activity) may represent the most effective method of slice positioning.

3-D imaging. The high temporal resolution of EPI sequences can be applied to the acquisition of additional spatial regions. With hardware capable of handling the high-duty cycle, up to 15 slices per second can be imaged, providing a complete brain volume scan in approximately 2 seconds.[204] While the exact anatomic location of activation in response to a stimulus is often unknown, neuroanatomic experience typically reduces location uncertainty to within only a few slice thicknesses. In cases of distinct focal sources, volumetric imaging may not be required. However, to observe contralateral or bilateral activations (e.g., somatomotor), resolve lateralization ambiguity (e.g., speech/language), or identify supplementary and as-

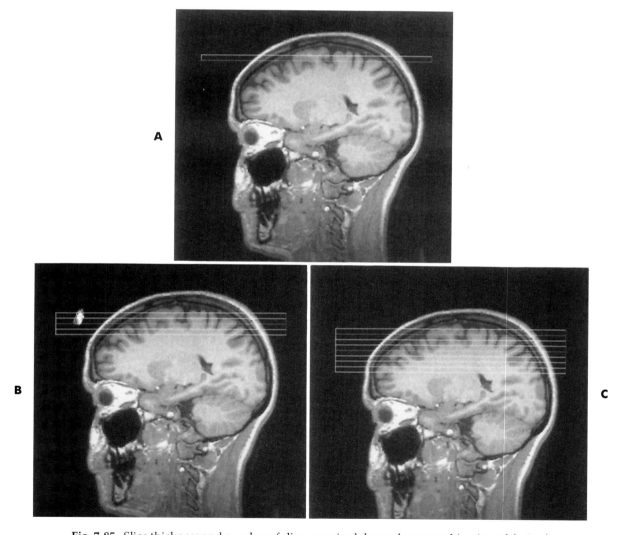

Fig. 7-85. Slice thickness and number of slices required depend on a combination of desired anatomic coverage, sequence temporal resolution, and uncertainly as to the expected location of activation. The slice coverage for single (**A**), four (**B**), and eight (**C**) 5 mm slices is shown.

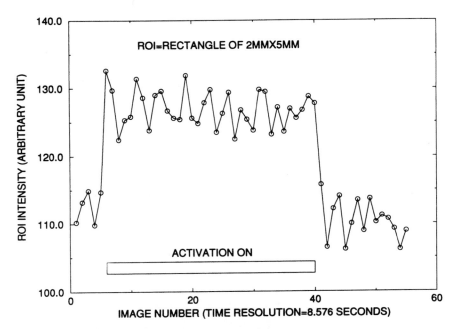

Fig. 7-86. The signal response is sustained throughout the 5 minutes of motor stimulation, allowing sufficient time for full 3-D data acquisition. (From Lai S et al: Magn Reson Med 30:387, 1993.)

sociation areas, large-scale FMRI coverage may be necessary.

Depending on the system capabilities, 3-D acquisitions can be used to observe longer sustained activations. Lai et al[211] have shown that motor stimulation durations of approximately 5 minutes show a sustained response (Fig. 7-86). Advantages of 3-D FMRI methods include a larger coverage of the brain and better SNR. Disadvantages include poorer temporal resolution and increased potential for motion sensitivity and subtraction artifacts. In addition, larger spatial coverage may require the use of larger and perhaps less efficient coils.

Flip angle. The choice of FLASH GRE flip angle is usually based on maximizing signal strength and minimizing inflow sensitivity. As discussed previously, sensitivity to signal from blood flowing into the imaging region increases with T1 saturation, which is determined by the sequence TR and flip angle.

With respect to imaging signal strength, the optimum flip angle, α, is defined by the familiar Ernst angle relation

$$\cos(\alpha) = e^{\left(\frac{-TR}{T1}\right)} \qquad (7\text{-}49)$$

which is dependent on both the sequence TR and the tissue T1. As shown in Fig. 7-87, the flip angle for optimum contrast increases with increasing TR/T1 ratio.[223] For a particular TR/T1 ratio, contrast will vary with flip angle, but the curves are flat enough that

angles near the peak of maximum contrast should also give acceptable results. In practice, one needs to know which TR to T1 curve applies for the subject; it may be easier to directly measure signal intensity in the image region of interest for a range of flip angles to determine the optimum flip angle rather than to measure local tissue T1 and calculate the optimum angle.

New FMRI Sequences

Because of the diversity of sequence requirements for FMRI, many different sequence methods can be applied to these examinations. In fact, as part of the development of this technology, a large number of imaging sequences previously developed for other applications have been, or are being, tested for effectiveness in FMRI studies. Principal FMRI sequence requirements typically include susceptibility weighting, imaging stability, and artifact insensitivity. In addition, imaging speed is often an important consideration.

Most of the current requirements for FMRI appear to be fulfilled by some variant of EPI. However, these requirements are evolving rapidly, and it is not clear that EPI will continue to represent the preferred method of performing robust and accurate FMRI examinations. For example, it has been suggested[204] that an approach to combine the advantages of both gradient echo and spin echo features may be to use some variant of combined gradient and spin echo acquisition such as GRASE.[224] Issues of activation mechanism/signal origin and characterization of

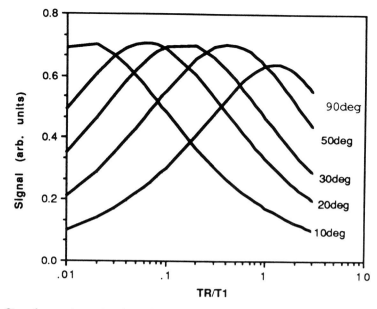

Fig. 7-87. Signal-to-noise ratio plotted as a function of the TR/T1 ratio assuming a constant total scan time for various flip angles, showing discrete maxima. Note that the smaller the TR/T1 ratio, the lower the optimum flip angle. (From Wehrli FW: Magn Reson Q 6[3]:171, 1990.)

sources of artifactual signal change will continue to influence the direction of FMRI sequence design.

EPI is known to have extensive hardware requirements. As these capabilities become more commonplace and the requirements of alternative methods become more demanding, imaging system instrumentation may become a less significant issue. Issues regarding optimum FMRI field strength (i.e., 1.5 versus 4.0 T) will continue to be clarified but will only define a significant clinical instrumentation requirement if the availability of 4.0 T systems increases substantially or if the tide of evidence turns away from indicating that studies at 1.5 T can be clinically useful. For the broadest clinical application of this technology, it is desired that FMRI be effectively performed on the installed base of clinical MRI scanners. Continuing sequence developments provide appropriately weighted images at rates approaching those of EPI but are able to be performed on conventional imagers.

Interleaved echoes. Increasing the T2* sensitivity of GRE sequences typically entails increasing TE, which leads to increased TR and imaging times. New FMRI sequences attempt to preserve or increase T2* weighing while reducing overall imaging times. The long TE times required for conventional GRE imaging sequences mean that there is a significant amount of underutilized sequence time spent waiting for susceptibility sensitivity to accumulate. One approach to improve imaging efficiency is to use "echo shifting,"[225] whereby the excitation and gradient echo formation are separated by more than one TR period.

Such a sequence is diagrammed in Fig. 7-88, showing that the sequence TE is longer than the sequence TR. The gradient recalled echo from spins excited by the first RF pulse is refocused in the second TR period. The shifted echo is realized by bringing spins in phase at the desired delayed echo time with respect to each principal gradient and dephasing other possible gradient and spin echoes. This technique can be extended[226] to refocus the echo signals after more than one TR period in order to increase T2* weighting and to incorporate segmented Fourier space acquisition.[227] Additional extensions to 3D acquisition have also been demonstrated.[228]

T2* magnetization preparation. Magnetization preparation pulses applied before the image acquisition have been long used by ultrafast imaging sequences.[229,230] Perman and Gado[156] demonstrated a "driven equilibrium" 90_x-θ-90_{-x} sequence as a preparation pulse scheme where T2*-dependent dephasing evolves during θ. Unfortunately, this method results in intensity modulations from intervoxel phase differences caused mainly by background inhomogeneities of the main B_0 field. The high sensitivity to background B_0 inhomogeneities leads to large phase shifts in the signal. One approach to overcoming this problem was employed by Hu and Stillman[231] in using a crusher gradient pulse during the preparation period. Kim et al[232] applied this approach using a segmented BIR-4 adiabatic pulse for excitation. They also suggested that the intensity modulation caused by B_0 inhomogeneities could be eliminated by creating

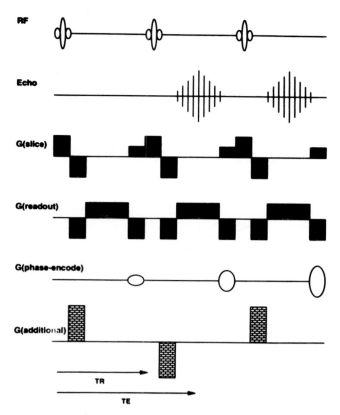

RF

Echo

G(slice)

G(readout)

G(phase-encode)

G(additional)

TR

TE

Fig. 7-88. Echo-shifted sequences have TEs greater than the TR. The echo is formed after one or more intervening RF pulses. (From Moonen CTW et al: Magn Reson Med 26:184, 1992.)

a phase-shifted image, which is combined with the first image in quadrature. This approach has been extended by Bendel,[233] using the quadrature combination of two phase-cycled acquisitions to eliminate background shifts from inhomogeneity. Hu and Kim[234] demonstrated a T2*-weighted magnetization preparation technique that is insensitive to static field inhomogeneity but requires only a single acquisition (Fig. 7-89).

K-space substitution. Efforts to develop sequences that allow the production of rapid (subsecond) images on clinical instrumentation have led to several interesting approaches for improving image temporal resolution during bolus injection experiments. One approach is to rapidly obtain a limited selection of Fourier space samples and supply the missing data (i.e., lines in Fourier space) from a complete acquisition obtained once before the start of dynamic imaging.[235-237] This technique typically obtains the lower spatial frequency lines in Fourier space and uses the high-frequency information from a single reference image (Fig. 7-90). While the images can be acquired faster (on the order of one-fourth the time) and have a better appearance than those acquired without adding the reference information, the dy-

namic information content is not improved by added spatial frequencies, and only changes in low image spatial frequencies can be observed. This limits this technique to observation of changes in relatively large and uniform image regions.

Processing Procedures

In general, FMRI procedures require a comparison between the results of two separate acquisitions, obtained both with and without neural activation. FMRI processing procedures attempt to optimally compare these data sets and form an image by superimposing the identified activity onto corresponding MR anatomic images. FMRI data processing often involves identification of small activation-induced signal differences between image sets. These small changes, particularly at 1.5 T, are within the range of those contributed by a number of potential artifactual sources. In order to increase the SNR of the images, and thus the image differences, data averaging of multiple acquisitions is typically employed, which, given limited stimulation durations, gives rise to the cyclic stimulation/rest (ON/OFF) nature of raw FMRI data sets. This section is intended to introduce how this series of acquired images gets processed into a set of spots (representing activated regions) to be superimposed on an anatomic image.

As the number of images and the time of the imaging session increase, nonstimulus processes such as bulk patient motion and pulsatile blood or CSF motions can lead to artifactual signal changes. Simple difference image formation is highly susceptible to these artifacts. The purpose of processing is to desensitize the resulting functional image to these nonactivation-related sources of signal variation in order to accurately map the activated regions on a corresponding anatomic image.

Data processing of FMRI results is perhaps the most fragmented part of the field, with many interesting approaches and little standardization. In addition to the basic subtractions and t-tests, the processing procedures range from ANOVA,[238] Z mapping,[239] power spectrum analysis,[240,241] time domain phase shifts,[242] and frequency domain phase shifts[243] on up to sophisticated particle clustering analyses.[244] Unfortunately, imprecise application of exotic procedures may lead to erroneous interpretations of FMRI data. These methods will need a great deal of validation testing before they can be used in a clinical setting.

The variety of processing procedures, in addition to dependence on the multitude of sequence and experimental details, makes it very difficult to objectively compare results between institutions. This is particularly the case with time course data from a selected image region of interest (ROI). While time courses from selected ROIs are useful for displaying the

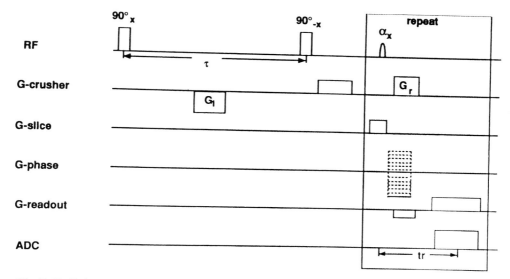

Fig. 7-89. Pulse sequence showing the T2* contrast preparation period and its combination with a turbo-FLASH sequence. (From Hu X, Kim SG: Magn Reson Med 30:512, 1993.)

temporal responses to the stimulation, the results obtained are surprisingly dependent on the location and size of the ROI. In general, it is preferable to perform temporal processing on a pixel-by-pixel basis to eliminate this arbitrary spatial positioning dependence.

Subtraction. The processing of initial FMRI results involved only the subtraction of the means of the two data sets. Typically, the average of the resting images is subtracted from each of, or the mean of, the activated images so that activation differences will be positive. This simple approach is susceptible to noise, particularly for small changes in large signals, and offers no resistance to the effects of motion between activation and rest. Testing with interpolated data sets confirms that even subpixel movements can lead to quite noticeable appearances in difference images. This method is also very sensitive to variations in image and pixel intensity. Regions of activation are identified only by heuristically applying a threshold to the difference image.

The data subtraction can also be done during data acquisition. While most procedures acquire entire image data sets during stimulus on and off periods, Hijnal et al[245] acquired a single image encode signal during each period using an inversion recovery sequence. Subtraction of data from successive TR cycles leads to the production of images that display only the signal difference between the two cycles and show a reduced sensitivity to motion artifact. Furthermore, by acquiring different images in which the ordering of the ON and OFF stimulation pairs has been reversed, an image representing twice the ON/OFF difference can be produced.

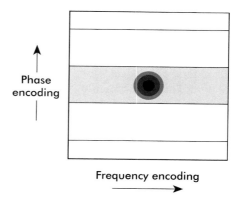

Fig. 7-90. K-space substitution techniques typically only acquire low spatial frequency information for each repeated image and fill in the remaining high-frequency lines using a single reference image. (From Jones RA et al: Magn Reson Med 29:830, 1993.)

Stimulation time course. While the image data sets can be identified as being obtained during either ON or OFF periods, that information is not effectively used during simple subtraction. The a priori knowledge of the stimulation time course represents a powerful source of information for identifying responses that are specifically the result of the stimulation. Processing procedures more sophisticated than subtraction use this information in different ways and to different extents.

FMRI data analysis can often be cast in terms of a classic treatment/response model that considers the stimulation or task as being a treatment. The goal is to examine the data to see whether the treatment had a significant effect on the outcome (pixel intensity). Complications with this simple model can arise if the data are obtained under nonequilibrium conditions. For images acquired at rates comparable to the hemodynamic response times, data may be recorded during the transitions between states. Furthermore, given the latencies of these responses to the abrupt introduction or removal of the stimulus, complete "mislabeling" of the data in regard to treatment may be made if data are acquired before the response begins (Fig. 7-91). Often these transitional points are omitted from the analysis or acquisition time delays are inserted to allow for reequilibration. Images synchronized with the stimulation presentation but acquired over significantly longer times can often neglect the transitional effects.

Statistical tests. In considering a treatment/response model, one can apply a number of long-established statistical tests. While a complete tutorial on statistical methods is beyond the scope of this section, effective FMRI image interpretation requires some introduction to methods encountered in FMRI reports. For this processing, the pixel data from the temporal series of images can be pooled over both ON and OFF periods, or the repeated nature of the ON/OFF pairings can be considered as repeated experiments on the same subject. Statistical tests have a particular advantage over simple subtraction in that they define an objective and quantitative measure for assessing the significance of changes between image data acquisitions.

t-test. The most commonly reported procedure is the Student's t-test, which determines if the two sets of acquired pixels (since the processing is done for each image pixel) represent samples from one population (no difference between the sets) or from two populations (resulting from the treatment). Even though it requires two passes through each image pixel, this is not a particularly computationally expensive procedure. Reports using the related z-test are occasionally seen, but the t-test is more appropriate for sample sizes (amount in OFF and ON groups) of less than 30. These results become identical for higher sample sizes (the shape of the t-distribution approaches the normal shape assumed by z).

Simply stated, the t-value is the difference of the sample means divided by the standard error of difference of sample means. There are actually three different formulas for computing the t-value, depending on the nature of the data and the experiment, and the one used should be specified. There is a "pooled" formula for use when assumptions of equal sample variances are met, a "separate" formula for use with unequal group variances (e.g., when activated pixels show more fluctuation), and a "paired" formula for use when the data of the two groups are correlated. This last situation is typical of FMRI, where the same subject is imaged both with and without the treatment. In this case the emphasis is on testing the significance of the average *change* with treatment instead of the difference in average responses with and without treatment. This approach reduces the variability in the observations caused by differences between individuals and yields a more sensitive test.[246]

The size of the image data set used in this analysis is reflected in the number of "degrees of freedom," which is simply $df = (n_1 + n_2) - 2$, where n_1 and n_2 are the number of samples in each group. The

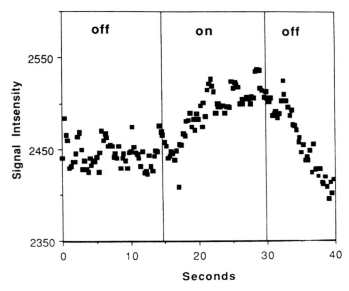

Fig. 7-91. For high temporal resolution measurements, transition time points require special consideration with respect to stimulated/nonstimulated labeling. (From Belliveau JW et al: Invest Radiol 27:S59, 1992.)

significance of any difference between groups is obtained by indexing into a table of a t-distribution using the calculated *t* and *df* values. The "significance" is a number between 0 and 1 and is the probability that the observed difference between groups could be obtained by chance. For example, a significance value of 0.01 means that, given the measurement characteristics, there is only one chance in 100 that the difference could occur by chance. FMRI images are formed by applying a low significance threshold as a mask to the difference or t-value image data and superimposing these locations on top of an anatomic image.

Information as to whether a "one-tailed" or "two-tailed" t-test was performed should also be included with the reported data. This choice arises from assumptions about the underlying mechanism. A one-tailed test is most often performed since it can be assumed that increasing neural activity leads to increasing pixel intensity. For a given pair of *t* and *df* values, the significance value for a one-tailed test will be half of that of the two- tailed test (twice as significant). This is because the likelihood of the activated pixels being significantly larger *or* smaller than nonactivated is twice the likelihood of the

activated pixels just being larger than nonactivated ones.

ANOVA. The analysis of variance (ANOVA) statistical tests is the generalization of the t-test, allowing consideration of multiple factors contributing to the measured image intensities. For FMRI studies, additional factors (other than the applied stimuli) can be additional contrast mechanisms or sources of artifactual signal change. It would be statistically incorrect to consider the different factors as defining multiple groups (e.g., right and left motor stimulation in addition to ON and OFF) and then simply use a pairwise application of the t-test to test between the different group combinations. For a single factor under consideration, the significance results from a (one-way) ANOVA will be identical to those from a t-test.

FMRI image formation from ANOVA processing is similar to that from the t-test, but the thresholded significance of a particular factor with respect to determining pixel intensity can be selected for use as the mask. Sanders et al[247] compared this approach with subtraction and t-test processing (Fig. 7-92) and found that system instability and other nonstimulus

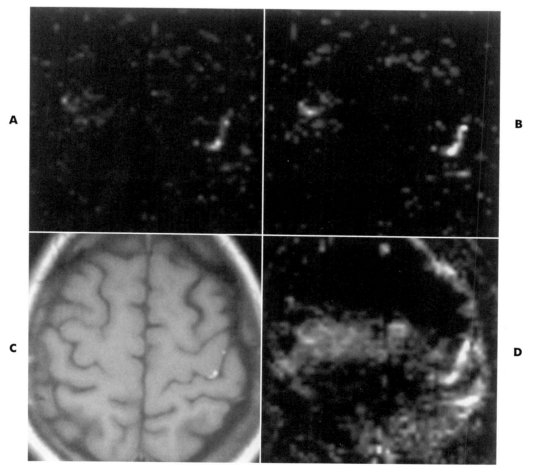

Fig. 7-92. Comparison between **A,** ANOVA; **B,** t-test; and **D,** subtraction processing of the motor activation data set. Corresponding anatomy is shown in **C.**

contributions to the observed signal changes could be reduced using ANOVA analysis.

Cross-correlation. The above statistical tests do not take particular advantage of the time course of the stimulus presentation used. The images are labeled as to whether they were obtained during stimulation or not, but the processing does not consider the specific (cyclic) ordering of the experiment—for example, four images per stimulus period, two periods per cycle, and four ON/OFF cycles. A repeated measures ANOVA would emphasize more of the temporal relation of intensity with stimulus, but the strict periodicity requirements may restrict the flexibility of stimulus presentation. An alternative approach using cross-correlation analysis of the pixel intensity variations with respect to the time course of the stimulus has been employed by Bandettini et al.[196,248] After some preprocessing steps, a "cross-correlation" image is computed by taking the dot product of the measured pixel intensity time course and a vector created to represent the stimulation time course. The correlation values are given arbitrary threshold values to em-phasize signal changes with the same timing as the stimulus and are mapped onto a corresponding T1 image. Fig. 7-93 shows some results from cross-correlation processing in comparison with those from simple subtraction.

Phase shifts. The complex nature of the MR image is typically ignored by the formation of magnitude reconstructed images. However, the phase image has long been known to be highly sensitive to changes in blood flow and signal characteristics. Binder et al[242] demonstrated the use of phase shifts, in conjunction with periodic stimulation protocols, to identify activation-induced changes. However, the sensitivity of image phase to other influences such as system instabilities and unwanted motion may limit this approach.

Registration with MR. The procedure of mapping FMRI activations onto anatomic images is straightforward when the anatomic (often T1-weighted) image data are obtained during the same session without intervening patient motion. Even in cases of varying

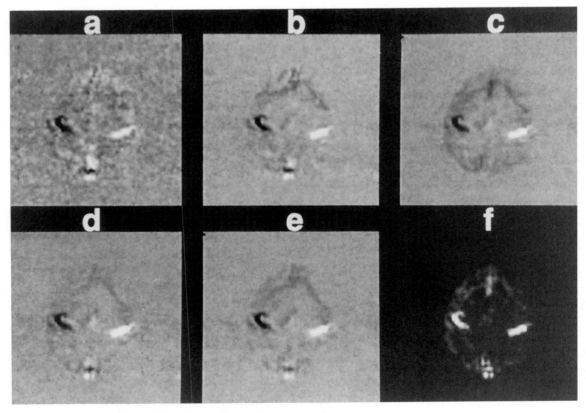

Fig. 7-93. Cross-correlation processing employs a vector constructed from the stimulation time course and provides improved FMRI results relative to image subtraction methods. **A,** Single subtraction image between peak right and peak left images. **B,** Subtraction image between average right and average left images. **C to E,** Different cross-correlation images. **F,** Spectral density image. (From Bandettini PA et al: Magn Reson Med 30:161, 1991.)

image FOV and slice orientation, registering different data sets from the same session can be performed by simple geometric transformations that are referenced to the fixed scanner geometry used for both acquisitions. In cases of motion or in registering FMRI data to previously acquired data, the two data coordinate systems can be related if identification of landmark structures can be made in both data sets. One data set can be mapped to the other by using either the identified transformation between fiducial points or by a computed correlation between 2D[249] or 3D[250] structures. Application of registration procedures to the unprocessed FMRI image data set may also be used to reduce the effects of bulk motion during the study.

APPLICATIONS

A number of significant issues remain regarding the exact mechanism leading to observed signal changes, and an increasing number of institutions are joining the effort to resolve these questions. However, FMRI technology has progressed to the point where the focus is being turned from demonstration and characterization of basic capabilities and toward the development of specific research or clinical applications. The initial applications of FMRI have involved identifying basic sensory or motor responses, and a substantial body of similar previous PET studies allowed for rapid progress during this stage. Subsequently, the limits of this technique in probing more subtle evoked or cognitive responses have begun to be tested. This process should continue while instrumentation and procedural improvements allow the observation of increasingly smaller activation-induced changes.

Most FMRI protocols use a sequential task-activation paradigm, alternating between resting and activated states. This alternation is intended to avoid accommodation or fatigue toward the stimulus. The number of ON/OFF cycles is determined by the required image SNR. ON/OFF labeling of the images in the data set is typically performed by the cuing of activity or the synchronization of continuous acquisitions to the presentation of the stimuli.

Vision

The cerebral cortex involved in vision constitutes a large part of the brain, up to a third in primates, reflecting the importance of vision in everyday activities.[251] In particular, the primary visual cortex along the calcarine fissue at the occipital pole has been the focus of much of the initial investigations because of the large evoked responses and the relatively well-known retinotopic organization. The distinctive structure of the calcarine fissure can be readily identified from sagittal localizing images for accurate slice

placement. There have also been a large number of previous studies to draw upon.

Procedures. Initial procedures have generally followed those established by Belliveau et al,[252-254] who drew on PET stimulation paradigms previously used by Fox et al.[2,153] These studies typically used LED goggles, with each eyepiece containing an array of red LEDs. Kwong et al[13] found that the maximal elicited response resulted from an 8 Hz stimulation, in agreement with previous PET reports[254,255] (Fig. 7-94). The dependence on stimulus rate is an important consideration in the design of stimulation paradigms so that factors in addition to presentation or scene change frequency can be isolated and investigated.

The types of potential stimuli are severely limited by the small LED arrays of the goggles. Computer-

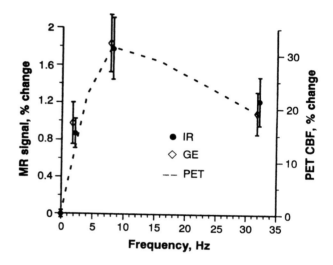

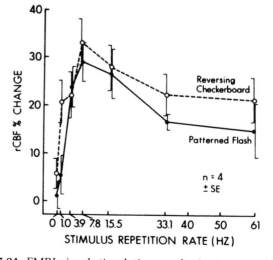

Fig. 7-94. FMRI visual stimulation results *(top)* are similar to the results obtained by PET studies *(bottom)* and show that maximal response is obtained using a 7.8 Hz presentation frequency. (**A** from Kwong KK et al: Proc Natl Acad USA 89:5675, 1992; **B** from Fox PT, Raichle ME: Ann Neurol 18:303, 1985.)

generated patterns projected into the visual field of the subject allow for more freedom in stimulus design. Fiberoptic cabling can be used if direct projection is impractical. A number of commercial systems are available, designed for reducing patient anxiety in clinical imaging, that provide audio-video to subjects within the confines of the magnet. These systems have been adapted for the magnetic field environment and can be employed for visual and auditory stimulus.

Results. Visual information is transferred from retina to the lateral geniculate nucleus and then to the visual cortex. Results obtained at 4.0 T using a FLASH

sequence clearly show activation in the primary visual cortex (Fig. 7-95). An initial report by Frahm et al[256] has indicated that changes at the level of the lateral geniculate nucleus can be detected during photic stimulation.

Vision is known to have a topographic organization, and this has been demonstrated by several studies including those by Belliveau et al[257] demonstrating lateralized activation from alternating hemifield stimulation (Fig. 7-96). This work has been extended by Schneider et al[258] on a conventional 1.5 T scanner using a variety of stimulus patterns. These authors further showed that such mapping across multiple subjects could be effectively combined to

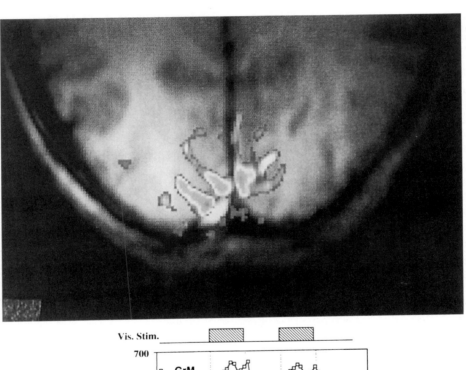

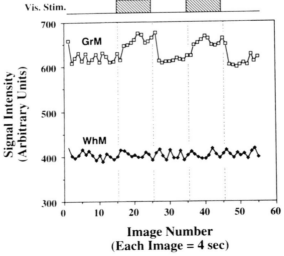

Fig. 7-95. Visual mapping results at 4.0 T clearly demonstrate activation of gray matter regions of primary visual cortex. (From Menon RS et al: Invest Radiol 27:S47, 1992.)

identify common visual topologies. Preliminary reports[212] also indicate that extrastriate cortex activation (V5) can be identified.

With the establishment of robust FMRI visual stimulation and examination methods, studies of visual system defects are enabled. A preliminary study by Sorensen et al[259] demonstrated that FMRI can delineate deficits in cerebrovascular activation of visual cortex that are consistent with the areas expected based on current understanding of clinical visual field deficits.

Motor/Somatosensory

Another robust activation often used in the development of FMRI techniques is that of the primary motor and sensory areas located on precentral and postcentral gyri extending laterally from the midsagittal plane.

In previous PET work,[260,261] it has been shown that repetitive contralateral hand squeezing will activate the primary motor region, M1. This is routinely observed with FMRI (Fig. 7-97). At least three reports[262-264] have identified cerebellar activations from isotonic hand flexion/extension or electrical stimulation of the wrist, consistent with previous PET observations.[265] Other investigations[266,267] have confirmed the expected result that handedness leads to asymmetric motor activation patterns. Rao et al[268] have mapped the primary motor cortex locations for fingers, toes, elbows, and tongue. Other effects asso-

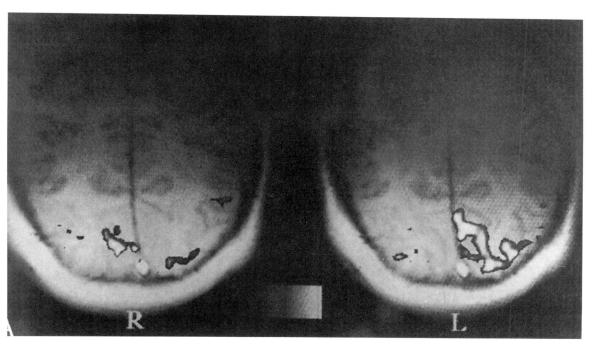

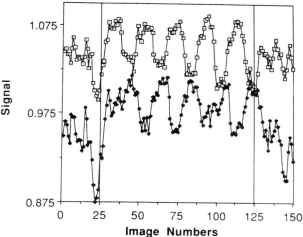

Fig. 7-96. Lateralized activation patterns resulting from alternating hemifield visual stimulation. (From Belliveau JW et al: Invest Radiol 27:S59, 1992.)

ciated with motor function are often seen, particularly in sensory, parietal, and associative cortex.

Procedures. A particular advantage that motor studies enjoy is that problems with effective stimuli presentation within the confines of the MR magnet (and magnetic field) are avoided when using a simple

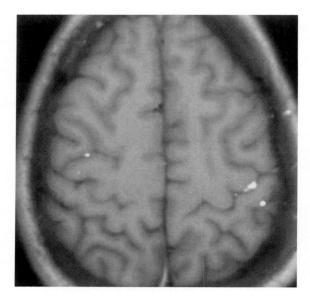

Fig. 7-97. Right hand motor activation results from a 1.5 T clinical instrument using FLASH sequences.

hand flexion or finger tapping paradigm. Because strong finger movement responses, on the order of 4.3%,[196] are elicited in activated cortex, motor studies are often employed during technique development. The characteristics of motor responses have been extensively studied.

Duration dependency. Lai et al[211] studied signals after 5 minutes of finger tapping. Since the measured response lasted continuously even during long time intervals, they concluded that poor imaging temporal resolution was nearly irrelevant in this type of FMRI. Bandettini et al[269] also studied stimulus duration dependencies. Subjects were instructed to tap their fingers for durations ranging from 0.5 second to 6 minutes. These results (Fig. 7-98) also indicate that the response is quite stable even for long stimulus durations. Even very abrupt (0.5 second) finger activity durations resulted in signal enhancement after 2 or 3 seconds, which continued for 3 to 5 seconds before returning to baseline.

Switching frequency. The stimulus switching frequency characteristics have also been studied by Bandettini et al.[269,270] In these experiments, subjects cycled between periods of finger activity and resting for period durations ranging from 1 to 25 seconds (0.5 to 0.02 Hz). The results, shown in Fig. 7-99, show that hemodynamic responses can follow switching fre-

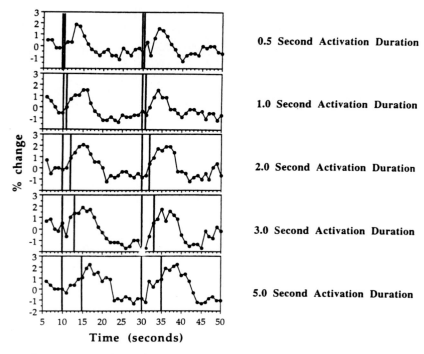

Fig. 7-98. Time courses from the same motor cortex location during finger movement activations ranging from 0.5 to 5 seconds in duration. (From Bandettini PA: Functional MRI of the brain: a workshop, SMRM, June 1993, p 144.)

quencies higher than approximately 0.16 Hz. A frequency of 5 Hz and ON/OFF durations of 8 seconds were found to be best for finger tapping motor studies.

Auditory

There is a known tonotopic organization of blood flow responses to different tonal frequencies, and activation of primary auditory cortex occurs in the hemisphere contralateral to the stimulation.[271] FMRI

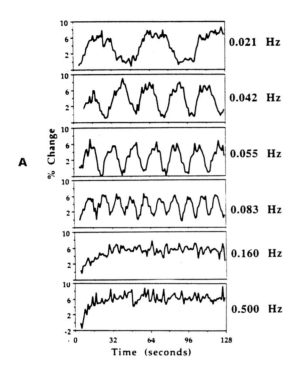

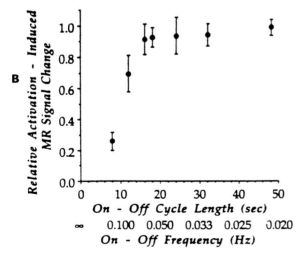

Fig. 7-99. A, Time courses from the same motor cortex location for ON/OFF switching frequencies ranging from 0.021 to 0.5 Hz. **B,** Relative signal change in the motor cortex relative to ON/OFF activation frequency. (From Bandettini PA: Functional MRI of the brain: a workshop, SMRM, June 1993, p 144.)

auditory experiments have not been actively pursued because it was anticipated that the loud and repetitive sounds from the imaging gradients would saturate the receptor system and small stimulus responses would not be visible. However, it has been shown[272,273] that mapping of auditory responses is possible with FMRI. The reported results indicate that auditory responses from specific tonal stimuli can be obtained despite the sounds produced by the imaging sequence gradient activity.

Speech/Language

The classic model of language-related functional neuroanatomy places the motor output of language in the left inferior frontal gyrus (Broca's area) and the reception and perception of language in the left posterior temporal lobe (Wernicke's area). Currently, language-related functional mapping for neurosurgical planning relies on two highly invasive procedures: the Wada test (intracarotid amytal injection) and direct intraoperative cortical stimulation.[274] The limited spatial resolution and SNR of PET or SPECT restrict their use in these cases where determination of hemispheric language dominance is required.

Language lateralization is potentially an important application for FMRI. Hinke et al[274] (at 4.0 T) demonstrated that language could be lateralized in six of eight subjects during internal speech word generation. Bandettini and colleagues[269] (at 1.5 T) studied the response of signals in the anterior and posterior superior temporal gyri (STG) to words presented at rates from 0.33 to 1.67 Hz. The linear response is shown in Fig. 7-100. Rao et al[275] found bilateral activation of the STG during passive word listening, and Balmire et al[276] observed activation in the left frontal area during an overt word production task. Additional studies[277,278] have identified activations resulting from word generation tasks. Covert word production was examined by Rueckert et al,[279] who found significant activation (2% to 6% changes) in Broca's area. Activity was also found in motor and premotor regions roughly corresponding to the face.

Preliminary reports from Binder et al[280] indicate that the time course of FMRI signal change in polymodal frontal cortex during a cognitive task (language processing) differs from that seen in sensory cortex during a sensory discrimination task (auditory). These findings suggest that activity periods of at least 20 seconds are required for maximal signal change to be observed in polymodal cortex.

Mental Tasks

Visual perception occurs when one encodes physically present stimuli. Visual mental imagery occurs when one has a short-term memory representation of a stimulus that is not physically present. PET and other

Left Anterior STG

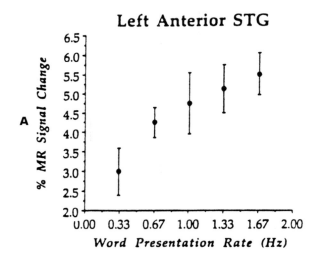

Left Posterior STG

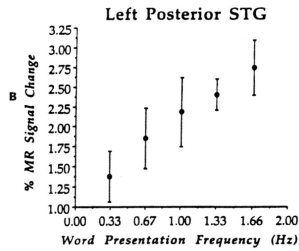

Fig. 7-100. Signal change dependence on word presentation frequency in the **A**, left anterior and **B**, left posterior superior temporal gyrus. (From Bandettini PA: Functional MRI of the brain: a workshop, SMRM, June 1993, p 144.)

studies support the theory that imagery and perception share common neural mechanisms.[281,282]

Preliminary FMRI results also support this theory by showing activation of primary visual cortex during mental imagery tasks. LeBihan et al[71] found that for the same sequence, visual perception resulted in an average signal increase of 2.8% ± 1.1% within the calcarine tissue. The response to the imagined stimulus was somewhat less, at 1.5% ± 0.6%, with two of the seven subjects showing no response. Background variation was 0.2%. Subject attention state was noted to be an important factor in these studies.

Several groups[283,284] identified activation in motor, premotor, and somatosensory cortex with mental rehearsal of complex finger movements. This finding is inconsistent with at least one radiotracer study,[285] where no precentral motor activity was observed during planning of complex motor tasks.

Blamire et al[286] also consistently observed changes associated with a spatial memory task. Cohen et al,[287] using a spiral scanning sequence at 1.5 T, observed activation in several areas, including the dorsolateral prefrontal cortex and along the inferior surface of the middle frontal gyrus, in response to a working memory task.

Epilepsy

A preliminary study from Connelly et al[288] has nicely demonstrated the clinical utility of FMRI in a single case of focal epilepsy in a 4-year-old boy. This examination found changes in some gyri in structurally abnormal areas that were consistent with corresponding SPECT results.

Stroke

Hees et al has described preliminary results examining linewidth (susceptibility broadening) and regional CBV changes with stroke in a pig model. The results showed that these parameters are sensitive to ischemic insult and are encouraging for the application of these techniques for stroke detection and assessment.

Pain

Slightly painful stimuli resulted in image phase changes[289] and frontal activation.[290] The results are consistent with painful heat stimulation resulting in the activation of regions around the postcentral sulcus, perhaps with some interconnection to motor regions near the central sulcus.

Obsessive Compulsive Personality Disorders

Obsessive compulsive personality persons responding to "disgusting" stimuli[291] showed changes in the orbital gyrus and dorsolateral prefrontal cortex in addition to changes in the temporal lobe. These changes are consistent with previous PET reports.[292,293] This study by Breiter et al indicates that FMRI can be used in the determination of the functional circuitry of these types of disorders.

Chemical Stimulation

Another interesting application for MR functional imaging was demonstrated by Cuenod et al.[294] This study evaluated the feasibility of imaging the brain response to neuroreceptor stimulation by pharmacologic agents with MRI and found a good correlation between the anatomic locations of increased MRI signal in subject monkeys and the sites of increased glucose metabolism in previous reports using rats. The initial results from this study are encouraging for the application of FMRI to monitoring responses to pharmacologic interventions.

A preliminary study by Wenz et al[295] observed small

but not significant changes in five schizophrenic persons using neuroleptic drugs as compared to normal persons. This study is encouraging in that it indicated the feasibility of following the effects of drug treatment with FMRI using clinically available instrumentation.

Alzheimer's Disease

Mattay et al[296] tried to detect changes in bolus injections with visual stimulation in six patients with Alzheimer's disease but could not detect anything other than the normal activations. This does not confirm previous reports that there is 40% decrease in flow with Alzheimer's disease.

VALIDATION/OTHER MODALITIES

A central issue for this technology is how the observed activation locations relate to the "actual" site of neural activity. This question is likely to have a different answer for each of the different sequences and magnetic field strengths used for these measurements. Now that techniques are available for routine acquisition of functional MR images, initial reports are available from a number of correlative studies comparing FMRI results with those from other modalities.

Hemodynamic Methods

The foundations of FMRI are built on PET observations of the relationships between activation-induced local flow and oxygenation patterns. Sharing the same basic hemodynamic mechanisms, correlative studies with PET are a logical study direction. Rosen et al[8] found that their bolus injection CBV results corresponded well to PET findings. Buchbinder et al[297] reported on comparison Gd-DPTA CBV mapping in six subjects and observed features similar to those from ^{11}CO and ^{18}FDG PET methods. While a number of PET studies comparing BOLD FMRI results are known to be under way, there have been few preliminary reports.

Electrophysiologic Methods

Electrophysiologic studies more directly measure neural activation since they are based on the detection of electromagnetic field patterns associated with neural current flow. However, as described more fully elsewhere in this book, localizing this activity using external detection of these patterns by arrayed detector systems requires a number of modeling assumptions. While multiple or distributed source localization procedures are available (but can be computationally expensive), the more commonly employed single dipole source model of activated neural populations results in the estimation of a single location of activity. In comparisons with these locations it may be difficult to assign a single location (or even a small number of points) as representing the distributed activity seen in FMRI results. Single source locations are appropriate for electrophysiologic procedures because the millisecond temporal resolution of the measurements allows the dipole locations to move over time, reflecting the activation dynamics of different neural populations. The distributed hemodynamic responses identified by FMRI represent a time-averaged (and delayed/dampened) view of neural activation. However, given an appropriate procedure of selecting points of FMRI activity (e.g., by clustering analyses), a comparison with electrophysiologic measurements offers insights into both the accuracy and the underlying mechanism of FMRI.

ECoG. A number of studies are under way for comparing FMRI localizations with those of the current "gold standards" of functional localizations: intraoperative electrocorticographic (ECoG) recording of somatosensory evoked responses and the production of motor responses from direct cortical stimulation. While widely employed when functional localization is clinically indicated, these techniques have the drawbacks of substantially lengthening surgical time (and associated infection risks) and being dependent on the craniotomy location and exposure. Since they provide information only after committing to a particular approach, there is little flexibility for using the information. Finally, corticography results are not always easily interpretable, especially when there is only limited exposure of the critical regions. These reasons, along with a defined need for functional localizations, have provided impetus for the development of noninvasive mapping methodology such as FMRI.

Very preliminary reports from three studies[298-300] have been presented comparing FMRI and intraoperative ECoG, but these were weakened by having very few patients (N = 1, 2, and 3, respectively) and no rigorous way for registration of the data. The first study reported that FMRI was within 3 mm while the second and third reports did not provide a number. As mentioned in the introduction to this chapter, the use of FMRI for presurgical planning will be an early application of this technology. These preliminary reports have supported that contention. Further studies with more patients and better procedures to register ECoG and FMRI data are under way in order to better determine whether FMRI using clinically available instrumentation is suitable for clinical presurgical mapping.

MEG. Magnetoencephalography (MEG) directly measures neural activation rather than the indirect effects on blood flow that form the basis of FMRI. Sanders et al[301] reported their preliminary results comparing FMRI localizations with those using a large array MEG biomagnetometer. Their results indicate that the localization performed on conventional imaging systems and using GRE sequences agrees to

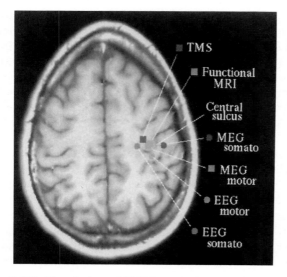

Fig. 7-101. Correlation of FMRI motor function localization with that of EEG, MEG, and transcranial magnetic stimulation (TMS) in a normal volunteer. (Reproduced in full color in color insert.)

within 10 mm with the localization from electrophysiologic measurements (Fig. 7-101). These results suggest that while FMRI localization at 1.5 T may reflect changes in vessels larger than capillaries, it does not necessarily mean that those changes occur particularly remote from the site of activated tissue. Considering that these results were performed on standard clinical instrumentation and used relatively simple determination of the point of FMRI localization (weighted average of activation over a large multislice ROI), the agreement to within 1 cm indicates that it is likely that 1.5 T FMRI localization will prove to be accurate enough for clinical utility.

Optical Methods

Optical imaging of activity-dependent intrinsic signals is based on the interaction between light and brain tissue. When the brain is illuminated, active areas reflect less light than nonactive areas; the more an area is active, the less light is reflected.[302] These small, light intensity changes occur with a slow temporal profile and have rise times of approximately 2 seconds after activation.[303] This technique has excellent spatial resolutions of approximately 50 μm but is limited to the cerebral surface. Different parts of the visible spectrum reflect changes in different physiologic responses to activation, such as changes in CBF and

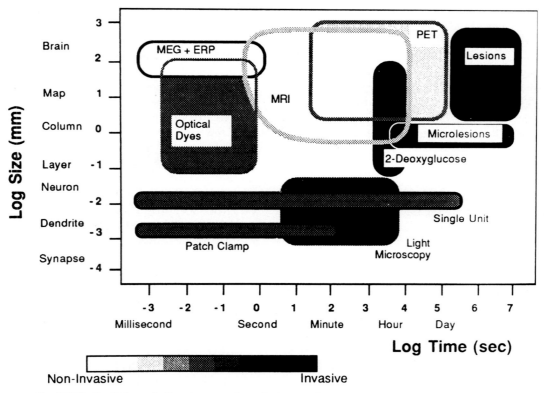

Fig. 7-102. Spatial resolution, temporal resolution, and invasiveness of available techniques for the study of brain function. (From Belliveau JW et al: Invest Radiol 27:559-565, 1992.)

oxy-deoxyhemoglogin levels. Examination of these absorbance characteristics is referred to as near infra-red spectroscopy (NIRS).

In visual stimulation studies employing both optical imaging and FMRI, Kato et al [304] obtained NIRS results supporting the mechanism that MR signal changes are the result of changes in oxygenation levels. However, these measurements indicated that while the level of oxygenated hemoglobin goes up with activation, deoxyhemoglobin levels decrease only slightly after stimulation.

Turner et al[203] performed a number of correlative optical studies on cats. In these studies, the Hb absorbance difference peak is observed as a clear feature at 582 nm, the amplitude of which is related to the mean concentration of deoxyhemoglobin in the FOV of the optic probe, providing a linear measure of oxygen saturation if volume changes are small. These optical measurements are also sensitive to blood volume changes. The results indicate that during periods of little volume change there is good agreement between the MRI data for changes of R2* and changes in oxygen saturation. When the blood volume changes, the MRI and optical results diverge, indicating that R2* depends on both blood volume and oxygenation. An explanation of these results suggested by the authors is that $\Delta R2^*$ depends on the voxel density of deoxyhemoglobin, which can be altered by changes in tissue blood volume and hematocrit as well as by changes in oxygen saturation.

· · ·

FMRI technology is now joining the arsenal of modalities used to address questions regarding the detailed relationship between neurophysiology and anatomy. Even if questions remain as to details of the underlying mechanisms and artifact sources, FMRI has demonstrated that it has a strong potential for becoming a successful clinical tool.

An issue related to the mechanism is the necessary and sufficient hardware requirements for successful study. The resolution to this issue may have the biggest impact on the clinical future of this technique. Specifically, will FMRI studies "work" on available clinical instruments or will they require dedicated specialized (i.e., expensive) hardware? This latter case may in fact relegate FMRI to a role similar to that of PET, where the full application of the functional imaging technology is limited to a few sites, with its use being primarily a research tool. A more likely scenario, based on the number of successful studies performed on conventional scanners, is that FMRI will follow a PET/SPECT development model whereby effective techniques developed on the limited number of specialty systems (i.e., PET) are implemented by the cheaper and more readily available clinical systems (i.e., SPECT) as procedural and hardware platform improvements allow.

The relationship among spatial resolution, temporal resolution, and invasiveness of the currently available techniques for studying brain function is illustrated in Fig. 7-102.[257] This comparison indicates that while there is some overlap in capabilities and applications, the strengths of each of the available functional imaging modalities are sufficiently unique that FMRI will not completely supersede any alternative. This also indicates that there is a tremendous potential for FMRI to be used in conjunction with other techniques to provide a fuller description of neurophysiology than would be available from either technique used in isolation.

REFERENCES

1. Sobel DF, Gallen CC, Schwartz BJ et al: Locating the central sulcus: comparison of MR anatomic and magnetoencephalographic functional methods, AJNR 14:915-925, 1993.
2. Fox PT, Mintun MA, Raichle ME et al: Mapping the human visual cortex with positron emission tomography, Nature (London) 323:806-809, 1986.
3. Fox PT, Raichle ME: Focal physiological uncoupling of cerebral blood flow and oxidative metabolism during somatosensory stimulation in human subjects, Neurobiology 83:1140-1144, 1986.
4. Belliveau JW, Kennedy DN, McKinstry RC et al: Functional mapping of the human visual cortex by magnetic resonance imaging, Science 254:716-719, 1991.
5. Fox PT, Raichle ME, Mintun MA et al: Nonoxidative glucose consumption during focal physiologic neural activity, Science 241:462-464, 1988.
6. Frostig RD, Lieke EE, Ts'o DY et al: Cortical functional architecture and local coupling between neuronal activity and the microcirculation revealed by in vivo high resolution optical imaging of intrinsic signals, Proc Natl Acad Sci USA 15:6082-6086, 1990.
7. Belliveau JW, Rosen BR, Kantor HL et al: Functional cerebral imaging by susceptibility-contrast NMR, Magn Reson Med 14:538-546, 1990.
8. Rosen BR, Belliveau JW, Aronen HJ et al: Susceptibility contrast imaging of cerebral blood volume: human experience, Magn Reson Med 22:293-299, 1991.
9. Thulborn KR, Waterton JC, Matthews PM et al: Oxygenation dependence of the transverse relaxation time of water protons in whole blood at high field, Biochim Biophys Acta 714:265-270, 1982.
10. Brooks RA, DiChiro G: Magnetic resonance imaging of stationary blood: a review, Med Phys 14:903-913, 1987.
11. Ogawa S, Lee T, Nayak AS et al: Oxygenation-sensitive contrast in magnetic resonance imaging of rodent brain at high magnetic fields, Magn Reson Med 14:68-78, 1990.
12. Ogawa S, Lee T: Magnetic resonance imaging of blood vessels at high fields: in vivo and in vitro measurements and image simulation, Magn Reson Med 16:9-18, 1990.
13. Kwong KK, Belliveau JW, Chesler DA et al: Dynamic magnetic resonance imaging of human brain activity during primary sensory stimulation, Proc Natl Acad Sci USA 89:5675-5679, 1992.
14. Turner R, LeBihan D, Moonen CTW et al: Echo-planar time course MRI of cat brain oxygenation changes, Magn Reson Med 22:159-166, 1991.

15. Pochobradsky J: Optimal field for detection of magnetically labeled blood, J Magn Reson 48:63-75, 1982.

16. Ogawa S, Lee TM, Barrere B: The sensitivity of magnetic resonance image signals of a rat brain to changes in the cerebral venous blood oxygenation, Magn Reson Med 29:205-210, 1993.

17. Heistad DD, Kontos HA: Cerebral circulation. In Shepard JT, Abboud FM (eds): Handbook of physiology Vol III, Section 2, Bethesda, MD, 1983, American Physiological Society.

18. Hudlicka O: Development of microcirculation: capillary growth and adaptation. In Renkin EM, Michel CC (eds): Handbook of physiology, Vol IV, Section 2, Bethesda MD, 1984, American Physiological Society.

19. Bassingthwaighte JB: Microcirculatory considerations in NMR flow imaging, Magn Reson Med 14:172-178, 1990.

20. Pawlik G, Rackl A, Bing RJ: Quantitative capillary topography and blood flow in the cerebral cortex of cats: an in vivo microscopic study, Brain Res 208:35-58, 1981.

21. Weiss HR, Buchweitz E, Murtha TJ et al: Quantitative regional determination of the total and perfused capillary network in the rat brain, Circ Res 51:494-503, 1982.

22. Brooks Battocletti JH, Sances A, Larson SJ et al: Nuclear magnetic relaxation in blood, IEEE Trans Biomed Eng 22:12-18, 1975.

23. Fenstermacher JD: The flow of water in the blood-brain-cerebrospinal fluid system, Syllabus, SMRM FMRI Workshop, Arlington VA, 1993, pp 9-17.

24. Koenig SH, Spiller M, Brown RD et al: Relaxation of water protons in the intra- and extracellular regions of blood containing Gd(DTPA), Magn Reson Med 3:791-795, 1986.

25. Brightman MW, Reese TS: Junctions between intimately apposed cell membranes in the vertebrate brain, J Cell Biol 40:648-677, 1969.

26. Reese TS, Karnovsky MJ: Fine structural localization of a blood-brain barrier to exogenous peroxidase, J Cell Biol 34:207-217, 1967.

27. Westergaard E, Brightman MW: Transport of proteins across normal cerebral arterioles, J Comp Neurol 152:17-44, 1973.

28. Eichling JO, Raichle ME, Grubb RL et al: Evidence of the limitations of water as a freely diffusible tracer in brain of the rhesus monkey, Circ Res 35:358-364, 1974.

29. Paulson OB, Hertz MM, Bolwig TG et al: Filtration and diffusion of water across the blood-brain barrier in man, Microvasc Res 13:113-124, 1977.

30. Moonen CTW, Pekar J, DeVeeschouwer MHM et al: Restricted and anisotropic displacement of water in healthy cat brain and in stroke studied by NMR diffusion imaging, Magn Reson Med 19:327-332, 1991.

31. Fenstermacher JD, Rapoport SI: Blood-brain barrier. In Renkin EM, Michel CC (eds): Handbook of physiology, ch. 21, Bethesda MD, 1984, American Physiological Society.

32. Fenstermacher J, Nakata H, Tajima A, et al: Functional variations in parenchymal microvascular systems within the brain, Magn Reson Med 19:217-220, 1991.

33. Purves MJ: The physiology of the cerebral circulation, New York, 1972, Cambridge University Press.

34. Suzuki K: Chemistry and metabolism of brain lipids. In Siegel GJ, Albers RW, Katzman R, Agranoff BW (eds): Basic neurochemistry, Boston, 1981, Little, Brown.

35. Rosen BR, Belliveau JW, Buchbinder BR et al: Contrast agents and cerebral hemodynamics, Magn Reson Med 19:285-292, 1991.

36. Bereczki D, Wei L, Otsuka T et al: Hypoxia increases velocity of blood flow through parenchymal microvascular systems in rat brain, J Cereb Blood Flow Metab 13:475-486, 1993.

37. Intaglietta M, Endrich BA: Experimental and quantitative analysis of microcirculatory water exchange, Acta Physiol Scand (Suppl) 463:59-66, 1979.

38. Arfors KE, Bergqvist D, Intaglietta M et al: Measurement of blood flow velocity in the microcirculation, Ups J Med Sci 80:27-33, 1975.

39. Johnson PC: Principles of circulatory control. In Johnson PC (ed): Peripheral circulation, New York, 1978, Wiley.

40. Fung YC: Stochastic flow in capillary blood vessels, Microvasc Res 5:34-48, 1973.

41. Lassen NA: Brain. In Johnson PC (ed): Peripheral circulation, New York, 1978, Wiley.

42. Kobayashi S, Waltz AG, Rhoton AL: Effects of stimulation of cervical sympathetic nerves on cortical blood flow and vascular reactivity, Neurology 21:297-302, 1971.

43. Meyer MW, Klassen AC: Regional brain blood flow during sympathetic stimulation. In Langfitt TW, McHenry LC, Reivich M, Wollman H (eds): Cerebral circulation and metabolism, New York, 1975, Springer Verlag, p 459.

44. Salanga VD, Waltz AG: Regional cerebral blood flow during stimulation of seventh cranial nerve, Stroke 4:213-217, 1973.

45. Johnson PC: The microcirculation and local and humoral control of the circulation. In Guyton AC, Jones CE (eds): Cardiovascular physiology, Physiology Series One, London, 1974, Butterworths.

46. Kuchinsky W, Wahl M, Bosse O et al: Perivascular potassium and pH as determinants of local pial arterial diameter in cats: a microapplication study, Circ Res 31:240-247, 1972.

47. Rubio R, Berne RM, Bockman EL et al: Relationship between adenosine concentration and oxygen supply in rat brain, Am J Physiol 228:1896-1902, 1975.

48. Wahl M, Kuchinsky W: The dilatory action of adenosine on pial arteries of cats and its inhibition by theophylline, Pflugers Arch 362:55-59, 1976.

49. Bean JW, Lignell J, Coulson J: Regional cerebral blood flow, O_2, and EEG in exposure to O_2 at high pressure, J Appl Physiol 31:235-242, 1971.

50. Ingvar DH, Sjolund B, Ardo A: Correlation between dominant EEG frequency, cerebral oxygen uptake and blood flow, Electroencephalogr Clin Neurophysiol 43:268-276, 1976.

51. Paulson OB, Sharbrough FW: Physiologic and pathophysiologic relationship between the electroencephalogram and the regional cerebral blood flow, Acta Neurol Chicago 50:194-220, 1974.

52. Fitzpatrick JH, Gilboe DD, Drewes et al: Relationship of cerebral oxygen uptake to EEG frequency in isolated canine brain, Am J Physiol 231:1840-1846, 1976.

53. Raichle ME, Brubb RL, Gado MH et al: Correlation between regional cerebral blood flow and oxidative metabolism, Arch Neurol Chicago 33:523-526, 1976.

54. Mangold R, Sokoloff L, Conner E et al: The effects of sleep and lack of sleep on the cerebral circulation and metabolism of normal young men, J Clin Invest 34:1092-1099, 1955.

55. Olesen J: Contralateral focal increase of cerebral blood flow in man during arm work, Brain 94:635-646, 1971.

56. Raichle M: Sensori-motor area increase of oxygen uptake and blood flow in the human brain during contralateral hand exercise: preliminary observations by the O^{15} method. In Ingvar DH, Lassen NA (eds): Brain work: the coupling of function, metabolism, and blood flow in the brain, Copenhagen, 1975, Munksgaard.

57. Leniger-Follert E, Lubbers DW: Behavior of microflow and local PO_2 of the brain cortex during and after direct electrical stimulation: a contribution to the problem of metabolic regulation of microcirculation in the brain, Pflugers Arch 366:39-44, 1976.

58. Fox PT, Raichle ME: Focal physiological uncoupling of cerebral blood flow and oxidative metabolism during somatosensory stimulation in human subjects, Proc Natl Acad Sci USA 83:1140-1144, 1986.

59. Meldrum RS, Nilsson B: Cerebral blood flow and metabolic rate early and late in prolonged epileptic seizures induced in rats by bicuculline, Brain 99:523-541, 1976.

60. Plum F, Duffy TE: The couple between cerebral metabolism and blood flow during seizures. In Ingvar DH, Lassen NA (eds): Brain work: the coupling of function, metabolism and blood flow in the brain, Copenhagen, 1975, Munksgaard, p 197-214.

61. Lassen NA: Cerebral blood flow and oxygen consumption in man, Physiol Rev 39:183-238, 1959.

62. Fieschi C, Battistini N, Lenzi GL et al: Metabolic and functional control of cerebral blood flow. In Ingvar DH, Lassen NA (eds): Brain work: the coupling of function, metabolism and blood flow in the brain, Copenhagen, 1975, Munksgaard, p 361.

63. Nicholson C: Diffusion of ions and macromolecules in the brain, Syllabus pp 1-7, SMRM FMRI Workshop, Arlington, VA, 1993.

64. Francois-Dainville E, Buchweitz, Weiss H: Effect of hypoxia on percentage of arteriolar and capillary beds perfused in the rat brain, J Appl Physiol 60:280-288, 1986.

65. Grubb BR: Blood flow and oxygen consumption in avian skeletal muscle, J Appl Physiol 60:450-455, 1981.

66. Hahn EL: Spin echoes, Phys Rev 80:580-594, 1950.

67. Carr HY, Purcell EM: Effects of diffusion on free precession in nuclear magnetic resonance experiments, Phys Rev 94:630-638, 1954.

68. Stejskal EE, Tanner JE: Spin diffusion measurements: spin echoes in the presence of a time-dependent field gradient, J Chem Phys 42:288-292, 1965.

69. LeBihan D, Breton E, Lallemand D et al: MR imaging of intravoxel incoherent motions: application to diffusion and perfusion in neurologic disorders. Radiology 161:401-407, 1986.

70. Hazelwood DG, Rorschach HE, Lin C: Diffusion of water in tissues and MRI, Magn Reson Med 19:214-216, 1991.

71. LeBihan D, Basser PJ, Mattiello J et al: Assessment of NMR diffusion measurements in biological systems: effects of micro-dynamics and microstructure, SMRM FMRI workshop, Arlington, VA, 1993, pp 19-25.

72. LeBihan D, Breton E, Lallemand D et al: Separation of diffusion and perfusion in intravoxel incoherent motion MR imaging, Radiology 168:497-505, 1988.

73. Stejskal EO: Use of spin echoes in a pulsed magnetic field gradient to study anisotropic restricted diffusion and flow, J Chem Phys 43:3597-6303, 1965.

74. Tanner JE, Stejskal EO: Restricted self-diffusion of protons in colloidal systems by the pulsed-gradient spin-echo method, J Chem Phys 49:1768-1777, 1968.

75. Moseley ME, Kucharczyk J, Asgari HS et al: Anisotropy in diffusion-weighted MRI, Magn Reson Med 19:321-326, 1991.

76. Rosen BR, Belliveau JW, Chien D: Perfusion imaging by nuclear magnetic resonance, Magn Reson Q 5:263-281, 1989.

77. Zhong J, Gore JC: Studies of restricted diffusion in heterogeneous media containing variations in susceptibility, Magn Reson Med 19:276-284, 1991.

78. Merboldt KD, Haenicke W, Frahm J: Self-diffusion NMR imaging using stimulated echoes, J Magn Reson 64:479-486, 1985.

79. Merboldt KD, Hanicke W, Frahm J: Diffusion imaging using stimulated echoes, Magn Reson Med 19:233-239, 1991.

80. Hazelwood DF: In Drost-Hansen W, Clegg JS (eds): Cell associated water, New York, 1976, Academic Press, p 165.

81. Moseley ME, Cohen Y, Mintorovitch J et al: Diffusion-weighted MR imaging of anisotropic water diffusion in cat central nervous system, Radiology 176:439-445, 1990.

82. LeBihan D, Turner R: Intravoxel incoherent motion imaging using spin echoes, Magn Reson Med 19:221-227, 1991.

83. Lorenz CH, Pickens DR, Puffer DB et al: Magnetic resonance diffusion/perfusion phantom experiments, Magn Reson Med 19:254-260, 1991.

84. Henkelman RM: Does IVIM measure classical perfusion, Magn Reson Med 16:470-475, 1990.

85. LeBihan D, Turner R: The capillary network: a link between IVIM and classical perfusion, Magn Reson Med 27:171-178, 1992.

86. Young IR, Hall AS, Bryant DJ et al: Assessment of brain perfusion with MR imaging, J Comput Assist Tomogr 12:721-727, 1988.

87. Young IR, Doran MD, Hajnal JV: Applications of the intravoxel coherent motion technique to the central nervous system, Magn Reson Med 19:266-269, 1991.

88. Chenevert TL, Pipe JG, Williams DM et al: Quantitative measurement of tissue perfusion and diffusion, Magn Reson Med 17:197-212, 1991.

89. Chenevert TL, Pipe JG: Effect of bulk tissue motion on quantitative perfusion and diffusion magnetic resonance imaging, Magn Reson Med 19:261-265, 1991.

90. Detre JA, Williams DS, Leigh JS et al: Perfusion imaging, Magn Reson Med 23:37-45, 1992.

91. Williams DS, Detre JA, Leigh JS et al: Magnetic resonance imaging of perfusion using spin inversion of arterial water, Proc Natl Acad Sci USA 89:212-216, 1992.

92. Detre JA, Leigh JS: Quantitative NMR imaging of perfusion in rat brain, Proceedings of 9th SMRM Annual Meeting, New York, 1990, p 1289.

93. Raichle ME, Eichling JO, Straatmann MG et al: Blood-brain barrier permeability of ^{11}C-labeled alcohols and ^{15}O-labeled water, Am J Physiol 230:543-552, 1976.

94. Mintun MA, Raichle ME, Martin WRW et al: Brain oxygen utilization measured with ^{15}O radiotracers and positron emission tomography, J Nucl Med 25:177-187, 1984.

95. deRoos A, Doornbos J, Baleriaux D et al: Clinical applications of gadolinium-DTPA in MRI. In Kressel HY ed: Magnetic resonance annual, New York, 1988, Raven Press, pp 113-145.

96. Runge VM, Clanton JA, Price AC et al: The use of Gd DPTA as a perfusion agent and marker of blood brain barrier disruption, Magn Reson Imag 3:43-55, 1985.

97. Wolf GL: Current status of MR imaging contrast agents: special report, Radiology 172:709-710, 1989.

98. Weinmann HJ, Brasch RC, Press WR et al: Characteristics of gadolinium-DTPA complex: a potential NMR contrast agent, AJR 142:619-624, 1984.

99. Villringer A, Rosen BR, Belliveau JW et al: Dynamic imaging with lanthanide chelates in normal brain: contrast due to magnetic susceptibility effects, Magn Reson Med 6:164-174, 1988.

100. Kantor HL, Rzedzian RR, Berliner E et al: A new NMR marker of coronary stenoses: the utility of dysprosium-DTPA in high speed cardiac imaging, Proceedings of 8th SMRM Annual Meeting, San Francisco, 1988, p 803.

101. Rozenman Y, Zou X, Kantor HL: Signal loss induced by superparamagnetic iron oxide particles in NMR spin-echo images: the role of diffusion, Magn Reson Med 14:31-39, 1990.

102. Chu SCK, Xu Y, Balschi JA et al: Bulk magnetic susceptibility shifts in NMR studies of compartmentalized samples: use of paramagnetic reagents, Magn Reson Med 13:239-262, 1990.

103. Weinman HJ, Brasch RC, Press WR et al: Characteristics of gadolinium-DTPA complex: a potential NMR contrast agent, Am J Roentgenol 142:619-624, 1984.

104. Runge VM, Clantan JA, Herzer WA et al: Intravascular contrast agents suitable for magnetic resonance imaging, Radiology 153:171-176, 1984.

105. Gadian DG, Payne DJ, Bryant IR et al: Gadolinium-DTPA as a contrast agent in MR imaging—theoretical projections and practical observations, Comput Assist Tomogr 9:242-251, 1985.

106. Larsson HBW, Stubgaard M, Frederiksen JL et al: Quantitation of blood-brain barrier defect by magnetic resonance imaging and gadolinium-DTPA in patients with multiple sclerosis and brain tumors, Magn Reson Med 16:117-131, 1990.

107. Fisel RC, Ackerman JL, Buxton RB et al: MR contrast due to microscopically heterogeneous magnetic susceptibility: numerical simulations and applications to cerebral physiology, Magn Reson Med 17:336-347, 1991.

108. Glasel JA, Lee KH: On the interpretation of water nuclear magnetic resonance relaxation times in heterogeneous systems, J Am Chem Soc 96:970-978, 1974.

109. Fung BM, McGaughy TW: Magnetic relaxation in heterogeneous systems, J Magn Reson 43:316-323, 1981.

110. Solomon I: Relaxation processes in a system of two spins, Physiol Rev 99:559-565, 1955.

111. Bloembergen N, Purcell EM, Pound RV: Relaxation effects in nuclear magnetic resonance absorption, Physiol Rev 73:679-712, 1948.

112. Bloembergen N: Proton relaxation times in paramagnetic solutions, J Chem Phys 27:572-573, 1957.

113. Rosen BR, Belliveau JW, Vevea JM et al: Perfusion imaging with NMR contrast agents, Magn Reson Med 14:249-265, 1990.

114. Gillis P, Koenig SH: Transverse relaxation of solvent protons induced by magnetized spheres: application to ferritin, erythrocytes, and magnetite, Magn Reson Med 5:323-345, 1987.

115. Majumdar S, Gore JC: Studies of diffusion in random fields produced by variations in susceptibility, J Magn Reson 78:41-55, 1988.

116. Case TA, Durney CH, Ailion DC et al: A mathematical model of diamagnetic line broadening in lung tissue and similar heterogeneous systems: calculations and measurements, J Magn Reson 73:304-314, 1987.

117. Hardy P, Henkelman RM: On the transverse relaxation rate enhancement induced by diffusion of spins through inhomogeneous fields, Magn Reson Med 17:348-356, 1991.

118. Weisskoff RM, Boxerman JL, Zuo CS et al: Endogenous susceptibility contrast: principles of relationship between blood oxygenation and MR signal change, Syllabus of SMRM FMRI Workshop, Arlington, VA, 1993, pp 103-110.

119. Lassen NA, Perl W: Tracer kinetic methods in medical physiology, New York, 1979, Raven Press.

120. Zierler KL: Theoretical basis of indicator dilution methods for measuring flow and volume, Circ Res 10:393-407, 1982.

121. Stewart GN: Researches on the circulation time in organs and on the influences which affect it, J Physiol 15:1-89, 1893.

122. Hamilton WF, Moore JW, Kinsman JM et al: Simultaneous determination of the pulmonary and systemic circulation times in man and of a figure related to the cardiac output, Am J Physiol 84:338-344, 1928.

123. Axel L: Cerebral blood flow determination by rapid-sequence computed tomography, Radiology 137:679-686, 1980.

124. Beringer WH, Axel L, Norman D et al: Functional imaging of the brain using computed tomography, Radiology 138:711-716, 1981.

125. Lassen NA, Henriksen O, Sejrsen P: Indicator methods for measurement of organ and tissue blood flow. In Shepherd JT, Abboud FM (eds): Handbook of physiology, Vol III, Section 2, Bethesda, MD, 1983, American Physiological Society.

126. Starmer CF, Clark DO: Computer computations of cardiac output using the gamma function, J Appl Physiol 28:219-220, 1970.

127. Thompson HK, Starmer CF, Whalen RE et al: Indicator transit time considered as a gamma variate, Circ Res 14:502-515, 1964.

128. Meier P, Zierler KL: On the theory of the indicator-dilution method for measurement of blood flow and volume, J Appl Physiol 6:731-744, 1954.

129. Zierler KL: Circulation times and the theory of indicator-dilution methods for determining blood flow and volume. Handbook of physiology, Vol I, Section 2, Bethesda, MD, 1962, American Physiological Society.

130. Zierler KL: Equations for measuring blood flow by external monitoring of radioisotopes, Circ Res 16:309-321, 1965.

131. Weisskoff RM, Chesler D, Boxerman JL et al: Pitfalls in MR measurement of tissue blood flow with intravascular tracers: which mean transit time? Magn Reson Med 29:553-559, 1993.

132. Lassen NA: Cerebral transit of an intravascular tracer may allow measurement of regional blood volume but not regional blood flow, J Cereb Blood Flow Metab 4:633-634, 1984.

133. Gore JC, Majumdar S: Measurement of tissue blood flow using intravascular relaxation agents and magnetic resonance imaging, Magn Reson Med 14:242-248, 1990.

134. Lauffer RB: Paramagnetic metal complexes as water proton relaxation agents for NMR imaging: theory and design, Chem Rev 87:901-927, 1987.

135. Alsaadi BM, Rossotti FJC, Williams RJP: Hydration of complex-one complexes of lanthanide cations, J Chem Soc 11:2151-2154, 1980.

136. Strich G, Hagan PL, Gerber KH et al: Tissue distribution and magnetic resonance spin lattice relaxation effects of gadolinium-DTPA, Radiology 154:723-726, 1985.

137. Perman WH, Gado GH, Larson KB et al: Simultaneous MR acquisition of arterial and brain signal-time curves, Magn Reson Med 28:74-83, 1992.

138. Villringer A, Rosen BR, Lauffer RB et al: Magnetic susceptibility-induced signal attenuation of rat brain using paramagnetic chelates, Abstract, 5th SMRM Annual Meeting, Montreal, Canada, 1986, pp 21-22.

139. Gore JC, Majumdar S: Measurement of tissue blood flow using intravascular relaxation agents and magnetic resonance imaging, Magn Reson Med 14:242-248, 1990.

140. White DL, Aicher KP, Tzika A et al: Iron-dextran as a magnetic susceptibility contrast agent: flow-related contrast effects in the T2-weighted spin-echo MRI of normal rat and cat brain, Magn Reson Med 14:14-28, 1992.

141. Packer KJ; The effects of diffusion through locally inhomogeneous magnetic fields on transverse nuclear spin relaxation in heterogeneous systems: proton transverse relaxation in striated muscle tissue, J Magn Reson 9:438-443, 1973.

142. Robertson B: Spin-echo decay of spins diffusing in a bounded region, Physiol Rev 151:273-277, 1966.

143. Albert MS, Huang W, Lee JH et al: Susceptibility changes following bolus injections, Magn Reson Med 29:700-708, 1993.

144. Albert MS, Huang W, Lee JH et al: Susceptibility-induced contrast enhancement during the rapid repetition of dilution bolus injections, Proceedings of 11th SMRM Annual Meeting, Berlin, Germany, 1992, p 1124.

145. Buxton RB, Wechsler LR, Alpert NM et al: The measurement of brain pH using $^{11}CO_2$ and positron emission tomography, J Cereb Blood Flow Metab 4:8-16, 1984.

146. Phelps ME, Huang SC, Hoffman EJ et al: Tomographic measurement of local cerebral glucose metabolic rate in human with (^{18}F)2-fluoro-2-deoxy-D-glucose: validation of method, Ann Neurol 6:371-388, 1979.

147. Subramanyam R, Alpert NM, Hoop B et al: A model for regional cerebral oxygen distribution during continuous inhalation of $^{15}O_2$, $C^{15}O$, and $C^{15}O_2$, J Nucl Med 19:48-53, 1978.

148. Gur D, Good WF, Wolfson SK et al: In vivo mapping of local cerebral blood flow by xenon-enhanced computed tomography, Science 215:1267-1268, 1982.

149. Drayer BP, Wolfson SK, Reinmuth OM, et al: Xenon enhanced CT for analysis of cerebral integrity, perfusion, and blood flow, Stroke 9:123-130, 1978.

150. Grubb RL, Raichle ME, Eichling JO et al: The effects of changes in Pa_{CO_2} on cerebral blood volume, blood flow and vascular mean transit time, Stroke 5:630-639, 1974.

151. Smith AL, Neufeld GR, Ominsky AJ et al: Effect of arterial carbon dioxide tension on cerebral blood flow, mean transit time, and vascular volume, J Appl Physiol 31:701-707, 1971.

152. Greitz T: Normal cerebral circulation time as determined by carotid angiography with sodium and methylglucamine diatrizoate (Urografin), Acta Radiol [Diag] 7:331-336, 1968.

153. Fox PT, Miezin FM, Allman JM et al: Retinotopic organization of human visual cortex mapped with positron-emission tomography, J Neurosci 7:913-922, 1987.

154. Lueck CJ, Zeki S, Friston KJ et al: The colour centre in the cortex of man, Nature 340:386-388, 1989.

155. Edelman RR, Mattle HP, Atkinson DJ et al: Cerebral blood flow: Assessment with dynamic contrast-enhanced T2*-weighted MR imaging at 1.5T, Radiology 176:211-220, 1990.

156. Perman WH, Gado M, Sandstrom JC: A method for increasing susceptibility contrast weighting for echo planar, snapshot FLASH and spin echo imaging, Proceedings of 9th SMRM Annual Meeting, New York, 1990, p 1302.

157. Kent TA, Quast MJ, Kaplan BJ et al: Cerebral blood volume in a rat model of ischemia at 4.7 T, AJNR 10:335-338, 1989.

158. Schmiedl U, Ogan M, Paajanen H et al: Albumin labeled with Gd-DTPA as an intravascular, blood pool-enhancing agent for MR imaging: biodistribution and imaging studies, Radiology 162:205-210, 1987.

159. Moseley ME, Chew WM, White DL et al: Hypercarbia-induced changes in cerebral blood volume in the cat: a 1H MRI and intravascular contrast agent study, Magn Reson Med 23:21-30, 1992.

160. Tyler JL, Diksic M, Villemure J-G et al: Metabolic and hemodynamic evaluation of gliomas using positron emission tomography, J Nucl Med 28:1123-1131, 1987.

161. Ianotti F, Fieschi C, Alfano B et al: Simplified, noninvasive PET measurement of blood brain barrier permeability, J Comput Assist Tomogr 11:390-397, 1987.

162. Conlon T, Outhred R: Water diffusion permeability of erythrocytes using an NMR technique, Biochim Biophys Acta 288:354-361, 1972.

163. Lipschitz-Farber C, Degani H: Kinetics of water diffusion across phospholipid membranes. 1H- and 17O-NMR relaxation studies, Biochim Biophys Acta 600:291-300, 1980.

164. Tofts PS, Kermode AG: Measurement of the blood-brain barrier permeability and leakage space using dynamic MR imaging. 1. Fundamental concepts, Magn Reson Med 17:357-367, 1991.

165. Bullock PR, Mansfield P, Gowland P et al: Dynamic imaging of contrast enhancement in brain tumors, Magn Reson Med 19:293-298, 1991.

166. Pauling L, Coryell C: The magnetic properties and structure of hemoglobin, Proc Natl Acad Sci USA 22:210-216, 1936.

167. Cho ZH, Ro YM, Lim TH: NMR venography using the susceptibility effect produced by deoxyhemoglobin, Magn Reson Med 28:25-38, 1992.

168. Bryant RG, Marill K, Blackmore C et al: Magnetic relaxation in blood and blood clots, Magn Reson Med 13:133-144, 1990.

169. Koenig SH, Brown RD, Lindstrom TR: Interactions of solvent with the heme region of methemoglobin and fluoromethemoglobin, Biophys J 34:397-408, 1981.

170. Koenig SH, Brown RD: Relaxation of solvent protons by paramagnetic ions and its dependence on magnetic field and chemical environment: implications for NMR imaging, Magn Reson Med 1:478-495, 1984.

171. Weisskoff RM, Kiihne S: MRI susceptometry: image-based measurement of absolute susceptibility of MR contrast agents and human blood, Magn Reson Med 24:375-383, 1992.

172. Brooks RA, Brunetti A, Alger JR et al: On the origin of paramagnetic inhomogeneity effects in blood, Magn Reson Med 12:241-248, 1989.

173. Brindle KM, Brown FF, Campbell ID et al: Application of spin-echo nuclear magnetic resonance to whole-cell systems: membrane transport, Biochem J 180:37-44, 1979.

174. Gomori JM, Grossman RI, Yu-Ip C et al: NMR relaxation times of blood: dependence on field strength, oxidation state, and cell integrity, J Comput Assist Tomogr 11:684-690, 1987.

175. Wright GA, Hu BS, Macovski A: Estimating oxygen saturation of blood in vivo with MR imaging at 1.5 T, J Magn Reson Imaging 1:275-283, 1991.

176. Intaglietta M, Johnson PC: Principles of capillary exchange. In Johnson PC (ed.): Peripheral circulation, New York, 1978, Wiley.

177. Dumke PR, Schmidt CF: Quantitative measurements of cerebral blood flow in the macaque monkey, Am J Physiol 138:421-431, 1943.

178. Duhling BR, Berne RM: Longitudinal gradient in periarteriolar oxygen tension, Circ Res 27:669-678, 1970.

179. Pykett IL, Rosen BR: Nuclear magnetic resonance: in vivo chemical shift imaging, Radiology 149:197-201, 1984.

180. Dixon WT: Single proton spectroscopic imaging, Radiology 153:189-194, 1984.

181. Wedeen VJ, Meuli RA, Edelman RR et al: Projective imaging of pulsatile flow with magnetic resonance, Science 230:946-948, 1985.

182. Young IR, Khenia S, Thomas DGT et al: Clinical magnetic susceptibility mapping of the brain, J COMPUT Assist Tomogr 11:2-6, 1987.

183. Wendt RE, Willcott MR, Nitz W et al: MR imaging of susceptibility-induced magnetic field inhomogeneities, Radiology 168:837-841, 1988.

184. Turner R, Jezzard P, Wen H et al: Functional mapping of the human visual cortex at 4 and 1.5 Tesla using deoxygenation contrast EPI, Magn Reson Med 29:277-279, 1993.

185. Frahm J, Merboldt KD, Hanicke W et al: Temporal and spatial resolution: concepts, sequences, and applications, Syllabus, SMRM FMRI Workshop, Arlington, VA, 1993.

186. DeLaPaz RL, New PFJ, Buonanno FS et al: NMR imaging of intercranial hemorrhage, J Comput Assist Tomogr 8:599-607, 1984.

187. Gomori JM, Grossman RI, Goldberg HI et al: Intracranial hematomas: imaging by high-field MR, Radiology 157:87-93, 1985.

188. Edelman RR, Johnson K, Buxton R et al: MR of hemorrhage: a new approach, Am J Neuroradiol 7:751-756, 1986.

189. Bradley WG, Schmidt PG: Effect of methemoglobin formation on the MR appearance of subarachnoid hemorrhage, Radiology 156:99-103, 1985.

190. Morin MG, Paulett G, Hobbs ME: Nuclear magnetic resonance chemical shift determinations by means of a concentric cylinder sample cell, J Phys Chem 60:1594-1596, 1956.

191. Cho ZH, Ro YM, Lim TH: NMR venography using the susceptibility effect produced by deoxyhemoglobin, Magn Reson Med 28:25-38, 1992.

192. Ogawa S, Lee TM, Kay AR et al: Brain magnetic resonance imaging with contrast dependent on blood oxygenation, Proc Natl Acad Sci USA 87:9868-9872, 1990.

193. Ogawa S, Menon RS, Tank DW et al: Functional brain mapping by blood oxygenation level-dependent contrast magnetic resonance imaging, Biophys J 64:803-812, 1993.

194. Jezzard P, LeBihan D, Cuenod C et al: An investigation of the contribution of physiological noise in human functional MRI studies at 1.5 Tesla and 4 Tesla, Proceedings of 12th SMRM Annual Meeting, New York, 1993, p 1392.

195. Weisskoff RM, Hoppel BE, Rosen BR: Abstracts, 10th SMRI Annual Meeting, Chicago, 1992.

196. Bandettini PA, Wong EC, Hinks RS et al: Time course EPI of human brain function during task activation, Magn Reson Med 25:390-397, 1992.

197. Frahm J, Bruhn H, Merboldt K et al: J Magn Reson Imaging 2:501, 1992.
198. Ogawa S, Tank DW, Menon R et al: Intrinsic signal changes accompanying sensory stimulation: functional brain mapping with magnetic resonance imaging, Proc Natl Acad Sci USA 89:5951-5955, 1992.
199. Menon RS, Ogawa S, Kim S et al: Functional brain mapping using magnetic resonance imaging: signal changes accompanying visual stimulation, Invest Radiol 27:S47-53, 1992.
200. DeYoe EA, Neitz J, Bandettini PA et al: Time course of event-related MR signal enhancement in visual and motor cortex, Proceedings of 11th SMRM Annual Meeting, Berlin, 1992, p 1824.
201. Blamire AM, Ogawa S, Ugurbil K et al: Dynamic mapping of the human visual cortex by high-speed magnetic resonance imaging, Proc Natl Acad Sci USA 89:11069-11073, 1992.
202. Bereczki D, Otsuka T, Wei L et al: Hypoxia increases velocity of blood flow through parenchymal microvascular systems in rat brain, J Cereb Blood Flow Metab 11(suppl 2): S72, 1993.
203. Turner R, Jezzard P, Heineman F: Quantitative studies of EPI BOLD contrast with animal models, Syllabus, SMRI FMRI Workshop, Arlington, VA, 1993, pp 121-128.
204. Turner R, Jezzard P, Hertz-Pannier L et al: Functional neuroimaging with EPI: sequence issues, Syllabus, SMRM FMRI Workshop, Arlington, VA, 1993, pp 163-169.
205. van Yperen GH, de Boer RW, Berkelbach van der Sprenkel JW et al: TSE and increased perfusion during activation of the motor cortex, Proceedings of 12th SMRM Annual Meeting, New York, 1993, p 171.
206. Fisel CR, Moore JR, Garrido L et al: A general model for susceptibility-based MR contrast, Proceedings of 8th SMRM Annual Meeting, Amsterdam, 1989, p 324.
207. Ogawa S, Tank DW, Menon R et al: Blood oxygenation level dependent T2* rate estimated with a simple biophysical model, Proceedings of 12th SMRM Annual Meeting, New York, 1993, p 618.
208. Hoppel BE, Baker JR, Weisskoff RM et al: The dynamic response of ΔR2 and ΔR2' during photic activation, Proceedings of 12th SMRM Annual Meeting, New York, 1993, p 1384.
209. Bandettini PA, Wong EC, Jesmanowicz A et al: Simultaneous mapping of activation-induced ΔR2* and ΔR2 in the human brain using a combined gradient-echo and spin-echo EPI pulse sequence, Proceedings of 12th SMRM Annual Meeting, New York, 1993, p 169.
210. Menon RS, Ogawa S, Tank DW et al: 4 Tesla gradient recalled echo characteristics of photic stimulation-induced signal changes in the human primary visual cortex, Magn Reson Med 30:380-386, 1993.
211. Lai S, Hopkins AL, Haacke EM et al: Identification of vascular structures as a major source of signal contrast in high resolution 2D and 3D functional activation imaging of motor cortex at 1.5T: preliminary results, Magn Reson Med 30:387-392, 1993.
212. Kwong KK, Chesler DA, Baker JR et al: Functional magnetic resonance imaging—MR movie of human brain activity, Syllabus, SMRM FMRI Workshop, Arlington, VA, 1993, pp 135-142.
213. Hajnal JV, White SJ, Pennock JM et al: Functional imaging of the brain at 1.0 T and 0.15 T using fluid attenuated inversion recovery (FLAIR) pulse sequences, Proceedings of 11th SMRM Annual Meeting, Berlin, 1992, p 1023.
214. Duyn JH, Moonen CTW, de Boer RW et al: Inflow versus deoxyhemoglobin effects in "BOLD" functional MRI using gradients echoes at 1.5T, Proceedings of 12th SMRM Annual Meeting, New York, 1993, p 168.
215. van Yperen GH, de Boer RW, Berkelbach van der Sprenkel JW et al: TSE and increased perfusion during activation of the motor cortex, Proceedings of 12th SMRM Annual Meeting, New York, 1993, p 171.
216. Feinberg DA, Mark AS: Human brain motion and cerebrospinal fluid circulation demonstrated with MR velocity imaging, Radiology 163:793-799, 1987.
217. Glover GH, Lee AT, Meyers CH: Motion artifacts in FMRI: comparison of 2DFT with PR and spiral scan methods, Proceedings of 12th SMRM Annual Meeting, New York, 1993, p 197.
218. Hajnal JV, Oatridge A, Schwieso J et al: Cautionary remarks on the role of veins in the variability of functional imaging experiments, Proceedings of 12th SMRM Annual Meeting, New York, 1993, p 166.
219. Hajnal JV, Myers R, Oatridge A et al: Artifacts due to stimulus correlated motion in functional imaging of the brain, Magn Reson Med 31:283-291, 1994.
220. Frahm J, Merboldt KD, Hanicke W: Functional MRI of human brain activation at high spatial resolution, Magn Reson Med 29:139-144, 1993.
221. Bandettini PA, Wong EC, Hinks et al: Quantification of changes in relaxation rates R2* and R2 in activated brain tissue, Abstract, 11th SMRM Annual Meeting, Berlin, 1992.
222. Baker JR, Cohen MS, Stern CE et al: The effect of slice thickness and echo time on the detection of signal change during echo-planar functional neuroimaging, Proceedings of 11th SMRM Annual Meeting, Berlin, 1992, p 1822.
223. Wehrli FW: Fast scan magnetic resonance: principles and application, Magn Reson Q 6:165-236, 1990.
224. Feinberg DA, Oshio K: Gradient-echo shifting in fast MRI techniques (GRASE imaging) for correction of field inhomogeneity errors and chemical shift, J Magn Reson 97:177-183, 1992.
225. Moonen CTW, Liu G, van Gelderen P et al: A fast gradient-recalled MRI technique with increased sensitivity to dynamic susceptibility effects, Magn Reson Med 26:184-189, 1992.
226. Liu G, Sobering G, Olson AW et al: Fast echo-shifted gradient-recalled MRI: combining a short repetition time with variable T2* weighting, Magn Reson Med 30:68-75, 1993.
227. Liu G, Sobering G, Duyn J et al: A functional MRI technique combining principles of echo-shifting with a train of observations (PRESTO), Magn Reson Med 30:764-768, 1993.
228. Duyn JH, Moonen CTW, Mattay VS et al: 3-Dimensional functional imaging of the human brain using echo-shifted FLASH, Proceedings of 12th SMRM Annual Meeting, New York, 1993, p 1386.
229. Haase A: Snapshot FLASH MRI: applications to T1, T2, and chemical shift imaging, Magn Reson Med 13:77-89, 1990.
230. Jones RA, Southon TE: A magnetization transfer preparation scheme for snapshot FLASH imaging, Magn Reson Med 19:483-488, 1991.
231. Hu X, Stillman AE: A new T2* weighting technique for perfusion imaging by dynamic susceptibility contrast, Abstract, 10th SMRM Annual Meeting, San Francisco, 1991, p 778.
232. Kim SG, Hu X, Ogawa S et al: T2* imaging with adiabatic pulse and turbo-flash at 4 Tesla, Abstract, 11th SMRM Annual Meeting, Berlin, 1992, p 1122.
233. Bendel P: Snapshot MRI with T2*-weighted magnetization preparation, Magn Reson Med 30:399-402, 1993.
234. Hu X, Kim SG: A new T2*-weighting technique for magnetic resonance imaging, Magn Reson Med 30:512-517, 1993.
235. Jones RA, Haraldseth O, Muller TB et al: K-space substitution: a novel dynamic imaging technique, Magn Reson Med 29:830-834, 1993.
236. Van Vaals JJ, Engels H, De Graaf RG et al: Method for accelerated perfusion imaging, Abstract, 11th SMRM Annual Meeting, Berlin, 1992, p 1139.
237. Pike GB, Fredrickson JO, Glover GH et al: Dynamic susceptibility contrast imaging using a gradient-echo sequence, Abstract, 11th SMRM Annual Meeting, Berlin, 1992, p 1131.
238. Sanders JA, Orrision WW: ANOVA tests for identification of

FMRI activation, Proceedings of 12th SMRM Annual Meeting, New York, 1993, p 1376.

239. LeBihan D, Jezzard P, Turner R et al: Practical problems and limitations in using Z-maps for processing of brain function MR images, Proceedings of 12th SMRM Annual Meeting, New York, 1993, p 11.

240. Weisskoff RM, Baker J, Belliveau J et al: Power spectrum analysis of functionally-weighted MR data: what's in the noise, Proceedings of 12th SMRM Annual Meeting, New York, 1993, p 7.

241. Noll DC, Schneider W, Cohen JD: Artifacts in functional MRI using conventional scanning, Proceedings of 12th SMRM Annual Meeting, New York, 1993, p 1407.

242. Binder JR, Jesmanowicz A, Rao SM et al: Analysis of phase differences in periodic functional MRI activation data, Proceedings of 12th SMRM, New York, 1993, p 1283.

243. Wen H, Wolff S, Berman K et al: Phase and magnitude functional imaging of motor tasks and pain stimuli, Proceedings of 12th SMRM Annual Meeting, New York, 1993, p 9.

244. Schneider W: Functional MRI mapping of individual stages of visual processing, Proceedings of 12th SMRM Annual Meeting, New York, 1993, p 56.

245. Hajnal JV, Collins AG, White SJ et al: Imaging of human-brain activity at 0.15 T using fluid attenuated inversion recovery (FLAIR) pulse sequences, Magn Reson Med 30:650-653, 1993.

246. Glantz SA: Primer of biostatistics, ed 2, New York, 1987, McGraw-Hill, p. 246.

247. Sanders JA, Orrison WW: ANOVA tests for identification of FMRI activation, Proceedings of 12th SMRM Annual Meeting, New York, 1993, p 1376.

248. Bandettini PA, Jesmanowicz A, Wong EC et al: Processing strategies for time-course data sets in functional MRI of the human brain, Magn Reson Med 30:161-173, 1993.

249. Woods RP, Cherry SR, Mazziota JC: Rapid automated algorithm for aligning and reslicing PET images, J Comput Assist Tomogr 16:620-633, 1992.

250. Diegert C, Sanders JA, Orrison WW: Practical, computer-aided registration of multiple three-dimensional magnetic resonance observations of the human brain, SPIE Neural and Stochastic Methods in Image and Signal Processing II, 2032:167-173, 1993.

251. Watson JDG: PET mappings of the visual cortex, SMRM FMRI workshop, Arlington, VA, 1993, pp 129-133.

252. Belliveau JW, McKinstry RC, Kennedy DN et al: J Cereb Blood Flow Metab 11(2): S5, 1991.

253. Belliveau JW, Kennedy DN, McKinstry RC et al: J Magn Reson Imaging 1(2):202, 1991.

254. Fox PT, Raichle ME: Stimulus rate determines regional blood flow in striate cortex, Ann Neurol 17:303-305, 1985.

255. Fox PT, Raichle ME: Stimulus rate dependence of regional cerebral blood flow in human striate cortex, demonstrated by positron emission tomography, J Neurophysiol 51:1109-1120, 1984.

256. Frahm J, Merboldt KD, Hanicke W et al: High-resolution functional MRI of focal subcortical activity in the human brain. Long-echo time FLASH of the lateral geniculate nucleus during visual stimulation, Proceedings of 12th SMRM Annual Meeting, New York, 1993, p 57.

257. Belliveau JW, Kwong KK, Kennedy DN et al: Magnetic resonance imaging mapping of brain function: human visual cortex, Invest Radiol 27:S59-65, 1992.

258. Schneider W, Noll DC, Cohen JD: Functional topographic mapping of the cortical ribbon in human vision with conventional MRI scanners, Nature 365:150-153, 1993.

259. Sorensen AG, Caramia F, Wray SH et al: Extrastriate activation in patients with visual field defects, Proceedings of 12th SMRM Annual Meeting, New York, 1993, p 62.

260. Dieber MP, Passingham RE, Colebatch JG et al: Cortical areas and the selection of movement: a study with positron emission tomography, Exp Brain Res 84:393-402, 1991.

261. Fox PT, Fox JM, Raichle ME et al: The role of cerebral cortex in the generation of voluntary saccades: a positron emission tomographic study, J Neurophysiol 54:348-369, 1985.

262. Ellermann JM, Flament D, Kim SG et al: Studies of human cerebellar function using multislice nuclear magnetic resonance imaging at high magnetic field. Proceedings of 12th SMRM Annual Meeting, New York, 1993, p 1401.

263. Bates SR, Yetkin FZ, Bandettini PA et al: Activation of the human cerebellum demonstrated by functional magnetic resonance imaging, Proceedings of 12th SMRM Annual Meeting, New York, 1993, p 1420.

264. Cuenod CA, Zeffiro T, Pannier L et al: Functional imaging of the human cerebellum during finger movement with a conventional 1.5 T MRI scanner, Proceedings of 12th SMRM Annual Meeting, New York, 1993, p 1421.

265. Fox PT, Raichle ME, Thach WT: Functional mapping of the human cerebellum with positron emission tomography, Proc Natl Acad Sci USA 83:1140-1144, 1986.

266. Kim SG, Hendrich K, Ellermann JM et al: Motor cortex and handedness studies by functional MRI at 4 Tesla. Proceedings of 12th SMRM Annual Meeting, New York, 1993, p 1395.

267. Berkelbach van der Sprenkel JW, Verheul J, de Boer RW et al: Functional imaging of dominance in senso motor cortex of the human brain, Proceedings of 12th SMRM Annual Meeting, New York, 1993, p 1424.

268. Rao SM, Binder JR, Hammeke TA et al: Somatotopic mapping of the primary motor cortex with functional magnetic resonance imaging, Proceedings of 12th SMRM Annual Meeting, New York, 1993, p 1397.

269. Bandettini PA: MRI studies of brain activation: dynamic characteristics, Syllabus, SMRM FMRI Workshop, Arlington, VA, 1993, pp 143-152.

270. Bandettini PA, Wong EC, DeYoe EA et al: The functional dynamics of blood oxygen level dependent contrast in the motor cortex, Proceedings of 12th SMRM Annual Meeting, New York, 1993, p 1382.

271. Lauter JL, Herscovitch P, Formby C et al: Tonotopic organization in human auditory cortex revealed by positron emission tomography, Hear Res 20:199-205, 1985.

272. Turner R, Jezzard P, LeBihan D et al: BOLD contrast imaging of cortical regions used in processing auditory stimuli, Proceedings of 12th SMRM Annual Meeting, New York, 1993, p 1411.

273. Singh M, Kim H, Kim T et al: Functional MRI at 1.5T during auditory stimulation, Proceedings of 12th SMRM Annual Meeting, New York, 1993, p 1431.

274. Hinke RM, Hu X, Stillman AE et al: The use of multislice functional MRI during internal speech to demonstrate the lateralization of language function, Proceedings of 12th SMRM Annual Meeting, New York, 1993, p 63.

275. Rao SM, Bandettini PA, Wong EC et al: Gradient-echo EPI demonstrates bilateral superior temporal gyrus activation during passive word presentation, Proceedings of 11th SMRM Annual Meeting, Berlin, 1992, p 1829.

276. Blamire AM, McCarthy G, Gruetter R et al: Echo-planar imaging of the left inferior frontal lobe during word generation, Proceedings of 11th SMRM Annual Meeting, Berlin, 1992, p 1834.

277. McCarthy G, Blamire AM, Bloch G et al: Echo planal MRI studies of frontal cortex during word generation, Proceedings of 12th SMRM Annual Meeting, New York, 1993, p 1412.

278. Cuenod CA, Bookheimer S, Pannier L et al: Functional imaging during word generation using conventional MRI scanner, Proceedings of 12th SMRM Annual Meeting, New York, 1993, p 1414.

279. Rueckert L, Appollonio I, Grafman J et al: Functional activation of left frontal cortex during covert word production, Proceedings of 12th SMRM Annual Meeting, New York, 1993, p 60.

280. Binder JR, Rao SM, Hammeke TA et al: Temporal characteristics of functional magnetic resonance signal change in lateral frontal and auditory cortex, Abstracts, 12th SMRM, New York, 1993, p 5.

281. Kosslyn SM, Alpert NM, Thompson WL: Visual mental imagery and visual perception: PET studies, SMRM FMRI Workshop, Arlington, VA, 1993, p 183-190.

282. Kaufman L, Schwartz B, Salustri C et al: Modulation of spontaneous brain activity during mental imagery, J Cogn Neurosci 2:124-132, 1992.

283. Bandettini PA, Rao SM, Binder JR et al: Magnetic resonance functional neuroimaging of the entire brain during performance and mental rehearsal of complex finger movement tasks, Proceedings of 12th SMRM Annual Meeting, New York, 1993, p 1396.

284. Fieldman JB, Cohen LG, Jezzard P et al: Functional neuroimaging with echo-planar imaging in humans during execution and mental rehearsal of a simple motor task, Proceedings of 12th SMRM Annual Meeting, New York, 1993, p 1416.

285. Roland PE, Larsen B, Lassen NA et al: Supplementary motor area and other cortical areas in organization of voluntary movements in man, J Neurophysiol 43:118-136, 1980.

286. Blamire AM, McCarthy G, Nobre AC et al: Functional magnetic resonance imaging of human pre-frontal cortex during a spatial memory task, Proceedings of 12th SMRM Annual Meeting, New York, 1993, p 1413.

287. Cohen JD, Forman SD, Casey BJ et al: Spiral-scan imaging of dorsolateral prefrontal cortex during a working memory task, Proceedings of 12th SMRM Annual Meeting, New York, 1993, p 1405.

288. Connelly A, Jackson GD, Cross JH et al: Functional magnetic resonance imaging of focal seizures, Proceedings of 12th SMRM Annual Meeting, New York, 1993, p 61.

289. Wen H, Wolff S, Berman K et al: Phase and magnitude functional imaging of motor tasks and pain stimuli, Proceedings of 12th SMRM Annual Meeting, New York, 1993, p 9.

290. Russel DP, Howland EW, Jones JR et al: High-resolution functional neuroimaging of noxious and innocuous sensory stimuli using a clinical scanner, Proceedings of 12th SMRM Annual Meeting, New York, 1993, p 1425.

291. Breiter HC, Kwong KK, Baker JR et al: Functional magnetic resonance imaging of symptom provocation in obsessive-compulsive disorder, Proceedings of 12th SMRM Annual Meeting, New York, 1993, p 58.

292. Baxter LR, Schwartz JM, Bergman KS et al: Caudate glucose metabolic rate changes with both drug and behavior therapy for obsessive-compulsive disorder, Arch Gen Psychiatry 49:681-689, 1992.

293. Swedo SE, Pietrini P, Leonard HL et al: Cerebral glucose metabolism in childhood-onset obsessive-compulsive disorder, Arch Gen Psychiatry 49:690-694, 1992.

294. Cuenod CA, Chang MCJ, Arai T et al: Local brain response to cholinergic receptor stimulation detected by MRI, Proceedings of 12th SMRM Annual Meeting, New York, 1993, p 1387.

295. Wenz F, Schad LR, Baudendistel et al: Effects of neuroleptic drugs on the signal intensity during motor cortex stimulation: functional MR-imaging performed with a standard 1.5T clinical imager, Proceedings of 12th SMRM Annual Meeting, New York, 1993, p 1419.

296. Mattay VS, Frank JA, Sunderland T et al: Dynamic contrast functional MRI in Alzheimer's disease during visual activation, Proceedings of 12th SMRM Annual Meeting, New York, 1993, p 1404.

297. Buchbinder BR, Belliveau JW, McKinstry RC et al: Functional MR imaging of primary brain tumors with PET correlation, Proceedings of 10th SMRM Annual Meeting, San Francisco, 1991, p 121.

298. Cao Y, Towle VL, Levin DN et al: Conventional 1.5T MRI localization of human hand sensorimotor cortex with intraoperative electrophysiologic validation, Proceedings of 12th SMRM Annual Meeting, New York, 1993, p 1417.

299. Jack CR, Thompson R, Butts RK et al: Sensory motor cortex: correlation of presurgical mapping with functional MR imaging and invasive cortical mapping, Radiology 190:85-92, 1994.

300. Connelly A, Gadian DG, Jackson GD et al: Presurgical identification of the motor cortex using functional MRI, Proceedings of 12th SMRM Annual Meeting, New York, 1993, p 1422.

301. Sanders JA, Lewine JD, George JS et al: Correlation of FMRI with MEG, Proceedings of 12th SMRM Annual Meeting, New York, 1993, p 1418.

302. Frostig RD: Optical measurements of brain oxygenation: coupling with high resolution imaging of brain function, SMRM FMRI workshop, 1993, p 898-894.

303. Grinvald A, Lieke E, Frostig RD et al: Functional architecture of cortex revealed by optical imaging of intrinsic signals, Nature 324:361-364, 1986.

304. Kato R, Takashima S, Kamada K et al: Advantage of near-infrared spectroscopy in the human functional MR imaging in brain, Proceedings of 12th SMRM Annual Meeting, New York, 1993, p 1409.

8

Clinical Electroencephalography and Event-Related Potentials

Jeffrey David Lewine
William W. Orrison, Jr.

Noninvasive neuroelectric techniques (electroencephalography [EEG] and event-related potentials [ERPs]) are some of the most important tools in the armamentarium of diagnostic procedures available to neurologists and psychiatrists.[1,2] Whereas EEG-based methods are generally not considered as true imaging techniques, EEG-derived information on brain function nevertheless provides an important complement to information on brain structure derived from computed tomography (CT) and magnetic resonance imaging (MRI). These later methods provide key insights into brain structure, but only electromagnetic techniques provide direct, real-time insight into neural processing.

In 1848, the German physiologist Dubois-Reymond demonstrated that an externally recordable electrical signal occurred concomitantly with passage of a nerve impulse along a peripheral nerve.[3] This discovery led the English physiologist Richard Caton to explore the possibility that nerve impulses flowing within brain cells might also produce detectable electrical signals. At the 1875 meeting of the British Medical Association, Caton reported his pioneering animal experiments, in which he demonstrated that "feeble currents of varying direction pass through the multiplier when the electrodes are placed on two points of the external

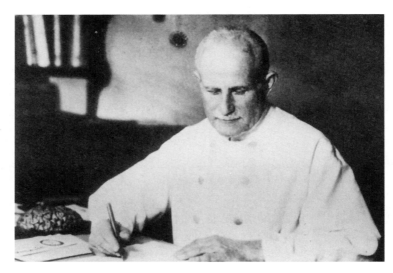

Fig. 8-1. Hans Berger, the "father" of human EEG. (From Blakemore C.: Mechanisms of the mind, Cambridge, 1977, Cambridge University Press, p 50.)

surface, or one electrode on the grey matter, and one on the surface of the skull." Caton demonstrated that the cerebral cortex had a tonic level of oscillatory electrical activity and that additional phasic electrical activity could be evoked in response to peripheral sensory stimulation.[4]

The diagnostic potential of EEG was first hinted at by the subsequent (1912) animal experiments of Kaufman, who discovered abnormal neuroelectric discharges in animals with experimentally induced epilepsy.[5] Despite these exciting developments in animal EEG, it was not until 1929 that Hans Berger, a German neuropsychiatrist, recorded the first human EEG (Fig. 8-1). As early as his original 1929 report, Berger described a posterior rhythm of 8 to 13 Hz (cycles per second). This "alpha" rhythm was prominent when the subject's eyes were closed, and it was greatly reduced with opening of the eyes.[6] During the next several years, Berger and others began to record the electroencephalogram (also abbreviated EEG) in various clinical populations, and following confirmation of Berger's work by Adrian and colleagues in the early 1930s,[7] there was an explosion of interest in neuroelectric phenomena. Of particular note were the ground-breaking studies of human epilepsy by Fredric Gibbs and his colleagues. His 1935 paper with Davis and Lennox demonstrated the 3 Hz spike/wave complexes associated with petit mal absence seizures[8] (Fig. 8-2). This work, in combination with subsequent studies of grand mal and psychomotor seizures, formed the foundation of clinical neurophysiology and signaled the beginning of a new era in the study of epilepsy. (Berger actually noted the presence of paroxysmal discharges associated with petit mal seizures in 1933, but these observations were just mentioned in passing and went mostly unnoticed.)

The importance of EEG and its applications in neurology, neurosurgery, and psychiatry were quickly established by Gibbs and other pioneers, including Donald Lindsley in the United States, Herbert Jasper, working first in the United States and then in Canada, and W. Grey Walter in England. EEG is now considered a routine clinical procedure of considerable diagnostic value and it is proving to be a very useful measure of brain physiology in neuroscientific research.

This chapter, as with others in this text, focuses on clinical applications of EEG and ERPs. Readers interested in the extraordinary uses of these techniques for exploring basic brain information processing and cognitive mechanisms should consult the excellent reviews of these types of studies in the *Handbook of Electroencephalography and Clinical Neurophysiology*.

There are two basic types of neuroelectric examinations: (1) EEG studies that involve inspection of spontaneous brain activity and (2) ERP studies that use signal-averaging techniques to extract (from the spontaneous EEG) neuroelectric activity that is time-locked to specific sensory, motor, or cognitive events. Hybrid techniques, such as those that examine event-related desynchronization or synchronization of the spontaneous EEG,[9,10] are mostly of interest in cognitive neuroscience and are not discussed in detail. Parameters of particular interest in EEG examinations include the gross morphology and topographic distribution of the recorded activity and the relative frequency content of the activity. Of special interest in clinical EEG examinations is the presence of epileptic discharges and paroxysmal slowing, which can be signs of gross brain pathology. ERP examinations are generally designed to assess the integrity of particular information-processing pathways (e.g., vision, audition). Parameters of interest include the waveform

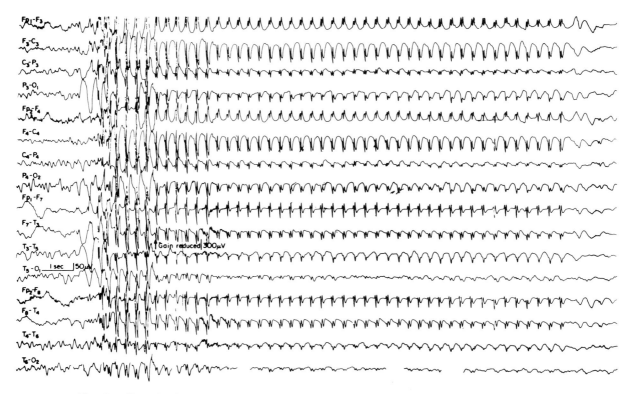

Fig. 8-2. Petit Mal absence seizure showing characteristic 3 Hz spike/wave complexes. (From Niedermeyer E: Epileptic seizure disorders. In Niedermeyer E, Lopes da Silva, editors: Electroencephalography—basic principles, clinical applications and related fields, ed 2, Baltimore, 1987, Urban and Schwarzenberg, p 416.)

morphology of average evoked responses, with definition of the latency and amplitude of various waveform components diagnostically useful.

NEUROELECTRIC RECORDINGS: BASIC PRINCIPLES AND TECHNIQUES
Neural Substrates of Scalp Neuroelectric Activity

Since the first recordings of the scalp EEG by Berger, tremendous effort has focused on defining the neural substrates of the scalp phenomenon. However, several factors make defining the relationship between the EEG and the brain difficult. There are two types of brain cells, neurons and glia, and both contribute to the EEG. Nerve cells display two distinct classes of neuroelectric events: graded synaptic potentials and action potentials. Glia are known to show slow changes in their resting membrane potentials, and these, along with the previously mentioned neuroelectric phenomena, all contribute to the scalp EEG.

As discussed in Chapter 2, graded synaptic potentials are the result of neurochemically induced, transient changes in the ionic permeability of the postsynaptic membrane. Consider, for example, an excitatory synapse on a dendrite that causes a transient increase in sodium permeability. When the sodium permeability increases, sodium ions move down their electro-chemical gradient into the cell. This transmembrane ionic current, in turn, causes intracellular current flow within the dendrite, directed away from the site of sodium influx. The intracellular current is characterized by an advancing accumulation of positive charges that results in outwardly directed transmembrane displacement currents down the length of the axon. The original transmembrane ionic current creates a deficit of positive charges in the local extracellular space. This is known as an *extracellular current sink*. The outwardly directed transmembrane displacement currents produce extracellular regions of excess positive charge—current sources. To complete the overall current pathway, extracellular volume currents flow from these current sources to the current sink. Thus, a complete pathway is made from the ionic transmembrane current, the intracellular current, the transmembrane displacement currents, and the extracellular volume currents (Fig. 8-3).

The extracellular current sinks and sources (and associated volume currents) cause an electrical potential distribution in the conductive media, with the magnitude of the potential decreasing with increasing distance from the neuron. The exact manner in which the potential changes within the media partly depends on the configuration of the relevant currents.

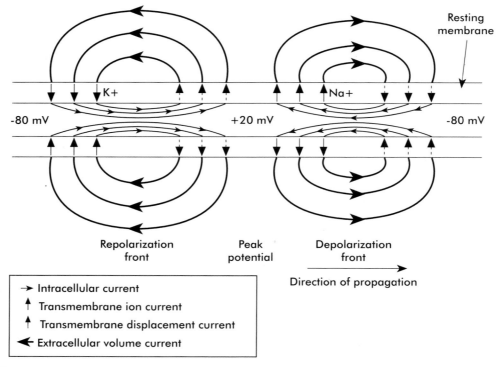

Fig. 8-3. Neuronal activity results in the formation of extracellular current sources and sinks. The overall continuous current pathway has four components: (1) the transmembrane ionic current, (2) the intracellular current, (3) the transmembrane displacement current, and (4) the extracellular volume current.

When viewed at the microscopic level, this pattern of current flow is rather complex, with multiple extracellular current sources distributed along the length of the dendrite. However, at the macroscopic level, when the electrical potential pattern is considered at a distance from the cell, most of this complexity has little effect in determining how the electrical potential changes with distance.[8] Specifically, the potential behaves as if it were produced by current flow between two poles. This "dipole approximation" applies at all points located at distances greater than a few lengths of the dendrite. An important feature of the dipole approximation is that it can be accurately applied to the potential pattern generated by focal populations of neurons, such as those that make up a cortical column. That is, the potential pattern generated by complex activation of the thousands of neurons that comprise a cortical column is, at a measuring distance of a centimeter or more, mostly dipolar.

For a dipole, the potential that it produces in a homogeneous surrounding medium decreases as the inverse square of the distance. For example, if the potential is 16 microvolts (μV) at 1 cm, it is 1 μV at 4 cm. If recording electrodes are located 1 and 4 cm from the source, the potential difference between these is thus 15 μV (Fig. 8-4). The electrical potential difference recorded between two electrodes reflects weighted contributions from all current sources within the medium, so strong activity at a distance can be somewhat influential.

Currents associated with individual action potentials are generally much stronger than synaptic currents, but postsynaptic potentials generally make the more significant contribution to the EEG.[11] Several factors contribute to this situation. First, the spatial extent of an action potential is quite small. A depolarization front is associated with intracellular current flow away from the soma, and a repolarization front is associated with intracellular current flow oriented toward the soma (Fig. 8-5). At a distance, the electrical potential generated by these two current components mostly cancel each other. Whereas synchronous activation of the dendrites of cells composing a restricted cortical sheet is common, the timing of action potentials is such that there is generally little synchrony across nearby axons. Although an individual action current may produce a significant potential at a distance, the net potential change generated by multiple action potentials across a population of axons is small.

Glial cells show neither action potentials nor synaptic potentials, but the transmembrane potential of glial cells has been shown to be highly dependent on the potassium content of the local extracellular media—potassium content that is greatly altered

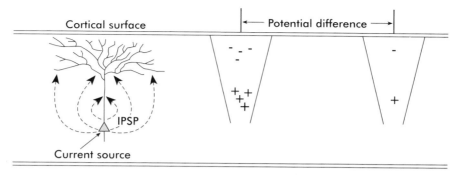

Fig. 8-4. The surface potential established by intracranial neural activity decreases with distance from the source. For dipolar sources, the potential falls as a function of the square of the distance. EEG measures potential differences between two recording sites.

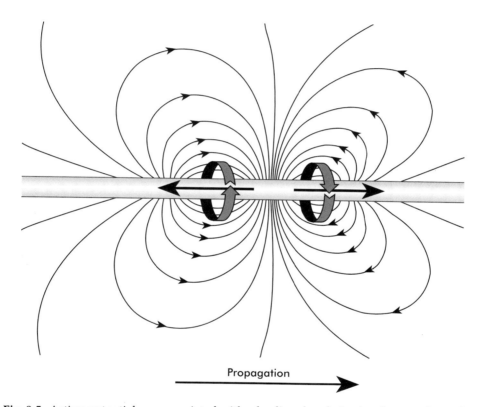

Fig. 8-5. Action potentials are associated with a leading depolarization front and a trailing repolarization front. The associated current configuration is quadrupolar, and at a distance, the electrical field generated by each of the opposing current components mostly cancel each other.

by neighboring neuronal activity.[12] If extracellular changes in potassium concentration occur at a relatively restricted location, potential gradients that give rise to intracellular and extracellular current flow may build up along the glial cell. These give rise to field potentials similar to those described for synaptic currents.

In his classic 1947 paper in the *Journal of Cellular and Comparative Physiology,* Lorente de No[13] described individual cell types (and cell ensembles) that

have open-field versus closed-field configurations (Fig. 8-6). The difference between these two categories relates to production of potential variations in the extracellular media outside of the dendritic extent of the cells. Open-field cells produce a varying potential in the media outside of the dendritic field, whereas closed-field cells do not. Closed-field cells and closed-field cell ensembles are electrically isotropic with symmetric dendritic morphology. Thus, at a distance, the potential effects from symmetric currents cancel.

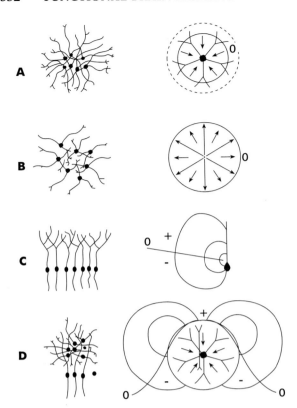

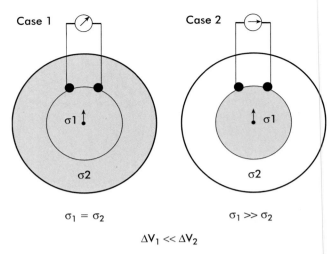

Fig. 8-7. Inhomogeneities in the conductive media cause significant perturbation of the electrical potential pattern. In case 1, the two concentric regions have equivalent conductivities, and the volume can be treated as an infinite homogeneous volume conductor. In case 2, the outer volume has essentially no conductivity, so the inner region must be treated as a bounded spherical volume. When the potential is measured at equivalent points on the surface of volume 1, the potential difference in case 2 is much higher than that in case 1.

Fig. 8-6. Examples of closed, open, and open-closed cell ensembles. **A** and **B** represent cell ensembles from the oculomotor nucleus and superior olive, respectively. Both configurations are closed, with a circular isopotential line (**O**) and current flow confined to within the nucleus. That is, no potential gradient is generated outside of the nucleus. **C** represents neurons from the accessory olive. The parallel array of pyramidal cells gives an open-field configuration, with the arrangement of sources and sinks permitting the spread of current throughout the extracellular media. **D** shows a combination of the above arrangements. (Modified from Lorente de No, 1947, and Hubbard et al, 1969; from Lopes da Silva F, Van Rotterdam A: Biophysical aspects of EEG and magnetoencephalogram generation. In Niedermeyer E, and Lopes da Silva F, editors: Electroencephalography—basic principles, clinical applications and related fields, ed 2, Baltimore, 1987, Urban and Schwarzenberg, p 30.)

The open-field configuration is anisotropic and produces significant potential variation throughout a conductive medium.

The specification of the potential pattern that a particular current configuration generates within a homogeneous conductive medium is relatively straightforward, as given by Maxwell's equations. However, the human head is not a homogeneous volume. There are local inhomogeneities within the brain and significant conductivity barriers between the brain, cerebrospinal fluid (CSF), skull, scalp, and air. Current flows along the path of least resistance, so these conductivity barriers can cause significant distortions in current pathways and the associated potential pattern. Consider a simple situation of two spherically concentric regions (Fig. 8-7). In case 1, imagine the two regions to have equal conductivities so that the overall media can be treated as homogeneous. In case 2, imagine the outermost region to be air, which has essentially no electrical conductivity, so all currents are restricted to the inner volume. If a dipole source is embedded within the innermost volume, and if the electrical potential difference is recorded between points at the inner surface of the outer volume, very different data are obtained from the two situations. In particular, the potential difference recorded in the inhomogeneous case is larger than that recorded in the homogeneous case. The extent to which the potential is larger depends on the position of the generative dipole. In some cases the difference may be as much as 300% as it is for a radially oriented dipole located at the center of the inner volume.[14]

Depending on the type of analysis being applied to a particular data set, detailed knowledge of the shape and electrical conductivity properties of the brain, skull, and scalp can be critical. For example, if analysis is simply focusing on the reactivity of the alpha rhythm, these issues are of minimal import. In contrast, if the goal of a study is to localize the spatial position of sensorimotor cortex, this information can be essential.

Recording Techniques

Noninvasive recording of neuroelectric activity is done by placing electrodes on the scalp surface. These

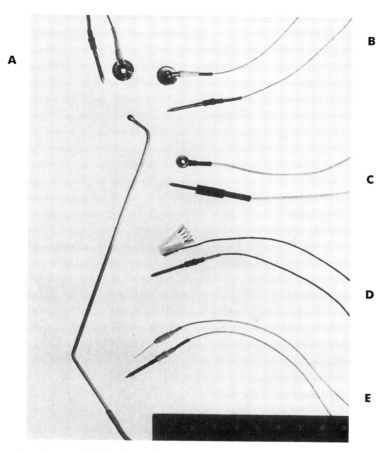

Fig. 8-8. Various types of EEG electrodes, shown with their connector plugs and part of their lead wire. **A**, Large metal cup electrode with central hole; **B**, large metal cup electrode without hole; **C**, small metal cup electrode with central hole; **D**, clip electrode (for ears); **E**, needle electrode; **F**, nasopharyngeal electrode. (From Fisch BJ: Spehlmann's EEG primer, ed 2, Amsterdam, 1991, Elsevier, p 22.)

electrodes usually are small metal disks or cups, although needle electrodes and other types are used occasionally (Fig. 8-8). A key factor in neuroelectric experiments is achieving good mechanical and electrical contact between the electrode and the scalp. The skin at the application site is typically abraded with an electrolytic gel. This removes upper layers of dead skin and allows for better electrical contact. The electrodes are coated with a conductive paste and applied to the scalp. An adhesive, suction, or pressure from caps or headbands is typically used to keep the electrodes in place.

Some care is needed in the selection of electrodes and conductive gels. Metals discharge positive ions into solution when they come into contact with electrolytic gels. Some of these discharged ions adhere closely to the electrode surface, a situation that causes an adjacent layer of oppositely charged ions to form. Therefore, an electrical double layer is formed.[15] However, the rates at which positive ions are discharged and the negative ion layer forms are often different, depending on the exact nature of the

electrode and the electrolyte. This results in an electrode half-cell potential, which can impede current flow from the scalp to the electrode. Real problems can arise if different metals are used for different scalp electrodes because different metals show different half-cell potentials. As a result, potential differences unrelated to neural activity may arise between electrodes. Although this is only a very significant problem in those rare situations when one is interested in especially low frequency and direct-current (DC) activity, it is generally best to use electrode/electrolyte combinations that result in minimal electrode polarization and small bias-potentials.

For standard clinical studies, electrode/scalp impedances should be maintained at less than 5000 ohms. The actual critical factors are the relative impedance of electrodes and the input resistance of the amplifiers to be used, not the absolute value of the electrode impedance. With the newest generation of very sensitive high-impedance (100 mega-ohm) amplifiers, good-quality recordings can be attained even with electrode impedances of 20,000 ohms.

International (10-20) Electrode Placement

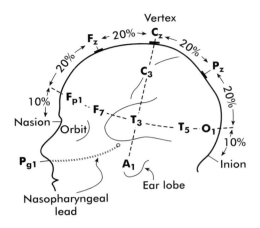

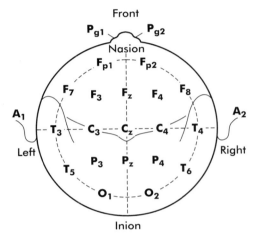

Fig. 8-9. Electrode locations in the international 10-20 system developed by Jasper. (Diagram courtesy of Grass Instruments Co, Quincy, Mass.)

Neuroelectric signals are recorded as potential differences between electrodes. The recorded signal therefore depends intimately on the positions of the individual electrodes and how they are paired. Most laboratories performing routine clinical evaluations use the international 10-20 system of electrode placement.[16] This system is based on 10% to 20% proportional distances between anatomic landmarks on the skull and head, with the proportional strategy providing for some standardization across head size. There are four critical landmarks: (1) the nasion, located at the bridge of the nose immediately beneath the forehead; (2) the inion, a bony protrusion located in the middle of the back of the head; and (3 and 4) the left and right preauricular points located at the depression of the bone in front of each ear canal. The standard recording array for adults consists of 21 electrodes plus a ground electrode (Fig. 8-9). Each electrode is given a letter name related to the general underlying cortical region (Fp, frontopolar; F, frontal; C, central; T, temporal; O, occipital; A, auricular) and

a subscript reflecting its position relative to the midline. Odd-numbered electrodes are over the left hemisphere, with even-numbered sites over the right. Additional electrodes are often added to obtain more fine-grain recordings over a region of particular interest.

Neuroelectric signals are always measured as the potential difference between two recording sites. Thus, the leads from each of two electrodes forming a recording pair are connected to opposite inputs of a differential amplifier. There are two common types of recording strategy: (1) referential/monopolar and (2) bipolar. In the *referential strategy*, potential differences are determined with respect to a single common electrode. This type of recording strategy is sometimes called "monopolar" (a misnomer). The major advantage of using a common reference is that this allows valid comparisons to be made with respect to the amplitude of the signal recorded in the different electrode-pair derivations. When using a referential montage, inferences on the location of the neuronal generators of signal components are based on amplitude differences. Specifically, the source is presumed to be nearest the electrode with the largest signal. However, the spatial pattern of the electrical field generated by an active patch of neurons depends on both the spatial location of the activity and the direction of the relevant current vectors. In some cases, the site of the signal maxima can be far removed from the actual site of neuronal activity.

The major disadvantage of the referential strategy is that no ideal, truly inactive, reference site exists. Ear electrodes are often used as references, but the electrical field at these sites can be greatly influenced by temporal lobe activity. Consider, for example, a case of right temporal lobe epileptic activity. Even though a T4 electrode may immediately overlie the focus, the signal in a T4-A2 derivation can be less than that in an F8-A2 derivation. Given the previous simple localization rules, this will lead to a mislocalization of the activity. Indeed, the entire spatial pattern of the recorded activity depends dramatically on the reference site.

One strategy for partly compensating for this situation is to use a common average reference. Average reference strategies often give good quality recordings, but they tend to smear spatial patterns, especially for large-amplitude signals. For example, when an average reference strategy is used, significant alpha activity (originating from occipital areas) may be seen at frontal Fp1 and Fp2 leads.

In *bipolar recording montages*, the potential difference between two scalp electrodes is displayed. Electrodes are generally paired in a chain with each successive electrode (except for those at the end) being represented in adjacent pairs. For example, a chain of five electrodes would be paired as follows:

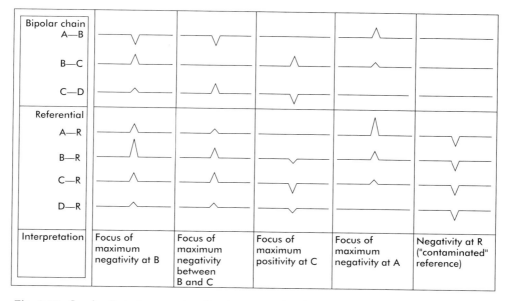

Fig. 8-10. Crude clinical source localization strategies for interpretation of EEG signals. In bipolar montages, the site of phase reversal is associated with the source. In referential montages, the site of signal maxima is associated with the source. (From Duffy FH, Iyer VG, Surwillo WW, Clinical electroencephalography and topographic brain mapping: technology and practice, New York, 1989, Springer-Verlag, p 92.)

1-2, 2-3, 3-4, 4-5. Note that the common electrode in adjacent pairs is connected to opposite sides of a differential amplifier, so the contribution of the common electrode is out of phase across pairs. As a consequence, if one of the common electrodes is located at a voltage maxima, the recorded activity in the two channels to which it contributes shows a polarity inversion. A phase reversal in a bipolar montage is therefore a sensitive indicator of the location of a voltage maxima (Fig. 8-10). To the extent that the dominant current vector for the underlying cortical activity is perpendicular to the skull surface, this provides for excellent localization of the activity. However, if the vector orientation is oblique, the location of the field maxima and minima may be removed from the actual location of the activity. For both monopolar and bipolar montages, care must be used in the application of simple amplitude and phase-reversal strategies of source localization.

SPONTANEOUS NEUROELECTRIC ACTIVITY OF THE NORMAL BRAIN

Given the complexity of the neuronal activities that contribute to scalp-recorded neuroelectric activity, it is somewhat surprising that the normal human EEG, both awake and at rest, is mostly characterized by rhythmic activity that is only occasionally punctated by transient discharges.[1,12,15,17-21] These various rhythms and discharges are distinguished and classified along multiple dimensions, including location, frequency, amplitude, morphology, perodicity, and behavioral/functional correlates. The exact mecha-

nisms responsible for many of the brain's characteristic rhythmic patterns remain somewhat elusive, but several lines of evidence converge to indicate the importance of interactions between cortical regions and supplying subcortical structures (especially the thalamus) in the generation of brain rhythms (Fig. 8-11).

Support for the role of the thalamus in modulation of certain cortical rhythms comes from four experimental findings derived mostly from animal research[22]:

1. Destruction of the thalamus obliterates sleep spindles and spindlelike activity that is induced by barbiturates, whereas lesions below the level of the thalamus have minimal effect on these types of activity.
2. Repetitive stimulation of the nonspecific medial and intralaminar thalamic nuclei produces rhythmic cortical activity that resembles widespread, barbiturate-induced spindle patterns.
3. Stimulation of the sensory-relay nuclei of the thalamus induces rhythmic activity patterns in the associated cortical sensory projection zones.
4. After isolation of the cortex from the thalamus, rhythmic activity persists in thalamic nuclei but is greatly reduced at the cortex.

These observations led to development of the *facultative pacemaker theory*, in which rhythmic activity is postulated as an inherent property of certain intrathalamic and interthalamic circuits that impose rhythmicity on the cortex via specific thalamocortical fibers arising from nonspecific association and specific

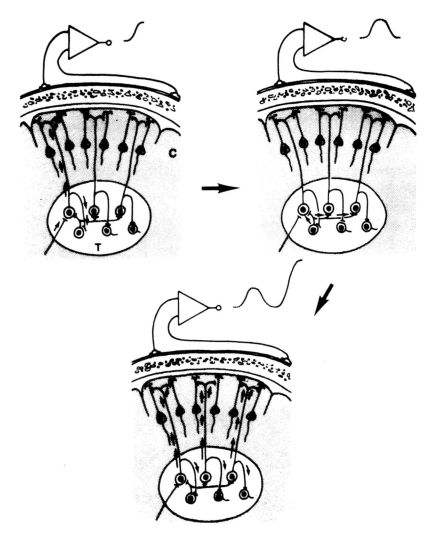

Fig. 8-11. Thalamocortical interactions play an important role in the generation of rhythmic EEG patterns. One model for these interactions is the facultative pacemaker theory, in which thalamocortical relay cells activate both the overlying cortex and the inhibitory interneurons within the thalamus. These interneurons synapse with relay cells and "clamp down" their activity. This, in turn, causes a release from inhibition and gives the thalamocortical cells an oscillatory output. (From Fisch BJ: Spehlmann's EEG primer, ed 2, Amsterdam, 1991, Elsevier, p 12.)

thalamic-relay nuclei.[22] Briefly, according to this theory, thalamocortical relay cells that send their main projection to the cortex also give rise to interthalamic collaterals that synapse with inhibitory thalamic interneurons. These, in turn, inhibit a large pool of relay neurons. When the period of inhibition is over, the disinhibited relay neurons rebound and generate a synchronized excitatory burst that initiates the next periodic cycle of inhibition and rebound.

Although widely accepted, several recent studies have called certain aspects of this theory into question.[21] First, most thalamic relay cells show very limited intrathalamic and interthalamic collateralization, and many of the thalamic nuclei contain very limited populations of inhibitory interneurons. Sec-

ond, cross-correlation studies show that rhythmic activity in one cortical zone is often more highly correlated with activity in other cortical zones than with similar thalamic activity. Corticocortical connections are more abundant than thalamocortical projections, and the emerging picture seems to be that a complex system of thalamocortical and corticocortical interactions are responsible for rhythmicity in the EEG. Thalamic input is critical, but cortical interaction modulate and fine-tune rhythm properties.[12]

Alpha Rhythm

The alpha rhythm (Fig. 8-12), is one of the most prominent normal adult brain rhythms and is identified by its frequency, spatial topography, behavioral

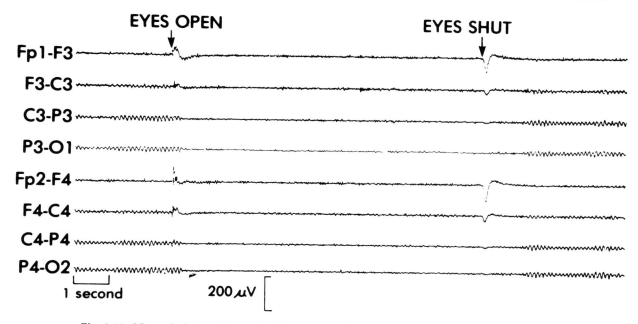

Fig. 8-12. Normal alpha pattern showing maximal activity at posterior leads and reactivity to eye opening. (From Aminoff MJ: Electroencephalography: general principles and clinical applications. In Aminoff MJ, editor: Electrodiagnosis In clinical neurology, ed 2, New York, 1986, Churchill Livingstone, p 27.)

correlates, and reactivity to stimuli.[17-22] The alpha rhythm is fully present only when a subject is mentally inactive, yet alert, with eyes closed. The rhythm is mostly defined by its frequency of 8 to 13 Hz and by its posterior distribution showing high amplitudes at occipital and parietal electrodes (in referential linked-ear montages) (Table 8-1). The alpha rhythm typically has a peak-to-peak amplitude of 20 to 60 μV. Alpha amplitude often waxes and wanes over 1 to 2-second intervals to form spindles or envelopes of activity (Fig. 8-13). The center alpha frequency for a particular individual is generally quite stable (within 0.5 Hz) across recording sessions, and generally little frequency difference exists in the alpha recorded over the two hemispheres.

An important functional characteristic of the alpha rhythm is its disruption by visual attentiveness. Just opening the eyes is generally sufficient to cause alpha blocking, which is a significant decrease in the signal versus an eyes-closed state (often by more than a factor of two). In most right-handed individuals, the alpha rhythm on the left is somewhat lower in magnitude (25%) than that on the right. This is suspected to reflect left hemispheric dominance for motor and language functions in these individuals.[18]

The frequency of the alpha rhythm shows certain developmental trends.[21,23,24] In small children, lower-frequency theta activity (4 to 7 Hz) tends to dominate, but by age 8 years, the alpha rhythm becomes dominant. In the progression to adulthood, the dominant alpha frequency often increases by a couple of cycles per second (e.g., from 8 to 10 Hz). With advancing age beyond 65, a decrease in alpha frequency can occur, although in healthy aged persons, the mean alpha frequency generally remains above 8 Hz, even at age 100.

Mu Rhythm

The alpha rhythm is not the only rhythm in the 8 to 13 Hz band. Mu is a 7 to 11 Hz rhythm seen in 10% to 20% of EEG recordings.[17-21] It is distinguished from alpha by its spatial topography showing maximal amplitude at central rather than occipital locations and by its lack of reactivity to opening and closing the eyes (Fig. 8-14). In contrast to alpha, mu shows blocking before movement of the contralateral hand.

Beta Activity

Beta activity is defined mostly by its frequency characteristics, that is, activity faster than 13 Hz (Table 8-1). Very fast activity around 40 Hz is often referred to as *gamma activity*. Beta activity is smaller in magnitude than alpha (1 to 10 μV). Beta topography is quite variable, although three dominant distributions have been described.[21,25]

A frontal beta rhythm is the most prominent type. It involves central-frontal leads, and this form of the rhythm is believed to be produced mostly by sensorimotor regions of the brain. As with mu rhythm, beta is often blocked by movement, intention to move, and tactile stimulation. A widespread beta rhythm can often be recorded simultaneously over most areas of

Table 8-1. Type of waves and rhythms in the human electroencephalogram and their approximate and relative specifications and distributions, including condition, when present and whether normal

Type of wave or rhythm	Frequency per second (range, Hz)	Amplitude or voltage (μV)	Region of prominence or maximum	Condition when present	Normal or abnormal
Alpha	8-13	5-100	Occipital and parietal	Awake, relaxed, eyes closed	Normal
Beta	18-30	2-20	Precentral and frontal	Awake, no movement	Normal
Gamma	30-50	2-10	Precentral and frontal	Awake	Normal, sleep deprived
Delta	0.5-4.0	20-200	Variable	Asleep	Normal
	0.5-4.0	20-400	Variable	Awake	Abnormal
Theta	4-7	5-100	Frontal and temporal	Awake, affective or stress	Normal (?), abnormal
Kappa	8-12	5-40	Anterior and temporal	Awake, problem solving (?)	Normal
Lambda	Positive-negative spike or sharp waves	5-100	Parietooccipital	Visual stimulation or eye opening	Normal (?)
K-complex	Positive sharp wave and other slow positive-negative waves	20-50	Vertex	Awake, auditory stimulation	Normal (?)
		50-100	Vertex	Asleep, variable stimulation	Normal
Sleep spindles	12-14	5-100	Precentral	Sleep onset	Normal

From Lindsley DB (unpublished data). In Thompson RF, Patterson MM: Bioelectric recording techniques Part B: electroencephalography and human brain potentials, New York, 1974, Academic Press, p 26.

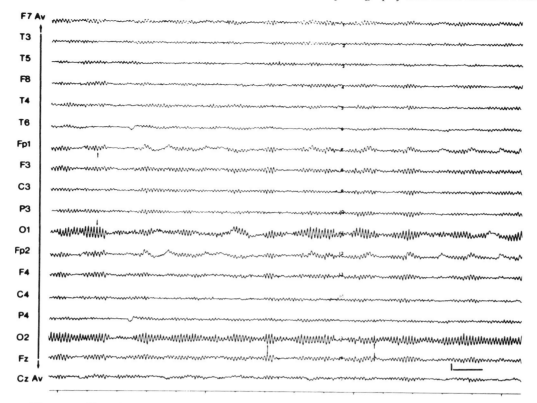

Fig. 8-13. The alpha rhythm is often characterized by periodic high-amplitude bursts known as *spindles*. These data were collected using an averaged reference montage that causes a smearing of the spatial topography of the rhythm. Note the activity at frontal electrodes, a consequence of the reference strategy, not the presence of alpha generators in frontal regions. (From Duffy FH, Iyer VG, Surwillo WW: Clinical electroencephalography and topographic brain mapping: technology and practice, New York, 1989, Springer-Verlag, p 102.)

the head, although it may be masked by other rhythms. This type of beta activity is often unreactive to any stimuli. A posterior beta rhythm, intermixed or alternating with alpha, is also common. This rhythm, as with alpha, often shows reactivity to eye opening.

Beta activity is generally symmetric between the hemispheres, and excessive asymmetry can be a sign of focal pathology. It is noteworthy that beta activity can be greatly influenced by pharmacologic agents (Fig. 8-15), especially benzodiazepines and barbiturates, both of which cause accentuation of the rhythm.[26]

Theta Rhythm

Although common in recordings from children, theta rhythm (4 to 7 Hz) is rare in the EEG of awake adults.[17-21] When present in awake normal adults, theta is most common over frontal and temporal regions. Focal or lateralized theta is often an indication of focal pathology, whereas diffuse theta is associated with a variety of generalized neurologic syndromes. Theta is a normal finding in the EEG of the drowsy transitions between awake and sleeping states, so it is imperative that the EEG always be interpreted within the behavioral context in which the recordings were

obtained. During drowsiness, alpha activity dissipates, and medium-amplitude (10 to 50 μV) theta activity may become prominent (Fig. 8-16). Increased beta activity and the appearance of beta spindles are other common features of the normal drowsy state.

Delta Activity

EEG activity less than 4 Hz is referred to as delta activity (Fig. 8-17). Delta is the dominant rhythm of the EEG in infants and is prevalent in deep stages of adult sleep. Prominent delta activity in the EEG of an awake adult is a significantly abnormal finding.[17-21] Polymorphic delta activity has been associated with several neurologic abnormalities, especially those involving metabolic anomalies and deafferentation of cortical areas. As outlined in subsequent sections, the activity may be diffuse or quite focal, depending on the nature of the pathology.

EEG of Sleep

As already mentioned, significant EEG changes occur during drowsiness and subsequent transitions through the stages of sleep.[17-21] In stage I sleep, the transition from the awake to drowsy state, the alpha

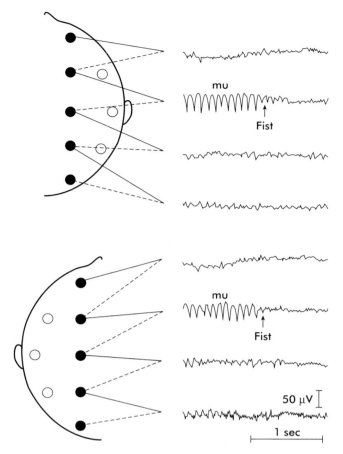

Fig. 8-14. When present, the mu rhtyhm is maximal in a central-frontal derivation. It is unreactive to eye opening and closing but highly reactive to movements, such as making a fist. (Modified from Fisch BJ: Spehlmann's EEG primer, ed 2, Amsterdam, 1991, Elsevier, p 220.)

rhythm disappears and medium-amplitude theta activity becomes dominant (Fig. 8-18). Periods of drowsiness may alternate with periods of wakefulness characterized by a return of alpha activity.

As one drifts into stage II sleep, several changes occur in the EEG (Fig. 8-19). The most prominent of these is the emergence of large-amplitude (75 + μV), bilaterally synchronous, and symmetric vertex waves at Cz, C3, and C4 electrodes. The exact morphology of vertex waves can be quite variable, ranging from sharp wave to spikelike configurations, so they are most clearly defined in terms of the previously mentioned spatial topography (Fig. 8-20). Frontal waves, with similar morphology to vertex waves but with a frontal midline distribution, may also occur. K-complexes are another prominent feature of stage II sleep. As in vertex waves, these are maximal at Cz, but they are larger in amplitude (often several hundred μV). K-complexes are typically diphasic, and they may last as long as 1 second. Sleep spindles are another stage II feature. Spindles are 1-second long bursts of 11 to 15 Hz activity with a wide distribution. They are often

preceded by vertex waves or K-complexes. Positive occipital sharp transients (POSTs) are, as the name suggests, positive occipital sharp waves that occur singly or in bursts during stage II sleep.

Stage III and stage IV sleep (Fig. 8-21), often referred to as *slow wave sleep*, are dominated by theta and delta activities. In stage III, large-amplitude (100 + μV) delta activity makes up more than 20% of the record. Irregular and semirhythmic theta activity is also prominent, with sleep spindles occurring only rarely. Stage IV is dominated by very-large-amplitude delta activity (300 + μV). The EEG during REM sleep has a very different EEG pattern that is most similar to an awake, eyes-open EEG dominated by relatively low-amplitude diffuse beta activity.

PATHOPHYSIOLOGIC SPONTANEOUS BRAIN ACTIVITY

Three major classes of EEG abnormalities are associated with cerebral dysfunction[17-21]: (1) nonparoxysmal abnormalities, (2) nonspecific paroxysmal activities, and (3) specific paroxysmal and epileptiform activities. *Nonparoxysmal abnormalities* refer to alterations, disruptions, or absence of normal spontaneous rhythms and the occurrence of intermittent focal or diffuse polymorphic discharges. *Paroxysmal abnormalities* are characterized by an abrupt onset and a subsequent cessation of a repetitive, rhythmic pattern of sharp or slow wave transients. *Epileptiform abnormalities* typically display paroxysmal characteristics and are identified by the morphology of the associated rhythmic events that have spike or spike and wave characteristics (Fig. 8-22).

Because the EEG is generally recorded for only a brief period (the recording time of a typical clinical EEG is less than 1 hour) and because the EEG only reflects synchronous activities of a restricted portion of the brain, a lack of abnormal slow wave or epileptiform activity does not necessarily mean that all is functioning well. In contrast, when such activities are present, they frequently reflect significant pathology.

Alterations in the frequency and/or symmetry of intrinsic patterns are often a sign of brain pathology. Frequency investigations are generally limited to specification of alpha frequency because this can generally be determined with a fair amount of precision. Recall that the alpha rhythm is defined by its behavioral reactivity (maximal in eyes closed but alert state), topography (maximal at occipital sites), and characteristic frequency (8 to 13 Hz). Alpha activity with appropriate reactivity and topography, but a center frequency less than 8 Hz is considered abnormal for adults (slow alpha is distinguished from theta by its reactivity and topology). Slowing of this type is considered a nonspecific abnormality and may be seen in a variety of metabolic, toxic, and infectious

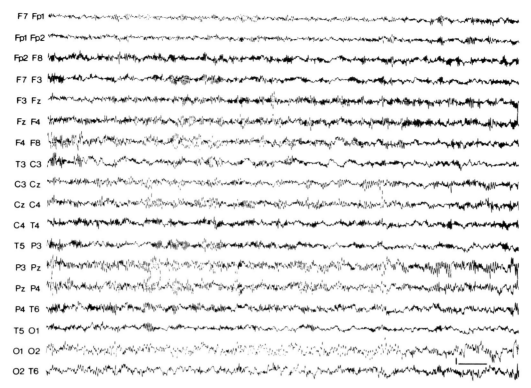

Fig. 8-15. Certain drugs cause significant changes in the EEG. For example, phenobarbital, given for the control of generalized seizures, often induces excessive diffuse beta activity in the EEG, as illustrated in this data set from a 5-year-old child. (From Duffy FH, Iyer VG, Surwillo WW: Clinical electroencephalography and topographic brain mapping: technology and practice, New York, 1989, Springer-Verlag, p 139.)

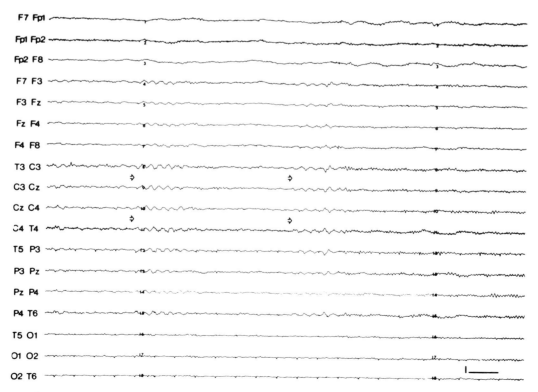

Fig. 8-16. Medium-amplitude theta and delta activity occurs in drowsiness. (From Duffy FH, Iyer VG, Surwillo WW: Clinical electroencephalography and topographic brain mapping: technology and practice, New York, 1989, Springer-Verlag, p 11.)

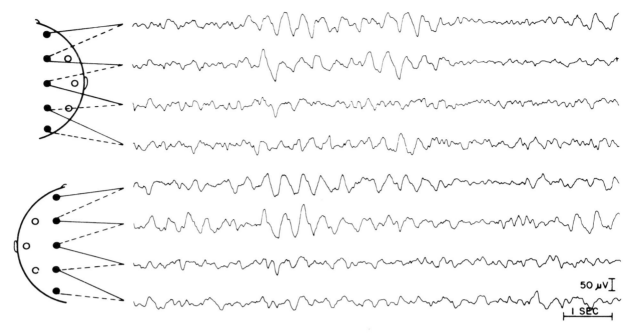

Fig. 8-17. Delta activity, when present in records from awake adults, is a sign of pathophysiology. This data set, derived from a patient with a severe head injury, shows frontal intermittent rhythmic delta activity. (From Fisch BJ: Spehlmann's EEG primer, ed 2, Amsterdam, 1991, Elsevier, p 442.)

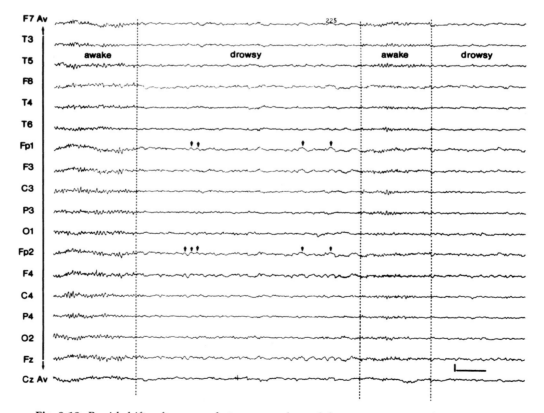

Fig. 8-18. Rapid shifts often occur between awake and drowsy states near sleep onset. The awake EEG is marked by alpha, whereas the drowsy EEG shows theta and delta activity. (From Duffy FH, Iyer VG, Surwillo WW: Clinical electroencephalography and topographic brain mapping: technology and practice, New York, 1989, Springer-Verlag, p 112.)

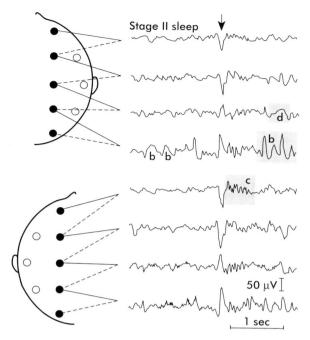

Fig. 8-19. Stage II sleep shows several characteristic features, including vertex waves *(arrow) (b)*, sleep spindles *(c)*, and 2 to 7 Hz slow waves *(d)*. (Modified from Fisch BJ: Spehlmann's EEG primer, ed 2, Amsterdam, 1991, Elsevier, p 232.)

conditions.[17-21] Asymmetries in alpha frequency (greater than 1.5 Hz) or amplitude (greater than 50%) are considered abnormal and are often indicative of a unilateral lesion, although the lesion is not necessarily in the occipital region. Unilateral loss of alpha reactivity to eye opening and closing is a significant finding, usually indicative of a lesion in the occipital lobe. A complete loss of alpha reactivity may be a sign of a brainstem lesion.

Abnormal nonparoxysmal activity is a common finding in several neurologic disorders. This activity generally takes the form of polymorphic delta or other rhythmic slow waves. Polymorphic delta is composed of 0.5 to 3.0 Hz waves in random sequential combinations, whereas rhythmic slowing is characterized by repetitive occurrence of activity at a particular wavelength. The amplitude of slow activity ranges from 10 μV to more than 500 μV. The more irregular, slower, and larger the activity, the greater is the underlying pathology. Polymorphic delta is usually associated with severe, acute, or ongoing injury to cortical neurons, such as may result from cerebrovascular accident (CVA, stroke) or a variety of other structural or metabolic disruptions of brain integrity.[17-21] More rhythmic discharges are thought to usually reflect physiologic dysfunction at a site distant from (but

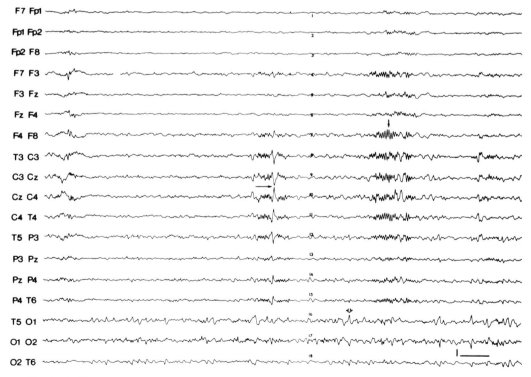

Fig. 8-20. Vertex waves *(horizontal arrow)* are one of the dominant features of stage II sleep. (From Duffy FH, Iyer VG, Surwillo WW: Clinical electroencephalography and topographic brain mapping: technology and practice, New York, 1989, Springer-Verlag, p 112.)

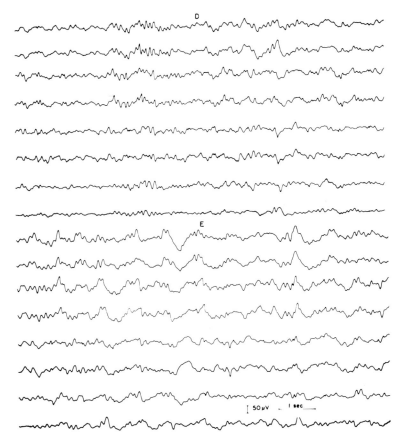

Fig. 8-21. Stage III and stage IV sleep (*D* and *E*) are characterized by large-amplitude theta and delta activities. (From Kooi KA, Tucker RP, Marshall RE: Fundamentals of electroencephalography, ed 2, New York, 1978, Harper and Row, p 53.)

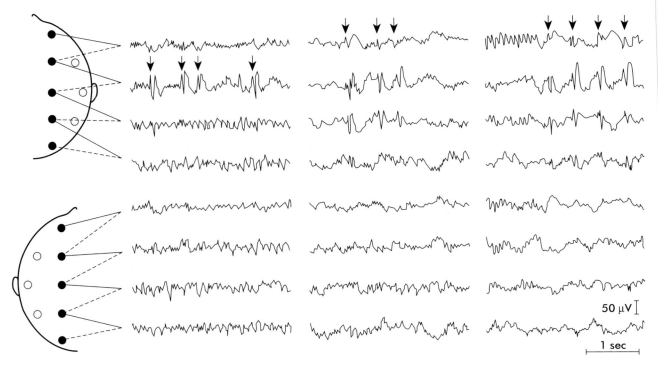

Fig. 8-22. Spike wave complexes are a common feature of the interictal EEG of patients with seizure disorders. (Modified from Fisch BJ: Spehlmann's EEG primer, ed 2, Amsterdam, 1991, Elsevier, p 320.)

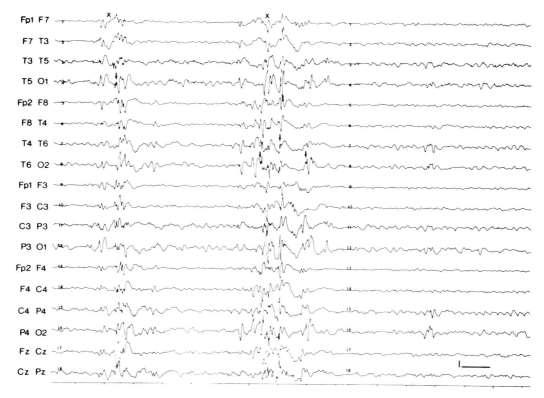

Fig. 8-23. Multiple spikes and sharp wave complexes punctate this record from a 3-year-old child with recurrent tonic-clonic and myoclonic seizures. (From Duffy FH, Iyer VG, Surwillo WW: Clinical electroencephalography and topographic brain mapping: technology and practice, New York, 1989, Springer-Verlag, p 166.)

connected to) the region of primary pathology. For example, monorhythmic frontal delta activity is a common finding in many cerebral pathologic states, including those that have only indirect effects on the frontal lobes. Subcortical damage can also cause rhythmic slowing.

Nonspecific paroxysmal discharges are a series of discharges appearing and disappearing abruptly and having a different frequency, morphology, or amplitude than that demonstrated in the background EEG. Bursts of high-voltage (greater than 100 μV) slow waves is the most common EEG sign of cerebral dysfunction. Paroxysmal slowing is found in a variety of neurologic conditions, ranging from cerebrovascular disorders to epilepsy to Alzheimer's dementia. The exact generative mechanisms remain unclear, but ischemia and deafferentation are known causes.

EEG, in combination with behavioral sequelae, is the defining diagnostic tool for epilepsy. An epileptic seizure is defined as a sudden disturbance in consciousness, mental functions, or motor, sensory, or autonomic activity caused by abnormal discharges by a population of brain cells.[27] Seizures typically last only a few minutes and may be generalized, involving most of the brain, or quite focal, involving only a small brain area. Because epileptic attacks occur relatively

infrequently, seizure (ictal) activity rarely is recorded during a routine EEG. In some patients, certain activating procedures, including hyperventilation, photic stimulation, or pharmacologic manipulations, may be used to precipitate a seizure. Many seizure patients undergo long-term (several days) continuous video EEG monitoring for the purpose of recording spontaneous seizures. Unfortunately, in some patients, muscle and movement artifacts may be so obscuring during a seizure that relatively little information is obtained. On the other hand, many epileptic patients have an abnormal interictal EEG that can be instrumental in diagnosis.

Two specific paroxysmal discharges are associated with the ictal and interictal EEG of epileptic patients: spikes and sharp waves (Fig. 8-23). Spikes are deflections of less than 70 msec that may be multiphasic. The surface negative phase (ear reference) usually, but not always, dominates the event. Sharp waves are similar to spikes but of longer duration (80+ msec). Spikes and sharp waves may occur sequentially or in an independent manner. Sharp waves tend to have a more widespread distribution and in some cases reflect a discharge secondary to a primary spike discharge. Spikes are often followed by sharp waves or slow wave events.

EEG: focal motor seizure, left arm and hand

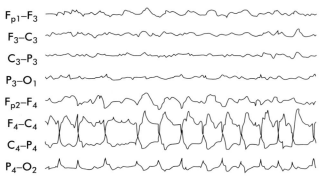

Repetitive sharp waves over right central region

Fig. 8-24. Simple partial seizures show focal discharge patterns. In this case of motor seizures involving the left upper extremities, EEG signs are maximal over the right central region. (From Netter FH: The CIBA collection of medical illustrations. Nervous system. Part II, New Jersey, 1986, CIBA, p 45).

Epilepsy

The most widely used classification scheme for epileptic disorders is that devised by the Commission on Classification and Terminology of the International League Against Epilepsy.[28] There are two main categories of seizures: partial and generalized. They are defined by specific relationships between behavior and EEG activity. Also, an additional category of unclassified epileptic seizures includes certain types of neonatal seizures that are poorly understood.

The defining characteristic of a *partial seizure* is that the first clinical and EEG signs of the seizure indicate initial involvement of a focal neuronal population, although generalization can be quite rapid. If consciousness is not impaired during the seizure, the seizure is classified as simple partial. In contrast, complex partial seizures involve a definitive impairment of consciousness.

Simple partial seizures may manifest with motor, sensory, autonomic, and psychic symptoms. Any portion of the body may be involved in a focal motor seizure, depending on the site of origin in the motor strip. Sometimes the seizure activity spreads to produce sequential body movements.

Somatosensory seizures generally arise from the postcentral gyrus and are characterized by tingling, pins-and-needle sensations, or numbness. Other types of sensory seizures manifest with visual, auditory, olfactory, gustatory, or vertiginous sensations. The complexity of manifestations in visual and auditory seizures is quite variable. For example, visual seizures can be associated with anything from simple light flashes to complex visual hallucinations. Autonomic seizures may manifest in any of several ways, including vomiting, sweating, and incontinence.

Psychic disturbances of higher cognitive functions are most frequently associated with complex partial seizures involving the temporal lobes, but they occasionally occur without a true disruption of consciousness. Common manifestations include dysphasia, déjà-vu sensations, disturbances of cognitive state, illusions, and emotive/affective changes.

Electrographically, simple partial seizures manifest as paroxysmal (bursting) patterns of spikes and sharp waves over contralateral regions associated with the impaired functions (Fig. 8-24). Abnormal neuroelectric activity is not always recordable at the scalp, especially for autonomic-type seizures. The interictal EEG is often characterized by localized epileptiform discharges.

Complex partial seizures may begin with simple symptomatology or may manifest with disruption of consciousness at the onset. Automatisms (repetitive movements such as chewing, lip smacking, and scratching that seem purposeful in themselves but are inappropriate in the actual situation) are a common finding. The interictal EEG is characterized by unilateral or bilateral asynchronous discharges, usually in temporal or frontal regions. Partial complex seizures often show rapid generalization with tonic-clonic features.

Generalized seizures may be either convulsive or nonconvulsive. There are five main types: (1) absence, (2) myoclonic, (3) clonic, (4) tonic, and (5) tonic-clonic. One of the most common types of nonconvulsive seizures is the *petit mal absence seizure*. This is more common in children than adults and is characterized by an impairment of consciousness without a loss of muscle tone or posture. Clinical manifestations include momentary apparent inattentiveness, an empty stare, and/or interruption of speech and movement. Automatisms and clonic 3 Hz movements are common. The interictal EEG is often normal, with occasional runs of paroxysmal spikes or spike and wave complexes. The ictal EEG is generally characterized by continuous, 3 Hz spike and slow wave complexes bilaterally, maximal at frontocentral locations (Fig. 8-25). Atypical absence seizures generally show a more heterogeneous EEG pattern both ictally and interictally.

Myoclonic seizures are another type of generalized seizure. These are characterized by myoclonic jerks involving mainly flexor muscles on both sides of the body. The massive contractions may occur at either regular or irregular intervals. Both the ictal and the interictal EEG are characterized by polyspike and wave activity or spike and wave or sharp and slow wave activity.

Clonic seizures consist of rhythmic myoclonic movement that last a minute or more. Febrile seizures in childhood often manifest with clonic charateristics.

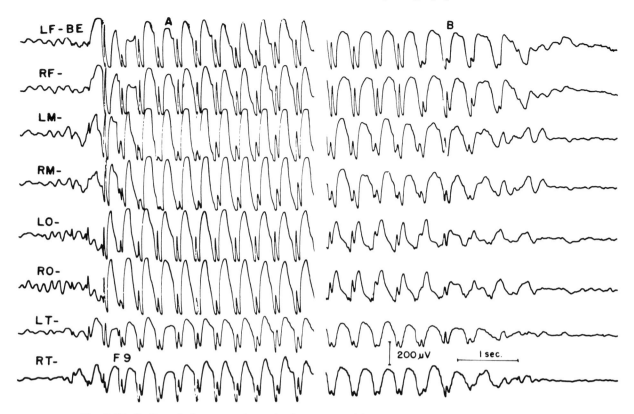

Fig. 8-25. Petit mal absence seizure is characterized by generalized 3 Hz spike and wave complexes. (From Kooi KA, Tucker RP, Marshall RE: Fundamentals of electroencephalography, ed 2, New York, 1978, Harper & Row, p 128.)

The interictal EEG often shows diffuse spike and wave discharges. Ictal activity is generally a mixture of both fast activity (greater than 10 Hz) and slow waves, with occasional spike and wave discharges.

Tonic seizures may last up to 1 minute and involve contraction of the axial musculature of the entire body. The interictal EEG shows runs of rhythmic discharges of sharp and slow waves against a mostly normal background. Ictal EEG generally shows low-voltage fast activity or a 9 to 10 Hz rhythm.

Tonic-clonic, or *grand mal, seizures* are the most common form of generalized seizure in adults (Fig. 8-26). Generalized bilaterally synchronous spike discharges or paroxysmal slow wave activity is often observed interictally. Tonic-clonic seizures generally begin suddenly with a loss of consciousness. During the initial tonic phase of the seizure, most of the body's muscles contract intensely. After about 20 seconds, the tonic phase gives way to rhythmic, sometimes violent clonic jerking motions of the entire body. This phase lasts for 30 to 40 seconds and leaves the patient in a deep stupor from which recovery progresses through the stages of sleep to a state of confusion and finally to mental alertness. The earliest change in the ictal EEG is often the appearance of low-voltage fast activity. This slows and increases in amplitude during the tonic

phase. The distribution becomes quite broad, and multiple spike or repetitive sharp wave discharges with a frequency of about 10 Hz may become prominent. In the clonic phase, there is a buildup of rhythmic slow activity with associated spike or polyspike discharges. The seizure is generally followed by a transient period of low-amplitude activity and then irregular polymorphic slowing that may persist for several hours.

Brain Tumors

EEG abnormalities in patients with brain tumors are a very common finding.[17,29] Abnormalities are seen in almost 90% of tumor patients. The probability of a positive finding in a particular patient reflects both the type and the location of the intracranial mass.[29] Focal slowing is the most common finding (Fig. 8-27), although seizure activity and disruption of spontaneous patterns have been reported in 10% to 30% of patients. In general, the most rapidly expanding types of lesions (e.g., abscesses, metastatic carcinomas, glioblastomas) produce the most severe abnormalities and they do so in a higher percentage of patients than do slowly expanding lesions. Supratentorial lesions are more likely to produce abnormalities than extratentorial masses, although when meningiomas cause significant compression of underlying

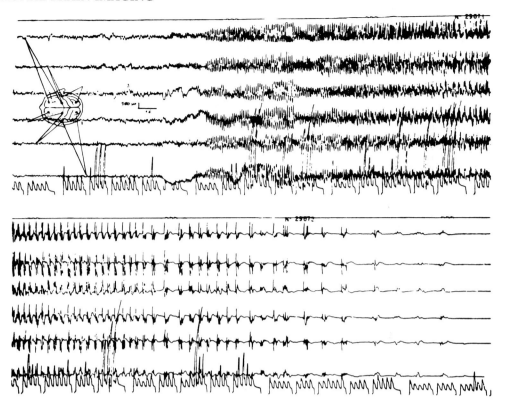

Fig. 8-26. Grand mal, tonic-clonic seizures show fast spiking during tonic phase (*upper tracings*) and repetitive bursts of spikes in the clonic phase (*lower tracings*). (From Gastaut H, Broughton R: Epileptic seizures, Springfield, 1972, Charles C Thomas.)

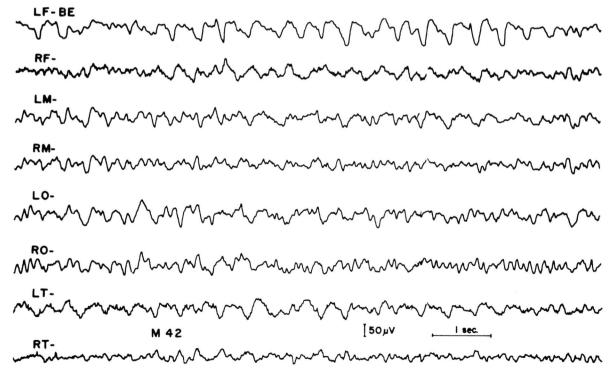

Fig. 8-27. Focal slowing is often associated with brain tumors, as shown in this patient with a deep left parietooccipital glioma. (From Kooi KA, Tucker RP, Marshall RE: Fundamentals of electroencephalography, ed 2, New York, 1978, Harper & Row, p 147.)

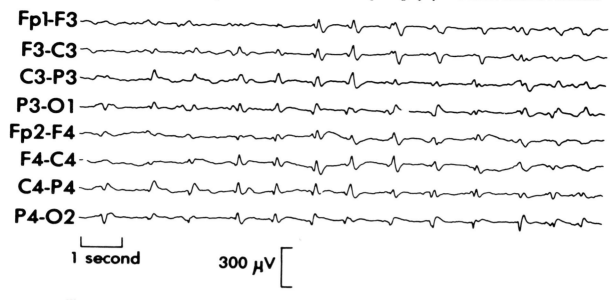

Fig. 8-28. Repetitive triphasic complexes is a characteristic finding of the EEG of patients with progressive Creutzfeldt-Jakob disease. (From Aminoff MJ: Electroencephalography: general principles and clinical applications. In Aminoff MJ, editor: Electrodiagnosis in clinical neurology, ed 2, New York, 1986, Churchill Livingstone, p 50.)

cortical areas, slowing is common. Slowly growing astrocytomas produce abnormalities in only 70% of patients, but along with oligodendrogliomas, they are the most likely type of mass lesion to cause epileptiform spikes and sharp waves.[17] When present, focal EEG slowing provides good data on tumor lateralization and localization. Lateralization is correct in about 90% of patients, with correct, more precise localization achieved in 80%. When multiple regions of focal slowing are detected, the best localizing sign relates to the irregularity of the activity. The less rhythmic the pattern, the more likely it is that active pathology is near the site, regardless of the amplitude of the activity.

Cerebrovascular Disease

Cerebrovascular disease, as with intracranial masses, often causes slowing, although the activity is generally somewhat more diffuse than that seen for neoplasms.[17,30] In patients with thrombosis of major vessels, polymorphic delta waves over the involved hemisphere are a common finding. Bilaterally symmetric, monorhythmic frontal delta activity is also common, as are diminished amplitude and desynchronization of the ipsilateral alpha rhythm. After acute nonhemorrhagic stroke, the EEG may show focal slowing, even when CT examinations are normal.[30] Small lacunar infarction of subcortical regions rarely causes significant EEG changes, whereas large lesions of the thalamus cause local rhythm changes in appropriate projection zones. In patients with mild atherosclerotic disease, the resting EEG is generally normal, but hyperventilation often brings

out lateralized abnormalities. Subdural hematomas have been associated with two differing types of EEG abnormalities. Some patients have a significant decrease in the amplitude of background activity on the side of the hematoma. In contrast, other patients show focal slowing against an otherwise normal amplitude pattern of background activity. The differential clinical significance of these two situations is presently unknown.

Trauma

EEG is often performed in patients with head injury in the hope of providing an index of the severity of the trauma, the likelihood of developing posttraumatic seizures, and the general prognosis for recovery.[17,31] In all these uses, it is important to note that the EEG changes typically associated with trauma (alpha slowing, focal slow waves, epileptiform discharges) are not diagnostically specific, so it is important to rule out nontraumatic etiologies. Furthermore, the correlation between clinical and neuroelectric findings is often poor when the EEG is recorded more than 3 months after the injury, especially in patients with mild trauma.

Coma

EEG is particularly useful in the evaluation of altered states of consciousness, such as those associated with coma, in which examination of EEG reactivity to stimuli provides insight in the depth of coma.[32] In light coma, stimulation results in an attenuation of background rhythms. This reactivity becomes inconsistent as the depth of coma increases.

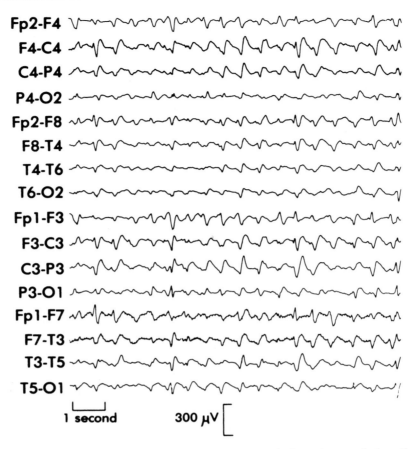

Fp2-F4

F4-C4

C4-P4

P4-O2

Fp2-F8

F8-T4

T4-T6

T6-O2

Fp1-F3

F3-C3

C3-P3

P3-O1

Fp1-F7

F7-T3

T3-T5

T5-O1

1 second   300 μV

Fig. 8-29. Triphasic and slow wave activity are prominent in hepatic encephalopathy. (From Aminoff MJ: Electroencephalography: general principles and clinical applications. In Aminoff MJ, editor: Electrodiagnosis in clinical neurology, ed 2, New York, 1986, Churchill Livingstone, p 64.)

In deep coma, slow wave activity dominates the EEG record, and there is often a paradoxical increase in slow wave activity in response to stimulation. As the depth of coma increases even further, there is a loss of all reactivity, and the amplitude of the EEG diminishes until it becomes flat.

Some comatose patients display an EEG dominated by 8 to 13 Hz activity that is similar to alpha, although generally unresponsive to stimulation. This "alpha coma" is most often associated with brainstem lesions and certain drug intoxications.

Dementias

During the progression to old age, intermittent temporal slowing often increases.[23,24] In senile and presenile dementia, this finding is often exaggerated, along with an increase in generalized slowing.[33] Creutzfeldt-Jacob disease is a rapidly progressing form of dementia with very characteristic EEG patterns (Fig. 8-28). At the onset of the disease, local slow waves may be present. These soon generalize, and the EEG becomes defined by periodic triphasic complexes.[34]

Metabolic Disorders

EEG is sometimes used to monitor cerebral function in patients with metabolic disorders, and in some cases, EEG anomalies become apparent before the appearance of gross clinical deficits. In most patients with metabolic dysfunction, the EEG shows diffuse rather than focal abnormalities, slowing of the alpha rhythm, and the appearance of increased theta and delta activity. Changes of this type have been found in many conditions, including hypoglycemia and hyperglycemia, Addison's disease, and hyperparathyroidism. In the latter case, spike and sharp wave discharges may also be seen. In patients with hepatic encephalopathy, a good correlation exists between clinical and neuroelectric findings. Initially, there is slowing of the alpha rhythm and eventual replacement of alpha dominance by theta and delta activity.[17,35] As the condition progresses, periodic triphasic complexes characterized by a large positive deflection flanked by smaller negative deflections are seen (Fig. 8-29).

EEG can also be useful in the evaluation of the

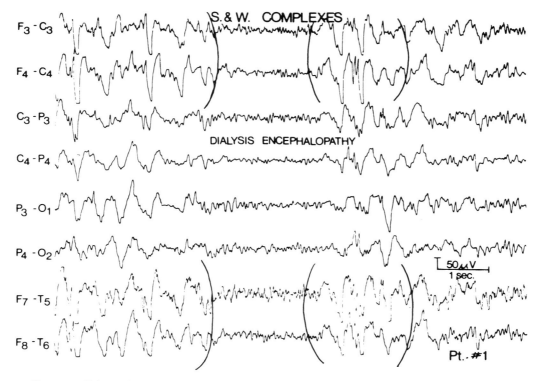

Fig. 8-30. Bilateral spike and wave complexes are seen in patients with encephalopathy from chronic dialysis. These are usually maximal and frontal sites. (From Hughes JR, Schreeder MT: EEG in dialysis encephalopathy, Neurology 30:1148-1154, 1980.)

consequences of renal insufficiency.[36] Initially, the EEG may be normal, but background slowing and the appearance of theta and delta activity are seen as the condition progresses. Triphasic complexes are an occasional finding, as are spike and spike-wave discharges. During hemodialysis, the EEG is characterized by generalized rhythmic delta activity of high voltage.[36] Progressive encephalopathy often occurs during chronic dialysis and is associated with bilaterally synchronous slow, sharp, triphasic, and spike-wave complexes (Fig. 8-30). Several studies have examined the relationship between EEG abnormalities (especially spike and wave discharges) and the presence or likely development of encephalopathy. In one study, such discharges were found in 80% of 26 patients with encephalopathy.[37] In a separate phase of this study, abnormal EEG findings were useful in predicting the presence versus absence of encephalopathy in 91% of 77 dialysis patients studied. Of particular note is the finding that in some cases, EEG abnormalities were seen several months before clinical manifestations of a progressing encephalopathy.

Psychiatric Dysfunction

Conventional EEG, in conjunction with other neuroimaging modalities, is often used in the evaluation of psychiatric patients, mostly for the purpose of ruling out gross neurologic abnormalities. For example,

temporal lobe epilepsy is associated with a number of psychic changes and it is important to distinguish patients who have versus those who do not have epileptogenic psychoses.[2] Even for patients without epileptiform activity, other mild EEG abnormalities usually are present. For example, an abnormal EEG is found in more than 60% of schizophrenic subjects, the most common abnormalities being alpha slowing, increased theta activity, and interestingly, significant asymmetries in spontaneous activity patterns.[38] New techniques involving quantitative EEG and brain electrical activity mapping (BEAM) are often used in the assessment of psychiatric dysfunction and are described in later sections of this chapter.

EVENT-RELATED AND STIMULUS-EVOKED POTENTIALS

Caton, in his early EEG experiments with rabbits, observed clear reactivity to peripherally applied sensory stimuli in the form of a cortical evoked response. Because the skull causes significant attenuation of the cortical electrical signal, neuroelectric signal changes associated with presentation of a stimulus are generally not readily apparent in the ongoing scalp EEG. In 1951, Dawson introduced the notion of signal summation as a means for extracting signal changes time-locked to presentation of a sensory stimulus.[39] Briefly, a sensory stimulus is presented repeatedly,

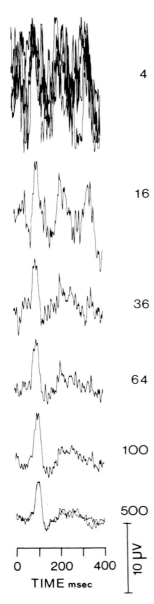

TIME msec

Fig. 8-31. Signal averaging enhances the signal-to-noise ratio in evoked potential experiments, as shown in this case of the auditory-evoked response. An average of as few as 16 trials allows identification of the prominent N100 component. (From Regan D: Human brain electrophysiology, Amsterdam, 1989, Elsevier, p 53.)

with recording epochs spanning the stimulus presentation time summated or, more often, averaged. The magnitude of time-locked signals increases as a direct function of the number of summated epochs, whereas the magnitude of non-time-locked activity increases as the square root of the number of epochs. Thus, the summation process increases the ratio of the time-locked signal to the non-time-locked noise. Consider a simple evoked response associated with presentation of a tone burst of 50 msec in duration. Individual epochs spanning the stimulus show little obvious

reactivity, but an averaging of as few as 16 events reveals the presence of a series of significant time-locked oscillations, the largest of which occurs approximately 100 msec after the stimulus (Fig. 8-31).

Evoked potential strategies represent the most powerful noninvasive neurophysiologic techniques for evaluating the integrity of human sensory processing systems.[40,41] Provided that a stable time point can be specified for signal averaging, the strategy is not limited to sensory applications. For example, movement onset (rather than stimulus presentation) can be used as a time mark for signal averaging to extract event-related activity preceding the movement.[42] Physiologic evidence of cognitive activity can also be extracted when the timing of a cognitive event (e.g., stimulus classification) relative to the time of stimulus presentation is relatively constant.[43]

Stimulus-evoked and event-related neuroelectric recording techniques represent an essential line of research, because only electromagnetic techniques provide the temporal resolution required for identification of the neural correlates of specific stages of information processing. A review of the relevant cognitive neuroscience literature surveying topics as expansive as attention, language, and memory is beyond the scope of this chapter. The interested reader is referred to two excellent reviews.[41,43] The present discussion focuses on direct and specific clinical applications of these techniques, especially in the assessment of basic sensory processing. For each of the three major sensory modalities—somatosensation, vision, and audition—associated evoked responses are characterized by a series of specific positive and negative deflections (recorded in standard referential montages), with the latency and amplitude of particular waveform peaks relatively invariant across normal subjects. That is, abnormal variants are often easily recognized, and in some patients, the specifics of evoked potential abnormalities are useful diagnostically.

Somatosensory Evoked Potentials (SEPs)

The recording of the SEP is now a common part of clinical neurophysiologic examinations, especially in patients with suspected multiple sclerosis (MS) or other conditions in which lesions of the central somatosensory pathways are suspected. In most instances, the activating stimulus is a small electrical current passed between surface electrodes placed above the median nerve at the wrist. The median nerve is a mixed nerve containing both motor efferent and sensory afferent fibers, including type Ia muscle afferents and type II cutaneous afferents. Stimulus pulse durations of a few hundred microseconds are typically used with current levels of 5 to 15 milliamperes. Stimulus magnitude is generally ad-

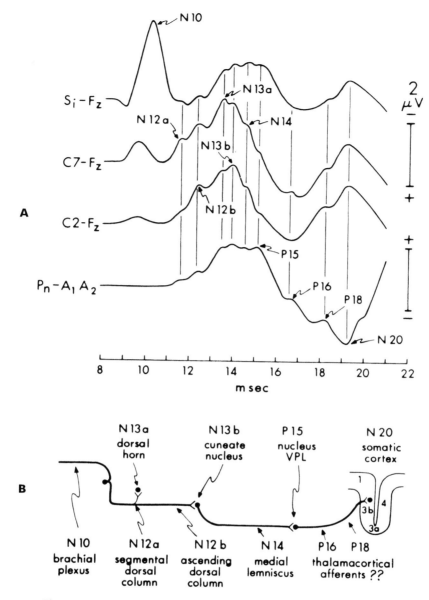

Fig. 8-32. The response evoked by electrical stimulation of the median nerve shows multiple components, many of which are generated below the level of the cerebral cortex. **A** shows waveforms recorded in different electrode derivations. **B** shows how Allison and his colleagues conceptualize the relationship between various waveform components and the somatosensory projection pathway. (From Allison TL: Development and aging changes in human evoked potentials. In Barber C, Blum T, Nodar R, editors: Evoked potentials III, Boston, 1987, Butterworth, pp 72-90.)

justed to produce a just noticeable twitch of the thumb. A stimulus repetition rate of 2 to 5 Hz is typical.

Several different recording strategies have been suggested. Some laboratories advocate the use of a noncephalic reference, but troublesome contamination of recordings from the heartbeat is common in these situations. More standard referential montages involving linked-ears, Cz, or Fz reference sites also are often used. The frequency spectrum of the evoked response is such that the low-pass filter on amplifiers should be set fairly high to avoid attenuation and distortion of various components of the evoked waveform. Faithful reproduction of all components of the median nerve response requires that the cutoff of the low-pass filter be no lower than 1.5 kHz. Multielectrode 10 to 20 arrays are typically employed with the C3/C4 electrode sites of greatest interest.

The scalp response is characterized by multiple components reflecting cortical, subcortical, and spinal cord activity, with different electrode derivations

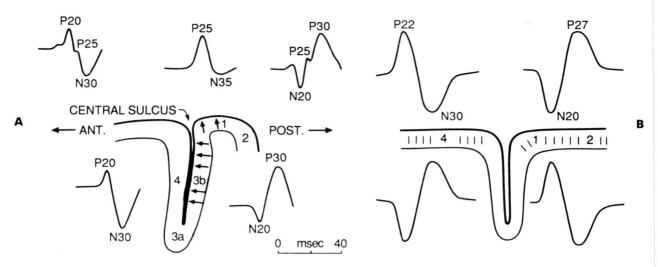

Fig. 8-33. There are two opposing models of the neural generators of the cortical somatosensory evoked potential: **A**, the tangential + radial model, and **B**, the dual radial model. (From Regan D: Human brain electrophysiology, Amsterdam, 1989, Elsevier, p 298.)

emphasizing different components. Fig. 8-32 shows example data for the early components of the waveform along with a putative view of the relationship between waveform components and generator sites.

The neural generators of the short-latency components of the human SEP have been strongly debated.[44,45] Available data on the latency of signals recorded at scalp electrodes over precentral versus postcentral sites indicate that multiple generators are active during the interval from 20 to 30 msec after the stimulus. Two alternative models have been proposed, the tangential + radial model and the dual radial model. The former emphasizes similarities in the timing of activity across electrodes, whereas the latter emphasizes differences. In the first model, activity is confined to the postcentral gyrus. Initially, tangential dipole-like sources in area 3b are active. This is followed by additional activation of radial sources in area 1. In the dual radial model, separate, radially oriented generators in the precentral and postcentral cortex are activated with slightly different time courses (Fig. 8-33). Several lines of recent evidence favor the tangential + radial model. For example, Allison and colleagues report monkey and human data in which removal of the primary motor cortex has no effect on the relevant activity, whereas ablation of the somatosensory cortex completely abolishes the relevant evoked signals.[46] On the other hand, Slimp and colleagues have reported some contradictory data.[47] Perhaps the strongest support for the tangential + radial model comes from the work of Wood and colleagues, who combined neuroelectric recordings with neuromagnetic recordings.[48] Magnetoencepha-

lographic (MEG) data provide unequivocal evidence that a tangential source in area 3b of the postcentral gyrus accounts for the N20-P30 complex (Fig. 8-34).

The resolution of this debate is important with respect to the general approach of attempting to localize generators of EEG and components of evoked potential signals. It is clear from the previously mentioned MEG results that radial sources do not alway underlie electrode sites recording maximal signals. Rather, the actual source may lie between positive and negative potential extrema, under an electrode that records relatively little signal.

SEPs play an important role in the investigation of the peripheral nervous system and the spinal cord. For example, SEPs can provide valuable information on the conduction velocity of distal nerve segments. In many patients, this information can be obtained by routine peripheral nerve conduction velocity studies, but in some, routine methods fail. For example, in patients with Charcot-Marie-Tooth disease, a form of hereditary motor-sensory neuropathy, the scalp SEP elicited by stimulation of the fingers can be recorded even when sensory nerve action potentials cannot be recorded from proximal nerve segments.

The most common use of SEPs is in the assessment of patients with suspected demyelinating diseases such as MS. SEPs can be useful in the identification of multiple lesion sites and can provide objective evidence of dysfunction when clinical findings fail to be definitive. Abnormalities in SEPs are found in about 80% of patients known to have MS. Abnormalities in patients suspected of having MS are more often found with stimulation of the tibial versus median nerve and

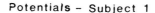

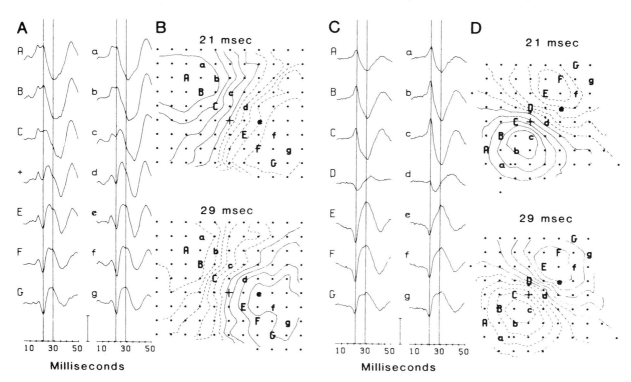

Fig. 8-34. Neuromagnetic data strongly support the tangential + radial hypothesis. There is a clear tangential component rotated 90 degrees from the electrical potential pattern, and results imply a common generator. (From Wood CC, Cohen D, Cuffin BN et al: Electrical sources in human somatosensory cortex: Identified by combined magnetic and potential recordings, Science 227:1051-1053, 1985.)

are apparent in 25% to 35% of patients without clinical signs.[49,50] It is noteworthy that SEPs appear to be more diagnostically sensitive than visual and auditory evoked potentials in this application. Abnormalities take several forms, including latency delays, absence of components, and altered waveform morphologies. Of particular interest is the N13 cervical component of the median nerve response, which is abnormal in approximately 40% of patients with suspected MS.[51] Left-right response asymmetries in terms of latency and amplitude generally provide a better diagnostic sign than absolute values per se.

Another important clinical use of SEPs is intraoperative monitoring of spinal cord surgery when there is significant risk of compromising the cord.[52] An additional neurosurgical use involves recordings of SEPs directly from the cortical surface for the purpose of mapping the location of sensorimotor cortex in patients undergoing resection of pathologic tissue in the vicinity of the frontal-parietal junction.[52]

One final clinical use of SEPs is in the assessment of head trauma and coma. The most noteworthy studies are those of Greenberg and colleagues, who studied multimodal evoked potentials in patients who were comatose subsequent to severe head injuries.[53] These investigators found a close association between the degree of abnormalities in scalp SEPs (recorded in response to median nerve stimulation) and clinical outcome. Furthermore, it was found that SEPs were diagnostically more sensitive than visual or auditory evoked responses.

Auditory Evoked Potentials (AEPs)

AEPs are used for clinical assessment of both peripheral and central auditory mechanisms.[54] As with SEPs, the very early components of AEPs reflect peripheral activities, whereas later components reflect central mechanisms. Components of AEPs are generally categorized along several dimensions, including latency (short, middle, long), presumed origin (cochlea, brainstem, cerebrum), and dependence on physical versus psychologic factors (exogenous versus endogenous). Short-latency, brainstem auditory evoked potentials (BAEPs) are most frequently studied, although other components may be of interest as well.

Early components of the response are best evoked by stimulation with loud (80 to 90 db) clicks generated

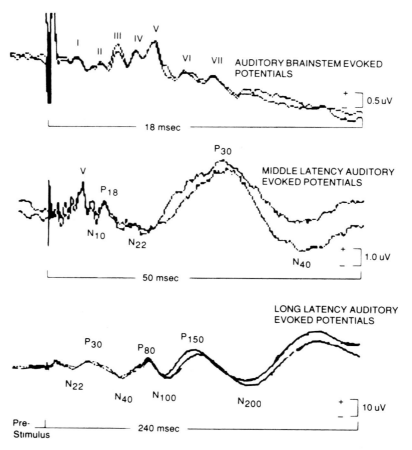

Fig. 8-35. Auditory evoked potentials in a normal adult showing brainstem and middle-latency and long-latency evoked components. (From McPherson D, Starr A: Auditory evoked potentials in the clinic. In Halliday AM, editor: Evoked potentials in clinical testing, ed 2, Edinburg, 1993, Churchill Livingstone, p 359.)

by applying a brief (less than 10 msec) square wave voltage to a calibrated earphone. The click has a broad power spectrum capable of activating a large portion of the basilar membrane. Tone bursts are used more often for examination of cortical activity. These activate restricted sections of the basilar membrane and are useful for examining frequency-specific activities. Fig. 8-35 illustrates the various components of AEPs. For recording of BAEPs, electrodes are typically placed at the vertex, the mastoids, and on the neck over the C7 spinal segment. Additional scalp electrodes (those of the International 10-20 system) are generally used in studies of cortical activity. As is the case for SEPs, the low-pass filter must be set high, greater than 1.5 kHz, for recording BAEPs (settings as low as 100 Hz can be used if only cortical activity is of interest). The magnitude of BAEPs is quite small with respect to the spontaneous EEG, and it is typically necessary to average several thousand epochs to extract reliable data. Long-latency cortical components can be extracted reliably with as few as 50 stimulus presentations. A stimulus repetition rate as high as 30/sec is acceptable for measurement of

BAEPs, but a much slower rate (1/sec) is required for undistorted recording of the long-latency AEP components.

The BAEP is characterized by six or sometimes seven deflections (I to VII) in the first 9 msec after the stimulus. Fig. 8-36 illustrates the suspected anatomic origins of these signals. For clinical purposes, waves I, III, and V are of greatest interest, since these reflect volume-conducted activity from the levels of the acoustic nerve, pons, and medulla, respectively.

Waves I and II are believed to reflect action potential activities of the eighth cranial nerve. Wave I primarily depends on activity associated with high-frequency stimulus components that activate hair cells along the base of the basilar membrane. Wave I occurs at the time of eighth nerve activity within the cochlea, whereas wave II occurs at the time when eighth nerve action potentials would be entering into the brainstem. Identification of wave I is particularly important because this defines an electrophysiologic time mark from which the latencies of other waves (generated more proximally) can be measured. Because it is generated distal to the brainstem, peripheral auditory

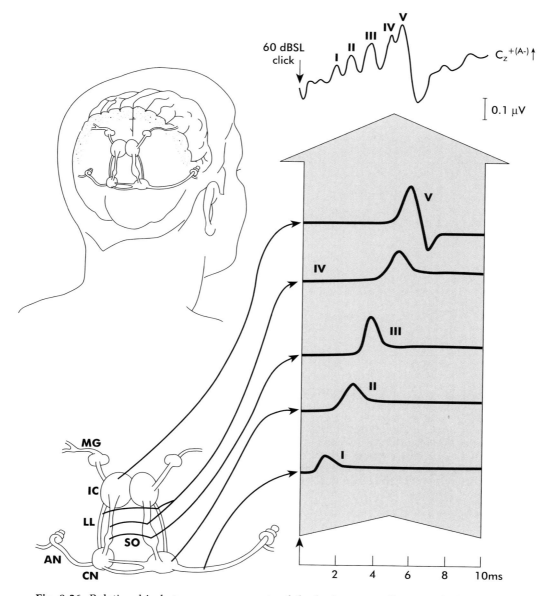

Fig. 8-36. Relationship between components of the brainstem auditory evoked response and the auditory projection pathways. *AN*, auditory nerve; *CN*, cochlear nucleus; *SO*, superior olive; *LL*, lateral lemniscus; *IC*, inferior colliculus; *MG*, medial geniculate. (Modified from Stockard JJ, Stockard E, Sharbrough FW: Nonpathologic factors influencing brainstem auditory evoked potentials, Am J EEG Technol 18:177, 1978.)

factors affect wave I in a manner similar to that found for subsequent waves, but central nervous system (CNS) diseases such as MS generally have minimal affect on wave I. Wave I is most readily identified in a Cz-ipsilateral mastoid derivation (as opposed to a contralateral mastoid derivation). High stimulus intensities and relatively slow repetition rates (less than 20/sec) provide the best signal-to-noise ratio (SNR). In contrast to wave I, wave II shows only minimal differences in ipsilateral versus contralateral mastoid derivations.

Wave III is believed to derive from synaptic activity in the superior olivary complex located at the level of the pons. It is best recorded in vertex to ipsilateral mastoid derivations and has a mean latency of 3.8 msec. Wave IV occurs with a mean latency of 4.5 msec, and it is believed to reflect activity in the lateral lemnisci. Wave V is the most easily identified of the BAEP components. Wave V is believed to reflect synaptic activity in the inferior colliculus. It is characterized by its latency (approximately 5.2 msec) and, more importantly, by its morphology and

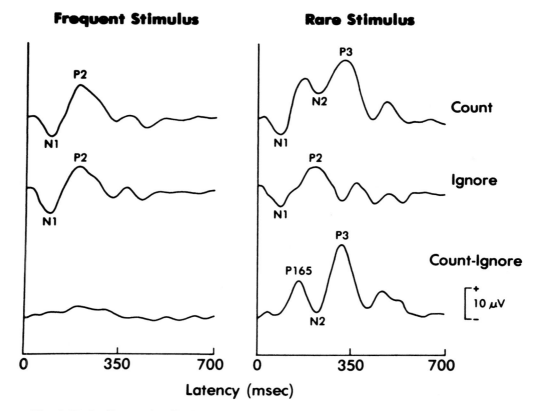

Fig. 8-37. Auditory stimuli give rise to exogenous N1 and P2 scalp components. If a sequence of stimuli is composed of two tones, one occurring on 80% of the trials and the other on 20% of the trials, the rare stimulus evokes an additonal P3 component if it is attended to. The P3 complex is believed to reflect mnemonic factors and the subjective probability of the rare event. P3 amplitude, latency, and topology have been shown to be abnormal is several neuropathologic and psychiatric conditions. (Modified from Goodin DS, Squires KC, Henderson BH, Starr A: An early event-related cortical potential, Psychophysiology 15:360, 1978.)

topography—a prominent positivity followed by a sharp negative deflection. Unlike prior components, wave V is attenuated relatively little by increasing the stimulus repetition rate. Even at rates as high as 100/sec, where other components cannot be easily identified, wave V remains prominent. Wave V is also less sensitive than other components to decreases in stimulus intensity, with significant activity remaining even when the stimulus intensity is near subjective threshold.[55]

There are three major clinical applications of BAEPs in adult neurology: (1) the detection of tumors in the region of the posterior fossa, (2) evaluation of coma, and (3) assessment of patients with suspected demyelinating diseases (e.g., MS).

The BAEP is considered abnormal and suggestive of a retrocochlear lesion when there is (1) a complete loss of all waveforms (in the absence of middle ear or cochlear disease), (2) absence of waveforms after wave I or III, (3) prolonged interpeak latencies, (4) significant left-right asymmetries in the wave I to V

interpeak latency, or (5) low amplitude of peak V relative to peak I.[15]

The BAEP is very sensitive to disruption by tumors in the region of the posterior fossa. Acoustic neuromas may cause complete loss of wave I on the side of the lesion or a significant increase in the I to III interpeak latency. Abnormalities of this type show a sensitivity to auditory neuromas of greater than 90%. Cerebellopontine tumors also disrupt the normal BAEP pattern, causing prolongation of the III to V interpeak latency, especially on the contralateral side. Intraaxial brainstem lesions (e.g., gliomas) generally cause bilateral increases in the III to V interpeak latency.

BAEPs are generally unaffected by drugs or metabolic dysfunction, so the BAEP provides a good index of the structural integrity of the brainstem of patients in a comatose state. Preserved wave I but absent or delayed later components are good indications of a structural lesion of the brainstem, and a total absence of all subsequent waves may be used as confirmatory

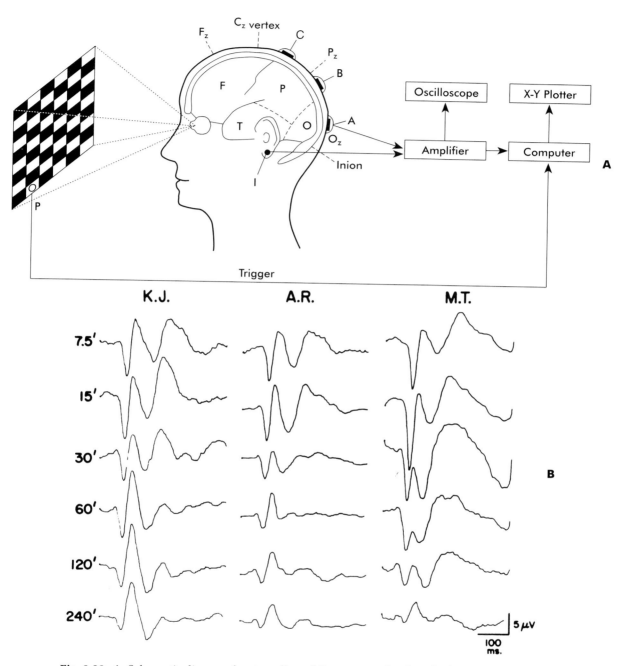

Fig. 8-38. A, Schematic diagram for recording of the pattern visual evoked response. Black checks turns white, and vice versa, to produce a pattern-reversing stimulus with signal-averaging time lock to the reversals. **B,** Example pattern-reversal VEPs from three normal subjects. Check size is shown to the left of the waveforms. The field size was 12 × 14 degrees; luminance, 2.0 log cd/m × ml; and contrast 85%. (**A** modified from Sokol S: The visually evoked potential: theory, techniques and clinical applications, Surv Ophthalmol 21:18, 1976; **B** from Sokol S: Visual evoked potentials. In Aminoff MJ, editor: Electrodiagnosis in clinical neurology, ed 2, New York, 1986, Churchill Livingstone, p 441.)

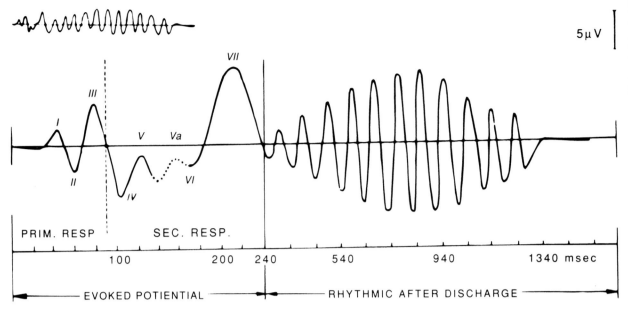

Fig. 8-39. Schematic representation of the flash visual evoked potential. (Modified from Ciganek L: The EEG response (evoked potential) to light stimulus in man, Electroenceph Clin Neurophysiol 13:163-172, 1961.)

evidence of brain death. In contrast, a normal BAEP pattern in a comatose patient implies that the coma is related to drug intoxication or severe metabolic dysfunction.[55]

Patients often have signs and symptoms traceable to a single CNS lesion, and clinicians must determine if these findings represent the first manifestations of a demyelinating process. Such a diagnosis is supported if other subclinical CNS lesions can be identified. As with SEPs, BAEP abnormalities are common in patients with MS. The "hit rate" is approximately 25% for patients suspected of having MS and 50% to 75% for patients known to have MS.[49]

The BAEP is often used to assess audiologic function and brainstem integrity in pediatric patients. Even a mild hearing loss during early development can lead to significant deficits in language development, so BAEP assessment of auditory functioning can be especially useful as an early diagnostic test, especially in children exposed to prenatal and early postnatal risk factors.[56] Behavioral assessment of audiologic function in early infancy is often difficult and unreliable, whereas the BAEP provides a sensitive measure of intact peripheral and brainstem pathways. However, a normal BAEP does not necessarily imply normal hearing and auditory perception.

Analyses of middle-latency and long-latency AEP components that reflect thalamic and cortical activities are done less often in routine clinical practice. Long-latency cortical components are often classified as exogenous versus endogenous. The characteristics of exogenous components are highly related to the physical characteristics of the eliciting stimuli. For example, components modulated by changing stimulus intensity are typically classified as exogenous. In contrast, the occurrence and morphology of some components is highly modulated by subjective factors and a subject's attentive state. For example, the N100 component of the AEP is an endogenous component that shows increasing amplitude with increasing signal intensity. If a sequence of two tones is played with the subjective probability of one tone being much higher than the probability of the other, the rare tone elicits an endogenous P300 (P3) response (Fig. 8-37) that reflects its low probability of occurrence, not its physical attributes.[57] Assessment of exogenous components can be useful in the identification of lesions in cortical projection pathways, whereas disruption of endogenous activity has been associated with various types of cognitive and psychiatric dysfunction.

Visual Evoked Potentials (VEPs)

VEPs recorded at the back of the scalp overlying the occipital lobe reflect overlapping cortical activity of multiple generator sites with little signal arising from subcortical zones. When full-field stimuli are used, the response mostly reflects activation of the occipital poles, which receive input from the fovea. The elicited activity is bilateral because each hemisphere receives input from the ipsilateral temporal retina and contralateral nasal retina and because of interhemispheric callosal projections. Half-field stimulation can be used to assess the retrochiasmal pathways more accurately. Two general classes of visual stimuli are typically used: *flashes* and *patterns*.[58,59] Pat-

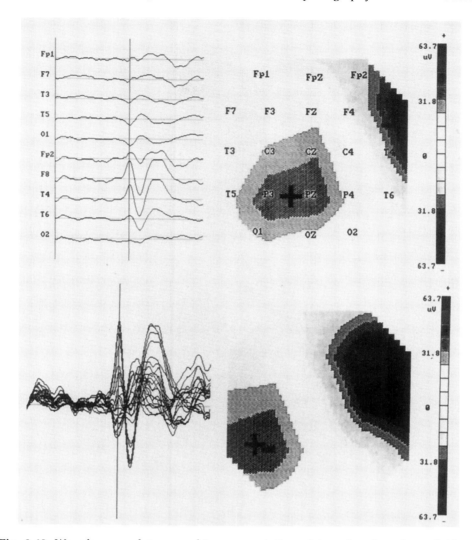

Fig. 8-40. Waveforms and topographic representation of type I scalp voltage fields at the peak of an averaged ($n = 8$) right temporal sharp wave. Upper map shows standard montage; lower map shows shifted oblique montage. (From Ebersole JS, Wade PB: Spike voltage topography and equivalent dipole localization in complex partial epilepsy, Brain Topogr 3:25, 1990.)

tern stimulation is generally obtained using a checkerboard pattern of black-and-white squares that periodically contrast-reverse without a change in overall luminance (Fig. 8-38). Several factors influence the pattern-reversal VEP, including the rate of pattern reversal, the size of the checks, the luminance level, and the check contrast. In some situations, it is useful to pattern-reverse restricted portions of a centrally fixated full-field pattern to assess topographic dysfunction, such as that associated with a restricted lesion of the visual cortex.

A pattern-reversal rate of 1 to 2/sec is useful for recording the transient VEP. In some patients, it is useful to use reversal rates greater than 10 Hz to elicit steady-state signals that are most appropriately analyzed in the frequency domain rather than the time domain. Low-pass filter settings should not be less

than 100 Hz for recording the response with reasonable fidelity.

The VEP waveform depends on the stimulus used to generate it, and there is considerable inter-individual variability in appearance. Fig. 8-39 shows the typical VEP elicited by a full-field flash stimulus. Waveform morphology is highly dependent on the stimulus intensity and the flicker rate. As stimulus intensity is decreased, the amplitude of the components decreases while their latencies increase. For the flash-VEP there are three main deflections: N70, P100, and N125 (N and P indicate negative and positive deflections at occipital leads referenced to linked ears, and the number indicates the response latency). The flash VEP is often followed by a time-locked burst of alpha activity.[60]

At slow reversal rates, the transient VEP evoked by

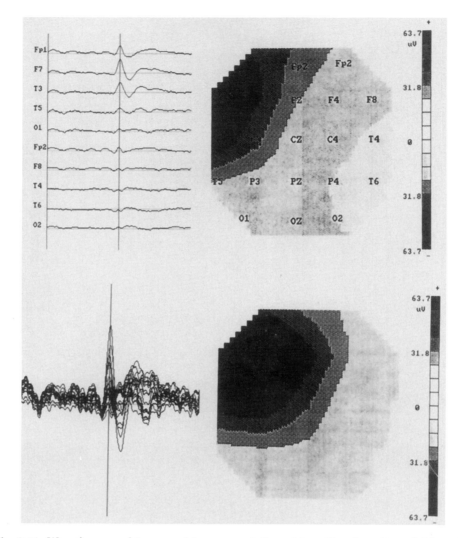

Fig. 8-41. Waveforms and topographic representation of type II scalp voltage fields at the peak of an averaged ($n = 8$) left temporal sharp wave. Upper map shows standard montage; lower map shows shifted oblique montage. (From Ebersole JS, Wade PB: Spike voltage topography and equivalent dipole localization in complex partial epilepsy, Brain Topogr 3:26, 1990.)

patterns is similar to that seen for flashes, although some of the earliest components of the response are absent. The pattern VEP typically has three components: N75, P100, and N145. Modulation of reversal rate, check size, and contrast can provide for a detailed assessment of visual functioning, although such manipulations are rarely carried out during routine clinical examinations. Excellent reviews of basic research and clinical research applications of pattern reversal VEPs are provided by Halliday[40] and Regan.[41] In most routine cases, slowly reversing, large checks of high contrast are used.

The latency of the P100 response of both flash and pattern VEPs is fairly stable across normal subjects, and latency delays of 30 msec or longer generally reflect significant pathology. Interocular latency dif-

ferences of 10 msec or longer also signify pathology.[41,58,59] In optic neuritis, the P100 component of the pattern evoked response is often delayed, even in the absence of a comparable delay in the flash evoked response. Abnormal responses to pattern stimulation are also closely associated with progressive MS which is often associated with early episodes of optic neuritis. As with other sensory evoked responses, abnormalities are found in 80% of patients with documented MS and 20% to 40% of patients with suspected MS.[49]

Evaluation of the VEP can also be of use in patients with suspected hysterical blindness, in which the presence of activity indicates an intact retinogeniculostriate pathway, although subsequent dysfunction of higher cortical processing centers is not easily ruled out by VEP methods.[58]

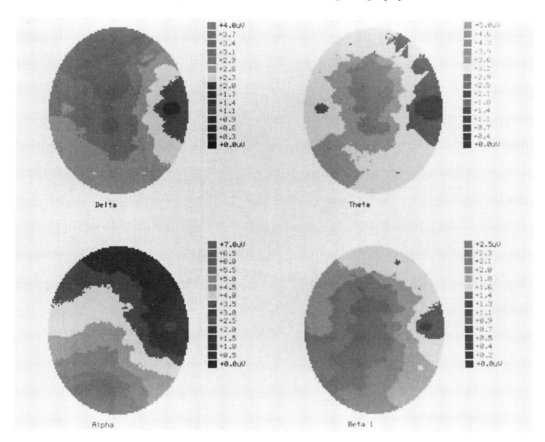

Fig. 8-42. Brain electrical activity map (BEAM) showing the spatial topography of spectral power for a schizophrenic patient. Note differences in the topography in the various frequency bands. (Reproduced in full color in color insert.)

ADVANCED ANALYSIS STRATEGIES
Topographic Mapping and Dipole Analyses

Recent developments in computer technology and signal processing have led to new strategies for the display, analysis, and interpretation of clinical EEG and evoked potential data. Of particular note is increased interest in the spatial pattern of activity (versus waveform morphology and the latency and amplitude of specific components). Consider first the standard clinical EEG. Routine EEG analysis provides for identification of electrode derivations where a signal is maximal or where a phase reversal is present, but data are rarely displayed in a way that allows a quantitative assessment of the spatial pattern of activity. However, computer algorithms now allow for easy display of the isopotential pattern at any instant in time. One of the best examples of the usefulness of this approach comes from the work of Ebersole and colleagues, who have been studying the electrical potential pattern associated with epileptic spikes arising from the temporal lobes.[61]

In this pioneering work, Ebersole has found two very common but different potential patterns in patients with complex partial seizures of suspected temporal/frontal origin. Type I patterns are characterized by surface negativity over the involved temporal lobe and a synchronous region of focal positivity over the contralateral parietal lobe (Fig. 8-40). Type II patterns also display a temporal negativity (although it tends to be broader and extends more toward the midline), but no focal positivity. Rather, there is a shallow positive gradient over the contralateral hemisphere (Fig. 8-41). These differing patterns imply differences in the orientation and position of the underlying neuronal generators.

To examine this latter point better, Ebersole has applied dipole modeling strategies to these data. Given knowledge of the electrical properties and geometry of the head, the surface potential pattern generated by a particular pattern of intracranial neuronal currents is uniquely specified by Maxwell's equations. However, the current pattern that generated a particular surface potential pattern cannot be specified uniquely because current elements may produce surface potentials that cancel each other. This *inverse problem* of specifying generative neuronal

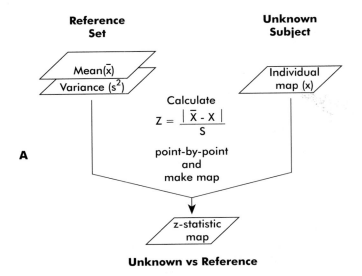

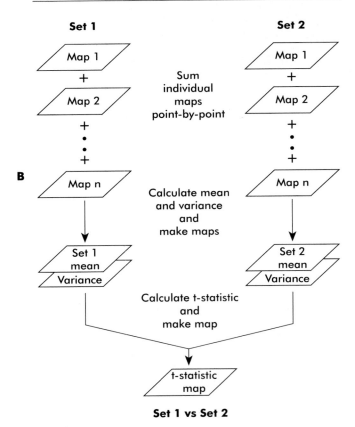

Fig. 8-43. **A,** Schematic showing generation of a significance probability map (SPM). At each electrode site of a patient data set, a Z score is determined with respect to a reference (normal) set. Standard spatial interpolation methods are used to provide a topographic Z map. **B,** T-statistical maps are used to show differences in field topography between populations. (From Duffy FH, Iyer VG, Surwillo WW: Clinical electroencephalography and topographic brain mapping: technology and practice, New York, 1989, Springer-Verlag, p 230.)

activity is ill-posed and unsolvable in its most general, unrestricted form.

However, by making assumptions about the conductive properties of the head and also the configuration of the generative currents, iterative procedures can be used to determine best-fitting source configurations.[62] In the analysis of neuroelectric data, the head is modeled as a spherical volume conductor of multiple concentric shells of differing but homogeneous electrical conductivity. A four-shell model is common with shells representing the brain, CSF, skull, and scalp. Currents associated with the neuronal activity of a focal population are mathematically modeled as though they were generated by a dipole source. Provided that the measured potential pattern mostly reflects activity from a single focal neuronal population, and also provided that the distance between scalp surface recording sites and the location of the neuronal activity is large relative to the spatial extent of the activated neuronal region, the dipole approximation is quite reasonable. Given these assumptions, mathematical procedures can be used to derive the position, orientation, and strength of the dipole that best accounts (in a least-squares sense) for the measured potential pattern.

To the extent that the conductivity and source model are accurate, the parameters of the best-sitting dipole source provide an indication of the location of the relevant neuronal population. On the other hand, realistic deviations from sphericity, an incorrect source model, inhomogeneities in the conductive media, and incorrect specification of the relative conductivities of the model shells all can cause significant inaccuracies in source modeling procedures.

Despite these caveats, Ebersole has used source modeling procedures with great utility. It is noteworthy that Ebersole has been most interested in the temporal stability of dipole positions, not the positions per se. This is important because simple dipole models are probably inadequate for characterization of temporal lobe epileptic spikes, so the absolute values of derived source parameters are probably inaccurate. Dipole modeling of type I events generally produces temporally stable solutions across the duration of the event, whereas type II patterns change rapidly over time. What makes this result and the data on the topography of the activity so exciting is the strong correlation between the presence of type I activity and mesial temporal lobe seizure onset, as assessed by invasive monitoring. Several patients with type I patterns have undergone temporal lobectomy/hippocampectomy with complete elimination of seizures. Noninvasive identification of type I activity may soon prove sufficient to indicate mesial temporal seizure origin without the need for dangerous and costly invasive monitoring. That is, by examination of spike/sharp

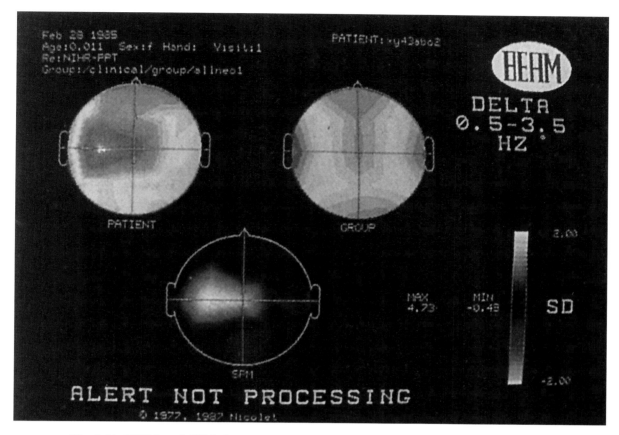

Fig. 8-44. BEAM and SPMs for a premature neonate (30 weeks) studied 42 weeks after gestation. The infant had a grade II intraventricular hemorrhage involving the left hemisphere. The BEAM map for delta activity is highly asymmetric relative to the average map for the control group. The SPM data show a statistically significant level of increased delta activity over the left hemisphere. (Reproduced in full color in color insert.) (From Duffy FH: Issues facing the clinical use of the brain electrical activity mapping. In Pfurtscheller G, Lopes da Silva FH, editors: Functional brain imaging, Toronto, 1988, Han Huber.)

wave topology and dipole modeling, EEG identification of mesial temporal epilepsy is greatly improved. Type II activity appears to be most closely associated with lateral temporal lobe epilepsy and inferior lateral frontal lobe epilepsy.

BEAM and Neurometrics

Topographic analysis of the spectral profile of spontaneous brain activity is another important emerging strategy of neuroelectric analysis. Brain electrical activity mapping (BEAM), pioneered by Duffy and colleagues,[63-65] and neurometric techniques, developed by John and colleagues,[66,67] are playing an increasing role in clinical neurophysiology. In a typical experiment, spontaneous brain activity is recorded from an international 10-20 referential montage, and the data at each electrode site are characterized by its spectral properties. Spatial power maps are then calculated for each of the standard frequency bands (e.g., delta, theta). Therefore, for each subject, a topographic map of power in each frequency band is generated (Fig. 8-42). A normative data base, complete with a measure of variability in the recorded power at each electrode, then can be generated from the data of multiple normal subjects. It is then possible to compare the data of a particular patient with the normative data set and identify sites of significant statistical anomaly. Significance probability maps (SPMs) that provide a spatial display of sites of statistically deviant activity can then be generated (Figs. 8-43 and 8-44). In this manner, pathologic activity profiles can be distinguished from normal profiles. Through application of discriminant functions and neural network strategies, it may be possible not only to identify pathologic activity profiles, but also to categorize these profiles by comparison of the particular patient data set with averaged data sets derived from various patient populations. As shown by the work of Prichep and John, neurometric analysis strategies are beginning to prove useful in the early identification and categorization of subjects with a wide range of neurologic and psychiatric disorders.[67]

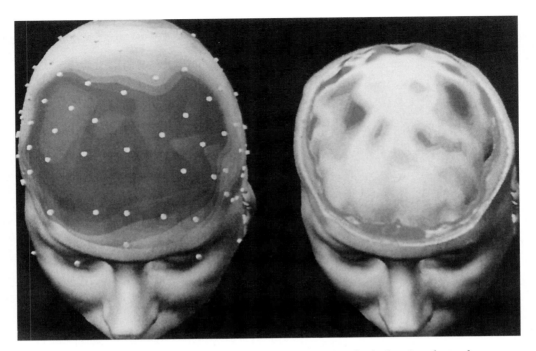

Fig. 8-45. Spatial deblurring of scalp data collected with a high-density electrode array provides increased spatial resolution of EEG data. Displayed data were collected in response to movements of one finger of each hand. In the scalp map, little detail is seen, but the deblurred image, projected just above the cortical surface, shows clear bilateral activity in the vicinity of the central sulcus. (Reproduced in full color in color insert.) (From Gevins A: High-resolution EEG enters imaging arena, Diagn Imaging Nov 1993, p 77.)

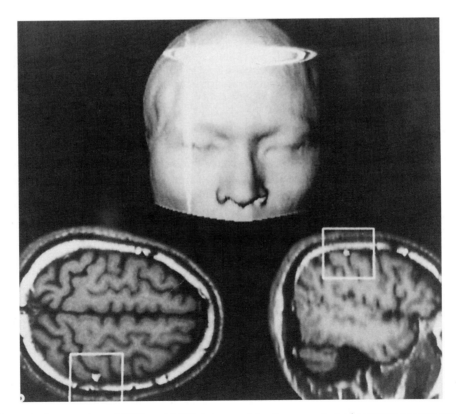

Fig. 8-46. Integration of EEG and MRI data provides for mapping of somatosensory cortex in individual subjects. EEG data collected during stimulation of the left index finger were analyzed with an equivalent dipole model. (Reproduced in full color in color insert.) (From Gevins A: High-resolution EEG enters imaging arena, Diagn Imaging, Nov 1993, p 78.)

High-Density Mapping and Spatial Deblurring

Despite the electrical conductivity barrier imposed by the skull causing significant smearing of the scalp surface potential relative to the cortical potential, routine EEG still significantly undersamples the spatial information available at the surface. Recent years thus have seen a move toward higher-density electrode arrays involving 32, 64, 128, or even 256 electrodes in some research applications. At present, the amount of time taken to place so many electrodes is a limiting factor in routine clinical practice, but application of 48 or 64 electrodes (a significant improvement over the standard 21) can now be accomplished in 30 minutes, and this provides for significant improvement in the spatial resolving power of EEG, especially when additional signal-processing techniques are employed. Of particular note are spatial deblurring techniques being developed by Gevins.[68] These methods integrate MRI-derived anatomic data into the EEG analysis procedure to determine the cortical potential pattern associated with the measured scalp pattern. In so doing, activities not easily resolvable by visual inspection of the scalp pattern are easily identified (Fig. 8-45). By deblurring the image, this method may prove very useful in giving epileptologists and surgeons a better picture of the activities they can expect to record using corticographic grids. Also, the usefulness of the described BEAM techniques and the efficiency of neurometric algorithms may be improved significantly by working with deblurred activity patterns.

Clearly, there is a move away from traditional waveform analyses of neuroelectric data to characterization of the spatial and temporal topography of activity. As structural MRI data become more closely integrated into EEG analysis strategies (Fig. 8-46), EEG becomes more and more a true imaging technique.

REFERENCES

1. Aminoff MJ: Electroencephalography: general principles and clinical applications. In Aminoff MJ, editor: Electrodiagnosis in clinical neurology, ed 2, New York, 1986, Churchill Livingstone.
2. Neyland TC, Reynolds CF, Kupfer DJ: Electrodiagnostic techniques in neuropsychiatry. In Yudofsk SC, Hales RE, editors: The American Psychiatric Press textbook of neuropsychiatry, ed 2, Washington, 1988, American Psychiatrc Press.
3. Dubois-Reymond E: Gesammelte Abhandlungen zur allgemeinen Muskel-und Nervephysikm, Leipzig, 1877, Veit.
4. Caton R: The electric currents of the brain, Br Med J, 2:278, 1875.
5. Kaufman PY: Electrical phenomena in cerebral cortex, Obzory Psikhiatrii Nevrologii i Eksperimental'noi Psikhlogii, 7-8:403, 1912.
6. Berger H: Uber das elektrekephalogramm des menschen, Arch Psychiatr Nervenkr 87:527-570, 1929.
7. Adrian ED, Mattews BHC: The Berger rhythm, potential changes from the occipital lobes of man, Brain 57:355-385, 1934.
8. Gibbs FA, Davis H, Lennox WG: The electroencephalogram in epilepsy and in conditions of impaired consciousness, Arch Neurol Psychiatry 34:1133-1148, 1935.
9. Pfurtsheller G, Aranibar A: Event-related cortical desynchronizations detected by power measurements of scalp EEG, Electroencephalogr Clin Neurophysiol 42:817-826, 1977.
10. Pfurtsheller G, Kimesch W: Topographical display and interpretation of event-related desynchronization during a visual-verbal task, Brain Topogr 3(1):85-94, 1990.
11. Goff WR, Allison T, Vaughan HG Jr: The functional neuroanatomy of event-related potentials. In Callaway E, Tueting P, Koslow S, editors: Event-related brain potentials in man, New York, 1978, Academic Press.
12. Niedermeyer E, Lopes da Silva F, editors: Electroencephalography—basic principles, clinical applications and related fields, ed 2, Baltimore, 1987, Urban and Schwarzenberg.
13. Lorente de No R: Analysis of the distribution of action currents of nerve in a volume conductor, Stud Rockefeller Inst Med Res 132:384-477, 1947.
14. Nunez PL: Electrical fields of the brain: the neurophysics of EEG, New York, 1981, Oxford University.
15. Duffy FH, Iyer VG, Surwillo WW: Clinical electroencephalography and topographic brain mapping: technology and practice, New York, 1989, Springer-Verlag.
16. Jasper HH: Report of the Committee on Methods of Clinical Examination in EEG: Appendix: The ten-twenty electrode system of the International Federation, Electroencephalogr Clin Neurophysiol 10:371-375, 1958.
17. Kooi KA, Tucker RP, Marshall RE: Fundamentals of electroencephalography, ed 2, New York, 1978, Harper & Row.
18. Kiloh LG, McComas AJ, Osselton JW et al: Clinical clectroencephalography, London, 1981, Butterworths.
19. Hughes JR: EEG in clinical practice, Boston, 1982, Butterworth.
20. Aminoff MJ, editor: Electrodiagnosis in clinical neurology, ed 2, New York, 1986, Churchill-Livingstone.
21. Fisch BJ: Spehlmann's EEG primer, ed 2, Amsterdam, 1991, Elsevier.
22. Andersen P, Adersson S: Physiological basis of the alpha rhythm, New York, 1968, Appleton-Century-Crofts.
23. Bennet DR: Electroencephalographic and evoked potential changes with aging, Semin Neurol 1:47-51, 1981.
24. Marsh GR, Thompson LV: Psychophysiology of aging. In Biren JE, Schaie KW, editors: Handbook of psychology of aging, New York, 1977, Reinhold van Nostrand.
25. Kozelk JW, Pedley TA: Beta and mu rhythms, J Clin Neurophysiol 7:191-208, 1990.
26. Fink M: EEG and human psychopharmacology, Am Rev Pharmacol 9:241-258, 1969.
27. Engle J, editor: Surgical treatment of the epilepsies, ed 2, New York, 1993, Raven.
28. Commission on Classification and Terminology of the International League Against Epilepsy: Proposal for classification of epilepsies and epileptic syndromes, Epilepsia 26:268-278, 1985.
29. Small JG, Bagchi BK, Kooi KA: Electro-clinical profile of 117 deep cerebral tumors, Electroencephalogr Clin Neurophysiol 13:193-207, 1961.
30. Gilmore PC, Brenner RP: Correlation of EEG, computed tomography and clinical findings: study of 100 patients with focal delta activity, Arch Neurol 38:371, 1981.
31. Rodin E: Contribution of EEG to prognosis after head injury, Dis Nerv Syst 28:598-601, 1967.
32. Bauer G: Coma and brain death. In Niedermeyer E, Lopes da Silva F, editors: Electroencephalography—basic principles, clinical applications and related fields, ed 2, Baltimore, 1987, Urban and Schwarzenberg.
33. Letemendia F, Pampiglione G: Clinical and electroencephalographic observations in Alzheimer's disease, J Neurol Psychiatry, 21:167-172, 1958.
34. Abbot J: The EEG in Jacob-Creutzfeldt's disease, Electroencephalogr Clin Neurophysiol 11:184-185, 1959.

35. McFarland HR, Kooi KA, Henley KS et al: Electroencephalographic frequency analysis in patients with hepatic encephalopathy, Univ Mich Med Center J 30:68-72, 1964.

36. Chokroverty S, Bruetman ME, Berger V et al: Progressive dialytic encephalopathy, J Neurol Neurosurg Psychiatry 39:411-419, 1976.

37. Hughes JR, Schreeder MT: EEG in dialysis encephalopathy, Neurology 30:1148-1154, 1980.

38. Abrams R, Taylor MA: Laboratory studies in the validation of psychiatric diagnoses. In Gruzelier JH, Flor-Henry P, editors: Hemispheric asymmetries of function in psychopathology, New York, 1979, Elsevier.

39. Dawson GD: A summation technique for detecting small signals in a large irregular background, J Physiol Lond 115:2P-3P, 1951.

40. Halliday AM, editor: Evoked potentials in clinical testing, ed 2, Edinburg, 1993, Churchill Livingstone.

41. Regan D: Human brain electrophysiology, Amsterdam, 1989, Elsevier.

42. Deecke L, Becker W, Grozinger B et al: Human brain potentials preceding voluntary limb movements, Electroencephalogr Clin Neurophysiol Suppl 33:87-94, 1973.

43. Gevins AS, Cutillo BA: Signals of cognition. In Lopes da Silva FH, van Leeuwen WS, Remond A, editors: Handbook of electroencephalography and clinical neurophysiology, vol 2, clinical applications of computer analysis of EEG and other neurophysiological signals, Amsterdam, 1986, Elsevier.

44. Allison T, Goff WR, Williamson PD et al: On the neural origin of early components of the human somatosensory evoked potential. In Desmedt JE, editor: Progress in clinical neurophysiology, vol 7, Basel, 1980, Karger.

45. Desmedt JE, Cheron G: Non-cephalic reference recording of early somatosensory potentials to finger stimulation in adult or aging normal man: Differentiation of widespread N18 and contralateral N20 from the prerolandic P22 and N30 components, Electroencephalogr Clin Neurophysiol 52:553-570, 1982.

46. Allison T, Wood CC, McCarthy G: Cortical somatosensory evoked potentials. II. Effects of excision of somatosensory and motor cortex in humans and monkeys, J Neurophysiol 66:64-82, 1991.

47. Slimp JC, Tamas LB, Stolov WC et al: Somatosensory evoked potentials after removal of somatosensory cortex, Electroencephalogr Clin Neurophysiol 37:663-669, 1985.

48. Wood CC, Cohen D, Cuffin BN et al: Electrical sources in human somatosensory cortex: identified by combined magnetic and potential recordings, Science 227:1051-1053, 1985.

49. Halliday AM: The comparative value of the different evoked potentials and other paraclinical tests in the diagnosis and prognosis of demyelinating disease. In Halliday AM, editor: Evoked potentials in clinical testing, ed 2, Edinburg, 1993, Churchill Livingstone.

50. Mastaglia FL, Black JL, Cala LA et al: Evoked potentials saccadic velocities and computerized tomography in diagnosis of multiple sclerosis, Br Med J 1:1315-1317, 1977.

51. Small DG, Matthews WB, Small M: The cervical somatosensory evoked potential in the diagnosis of multiple sclerosis, J Neurol Sci 35:211-224, 1978.

52. Jones SJ: Evoked potential in intraoperative monitoring. In Halliday AM, editor: Evoked potentials in clinical testing, ed 2, Edinburg, 1993, Churchill Livingstone.

53. Greenberg RP, Newlon PG, Hyatt MS et al: Prognostic implications of early multimodal evoked potentials in severely head-injured patients, J Neurosurg 55:227-236, 1981.

54. McPherson D, Starr A: Auditory evoked potentials in the clinic. In Halliday AM, editor: Evoked potentials in clinical testing, ed 2, Edinburg, 1993, Churchill Livingstone.

55. Stockard JJ, Stockard JE, Sharbrough FW: Brainstem auditory evoked potentials in neurology: methodology, interpretation, and clinical application. In Aminoff MJ, editor: Electrodiagnosis in clinical neurology, ed 2, New York, 1986, Churchill Livingstone.

56. Pictor TW, Taylor MJ, Duriex-Smith A et al: Brainstem auditory evoked potentials in pediatrics. In Aminoff MJ, editor: Electrodiagnosis in clinical neurology, ed 2, New York, 1986, Churchill Livingstone.

57. Donchin E, Ritter W, McCallum WC: Cognitive psychophysiology: the endogenous components of the ERP. In Callaway E, Tueting P, Koslow S, editors: Event-related brain potentials in man, New York, 1978, Academic Press.

58. Halliday AM: The visual evoked potential in the investigation of chiasmal and retrochiasmal lesions, field defects and systemic disease. In Halliday AM, editor: Evoked potentials in clinical testing, ed 2, Edinburg, 1993, Churchill Livingstone.

59. Sokol S: Visual evoked potentials. In Aminoff MJ, editor: Electrodiagnosis in clinical neurology, ed 2, New York, 1986, Churchill Livingstone.

60. Ciganek L: The EEG response (evoked potential) to light stimulus in man, Electroencephalogr Clin Neurophysiol 13:165-172, 1961.

61. Ebersole JS, Wade PB: Spike voltage topography and equivalent dipole localization in complex partial epilepsy, Brain Topogr 3(1):21-34, 1990.

62. Wood CC: Application of dipole localization methods to source identification of human evoked potentials, Ann NY Acad Sci 388:139-155, 1982.

63. Duffy FH, Burchfiel JL, Lombrosco CT: Brain electrical activity mapping (BEAM): a method for extending clinical utility of EEG and evoked potential data, Ann Neurol 5:309-321, 1979.

64. Duffy FH, Bartels PH, Burchfiel JL: Significance probability mapping: an aid to topographic analysis of brain electrical activity, Electroencephalogr Clin Neurophysiol 51:455-462, 1981.

65. Duffy FH: Topographic mapping of brain electrical activity, Boston, 1986, Butterworth.

66. John ER, Prichep LS, Easton P: Normative data banks and neurometrics: basic concepts, methods and results of norm construction. In Gevins AS, Remond A, editors: Handbook of electroencephalography and clinical neurophysiology, vol 1: methods of analysis of brain electrical and magnetic signals, Amsterdam, 1986, Elsevier.

67. Prichep LS, John ER: Neurometrics: clinical applications. In Lopes da Silva FH, van Leeuwen WS, Remond A, editors: Handbook of electroencephalography and clinical neurophysiology, vol 2, clinical applications of computer analysis of EEG and other neurophysiological signals, Amsterdam, 1986, Elsevier.

68. Gevins A: High-resolution EEG enters imaging arena, Diagn Imaging Nov. 1993, p 78.

Magnetoencephalography and Magnetic Source Imaging

Jeffrey David Lewine
William W. Orrison, Jr.

In the early 19th century, Hans Christian Oersted, a Danish physicist, discovered that electrical currents generate magnetic fields, with the direction of the magnetic field described by a simple right-hand rule. When the thumb of the right hand is pointed in the direction of current flow, the fingers curl in the direction of the surrounding magnetic field. This is as true for bioelectric currents, such as those flowing within neurons and muscle fibers, as it is for currents flowing within telephone and power lines. Biomagnetic fields directly reflect electrophysiologic events of the heart and brain, and they pass through the tissues of the body without distortion. Thus, their measurement and characterization can provide new insights into human physiology.

The first attempts to record biomagnetic data were in 1963 with the pioneering experiments of Baule and McFee.[1] Armed with a 2 million–turn, hand-wound induction coil, Baule and McFee made the first measurements of the magnetic signal generated by the human heart. Five years later, working in a specially designed magnetically shielded room constructed at the Massachussetts Institute of Technology (MIT), Cohen used a similar induction coil and signal-averaging techniques to measure the brain's alpha rhythm.[2]

The next major advance in biomagnetic technology came with the development of the point-contact SQUID (superconducting quantum interference device) by Zimmerman and colleagues.[3] Operating at liquid helium temperatures of −269° C, the SQUID achieved an unprecedented level of sensitivity to weak magnetic signals. The SQUID was first used in biomagnetic experiments inside of the shielded room at MIT in December 1969.[4] The initial experiments involved recording of a magnetocardiogram, but it soon became apparent that using SQUID technology in a shielded room made it possible to record a magnetoencephalogram without the need for signal averaging.[5] Furthermore, using signal-averaging techniques, the SQUID made it possible to measure stimulus-evoked neuromagnetic signals.[6-8]

Neuromagnetic recordings offer several advantages over alternative noninvasive imaging modalities. Mag-

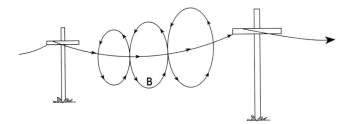

Fig. 9-1. All electrical currents, whether in telephone wires or brain cells, produce a magnetic field in the surrounding space.

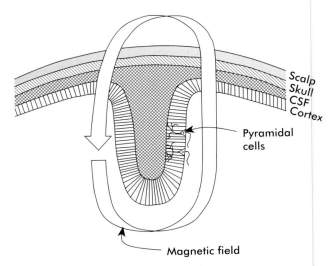

Fig. 9-2. The magnetic field outside of the head mostly reflects intracellular currents flowing in the apical dendrites of pyramidal cells oriented parallel to the skull surface.

netoencephalography (MEG), as with electroencephalography (EEG), provides for real-time, direct assessment of brain electrophysiology. MEG therefore provides an important complement to structural imaging modalities such as computed tomography (CT) and magnetic resonance imaging (MRI) and to hemodynamic and metabolic techniques such as functional MRI (fMRI), positron emission tomography (PET), and single-photon emission computed tomography (SPECT). MEG affords certain advantages over EEG. The most salient of these is that neuromagnetic signals penetrate the skull and scalp without significant distortion. The spatial resolution of MEG is higher than that for EEG, and mathematical analyses of the spatial pattern of the neuromagnetic field can offer accurate spatial localization of the neurons responsible for generating neuromagnetic signals. Of the available noninvasive neuroimaging techniques, MEG provides the best balance of temporal and spatial sensitivity to brain physiology.

During the past two decades, most MEG investigations have focused on basic research in sensory and cognitive neuroscience. However, with the recent development of large-array biomagnetometer systems capable of simultaneous recording of the magnetic signal over large portions of the head, clinical applications are moving to the forefront. This chapter, as in others within this book, focuses on clinical advances. The reader interested in basic work on sensory processing and cognition is referred to excellent review articles.[9-13] Before proceeding with a detailed description of research into and applications of biomagnetic principles, a brief tutorial of the biomagnetic technique is presented.

Just as current flow within a wire produces a magnetic field, so does current flow within neurons (Fig. 9-1). Because of biophysical properties, the neuromagnetic field recorded outside of the head mostly reflects the dendritic currents of pyramidal cells that are oriented parallel to the skull surface (Fig. 9-2).

The time-varying neuromagnetic field produced by current flow within neurons induces a current within

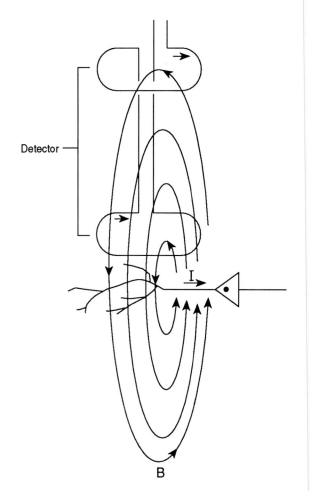

Fig. 9-3. Time-varying neuromagnetic signals induce an electrical current within the wire loops of the detection coil. For the axial gradiometer shown here, the upper and lower coil are wound in the opposite direction. The amount of current induced in the system therefore reflects the spatial gradient of the neuromagnetic field.

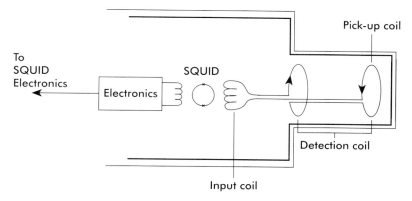

Fig. 9-4. The detection coil is inductively coupled to a superconducting quantum interference device (SQUID), which acts as a low-noise, high-gain, current-to-voltage converter.

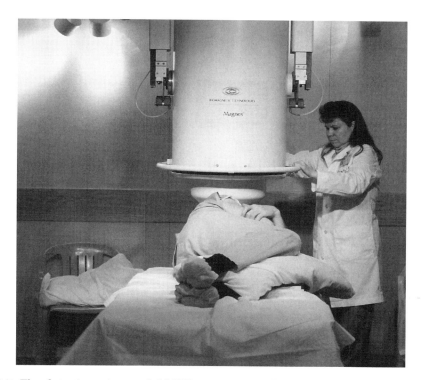

Fig. 9-5. The detection wires and SQUIDs are contained within a cryogenic dewar filled with liquid helium. During an experiment, the sensing array is positioned over brain regions of interest.

wire loops of a detection coil (Fig. 9-3). By coupling the detector to a SQUID, the induced current can be measured and the magnitude of the inducing magnetic field inferred (Fig. 9-4). The detection wires and SQUID must be maintained at superconducting tem-peratures. This is accomplished by immersing the sensors in a liquid helium bath contained within a cryogenically insulated dewar (Fig. 9-5). During an experiment, the dewar is positioned over regions of interest.

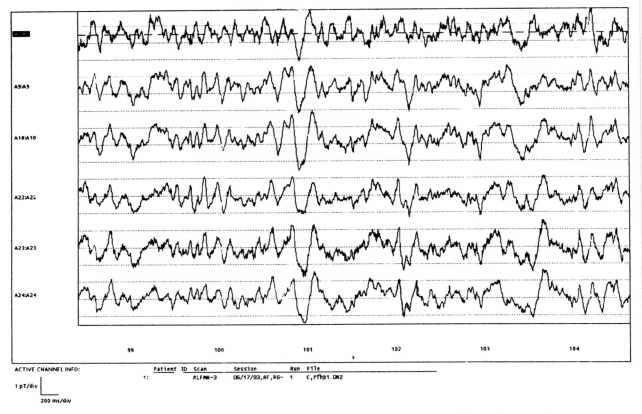

ACTIVE CHANNEL INFO:

Patient ID   Scan   Session   Run File
1:           RLFMA-3   06/17/93,AF,R6- 1   c,rfhp1.ON2

1 pT/div

200 ms/div

Fig. 9-6. Each MEG sensing channel (six are shown here) records a time-varying neuromagnetic signal that is similar in appearance to the EEG recorded at the scalp surface.

The recorded neuromagnetic signals are very similar in appearance to EEG signals that are recorded at the scalp surface (Fig. 9-6). There are two classes of MEG study: spontaneous and event related. For example, studies of epileptiform and abnormal low-frequency magnetic activity (ALFMA) involve analyses of *spontaneous* neuromagnetic signals, whereas studies of normal and abnormal functional organization and information processing generally take advantage of *event-related* signal-averaging techniques identical to those used in EEG investigations of evoked responses.

During an event-related experiment, such as for presurgical mapping of the spatial relationship between the primary somatosensory cortex and a tumor, the neuromagnetic field is recorded while the surface of a finger is repeatedly depressed by a pneumatically driven tactile stimulator. Data epochs spanning each stimulus are signal-averaged to extract time-locked signals from the background noise. Fig. 9-7 shows examples of averaged signals recorded with a 37-

channel biomagnetometer. Each waveform is a plot of signal magnitude versus time. About 50 msec after stimulus presentation (marked by the vertical line in each trace), a significant neuromagnetic response occurs in the averaged response, as indicated by the deflection in the waveforms. At each instant in time, the spatial pattern of neuromagnetic activity can be displayed as an isofield contour map. The map in Fig. 9-8 shows the spatial pattern of the magnetic field at the time of maximal response for the data of Fig. 9-7.

By mathematically modeling the field pattern, it is possible to infer (relative to a head-centered coordinate system) the location of those neurons that contribute to the recorded signal (Fig. 9-9). These mathematical models use simplifying assumptions about the shape and electrical properties of the head and also the configuration of the relevant neuronal currents. To the extent that these assumptions are valid, the inferred x, y, and z spatial position of the active cell population is accurate to within a few millimeters.

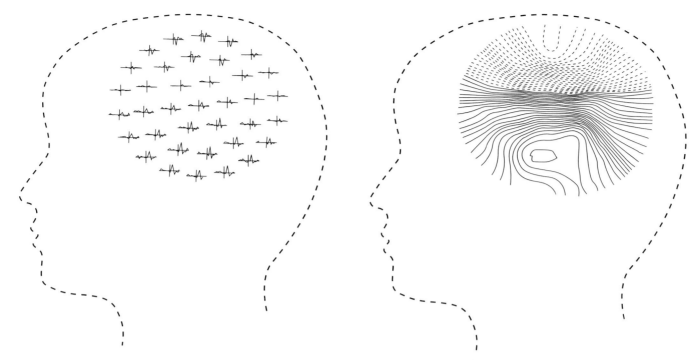

Fig. 9-7. Somatosensory evoked magnetic signals recorded with a 37-channel biomagnetometer system. The averaged waveforms were obtained in response to tactile stimulation of the contralateral index finger ($n = 256$). The vertical line represents the time of stimulus presentation. Approximately 50 msec after the stimulus, a large neuromagnetic response occurs.

Fig. 9-8. The isofield contour map shows the spatial pattern of the magnetic field at the time of maximal response (at 50 msec) to tactile stimulation of the contralateral index finger (data from Fig. 9-7). The field pattern is dipolar with clearly defined regions of entering (*solid lines*) and emerging (*dashed lines*) magnetic flux.

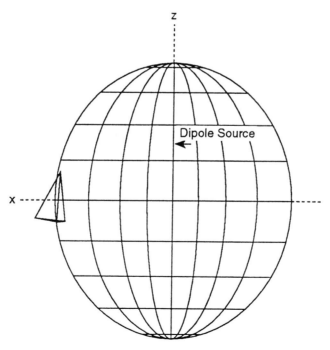

Fig. 9-9. By mathematical modeling of the magnetic field pattern, it is possible to infer the spatial location, orientation, and strength of the neuronal currents that generate the recorded data. The location is specified by *x, y,* and *z* coordinates in a head-centered coordinate system.

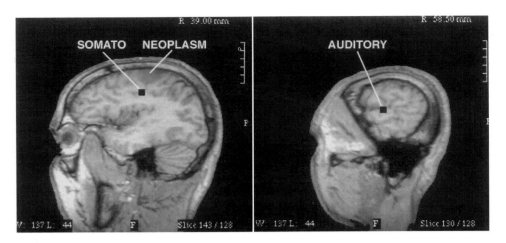

Fig. 9-10. The points used to define the MEG coordinate system (tragus of each ear and nasion) are readily identified on magnetic resonance (MR) images. Through a series of coordinate transformations, it is possible to identify the locations of MEG sources on appropriate MR images. The resultant magnetic source localization images provide a graphic representation of the spatial relationships among brain structure, function, and pathology.

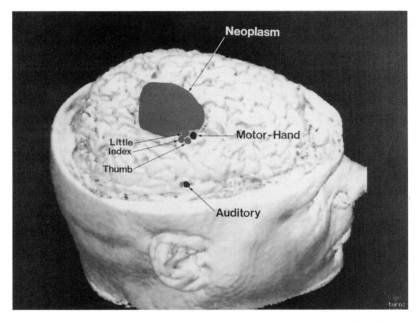

Fig. 9-11. Three-dimensional volumetric rendering of the data sets provides clinicians with concise structural and functional information.

One of the most significant advances in biomagnetism has been the development of magnetic source imaging (MSI), which combines MEG and MRI information into a merged graphic data set. MRI complements MEG functional imaging by providing exquisite resolution of brain anatomy and the structural boundaries of pathology. After identification of the points used to define the MEG coordinate space on MR images, it is possible to translate and rotate the coordinate axes so that MEG functional points can be marked with excellent precision on appropriate MR images. The resultant magnetic source localization images (Fig. 9-10) show the relationship between functional regions and pathology. In clinical practice, it is often useful to use computer reconstruction techniques that render the entire brain volume and display gross anatomy, pathology, and functional points in a single image (Fig. 9-11).

Overall, clinical applications of neuromagnetism can be divided into four basic types of examinations: (1) presurgical functional mapping, (2) characterization of epileptiform transients, (3) characterization of ALFMA, and (4) characterization of abnormal information processing. After a review of the basic principles of neuromagnetism and biomagnetic recording techniques, a review of clinical findings is provided.

NEUROPHYSIOLOGIC BASIS OF MAGNETOENCEPHALOGRAPHY

Two major classes of neuronal events can create an extracranial magnetic signal: the currents associated with postsynaptic potentials and those associated with action potentials.

For simplicity, let us first consider postsynaptic events associated with a simple excitatory synapse. After diffusion across the synaptic cleft, the neurotransmitter released from a presynaptic axon binds with receptor molecules embedded within the postsynaptic membrane. This results in a conformational change that causes, either directly or through an enzymatic cascade (e.g., the cyclic adenosine monophosphate [cAMP] second-messenger system), an increase in the membrane's permeability to positively charged sodium ions. As the positive ions enter the cell, they create a deficit of positive charges in the local extracellular space. The entering ions also cause repulsion of positive ions already within the cell and set up an axial intracellular current directed away from the region of the synapse. The intracellular current is characterized by an advancing accumulation of positive charges that causes outwardly directed transmembrane displacement currents down the length of the dendrite. The displacement currents, in turn, repel positive ions in the extracellular space and produce volume currents directed back toward the extracellular current sink near the synapse. The net volume current is equal but oppositely directed to the primary intracellular current.

In attempting to understand how external magnetic fields relate to neuronal activity, all these portions of the complete current pathway must be considered. That is, one must consider (1) transmembrane ionic and displacement currents, (2) intracellular currents, and (3) extracellular volume currents (Fig. 9-12). As given by the Biot-Savart law, each small portion of current produces a magnetic field, with the net magnetic field reflecting superposition of the field from all the current elements. It is therefore reasonable to assume that transmembrane, intracellular, and extracellular currents all make significant contributions to the extracranially recorded magnetic field. This, however, is generally incorrect, even though the Biot-Savart law holds. Consider, for example, the contribution of the transmembrane ionic and displacement currents. Swinney and Wikswo have shown that these currents contribute little to the extracranial magnetic field because they are radially symmetric around neuronal processes.[14] That is, the magnetic

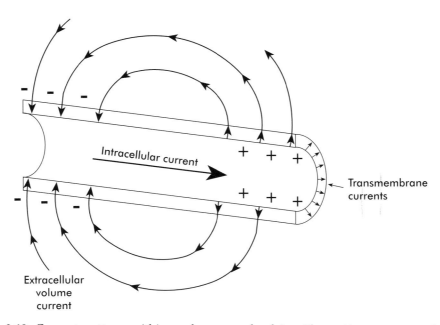

Fig. 9-12. Current pattern within and near a dendrite. The entire current path is continuous, with three parts: (1) transmembrane ionic and displacement currents, (2) intracellular currents, and (3) extracellular currents.

field from transmembrane current on one side of an axon or dendrite substantially cancels the magnetic field from oppositely directed currents around the other side of the cell.

The extent to which the extracranial neuromagnetic field reflects contributions from intracellular and extracellular currents depends on the spatial and temporal characteristics of the currents and the geometry and electrical conductivity properties of the head. To understand better how these factors interact in determining the extracranial neuromagnetic field, it is useful to consider the magnetic field generated by the simplest of current elements, the current dipole.

The *dipole* is defined by a positive and a negative charge with a primary current flowing in a straight line between these charges and return currents flowing in a dipolar pattern through the conductive medium (Fig. 9-13). The similarities between Figs. 9-13 and 9-12 should be obvious, indicating that the current dipole provides an excellent first-order representation of neuronal currents.

The exact orientation and configuration of currents associated with dendritic activity depend on the excitatory, versus the inhibitory, nature of the relevant synapse and its location along the dendritic shaft (Fig. 9-14). For example, a distal excitatory synapse gives rise to a dipolar current oriented toward the soma (Fig. 9-14,**B**), whereas a synapse located near the middle of the shaft (Fig. 9-14, **D**) induces a quadrupolar configuration of two nearby but oppositely oriented dipoles. This distinction between dipolar and quadrupolar currents is important because the magnitude of the magnetic field generated by a dipole decreases as a function of the square of the distance from the source, whereas a quadrupolar field decreases with the cube

of the distance. Therefore, magnetic fields measured at a distance more strongly reflect dipolar versus quadrupolar current components.

The neuromagnetic field associated with a single postsynaptic event is below the sensitivity of available detectors. The small magnitude of the currents associated with single postsynaptic events indicates that about 1 million synapses are synchronously active in the generation of magnetic signals of the strength typically recorded in evoked-response experiments. There are more than 100,000 pyramidal cells per square millimeter of cortex, each with thousands of synapses, so synchronous activation of as few as one synapse per thousand is probably adequate to generate a detectable extracranial signal.

The action potential is characterized by a leading edge of depolarization and a trailing edge of repolarization as it moves down an axon (Fig. 9-15). The current associated with the leading edge can be modeled by a current dipole oriented away from the cell body, whereas the currents associated with the repolarization front are modeled by a current dipole oriented toward the soma. Thus, one can conceive of the axonal impulse as a current quadrupole moving down the axon.[15,16] Given the thickness of the skull and scalp, synchronous activity in hundreds of thousands of axons would be required for generation of a measurable extracranial signal. However, the short duration and restricted spatial extent of the intracellular component of action currents make it extremely unlikely that sufficient temporal and spatial synchrony of events is generally obtained. Action potentials are therefore unlikely to make significant contributions to extracranial signals.

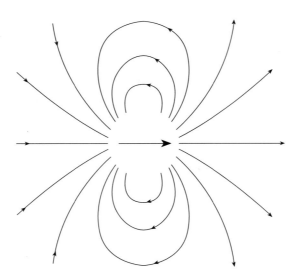

Fig. 9-13. The current pattern for a current dipole embedded in a conductive volume.

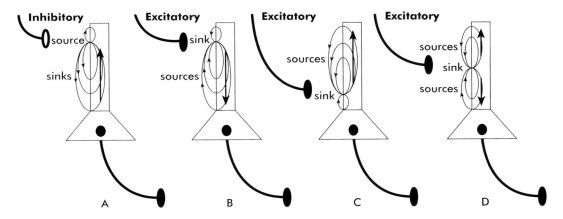

Fig. 9-14. Current configurations associated with inhibitory and excitatory synaptic activity at various points along a main dendritic shaft. Large arrows represent equivalent primary current configuration. (Modified from Lewine JD: Neuromagnetic techniques for the noninvasive analysis of brain function. In Freeman SE, Fukushima E, Greene ER, editors: Noninvasive techniques in biology and medicine, San Francisco, 1991, San Francisco Press.)

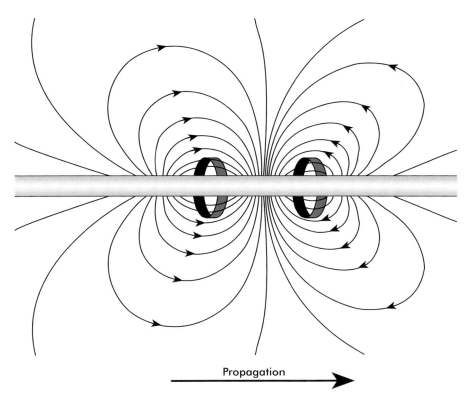

Propagation

Fig. 9-15. Current pattern associated with action potentials. (Modified from Lewine JD: Neuromagnetic techniques for the noninvasive analysis of brain function. In Freeman SE, Fukushima E, Greene ER, editors: Noninvasive techniques in biology and medicine, San Francisco, 1991, San Francisco Press.)

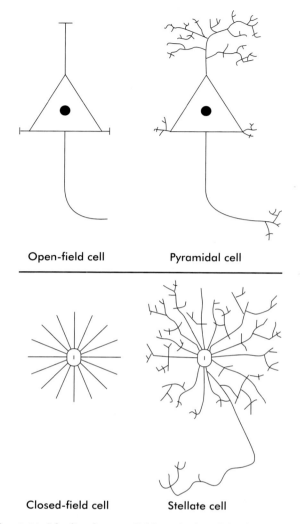

Open-field cell   Pyramidal cell

Closed-field cell   Stellate cell

Fig. 9-16. Idealized open-field and closed-field configurations and examples of nerve cells that fall into these categories. (Modified from Lewine JD: Neuromagnetic techniques for the noninvasive analysis of brain function. In Freeman SE, Fukushima E, Greene ER, editors: Noninvasive techniques in biology and medicine, San Francisco, 1991, San Francisco Press.)

When considering the magnetic field contribution of an individual neuron and the summated field generated by a neuronal ensemble, it is necessary to take into account the morphology of individual cells and the geometry with which the neurons are organized into cell clusters (Fig. 9-16). Some cells, such as stellate cells, have mostly symmetric dendritic configurations. As a consequence of this symmetry, dendritic activation produces electrical potential variations only within the region of the dendritic field. That is, the cells have a *closed-field* configuration, producing no potential variation at a distance.[17] These cells fail to

produce an external magnetic field because of symmetry in the pattern of dendritic currents.

Pyramidal cells, in contrast, have a highly asymmetric dendritic tree (typically characterized by an apical dendrite and multiple basilar dendrites). Synaptic activation of the apical dendrite causes electrical potential variations throughout the extracellular medium. That is, these cells have an *open-field* configuration. Pyramidal neurons constitute almost 70% of neocortical neurons, and the current flow in the apical dendrites of these cells is believed to be the dominant source of extracranial neuromagnetic signals.

Open-field and closed-field concepts also apply to cell ensembles. For example, many subcortical structures (e.g., vestibular nuclei) display mostly a closed-field configuration, even though they contain pyramidal cells. This is because the apical dendrites of the cells are arranged in a spherically symmetric fashion radial to the boundaries of the structure. Synchronous activation of the cells of these structures is therefore unlikely to produce a significant extracranial magnetic field because of mutual cancellation of the magnetic fields generated by the individual cells. In contrast, the neocortex, arranged into cortical columns and orthogonal laminae, possesses a mostly open-field structure.

If the conductive medium in which neurons are embedded is of infinite dimensions and uniform conductivity, only the primary current flowing within cells produces a measurable magnetic field. This is because the return current patterns are symmetric in such a way that the magnetic field generated by each return current element is canceled by the magnetic field generated by other current elements.

The medium in which neurons are embedded is not of infinite homogeneous conductivity. Therefore, in calculating neuromagnetic signals, it is important to consider boundary effects that distort the extracellular current pattern away from the symmetry seen in the unbounded situation (e.g., Fig. 9-17, **A**). In particular, on the side of higher electrical conductivity, the conductivity interface causes an increase in the current density parallel to the boundary. In evaluating the magnetic contribution of extracellular current pathways distorted by a conductivity boundary, it is useful to consider a mathematically equivalent but more tractable representation of the situation. Specifically, the conductivity boundary can be mathematically replaced by a distribution of current sources that have an equivalent effect. These secondary current sources must be placed at and oriented perpendicular to the original boundary. The magnitude of the secondary sources varies in such a way as to ensure continuity of the electrical potential. By definition, superposition of the magnetic field of the primary and secondary sources for the boundless situation is exactly equiva-

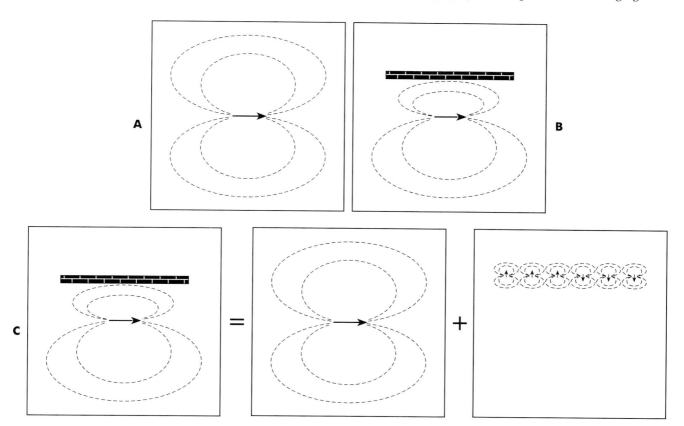

Fig. 9-17. A, The pattern of volume currents (*dashed lines*) from a primary dipolar impressed current (*arrow*) is symmetric in an infinite homogeneous medium. **B,** This pattern of symmetry is perturbed by electrical conductivity barriers. **C,** This perturbed current pattern is mathematically equivalent to that which would be produced in an infinite media by the original impressed current, plus the currents associated with secondary sources positioned at the conductivity barrier and oriented perpendicular to it. The magnetic field in this situation therefore reflects only the impressed current component of the primary and secondary sources.

lent to that generated by the dipole and its volume currents in the original bounded case.

This strategy greatly simplifies the evaluation of the magnetic field, because the changing of the original problem from bounded to nonbounded (through replacement of the boundary by secondary sources) allows volume currents to be ignored (because of symmetry).[18] The magnetic field therefore reflects only the primary current of the original and secondary sources. The primary current of secondary sources is always perpendicular to the conductivity boundary, so evaluation of the shape of the boundary provides information about the relative contribution of the secondary sources to the measured magnetic field.

To illustrate this point, consider the simplest of bounded cases, the conducting half-space. This consists of a flat surface of infinite extent with a uniform conductor on one side and an insulator on the other side (Fig. 9-17, **A**). Regardless of the orientation of the primary source, the secondary sources all align perpendicular to the conductivity boundary, with their resultant magnetic field tangential to it. Therefore, if one were to measure only the magnetic field perpendicular to the boundary, the secondary sources would make no contribution.[19] If the primary source is a dipole and it is also oriented perpendicular to the boundary, it also fails to produce a surface-normal magnetic field outside of the boundary. If, however, the dipole is not perpendicular to the boundary, the tangential current component of the primary source generates a magnetic field normal to the boundary. If measurements are made at an angle to the boundary, both primary and secondary sources may contribute to the measured signal.

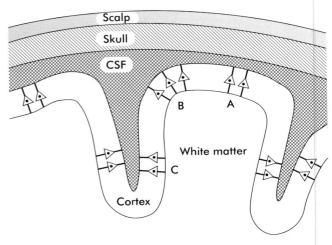

Fig. 9-19. Cells oriented perpendicular to the skull surface (**A**) fail to generate an extracranial magnetic field. Cells oriented parallel to the skull (**C**) produce a significant radial magnetic field. Cells of intermediate orientation (**B**) have both radial and tangential current components. To the extent that the head is spherical, only the tangential component of the total current generates an extracranial magnetic field. (Modified from Lewine JD: Neuromagnetic techniques for the noninvasive analysis of brain function. In Freeman SE, Fukushima E, Greene ER, editors: Noninvasive techniques in biology and medicine, San Francisco, 1991, San Francisco Press.)

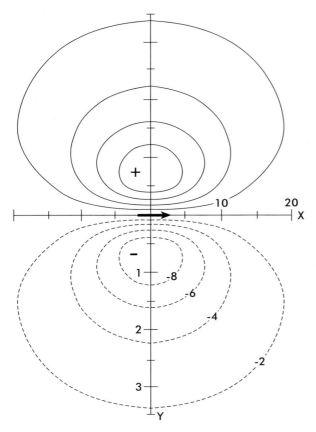

Fig. 9-18. Isofield contour map of the magnetic field generated by a dipole embedded in a half-space below the plane of measurement. The dipole (*arrow*) is located below the origin and oriented along the *x* axis. (Modified from Williamson SJ, Kaufman L: Analysis of neuromagnetic signals. In Gevins AS, Redmond A, editors: Handbook of electroencephalography and clinical neurophysiology, vol 1, Methods and analysis of brain electrical signals, Amsterdam, 1987, Elsevier.)

If the spatial pattern of the magnetic field normal to the boundary is measured selectively, and if it is known that the field is generated by a current dipole embedded within a half-space, the Biot-Savart law can be used to determine precisely the location, orientation, and strength of the primary current dipole. The magnetic field pattern generated by a dipole in a half-space is characterized by single regions of maximal emerging and entering flux. Fig. 9-18 shows an example of an isofield contour map generated by a dipole below the plane of measurement. The position of the dipole is halfway between the field maxima and minima and is oriented along the line of flux inversion (the zero cross). The depth of the dipole is proportional to the distance between regions of maximal ingoing and outgoing flux.

A more relevant situation is a current dipole embedded within a conducting sphere that provides a first-order approximation of the shape of the head. As for the half-space, the boundary perturbs the pattern of the volume currents. In characterizing the magnetic field, it is again convenient to replace the spherical boundary with a distribution of radially oriented secondary sources. The summated magnetic field produced by the secondary sources is complex, but as for the half-space, it is everywhere tangential to the original conductivity barrier. Thus, as long as only the magnetic field normal to the conductive space is considered, secondary sources do not contribute to the field. For the case of spherical symmetry, only the tangential current component of the primary source generates an external magnetic signal. This means that the normal component of neuromagnetic signals mostly reflects intracellular currents in dendrites oriented parallel to the skull surface (Fig. 9-19).

In practice, it is not always possible to make measurements exactly normal to a spherical surface. Under these circumstances, the contribution of secondary sources must be reconsidered. When doing this, it is useful to consider the radial component of the primary current (and its associated volume currents and secondary sources) separately from the tangential components. For a radial dipole, the magnetic field generated by the secondary sources exactly cancels the primary magnetic field. Therefore, regardless of what direction the field is measured in outside of the sphere, a radial dipole (and its volume currents) produces no magnetic field.

The situation for a tangential primary current is somewhat more complex because the magnetic field of the secondary sources is partly detected by nonradial sensors. The overall field depends on the measurement vector. Fortunately, the relevant biophysics has been worked out, and equations exist for exact forward calculation of the magnetic field that a tangential current dipole generates outside of a spherical conductive volume.[20] As for the half-space, the external magnetic field pattern can be used to determine the location, orientation, and the strength of the dipole, *given the knowledge that the external field pattern was generated by a dipole embedded within a sphere.* This important, italicized condition is the heart of the magnetic *inverse problem.* Calculation of the magnetic field produced by currents in a sphere involves a simple forward calculation. However, the inverse situation of specifying the exact currents that produced a particular field pattern is not simple, because an infinite number of current configurations (varying by magnetically silent sources) produce the same external field pattern. Given a particular magnetic field pattern but no simplifying constraints, it is not possible to provide a unique specification of the generative currents. Only by assuming something about the nature of the current configuration and conductive media (e.g., that a single current dipole is embedded within a sphere) does the problem become mathematically tractable. In this manner, the accuracy of inverse source modeling depends on the validity of the modeling assumptions (e.g., a current dipole in a sphere).

Real neuromagnetic measurements are invariably noisy and are typically made over a measurement surface that is not perfectly spherical. As a consequence, visual inspection of an isofield contour map can provide only coarse information of source location, and use of iterative computer algorithms is required to extract more precise source localization information.

Most of these algorithms are based on a dipole-in-a-sphere model of the magnetic field pattern. As previously discussed, this model treats the head as a uniform volume conductor with spherical symmetry, and it assumes that the magnetic field generated by the actual configuration of relevant neuronal currents can be equivalently represented as though it were produced by a point-source current dipole. Iterative dipole localization algorithms rely on least-squares minimization procedures. The interation process begins with postulation of a hypothetical current dipole at a particular location, orientation, and strength. The exact magnetic signal that this dipole would generate at each sensor is then calculated using the exact forward equations. These calculations must take into account the position, configuration, and orientation of the sensors, so it is essential to determine the precise position and orientation of the sensors relative to a head-centered coordinate frame. Generally, this is accomplished using a three-dimensional digitizer system.

The magnitude of the forward-calculated magnetic signal at each sensor is compared with the actual value recorded, and a mismatch term is calculated. This value is squared and summed across all sensors to generate an overall error term for the mismatch between the forward-calculated and the measured neuromagnetic field. The parameters of the hypothetical dipole are then changed and a new error term calculated. The algorithm works iteratively to find the parameters for the hypothetical dipole that generates the "best fit" (smallest error) between calculated and measured magnetic fields. Once the best-fitting dipole is identified, its location, orientation, and strength parameters are taken as indicative of the location, orientation, and strength of the relevant neuronal currents.

Caution must always be used in interpreting the results of these fitting procedures, because they are accurate only to the extent that the implicit assumptions of the model are correct. If, for example, the measured field actually reflects concurrent activation of two separated brain regions, but a single-dipole model is nevertheless used for inverse modeling, the location of the best-fitting dipole could be far removed from the site of any actual currents. In this situation, it is more appropriate to model the data by two dipoles. The quality of a dipole fit (e.g., the correlation between calculated and measured signals) can provide some information on the validity of a dipole model, but proper specification of model order (how many dipoles) is always problematic. Some investigators have begun to explore objective procedures (based on singular value decomposition and chi-square statistical strategies) for identification of model order, but this work is still in its initial phases.[11,21,22]

The scalp, skull, cerebrospinal fluid (CSF), and brain all display different electrical conductivities, so careful thought must be given to the use of a model that treats the head as a uniform spherical volume. Indeed, it is probably more appropriate to treat the scalp, skull, CSF, and brain as spherically concentric regions, each of homogeneous but different electrical conductivity. In calculating the electrical potential pattern produced on the scalp surface, this type of model is essential, and knowledge of the relative conductivities of the shells is critical. However, as long as the boundaries are spherically concentric, the external magnetic field is insensitive to the relative conductivities. Therefore, the simpler, single-shell model is generally adequate for evaluation of the magnetic field.[23]

Admittedly, the human head deviates somewhat from sphericity, most notably over temporal lobe regions. These deviations can result in incomplete cancellation between the magnetic fields of radial primary currents and their associated secondary sources. For some sources located under nonspherical regions, failure to take such deviations into account during inverse modeling can lead to localization errors of 1.0 cm or more. Computer algorithms that use more exact head shape information exist, but these are computationally very complex. The tradeoff between the benefits of increased accuracy and the cost of poor computational efficiency is currently under investigation in several laboratories.[24]

The assumption that the brain, skull, and scalp can each be treated as homogeneous conductive media is not fully valid. For example, neuronal and glial membranes impose nonspherical conductivity barriers in the extracellular space that cause volume currents to flow in highly convoluted and asymmetric pathways. However, because the extracellular current density is relatively low in comparison with intracellular current densities, this level of microcomplexity has only minimal effect on the extracranial field.[25]

Sensory events typically evoke synaptic activity in many thousands of cells within and across cortical columns. If the spatial extent of the evoked cortical activity is small (a few millimeters) relative to the distance at which the extracranial magnetic field is measured (a few centimeters), the magnetic field for the extended cortical source can be modeled as though it were generated by a point-source current dipole located a few millimeters deeper than the actual cortical sheet. That is, even though the actual pattern of current flow is that of a dipole sheet, first-order modeling of this activity by a single dipole still can provide very accurate localization of the "center of mass" of the activated region. Calculations by Okada suggest that the simplest evoked fields arising from the cortex reflect areas of activation on the order of 1 to 5 mm^3.[26]

Dipole strategy is successful because dipolar components of the magnetic field decrease in magnitude less rapidly with distance than higher-order terms, so even if the actual pattern of cortical currents is quite complex, provided that the extent of the activated region is small relative to the measuring distance, a simple dipole model is quite viable for localizing the activity. This is the key to the usefulness of the dipole model for source analysis, *not* the observation that the synaptic currents of individual neurons have a dipolar configuration.

The type of single-dipole analysis strategy described earlier is easily applied to the magnetic field pattern at a particular instant in time, and it provides excellent characterization of certain types of neuromagnetic activity, such as the early components of somatosensory evoked responses, and some epileptic discharges. Nevertheless, more sophisticated models that take into account the entire spatiotemporal data matrix are being developed in basic research laboratories. These algorithms will soon be available for use in the clinic, where they will prove to be especially useful in the characterization of certain epileptic conditions for which temporal definition of the pathways of seizure spread is critical.

Alternative procedures to dipole models (e.g., distributed current analysis procedures relying on linear estimation theory) are also being explored at several research sites, but at present, few specific clinical applications exist for these. Presently, dipole modeling is the mainstay of clinical applications, and although limited, it has proved to be unexpectedly useful in a number of clinical applications.

Table 9-1. Comparison of magnetic field strengths

Magnetic flux density (femotesla)	Source
10^{11}	
10^{10}	Earth's steady magnetic field
10^{9}	
10^{8}	Urban noise
10^{7}	
10^{6}	Magnetized lung contaminants
10^{5}	Abdominal currents
10^{4}	Cardiogram, oculogram
10^{3}	Epileptic and spontaneous activity
10^{2}	Corticol evoked activity
10	SQUID noise
1	Brainstem evoked activity

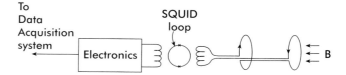

Fig. 9-20. Highly schematic diagram of typical SQUID input circuit. The neuromagnetic field induces currents in the magnetometer coils. This induces currents in the SQUID loop that are measured by the SQUID electronics.

BIOMAGNETIC RECORDING TECHNIQUES AND INSTRUMENTATION

Even the largest neuromagnetic signals (i.e., those associated with epileptic spikes) are only a few picotesla (10^{-12} T) in amplitude. This is six orders of magnitude smaller than the magnetic noise generated by power lines, cars, and elevators; eight orders of magnitude smaller than the Earth's steady magnetic field; and 12 orders of magnitude smaller than the 1.5 Tesla magnetic field of clinical MR imagers, which may be located less than a hundred feet from where neuromagnetic experiments are performed (Table 9-1).

Two significant problems arise in the evaluation of neuromagnetic signals: (1) the inherently small magnitude of the signal demands an extremely sensitive measuring device, and (2) these weak signals must be extracted from excessive background noise. As Dr. Christopher Gallen, director of the magnetic source imaging facility at the Scripps Clinic and Research Foundation in San Diego, is fond of saying, "Recording neuromagnetic signals is like listening for the footsteps of an ant in the middle of a rock concert." It is a significant scientific accomplishment that the hardware and signal-processing tools for accomplishing the task are now available for routine clinical use.

When a time-varying magnetic field passes perpendicular to the plane of a wire loop, it induces a small electrical current within the wire. The efficiency of this coupling partly depends on the number of turns in the detection coil and the electrical properties of the wire. As first shown in the late 1960s and early 1970s, it is possible to record neuromagnetic signals (the alpha rhythm) at room temperature using a 2 million–turn induction coil. However, the thermal noise of such a system renders it impractical for measuring the weaker neuromagnetic signals of clinical interest.

Sensitivity to very weak signals requires the use of cryogenic technologies. The simplest of modern-day neuromagnetic detectors consists of an induction loop of niobium wire, which is maintained in a superconducting state by immersing it in a liquid helium bath. When brought to extremely low temperatures (approximately $-258°$ C for niobium), certain materials become superconducting and lose their resistivity to the flow of electrical currents. This allows very small changes in magnetic flux (e.g., those associated with neuronal activity) to cause significant changes in the amount of current flowing within the wire. In modern biomagnetometers, the superconducting loop is inductively coupled to a SQUID that produces a voltage output proportional to the current flowing in the input coil (Fig. 9-20). That is, the SQUID acts as a high-gain current-to-voltage converter. It is important to note that the SQUID magnetometer is sensitive only to a change in the magnetic field, so the Earth's "steady" magnetic field has little effect on the SQUID output.

The SQUID consists of a ring of superconducting material interrupted by Josephson junctions. When a ring of superconducting wire is interrupted by a sizable resistive segment, it behaves as though the entire ring were made of resistive material. The current in such a ring dissipates quickly because energy is lost at the resistive section. However, if the ring is interrupted by only a microscopically thin section of nonsuperconducting material, the whole ring can still act as a superconductor, provided that the current is small enough. For currents less than the critical current of the Josephson junction, electrons can "tunnel" through the resistive segment without loss of energy.

A superconducting ring also acts as an induction coil, with any change in the magnetic field impinging on the ring, causing a change in the magnitude of current flowing in the ring. If the level of current in the ring is already at the critical current, a small change in the impinging magnetic field can cause the total current to exceed the critical value, a situation that causes a measurable voltage drop across the Josephson junction. Most large-array biomagnetometers use SQUIDs with two identical weak links (Josephson junctions) operated in a DC-biased mode.

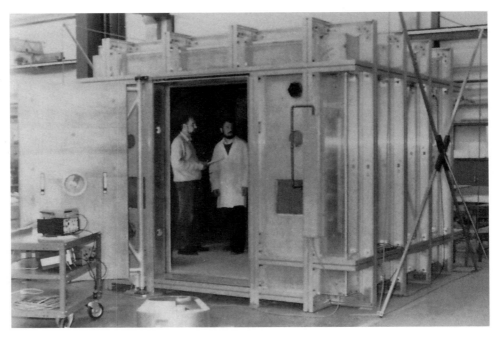

Fig. 9-21. Commercial magnetically shielded room showing first layer of mu-metal shielding and a rigid aluminum frame. (Courtesy of Vacuumschmelze, GmbH, Hanau, Germany.)

For these SQUIDs, a small DC current from the control electronics is applied to the ring to maintain the current crossing each junction just below the critical current level. The entire system works as follows:

1. Time-varying neuromagnetic fields induce currents in the detection coil that cause current flow in the input coil of the detection circuit.
2. These currents generate a magnetic field that influences the SQUID ring by induction.
3. The ring responds to this field with additional current to buck the field, so the critical current is exceeded and a detectable voltage drop occurs across the weak link.
4. This voltage drop is detected by the SQUID electronics, which in turn apply a feedback current to the ring to counterbalance the induced current.
5. The magnitude of the required feedback current is measured by the voltage produced across a resistor in the feedback circuit, and this serves as the output of the magnetometer system.

In this fashion, the SQUID electronics transforms a small, neuromagnetically induced current change in the input coil into a large-amplitude voltage signal.

The type of magnetometer system just described is so sensitive to magnetic signals that, if operated in an open hospital environment, it is overwhelmed by magnetic noise from power lines, elevators, and so on. Two technological developments help avoid this situation by suppressing much of the background noise.

Operating the magnetometer in a room with walls made of materials of high magnetic permeability partly shields the sensor from external magnetic fields. Just as different materials have differing electrical resistivity, they also have differing magnetic permeability. Most magnetically shielded rooms have one or more layers of an alloy known as mu metal (Fig. 9-21). The magnetic permeability of mu metal is 80,000 (compared with the permeability of 1 for air and other nonmetallic materials). The mu metal is typically mounted on an aluminum plate that serves as an eddy-current magnetic and radiofrequency shield. When an external magnetic flux impinges on the room, it takes the path of greatest permeability — through the walls around and away from the internally located sensor system. The shielding capability of the room varies as a function of the frequency characteristics of the noise. For a typical room, magnetic noise of less than 0.1 Hz is shielded by only 20 to 30 dB, whereas higher-frequency signals (e.g., 100 Hz) are attenuated by as much as 50 to 60 dB.

Even this level of attenuation is not fully adequate for making measurements with a simple magnetometer system, because the magnetic noise that makes it through the shielding is still several orders of magnitude larger than biomagnetic signals. Fortunately, by modifying the configuration of the detection circuit, it is possible to isolate neuromagnetic signals.

The strength of the magnetic field generated by a dipolar magnetic source decreases with the square of the distance from the source. This means that near a source, the spatial gradient of the field is steep, whereas far from the source, the gradient is shallow. For example, field strength of a dipolar source decreases by 75% when the measuring distance is increased from 2 to 4 cm, but it changes less than 1% when the distance changes an equivalent 2 cm from 1002 to 1004 centimeters. Therefore, by measuring the spatial gradient of the field rather than the overall magnitude of the field, it is possible to emphasize signals from sources near the detection system (e.g., neuronal sources) while deemphasizing the contribution from distant but stronger noise sources.

Most biomagnetometer systems have their detectors configured as axial first-order gradiometers. In these systems, the detector consists of two coil loops wound in opposition and connected in series (Fig. 9-22). A time-varying magnetic field passing through the detector induces oppositely directed currents within the lower pickup coil and the upper bucking coil. These currents partly cancel, with the net current reflecting the spatial gradient of the field. If the gradient is shallow (as it is far from a source), each coil experiences a nearly identical field—nearly identical currents are induced—and their cancellation is nearly complete. If the gradient is steep (as it is near a source), a significant mismatch occurs in the currents induced in the two coils, so there is a significant net output. If the distance between the two coils (the baseline) is less than 4 cm, when the detector is placed at the head

surface, the output of the gradiometer mostly reflects the magnetic field of nearby neuronal sources.

Early biomagnetometer systems typically employed second-order gradiometers (Fig. 9-23) that measured the second spatial derivative of the magnetic field. This provided even better rejection of far-field noise, but it also partly compromised the sensitivity of these systems to deep neuronal sources.

The vast majority of work in biomagnetism has been accomplished with axial gradiometer configurations. However, off-diagonal planar configurations are now finding more widespread use (Fig. 9-24). This type of gradiometer has several advantages over axial configurations, including its compact size and the availability of thin-film techniques for efficient fabrication. The spatial sensitivity pattern of planar gradiometers is narrower and shallower than that of their axial counterparts. That is, the planar sensor detects fields from a more spatially restricted area. However, because the baseline of planar gradiometers is gener-

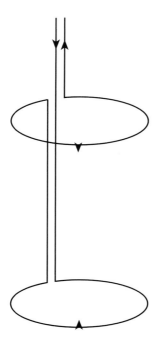

Fig. 9-22. Schematic of axial first-order gradiometer.

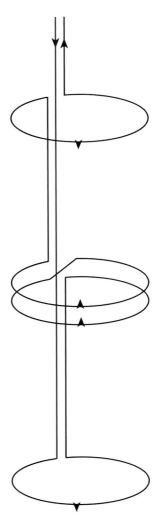

Fig. 9-23. Schematic of axial second-order gradiometer.

ally short, they are less sensitive to deeper sources than standard axial configurations. Regardless of the type of gradiometer employed, the number of detectors remains one of the most important aspects of a biomagnetometer system. Only through the use of large-array systems can clinical applicability be achieved.

Four companies offer large-array biomagnetometer systems: Biomagnetic Technologies, Inc. (BTi); Siemens; CTF Systems, Inc.; and Neuromag Ltd. Several custom-designed, large-array systems are also in rou-

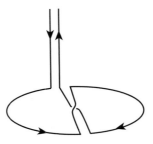

Fig. 9-24. Schematic of off-diagonal planar gradiometer.

tine use throughout the world, as are several small-array (one- to seven-channel) systems.

The Magnes system of BTi is presently the most common clinical system, with installations at nearly a dozen sites worldwide. Magnes (Fig. 9-25) consists of 37 first-order axial gradiometers arranged on a hexagonal grid with an intersensor spacing of about 2 cm. The diameter of the coil array is 14.4 cm. The sensors are contained in a cryogenic dewar that is easily moved over regions of interest. BTi has recently manufactured an inverted sensor system that can be used in conjunction with Magnes to provide for simultaneous bilateral recordings (Fig. 9-26).

Siemens also offers a 37-channel system, Krenikon. Krenikon, as with Magnes, consists of axial first-order gradiometers. The most fundamental difference between the Magnes and Krenikon systems is that the Magnes sensors are arranged along a spherical cap (radius of curvature, 10 cm) designed to allow for close positioning on a spherical head, whereas the Krenikon sensors are arranged on a flat plane, which also allows efficient use of the system in cardiac experiments (Fig. 9-27).

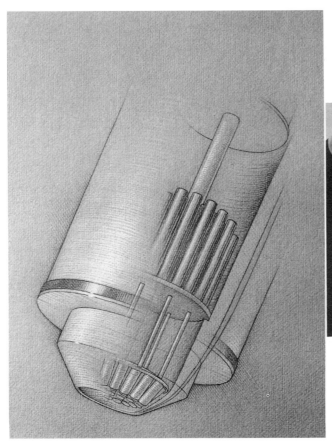

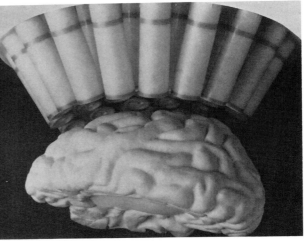

Fig. 9-25. The 37-channel Magnes biomagnetometer system of Biomagnetic Technologies, Inc. (BTi). (Courtesy of Biomagnetic Technologies, Inc, San Diego.)

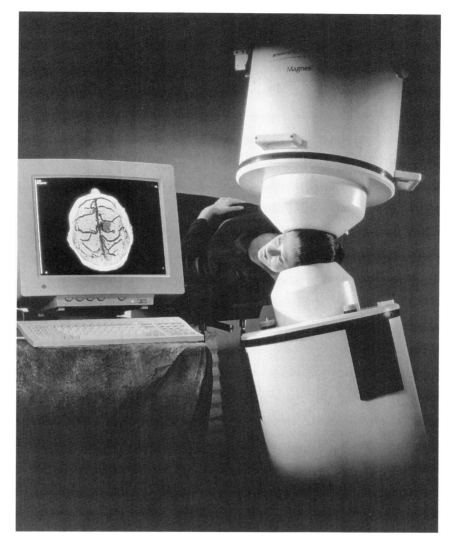

Fig. 9-26. Dual 37-channel units of BTi allow for simultaneous recording from the two hemispheres. (Courtesy of Biomagnetic Technologies, Inc., San Diego.)

Multichannel systems of the type just described cover a sufficiently large area of the head to be efficient in most routine clinical applications, such as localization of sensorimotor cortex and localization of focal epileptiform discharges. However, when an *a priori* estimate of the location of the relevant neuronal activity is not possible (e.g., in cases of cortical reorganization induced by a cerebrovascular accident), the dewar may need to be repositioned several times during the course of a study. Two companies, CTF Systems Inc. and Neuromag Ltd., therefore have focused efforts on the development of whole-head systems. Both companies have successfully solved several practical problems in the building of such a device, including the construction of an appropriately insulated, helmetlike dewar large enough to accommodate most patients.

The CTF whole-head system consists of 64 axial first-order gradiometers arranged on a semiregular grid (Fig. 9-28). The average center-to-center spacing between detectors is 4 cm, somewhat larger than ideal, but adequate for most routine clinical examinations. An interesting feature of the CTF system is the presence of 16 reference channels. Using electronics based on digital signal processors, data from the reference channels can be combined with data from the sensor channels to simulate second- and third-order gradiometers. This allows the system to be operated without a magnetically shielded room (although with reduced sensitivity to deep neuronal sources).

The whole-head system of Neuromag (Fig. 9-29) differs from most other neuromagnetometer systems in that it employs planar gradiometers. The system has

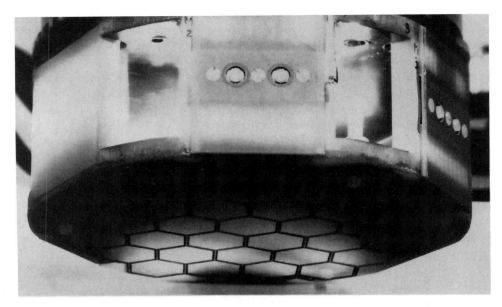

Fig. 9-27. The 37-channel Krenikon system of Siemens. Note the flat dewar bottom compared with the concave bottom of the BTi Magnes system. (Courtesy of Siemens, Erlangen, Germany.)

61 recording sites. Each site has two orthogonal sensors for independent measurement of the two tangential derivatives of the magnetic field. The separation between double sensor units is about 43 mm. This large spacing nevertheless provides adequate spatial sampling of the field, because simultaneous measurement of two planar gradients corresponds to an axial gradiometer sampling grid that is denser by a factor of 1.4.

CLINICAL APPLICATIONS
Presurgical Functional Mapping

In the neurosurgical treatment of brain neoplasms, vascular malformations, and epilepsy, precise localization of eloquent cortex is essential to minimize postoperative neurologic deficits yet allow for the maximal removal of nearby dysfunctional tissue.[27-29]

Empirical and clinical study have yielded some guidelines on the relationship between brain function and structure, especially for primary sensory and motor areas. However, individual variability in brain morphology and physiology often renders this general knowledge only modestly valuable in neurosurgical planning. A recent study by Sobel and colleagues compared two different neuroradiologists on the identification of the central sulcus from MR images.[30] For more than 20% of the 127 MRI sections examined, the radiologists disagreed by more than one sulcus. This situation undoubtedly becomes worse when the brain is distorted by structural pathology, and it is problematic because central sulcus identification is particularly salient in neurosur-

gical practice, because inadvertent damage to motor cortex can dramatically lower the quality of life after surgery.

The most widely accepted standard procedures for functional localization of sensorimotor cortex are direct electrical stimulation of motor cortex[31] and electrocorticographic (ECoG) monitoring of somatosensory evoked responses at the brain surface.[32,33] Unfortunately, these methods are not without drawbacks. Intraoperative monitoring may substantially lengthen surgical time and can increase the risk of infection. The quality of ECoG data often depends on the location and extent of the craniotomy,[34] and the data are not always easily interpretable. The greatest limitation of this procedure is that the crucial information is not available until after a particular surgical approach has been initiated. If detailed knowledge of the spatial relationship between the location of pathology and the location of cortex responsible for specific brain functions is available presurgically, it will facilitate risk assessment, craniotomy site selection, and decisions about how aggressively to resect pathologic tissue.

Functional mapping of sensorimotor cortex is now part of the routine clinical practice of several clinical MEG facilities.[35,36] Mapping of the auditory cortex is also prominent. For each of these modalities, it is possible to identify time points in the evoked neuromagnetic signal where the field pattern is believed to reflect activity of a focal neuronal population readily characterized by simple single-dipole models. Studies of the visual system are less commonplace because visual evoked fields generally have complex structures

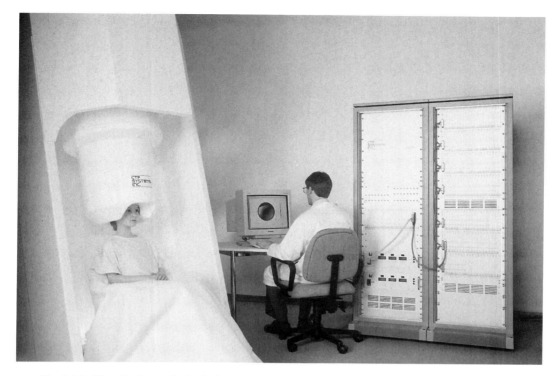

Fig. 9-28. The 64-channel whole-head system of CTF Systems, Inc. (Courtesy of CTF Systems Inc., Vancouver, British Colombia.)

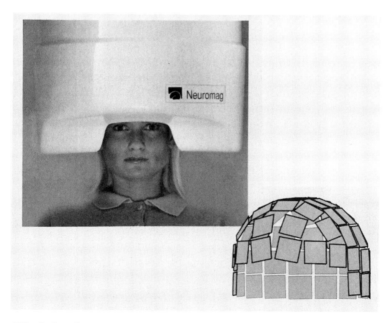

Fig. 9-29. Whole-head 122 planar gradiometer system of Neuromag Ltd. (Courtesy of Neuromag Ltd., Helsinki, Finland.)

indicative of concurrent activation of multiple visual cortical regions.

Mapping of the somatosensory cortex is generally considered the easiest and most straightforward of the MEG mapping procedures. Mapping of the face representation is generally accomplished by tactile or vibratory stimulation of the lower lip. The hand area can be assessed by tactile, vibratory, or electrical stimulation of the digits or, alternatively, by electrical stimulation of the median nerve. Electrical stimulation of the tibial nerve is typically used to localize the foot representation of primary somatosensory cortex. In all cases, the experiments take advantage of standard signal-averaging techniques. The stimulus is pre-

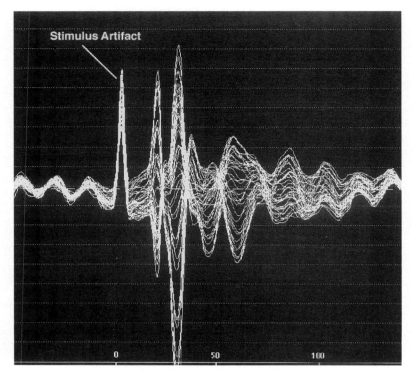

Fig. 9-30. Average neuromagnetic response ($n = 512$) to stimulation of the contralateral median nerve. Data were recorded with a Magnes system. Waveforms from all 37-channels are overlaid. There is an electrical artifact at time zero, followed by a series of neuromagnetic responses.

sented multiple times, and data epochs spanning the stimulus are averaged together to extract time-locked neuromagnetic signals from the background noise.

Fig. 9-30 shows an example set of neuromagnetic waveforms evoked by stimulation of the right median nerve of a normal subject. The data were collected at the Albuquerque Magnetic Source Imaging Facility using a 37-channel Magnes biomagnetometer system. The waveforms are characterized by a stimulus artifact associated with the applied electrical current and a sequence of subsequent neuromagnetic oscillations. Dipole modeling of the instantaneous magnetic field at the peak latency for each of the short-latency (less than 50 msec) neuromagnetic components is straightforward, with the best-fitting model generally providing an excellent account of the empirical data (r greater than 0.97). Source locations for each peak invariably fall within a few millimeters of each other, and in normal subjects, the sources consistently localize to the primary somatosensory cortex of the postcentral gyrus (as identified by structural methods). Later components of the waveform (at latencies greater than 70 msec) generally fail to be adequately characterized by single-dipole algorithms. Multiple-dipole modeling of these data indicates that these components reflect concurrent activation of primary somatosensory cortex and secondary somatosensory cortex (located

along the inferior parietal lobule). The exact latencies at which activation of primary somatosensory cortex dominates the neuromagnetic signal depend on the site and type of stimulation, but in all cases, components earlier than 50 msec seem to reflect activation of the primary cortical area.

For several patients, the availability of MEG somatosensory data has had a significant impact on surgical treatment. The MR images in Fig. 9-31 were obtained from a 35 year-old-male who initially experienced mild numbness and motor impairment of the right leg and foot. Three weeks after the onset of symptoms, the patient had several seizures. MRI revealed a large, left parietal neoplasm believed to be a high-grade astrocytoma. The tumor was unresponsive to radiation therapy. The patient was initially considered a poor surgical candidate because the tumor was believed to invade the sensorimotor strip. The lesion was quite large and caused significant distortion of the local neuroanatomy, especially near the midline (Fig. 9-32). This compromised conventional MRI methods for identification of the central sulcus. Each of four neuroradiologists shown the entire MRI series (available in all three planes) indicated difficulty in conclusive identification of the central sulcus. Nevertheless, each independently indicated that sulcus **B** was the most likely candidate and that the tumor would not be

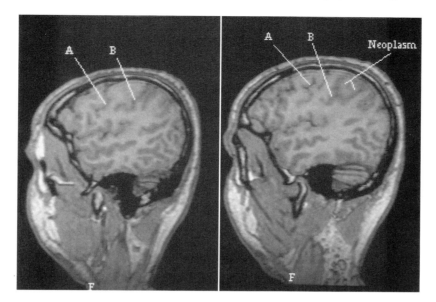

Fig. 9-31. Select MR images from a patient with a parietal neoplasm. The tumor was considered inoperable because neuroradiologists suspected suclus **B** to be the central sulcus. (From Benzel EC, Lewine JD, Bucholz RC et al: Magnetic source imaging: a review of the Magnes system by Biomagnetic Technologies Incorporated, Neurosurgery 33:252-259, 1993.)

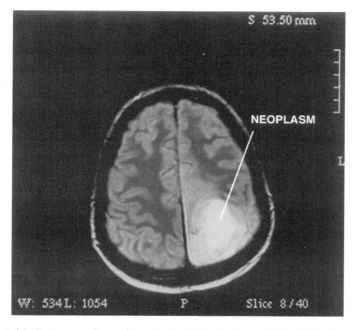

Fig. 9-32. Axial MR images show the extent of the lesion and the distortion of the local anatomy.

resectable without compromise of motor function. In contrast, MSI of responses to tactile stimulation of the digits of the right hand strongly implied that sulcus **A** was the central sulcus (Fig. 9-33). These later data were sufficient to convince a surgical team that a successful resection was possible. The patient was taken to surgery, where intraoperative monitoring of somatosensory evoked response confirmed the validity of

the MEG inference (Fig. 9-34). The neoplasm of this patient with an "inoperable tumor" by conventional neuroradiologic standards was resected without induction of motor deficits.

In several instances, there has been the opportunity to evaluate, with sterotaxic precision, noninvasive MEG inferences on the location of somatosensory cortex. Fig. 9-35 shows an example data set. In all cases,

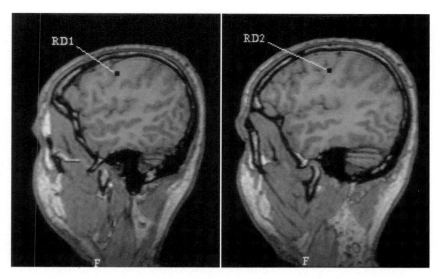

Fig. 9-33. Magnetic source localization images showing that the somatosensory responses to tactile stimulation of the contralateral digits localize along sulcus **A**, significantly anterior to the lesion. (From Benzel EC, Lewine JD, Bucholz RC et al: Magnetic source imaging: a review of the Magnes system by Biomagnetic Technologies Incorporated, Neurosurgery 33:252-259, 1993.)

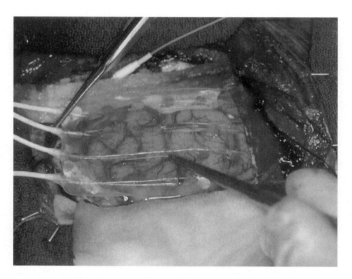

Fig. 9-34. Intraoperative electrocorticographic (ECoG) assessment of the somatosensory evoked potential to median nerve stimulation confirmed the noninvasive MEG inference that somatosensory and motor cortices were significantly anterior to the lesion. The neoplasm was resected without inducing functional deficits.

the agreement between invasive and noninvasive methods has been excellent, with the MEG median nerve source localizing within the brain tissue directly beneath the position identified by surface ECoG monitoring of the somatosensory evoked potential.[34,37]

Direct MEG studies of motor function are somewhat more difficult to execute because they require that the patient be able to make smooth, well-controlled movements of the hand. In the typical experiment, subjects flex or extend one or more digits

of the hand in a self-paced or visually cued manner. Either the EMG is used as a trigger or the movement is such that it triggers a photooptic switch. Signals are back-averaged to identify the primary motor field. Fig. 9-36 provides examples of motor waveforms recorded with a Magnes system. A slow dipolar shift in the magnetic signal begins a few hundred milliseconds before movement. This generally peaks 20 to 50 msec before movement onset and is followed by a large dipolar signal. Source modeling shows that the field peaking 20 to 50 msec before movement onset reflects

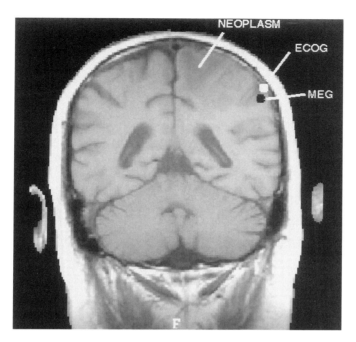

Fig. 9-35. Comparison of noninvasive MEG source localization and intraoperative ECoG surface localization of median nerve response in a patient in whom an intraoperative sterotactic wand system was used to localize the ECoG grid.

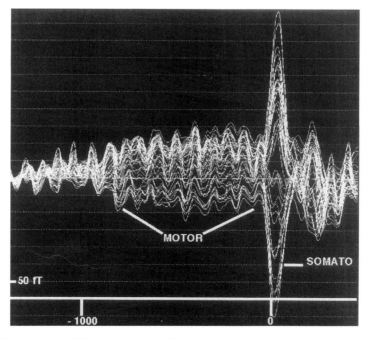

Fig. 9-36. Example of MEG waveforms related to movement of the contralateral thumb. Data were collected using a Magnes system. Data from all 37 channels are overlaid. The movement occurred at time zero. There is a slow shift preceding the movement, followed by a large postmovement somatosensory response.

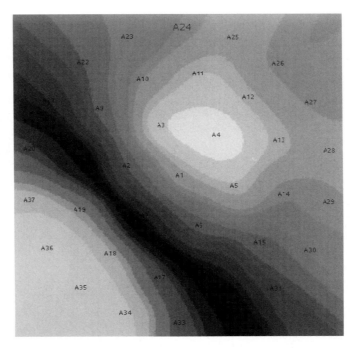

Fig. 9-37. The premovement field of the data in Fig. 9-36 has a dipolar source configuration.

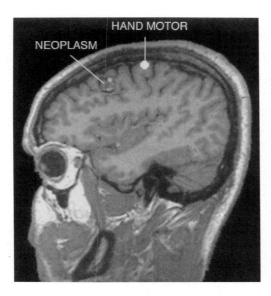

Fig. 9-38. Magnetic source localization image showing left thumb motor source for a patient with a right frontal lesion. (From Lewine JD, Orrison WW, Halliday A et al: MEG functional mapping in epilepsy surgery. In Cascino GD, Jack CR, editors: Neuroimaging in epilepsy: principles and practice, Boston, 1994, Butterworth and Heinemann.)

primary motor activation. The primary motor field is generally dipolar (Fig. 9-37), and its source localizes to the anterior bank of the central sulcus. The subsequent, often larger signal actually represents feedforward and feedback activation of somatosensory cortex. Fig. 9-38 shows the left thumb motor source for a

patient with a right hemispheric lesion. The data indicated that primary motor cortex was significantly posterior to the posterior margin of the lesion, which was subsequently resected without induction of motor deficits.

Because of the strong bilateral projections of the auditory system, unilateral compromise of primary auditory cortex is generally found to be significantly less devastating than compromise of motor cortex. However, given the proximity of primary auditory cortex to language areas, it is often useful to localize this region in neurosurgical patients. Presentation of a short-duration tone generally evokes a series of neuromagnetic oscillations that correspond to P50, N100, and P200 evoked potential components (Fig. 9-39). Additional longer-latency components may be identified in some stimulation paradigms. The N100 response is generally the strongest, and in standard paradigms, it is dipolar in configuration. N100 is believed to reflect activation of primary auditory cortex and concurrent activation of contiguous posterior association cortex.

Fig. 9-40 shows an interesting case in which an inferior parietal neoplasm caused distortion of the tonotopic map of auditory cortex. Normally, there is an orderly representation of tonal frequencies along the superior temporal surface, with higher-frequency tones mapping medial to lower-frequency tones.[38] In this patient, the response to a 3000 Hz tone was lateral to the response for a 1500 Hz tone. It is also noteworthy that right median nerve stimulation in this

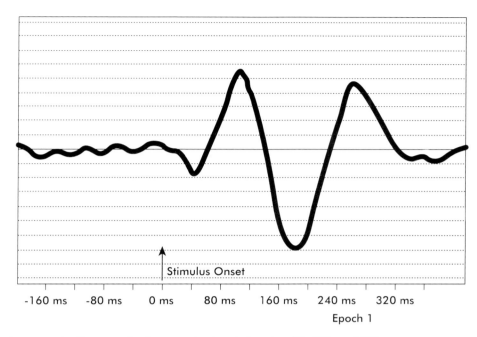

Fig. 9-39. Auditory evoked magnetic signal showing 50, 100, and 200 msec components corresponding to the P50, N100, and P200 of the auditory evoked potential.

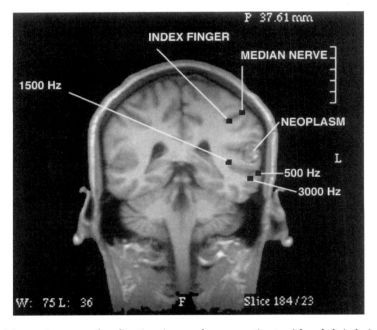

Fig. 9-40. Magnetic source localization image from a patient with a left inferior parietal neoplasm. The normal tonotopic organization of auditory cortex is distorted (the source for response to a 3000 Hz tone is lateral to that for a 1500 Hz tone), possibly because of cortical reorganization induced by a mass effect from the neoplasm.

patient failed to elicit those portions of the evoked signal typically associated with activation of secondary somatosensory areas on the left. This suggests that the neoplasm interfered with processing in this area, as expected from the inferior parietal location

of the neoplasm. Few presurgical studies of visual function have been performed because the magnetic field evoked by transient visual stimuli is generally too complex for standard dipole modeling. However, using very small, short-duration stimuli or small

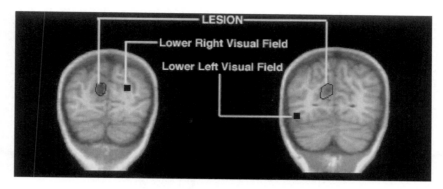

Fig. 9-41. Magnetic source localization images showing unusual visual response in right hemisphere.

checkerboard patterns undergoing rapid (greater than 10 Hz) contrast reversals, it is sometimes possible to isolate what appear to be dipolar visual responses.

Fig. 9-41 shows an interesting data set from a 9-year-old girl with a right occipital lesion. Stimulation of the right lower visual field with a small "X" evoked a sequence of neuromagnetic oscillations with a dipolar source at 200 msec. As is true for normal subjects, the source localized to the left parietal-occipital sulcus. Stimulation of the lower left quadrant (where visual field perimetry showed a moderate stimulus detection deficit) also evoked a response, but this localized to an uncharacteristic location along the right temporal-occipital gyrus. That is, the left and right hemispheric responses were highly asymmetric, with the unusual right hemispheric response perhaps reflecting some degree of cortical reorganization induced by the lesion.

Attempts to use evoked-response methods to evaluate a variety of cognitive functions (e.g., language, attention, memory) are underway at several research sites, but these types of studies have yet to be sufficiently developed and validated to the point where they can be used diagnostically in routine clinical practice.

It has been suggested that much less expensive EEG techniques can achieve functional mapping of primary areas as accurately and efficiently as MEG. In considering localization of the central sulcus, this could prove true for normal subjects, but the situation for patients is less clear. Indeed, the general lack of published reports of intraoperatively validated presurgical localization of central sulcus by scalp EEG suggests that the situation is not as straightforward as many critics of MEG argue. Only Sutherling and colleagues[34] have published relevant data, and none of the patients studied had lesions immediately adjacent to the central sulcus. This is an important consideration because tumors and other types of pathology generally have electrical conductivity prop-

erties that differ from surrounding healthy brain tissue. The physical phantom studies of Lewine et al.[39] suggest that this is likely to be much more problematic for EEG source localization procedures than it is for MEG procedures. Lewine and colleagues have recently evaluated one surgical patient in whom both MEG and high-density EEG data were obtained for presurgical mapping of sensorimotor cortex. MEG correctly identified the central sulcus (as confirmed by stereotactic ECoG), but EEG incorrectly implicated a more posterior sulcus near the lesion (Fig. 9-42).

One important recent advance in the presurgical mapping arena has been the refinement of techniques for display of the data. Of particular note are three-dimensional-rendering procedures that can provide surgeons with a more familiar view of the relationship between functional areas and pathology. Fig. 9-43 shows an interesting data set from a 28-year-old male with a recent history of seizures. MRI revealed the presence of a region of increased signal intensity near the presumed frontal-parietal border. MSI showed that sources for tactile stimulation of the digits of the hand and also movements of the hand localized just inferior to the mass. 3D rendering of the data set showed that the mass invaded superior portions of the sensorimotor strip. The MSI data were used to guide a biopsy away from central sulcus. The biopsy showed the presence of a low-grade glioma, which was treated with radiation therapy rather than more aggressive surgical intervention.

Current efforts in image processing are focusing on the integration of MR angiography data into the volume rendering because these will provide the operating team with visible, familiar, and effective landmarks during the surgical procedure.

Characterization of Epileptiform Transients

One of the oldest and most important clinical applications of MEG is the localization of epileptiform

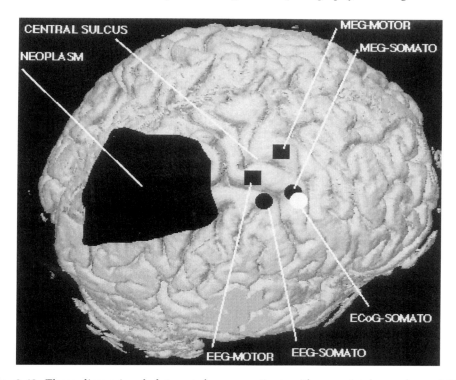

Fig. 9-42. Three-dimensional data set from a patient with a parietal neoplasm. MEG provides correct identification of the central sulcus (as confirmed by ECoG), whereas EEG incorrectly identifies a more posterior sulcus. (Modified from Lewine JD, Orrison WW, Halliday A et al: MEG functional mapping in epilepsy surgery. In Cascino GD, Jack CR, editors: Neuroimaging in epilepsy: principles and practice, Boston, 1994, Butterworth and Heinemann.)

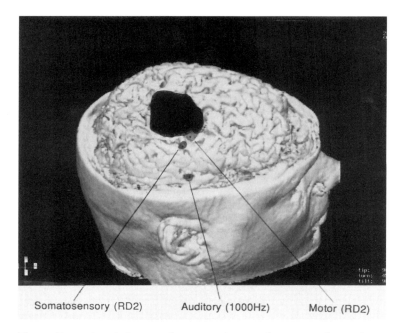

Fig. 9-43. Three-dimensional data set from a patient with a parietal neoplasm. The data show that neoplasm is too close the central sulcus for easy resection. (From Benzel EC, Lewine JD, Bucholz RC et al: Magnetic source imaging: a review of the Magnes system by Biomagnetic Technologies Incorporated, Neurosurgery 33:252-259, 1993.)

activity. Just under 1% of the population has epilepsy, and for almost 20% of these patients, anticonvulsant medications are contraindicated or ineffective in the control of seizures. In these patients, surgical treatment is considered. Effective surgical intervention requires accurate knowledge of the location of the relevant pathologic tissue. In some patients, obvious lesions account for the pathology, but even when a lesion is present, the site of an epileptic focus can be far removed. Neuroimaging by SPECT, PET, and other techniques is often used in the evaluation of epilepsy, and MEG is beginning to play a significant role.

The monitoring of a seizure with depth electrodes is considered the "gold standard" for localizing an epileptic focus before surgical resection.[40] Unfortunately, the implantation of the electrodes is a risky and expensive surgical procedure at the onset, and depth probes are not well tolerated by children. Relatively few hospitals have appropriate facilities for depth monitoring, so this has become a significant bottleneck in the surgical treatment of patients. Therefore, noninvasive evaluation is becoming increasingly important in the search for effective therapeutic and surgical interventions.

During the 1980s, MEG studies of epilepsy were performed at three major clinical research centers: University of California in Los Angeles (UCLA), National Institutes of Health (NIH), and University of Rome. This early work used available small-array systems (with seven or fewer channels) to characterize interictal epileptic spikes. Because a single dewar placement was not adequate to capture fully the spatial pattern of magnetic activity associated with an individual spike, special triggering, relative covariance, and signal-averaging techniques had to be developed to combine spatial data across separate spike events. Several excellent reviews of these innovative methods and early results are available,[41-44] so these studies are not discussed here. During the last few years, large-array systems have greatly improved the efficiency and accuracy of epilepsy examinations and have allowed for localization of individual epileptic events.[45-49] Fig. 9-44, shows sample MEG data obtained from a patient with a known right temporal lobe focus.

There are several important issues in the characterization of epileptic activity by MEG. First, MEG evaluations generally focus on interictal activity, although seizure onsets have been recorded occasionally. The debate on the necessity for ictal electrophysiologic observations (whether MEG or EEG) has yet to be resolved, but it is now clear that interictal MEG can be as informative as other interictal techniques such as PET and conventional EEG. Although it remains to be seen if MEG can provide an adequate alternative to ictal depth electrode recordings, interictal data obtained via MEG are already being used to guide the placement of depth probes.

Another issue concerns the validity of the single-dipole model in the characterization of epileptic spikes. In some patients, it is clear that multiple extended regions contribute to a spike, so a simple dipole model is inappropriate. However, some spikes are well characterized by single dipoles, and the relevant epileptic zone can be localized with considerable ease and accuracy, as confirmed by ECoG.[43,50-52] The challenge to the clinician is to be aware that the nondipolarity of a spike does not minimize its importance to the clinical picture.

A final issue of relevance is the usefulness of MEG versus surface EEG. The development of MEG has led to a focused effort on the refinement of source modeling tools for EEG.[53] As a consequence, the extent to which the high cost of MEG is justified has been challenged repeatedly.

To date, few studies have compared MEG and EEG source localizations directly. However, Ebersole and colleagues have recently initiated comparative studies in patients with temporal lobe epilepsy. These studies have already yielded several important results.[54-56] For example, it is now clear that some epileptic spikes prevalent in the EEG do not have simultaneous MEG counterparts. More surprising is the converse observation of epileptiform events in the MEG without correlates in simultaneous EEG data. Ebersole has also found that MEG data are often more easily modeled than corresponding EEG data, partly because of MEG's insensitivity to radial currents. In several patients in whom the location of the dominant epileptogenic zone was independently evaluated by depth probes, MEG source locations were found to be considerably more accurate than EEG source locations. This presumably reflects the significant impact that temporal lobe deviations from sphericity can have on standard EEG source modeling procedures.

MEG is proving particularly useful in the evaluation of patients when it is difficult to determine if the two hemispheres show independent spiking versus correlated spiking (with one side leading the other). Whereas an epileptic spike originating from one hemisphere often generates a strong EEG signal over the other hemisphere, this is generally not the case for MEG. When MEG data are collected over the two hemispheres simultaneously (using dual-probe or whole-head systems), quick visual inspection of the data is often adequate to determine the temporal relationship between spikes.

Despite these advantages of MEG over EEG investigations of temporal lobe epilepsy, in most patients, MEG merely serves to refine information already available from other imaging modalities. That is, MEG

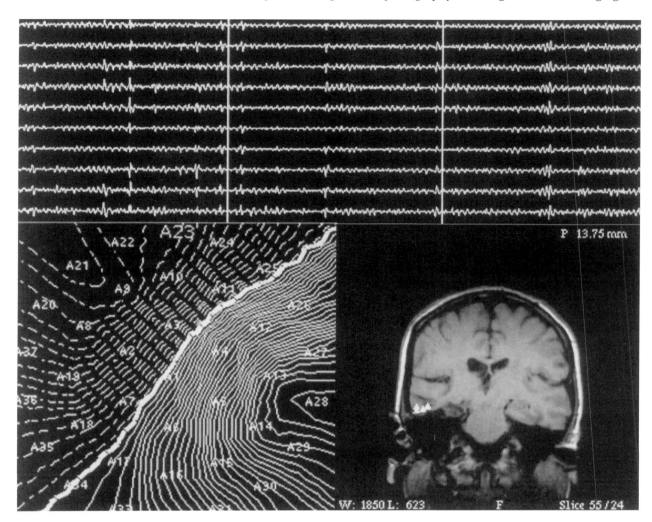

Fig. 9-44. MSI data set from a patient with right temporal lobe epilepsy (as confirmed by depth probes). Waveforms show example interictal spike that has a dipolar source configuration that localizes to the right temporal lobe. (From Lewine JD, Orrison WW, Halliday A et al: MEG functional mapping in epilepsy surgery. In Cascino GD, Jack CR, editors: Neuroimaging in epilepsy: principles and practice, Boston, 1994, Butterworth and Heinemann.)

rarely indicates one temporal lobe to be the dominant seizure focus in patients in whom other imaging modalities have suggested the opposite hemisphere.

In extratemporal lobe epilepsy, MEG often provides very important and previously unavailable information. This can be especially true in patients with frontal lobe epilepsy in whom traditional neuroimaging techniques often fail to reveal focal changes, even in patients subsequently shown to have focal seizures by depth probes (Fig. 9-45).

Perhaps the most exciting area of MEG epilepsy research involves pediatric patients. Children generally do not tolerate depth monitoring, so noninvasive imaging is critical. Unfortunately, children tend to have extratemporal conditions, and traditional neuroimaging studies often produce inconclusive or contradictory results. As illustrated in the following

case studies from the Albuquerque MSI facility, MEG can help to clarify the situation.

Case 1. The subject was a 14-year-old female with several nocturnal episodes of partial seizures characterized by lip quivering, disorientation, and partial aphasia. EEG revealed very active spiking in a pattern reminiscent of benign rolandic epilepsy, but there was some unexpected diffuse slowing on the EEG, and the spikes showed uncharacteristic, maximal positivity at the T4 electrode site. Thus, concern surrounded possible temporal lobe involvement. A Magnes system was used to collect MEG data sequentially over temporal and parietal sites, bilaterally. Simultaneous EEG revealed frequent right hemispheric spiking (maximal at T4) and diffuse right hemispheric slowing. MEG revealed neither spikes nor slow waves over the left

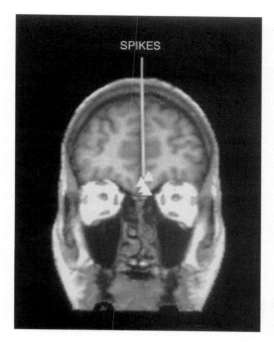

SPIKES

Fig. 9-45. Magnetic source localization images showing source locations (*triangles*) of interictal spikes of a patient with orbital-frontal epilepsy. (From Lewine JD, Orrison WW, Halliday A et al: MEG functional mapping in epilepsy surgery. In Cascino GD, Jack CR, editors: Neuroimaging in epilepsy: principles and practice, Boston, 1994, Butterworth and Heinemann.)

hemisphere, but more than 300 spikes were recorded over the right hemisphere (Fig. 9-46). All the spikes localized along the anterior bank of the central sulcus. Most of the activity was at an inferior location, just anterior to the site where tactile stimulation of the left lower lip elicited a response. Some activity spread superiorly along the precentral gyrus, but no spikes were found to be generated by the temporal lobe. Most of the deduced current dipoles pointed toward T4, a finding consistent with the EEG data. Slow wave sources also localized exclusively along the central sulcus, but with a considerable spread in the orientation of the sources (Fig. 9-47). This result is consistent with the diffuseness of the slow wave activity in the EEG. Overall, the data confirm the exclusive rolandic origin of the interictal epileptiform activity.

Case 2. The subject was a 5-year-old male with a history of uncontrolled partial-complex and tonic-clonic seizures. MRI revealed thickening of the cortical mantle at left parietal locations and a region of left parietal dysplasia (Fig. 9-48). EEG showed frequent interictal spikes maximal at left frontocentral sites. PET showed abnormal metabolism at left parietal sites, and SPECT showed decreased blood flow throughout the left hemisphere. The initial surgical recommendation was for a restricted resection near the structural lesion,

but a second independent set of physicians recommended complete left hemispherectomy. MEG revealed frequent dipolar interictal spiking at the suspect left parietal region without any evidence of spikes originating from temporal or frontal locations (Fig. 9-49). The dipole sources were oriented in an antero-posterior direction, pointing toward F3 and F7. Median nerve stimulation showed somatosensory cortex to be anterior to the lesion and spike focus (Fig. 9-50). The MEG data therefore supported the original recommendation for a restricted resection and significantly affected patient management.

Case 3. The patient was a 5-year-old male with a history of intractable simple-partial, complex-partial, and tonic-clonic left hemispheric seizures. EEG consistently showed a left temporocental epileptic focus. SPECT revealed cerebral hypoperfusion in the left temporal region, while PET showed decreased glucose metabolism in the left frontotemporal region. MRI and CT showed a region of dysplasia precentrally on the left.

Two years before MEG examination, the patient underwent a left frontal cortical excision of an epileptic region identified by ECoG. Initially, seizure control improved, but this was followed by a recurrence of complex-partial seizures. One year later, the child underwent repeat resection that extended the original site toward the central sulcus. Pathology from both surgeries revealed focal cortical dysplasia of the resected tissue. Postoperatively, the patient was seizure free for 17 days, but he then started to have recurrent complex-partial seizures six to eight times a day. He was referred to the Albuquerque MSI facility for motor mapping to determine if the previous resections could be extended more posteriorly without compromise of motor function. MSI revealed that the previous resections had come close to the inferior aspects of the precentral gyrus and that further posterior resection might compromise motor function.

More importantly, approximately 50 epileptic spikes were recorded during the experiment. These localized posterior to the central sulcus at a location superior and posterior to the original site of surgical intervention (Fig. 9-51). MRI was again performed after the MEG, with special attention to the region of the spike focus, and demonstrated structural pathology in the vicinity of the spike zone. No interictal spikes were recorded in the vicinity of the previous resection sites. MEG therefore revealed a new, potentially resectable spike focus at a location of previously unrecognized structural pathology.

Case 4. The patient was a 5-year-old male with Landau-Kleffner syndrome. In this condition, a rapid reduction in language skills occurs after age 4 years,

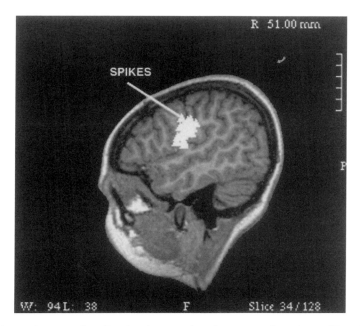

Fig. 9-46. Magnetic source localization images showing source locations of interictal spikes (*triangles*) of a patient with rolandic epilepsy. The orientations of the sources were such that EEG showed the spikes to be maximally positive at T3.

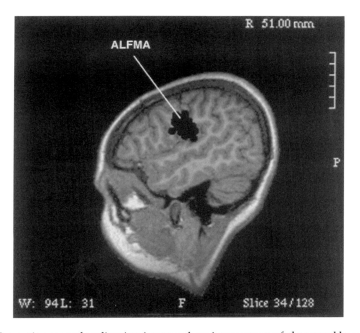

Fig. 9-47. Magnetic source localization images showing sources of abnormal low-frequency magnetic activity (ALFMA) in the delta band for a patient with rolandic epilepsy (same patient as in Fig. 9-46).

and frequent spiking emerges at left posterotemporal EEG leads. Landau-Kleffner syndrome is very amenable to surgical intervention, but the challenge is to decide how deep along the sylvian fissure to extend the series of subpial transections. MEG data were recorded sequentially over each hemisphere using a Magnes biomagnetometer. Three regions of dipolar

spikes were identified (Fig. 9-52). The region of most frequent activity was located in the left temporal lobe. It extended superiorly from Wernicke's area, up along the superior temporal gyrus, with an intense spike-generating zone 2 cm deep along the upper bank of the superior temporal gyrus. The second focus was at an inferior left frontal site believed to correspond to

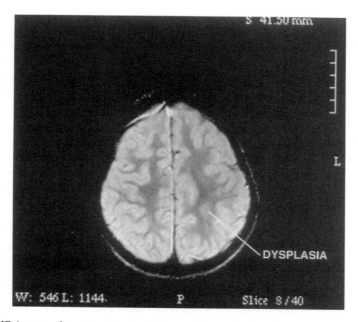

Fig. 9-48. MR images from a patient with complex-partial and tonic-clonic seizures. The data reveal cortical thickening in left parietal regions and an area of left parietal dysplasia. (From Lewine JD, Orrison WW, Halliday A et al: MEG functional mapping in epilepsy surgery. In Cascino GD, Jack CR, editors: Neuroimaging in epilepsy: principles and practice, Boston, 1994, Butterworth and Heinemann.)

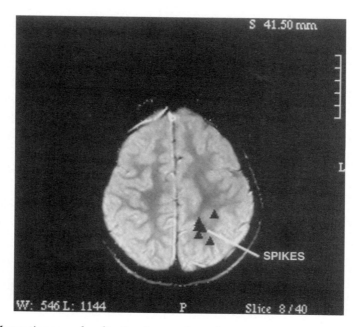

Fig. 9-49. Magnetic source localization images from the patient in Fig. 9-48. Interictal spikes were found to be generated in the region of structural anomalies.

Broca's area. Spike generators were also found throughout right auditory association areas. By analyzing the timing of the MEG spikes with respect to spikes observed in simultaneous EEG records, it became apparent that the MEG spikes in the left temporal area coincided with the lead edge of EEG spikes, whereas spikes in Broca's area and on the right trailed these by 20 and 25 msec, respectively. That is, the timing data demonstrated that the left temporal area was the triggering focus, with the activity in the other two areas reflecting propagation along known anatomic pathways.

Only a series of lateral subpial transections had been planned initially, but the MEG data indicated the

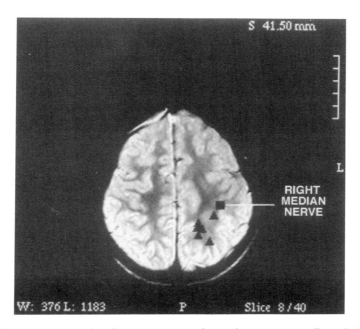

Fig. 9-50. Magnetic source localization images from the patient in Figs. 9-48 and 9-49 showing somatosensory cortex to be anterior to the spike-generating zone. (From Lewine JD, Orrison WW, Halliday A et al: MEG functional mapping in epilepsy surgery. In Cascino GD, Jack CR, editors: Neuroimaging in epilepsy: principles and practice, Boston, 1994, Butterworth and Heinemann.)

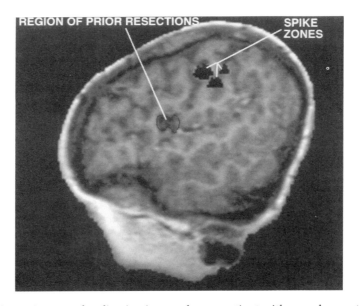

Fig. 9-51. Magnetic source localization images from a patient with complex-partial seizures despite previous resections of a precentral region of cortical dysplasia that was confirmed to be epileptogenic by ECoG. The data show a postcentral spike generation zone at a region found to be abnormal by MRI.

need for a more aggressive intervention along the superior temporal plane. Intraoperative ECoG confirmed the MEG data that indicated a significant epileptic focus 2 cm medial along the upper bank of the superior temporal gyrus. The surgery was success- ful, and the child began recovering several lost language skills.

In summary, as these cases illustrate, MEG evaluation of epileptiform activity can have a direct and positive effect on patient care. The expanding use of

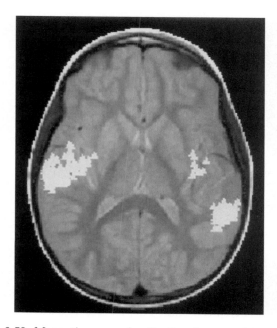

Fig. 9-52. Magnetic source localization images of interictal spike activity for the patient with Landau-Kleffner syndrome. Spikes in the left temporal regions were shown to trigger the left frontal and right temporal activity. (From Lewine JD, Orrison WW, Halliday A et al: MEG functional mapping in epilepsy surgery. In Cascino GD, Jack CR, editors: Neuroimaging in epilepsy: principles and practice, Boston, 1994, Butterworth and Heinemann.)

MEG in patients with complex epilepsy is offering new hope for this common but difficult disorder.

Characterization of Abnormal Low-Frequency Magnetic Activity (ALFMA)

The spontaneous EEG and MEG of normal healthy subjects is generally dominated by signals of 8 Hz or higher. However, in patients with neuropathology the amount of delta and theta power often increases in the 1 to 4 and 4 to 6 Hz bands, respectively (Fig. 9-53). Usually, this slowing of the spontaneous record is diffuse across recording sites (especially in the EEG), but in some circumstances, the slowing can be quite focal, especially in the MEG.[57-59]

Different laboratories have taken slightly different approaches to the analysis of ALFMA, but the basic strategies are similar. Briefly, spontaneous MEG signals are bandpass-filtered to emphasize low-frequency components in the theta or delta range. Slow wave events are then identified by visual inspection or through the use of automatic processing routines that identify large-amplitude signals. As might be expected, debate surrounds the appropriate parameters for automatic search routines. For example, the MSI facility at the Scripps Clinic and Research Facility considers only events with signal strengths greater than 400 femtotesla (fT) to be indicative of pathology. This strategy protects the analysis against false-positive results, but it compromises sensitivity to subtle pathology. In contrast, the group at the Albuquerque Magnetic Source Imaging Facility considers events with a signal strength as low as 200 fT to be potentially pathologic. This renders the analysis strategy more open to false-positive findings (10% to 15%), but it is also more open to identification of subtle pathophysiology.

Once a slow wave event is identified, standard dipole modeling strategies are applied to the signal. This also has caused considerable debate in the scientific community because spontaneous brain activity most assuredly reflects significant contributions from multiple brain regions. However, the neuromagnetic field generated by a region of focal pathology at times may be so large (greater than 200 fT) that it dominates the recorded signal. At these rare instants, the dipole model can prove to be quite appropriate and accurate.

Most work in the field has focused on ALFMA associated with ischemic changes,[57-61] but the domain is now being expanded to include conditions such as epilepsy,[61] trauma,[59] and psychiatric dysfunction.[62] Whereas source localizations for most stimulus-evoked signals are believed to be accurate to within a few millimeters, source localizations for ALFMA are probably accurate only to within a few centimeters. In part, this is because signal-averaging techniques are not used, so the background noise level is high. Another factor appears to be that ALFMA often reflects quite extended cortical regions. The dipole model still provides a reasonable statistical account of the data, but the dipole location is projected deep to the actual site of activation. Despite these caveats, the type of coarse localization obtainable by an ALFMA examination exceeds what is available through routine EEG monitoring.

Even in the most severe cases, more than 99% of the data is not well characterized by a single-dipole model, so it is ignored in standard analyses. It would be of interest to characterize better the more prevalent nondipolar signals, but at present, this is not possible in routine clinical practice. Regardless, the dramatically reduced, single-dipole data set can be remarkably informative.

Cerebrovascular disorders. Cerebrovascular disease is one of the most common causes of neurologic deficit. Patients in neurology clinics frequently complain of brief episodes of arm weakness, facial numbness, and/or speech loss. Many patients have recovered from the deficit by the time they are seen, and the physician's examination and radiologic examinations (MR or CT) are all normal. Some of these

Control Subject

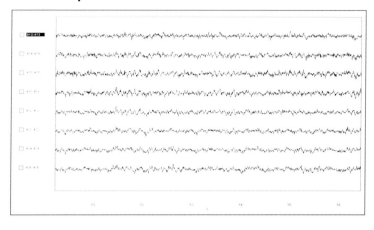

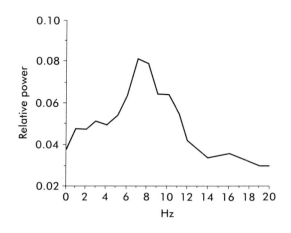

Trauma Subject

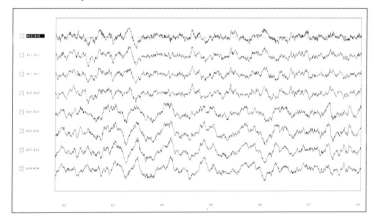

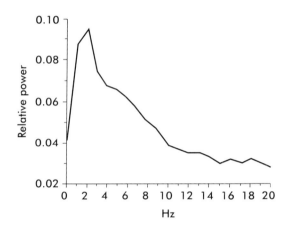

Fig. 9-53. Examples of MEG waveforms and power spectra from a normal control subject and a patient with head trauma. The data of the normal subject are dominated by alpha activity in the 8 to 12 Hz band, whereas the patient shows excessive delta bursting in the 1 to 4 Hz band.

episodes are transient ischemic attacks (TIAs) that indicate the patient should have an aggressive workup and possible carotid artery surgery to prevent cerebrovascular accident (CVA, stroke). Other episodes, however, are benign and should be treated conservatively. At present, clinicians have considerable trouble distinguishing between these two possibilities, so aggressive, expensive, and sometimes unnecessary workups are generally performed with all patients.

If ALFMA examinations can help to identify those patients at risk for CVA, MSI will become an important diagnostic tool that can perhaps guide preventive measures. Working initially with only a single-channel biomagnetometer, Vieth pioneered explorations of slow wave activity in cerebrovascular disease.[57] These early studies suggested that slow waves could sometimes be identified and localized in patients with TIAs,

even after neurologic deficits had cleared. Subsequent studies have confirmed these observations using large-array biomagnetometer systems.[58-60,63] It has also been shown that in patients with cortical CVA, slow wave activity selectively originates from the tissues along the margin of the lesion, a result believed to be indicative of the ischemic penumbra. This ability to define both the region of infarct and the surrounding penumbra of ischemic tissue might aid in evaluating the likelihood of functional recovery and planning therapeutic intervention.

Fig. 9-54 shows example Magnes data collected from a 56-year-old male patient who had right-sided numbness and partial aphasia 3 weeks before MSI examination. At the time of the MSI examination, symptoms were continuing to clear, but they had not completely resolved. Three minutes of continuous MEG data were recorded at each of eight sequential

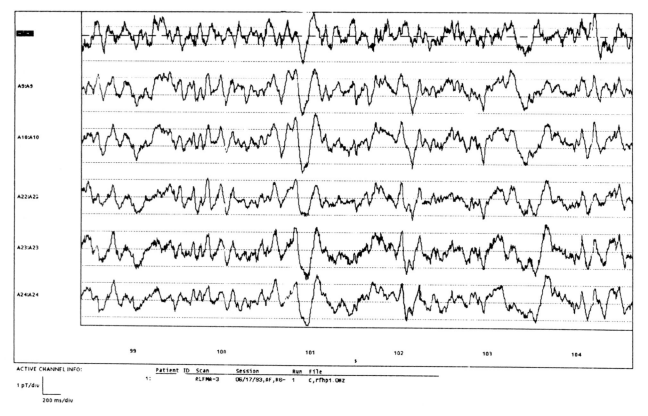

Fig. 9-54. MEG data from a patient with a cortical infarct. The data are characterized by ALFMA in the delta band.

dewar placements positioned to provide for a whole-head examination. Slowing was observed over the left hemisphere only. Sources of dipolar ALFMA localized exclusively to a region of ischemic change identified by MRI (Fig. 9-55).

In a recent study of five patients with TIA but no structural changes (as assessed by MRI), ALFMA was found for two, even several days after the original functional deficits had cleared (no ALFMA was found for any of five age-matched and gender-matched control subjects).[59] In a separate study Rieke and colleagues had the opportunity to study a patient before and after thromboendarterectomy.[63] In this patient, the amount of slowing was significantly reduced after intervention.

Overall, ALFMA is found in about 50% of patients with subcortical infarcts and more than 80% of patients with cortical lesions.[59] In patients with large infarcts and persistent neurologic and neuropsychologic deficits, extensive ALFMA may be persistent, even after 11 years (Fig. 9-56).

Epilepsy. Although the very first MEG study of epilepsy[5] focused on hyperventilation-induced changes in slow activity, most subsequent work in epilepsy has focused on characterization of epileptic

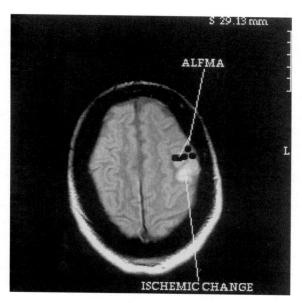

Fig. 9-55. Magnetic source localization images showing relationship between ALFMA source and a region of cerebral ischemia.

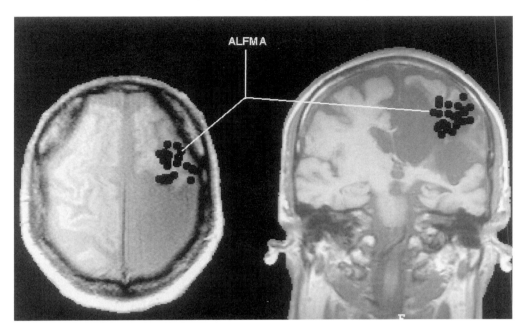

Fig. 9-56. Magnetic source localization images showing clustering of ALFMA sources along the margins of a large cortical infarct.

spikes. A limitation of this approach is that it is useful only for patients who have fairly frequent interictal spiking. Recent work at several MEG sites[64,65] indicates that ALFMA analyses offer an attractive alternative approach because focal slowing is generally seen even in patients without interictal spiking (Fig. 9-57).

In a study of 50 unselected patients with epilepsy, Lewine and colleagues found focal slow wave activity in 80%, whereas spiking was found in only 30%.[59,65] Similar percentages have been observed in work at the Scripps Clinic and Research Foundation. Multiple ALFMA foci are observed in more than 50% of patients, but one focus is generally much more intense than others. The location of the most intense focus agrees, in about 80% of patients, with the side and lobe of pathology, as identified by video EEG monitoring.[64,65] This predictive accuracy of phase II video findings by slow wave MEG examination far exceeds that evidenced by more traditional structural (MRI, CT) and functional (PET, SPECT) methods.[64] In several patients, ECoG has confirmed the validity of slow wave localizations and their relevance to epileptic pathology.[66]

Intracranial masses. In the surgical resection of brain neoplasms, it is important to remove the tumor as completely as possible. However, there is an equal desire not to remove healthy brain tissue aggressively. As shown in work at both the Scripps and Albuquerque MSI sites, ALFMA sources are found in about 70% of patients with neoplasms.[36,59] Sources of ALFMA rarely localize within the tumor. Rather, they are

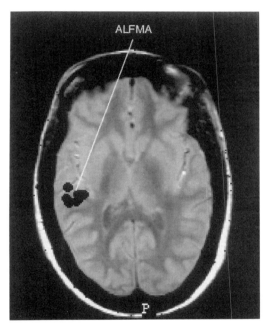

Fig. 9-57. Magnetic source localization images showing ALFMA sources in the right temporal lobe of an epileptic patient who does not have frequent interictal spiking. Video EEG confirmed that this patient's seizures originated in the right temporal lobe. (From Lewine JD, Orrison WW, Halliday A et al: MEG functional mapping in epilepsy surgery. In Cascino GD, Jack CR, editors: Neuroimaging in epilepsy: principles and practice, Boston, 1994, Butterworth and Heinemann.)

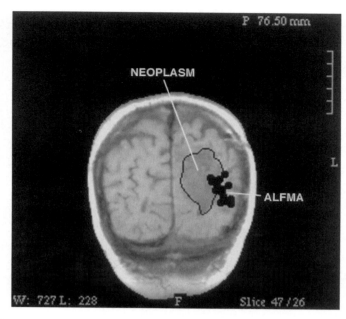

Fig. 9-58. Magnetic source localization image showing ALFMA sources to cluster around the margin of a neoplasm.

found in the immediately adjacent cortex that is compressed by the intruding mass (Fig. 9-58). It remains to be fully determined if the ALFMA-generating tissue is sufficiently pathologic that it should be surgically excised along with the tumor, or if the presence of ALFMA indicates viable tissue that will return to normal functioning once compression by a tumor is alleviated. Preliminary data are most consistent with the later interpretation, but additional cases are required (Lewine, unpublished observations).

Traumatic brain injury. Head trauma causes more than 50,000 deaths annually and leads to hundreds of thousands of hospitalizations. In patients who survive, various posttraumatic syndromes characterized by neurologic or psychologic dysfunction often follow. In many patients, radiologic imaging reveals contusions, deep white matter lesions, and other pathology, but the long-term neurophysiologic consequences of these remain undetermined. Also, some patients show no positive radiologic findings even when psychologic deficits exist. This situation is exceptionally problematic when it comes to (1) predicting long-term outcome, (2) deciding among therapeutic alternatives, and (3) making decisions about a person's fitness to return to work. To the extent that MSI can better characterize neurophysiologic dysfunction, it will make a significant impact on the care and treatment of patients with traumatic brain injury.

ALFMA activity has been examined in both moderate[67] and mild head trauma.[59] The most extensive study of ALFMA in head trauma has focused on patients with mild traumatic brain injury who did not require extended posttraumatic hospitalization.[59] In this study of 30 such patients, MRI pathology was found in only six, whereas ALFMA was identified in 18. Sources of ALFMA generally localized pathophysiologic activity to sites coup or contrecoup to the trauma. Also, a predictable relationship existed between specific symptoms and the locations of ALFMA sources (Fig. 9-59). In a subset of 14 patients who had additional EEG examinations, only three showed abnormal EEG findings, whereas seven showed significant ALFMA. In four patients, each examined with MEG, EEG, and MRI, MEG was the only modality to provide objective evidence of brain dysfunction. Whereas the sensitivity of the ALFMA examination to the pathophysiologic sequelae of mild traumatic brain injury is less than 100%, it appears to be more than double that afforded by any other noninvasive imaging modality. Of the 30 patients examined in this study, six patients with ALFMA during initial examination underwent two or more sequential examinations (spaced at 1-month intervals). The persistence or alleviation of ALFMA correlated with the persistence or alleviation of symptoms (Figs. 9-60 and 9-61).

Other conditions. Several MEG facilities are engaged in ALFMA investigations of other clinical conditions, including psychiatric dysfunction, demen-

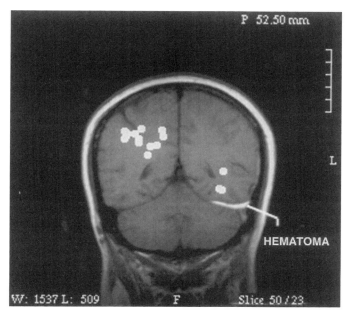

Fig. 9-59. Magnetic source localization image showing ALFMA sources (*circles*) in a patient with recent head trauma to a right parietal location. MRI shows a contrecoup left temporal hematoma. ALFMA is found at both coup and contrecoup sites.

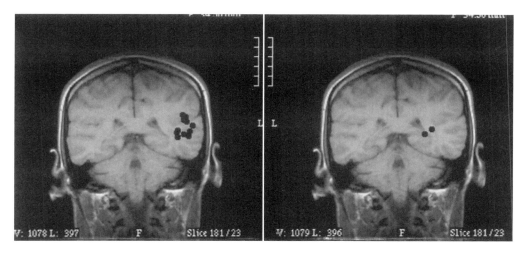

Fig. 9-60. Magnetic source localization images from a trauma patient showing a reduction of ALFMA with temporal improvement of symptoms. Data in **A** were collected 1 month after trauma, at a time of severe memory impairment. Data in **B** were obtained 3 months later after improvement in symptomatology but incomplete resolution.

tia, substance abuse, and learning disabilities. At present, most of this work is still in very preliminary stages, but many initial results are encouraging (Figs. 9-62 and 9-63).

It should be noted that special care must be taken in ALFMA examinations of prepubescent children because 50% of normal children have dipolar, high-amplitude alpha activity that is not adequately suppressed by standard 1 to 6 Hz digital filtering techniques. It is therefore important to demonstrate specifically that putative sources of ALFMA are not mischaracterizations of normal spontaneous rhythms.

Overall, the ALFMA examination appears to be very sensitive to a variety of pathophysiologic conditions, although there seems to be little specificity with respect to particular conditions. On the other hand, additional analyses of waveform morphology and bursting patterns may soon provide better diagnostic specificity and new insights into the exact pathologic mechanisms that create ALFMA.

Recently, there have been some clinical investigations of spontaneous brain activity in other frequency

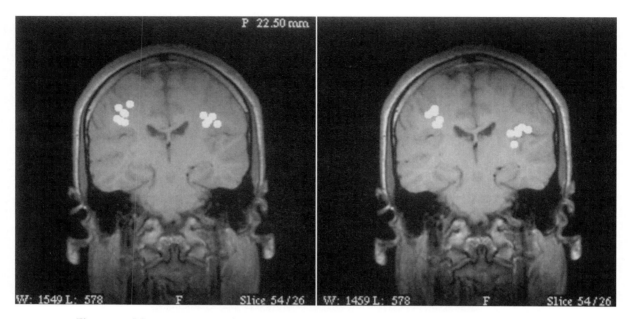

Fig. 9-61. Magnetic source localization images from a trauma patient with a stable posttraumatic attention deficit disorder. The two images were obtained 6 months apart.

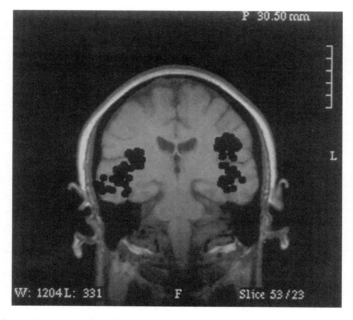

Fig. 9-62. Magnetic source localization images showing ALFMA activity (*circles*) in a schizophrenic patient with active auditory hallucinations that were uncontrolled by medication.

bands. For example, Grummich et al. have shown that beta sources, such as sources of ALFMA, often cluster around the margins of neoplasms.[68] Another interesting set of data comes from the work of Barckley and colleagues, who have described the presence of DC shifts in the magnetic field associated with migraines.[69,70] These investigators have also described migraine-associated suppression of electrocerebral rhythms, and they argue that a migraine with aural attack may be related to a form of spreading depression similar to that seen in experimental animals.[71,72]

Characterization of Abnormal Information Processing

One of the most promising areas of clinical research is in the characterization of abnormal information

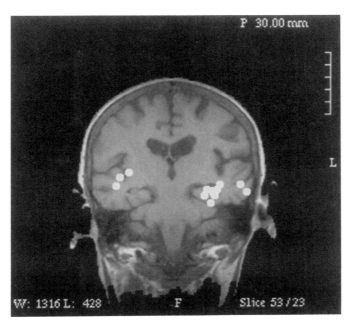

Fig. 9-63. Magnetic source localization images showing ALFMA activity (*circles*) in a patient with Alzheimer's disease and a moderate memory impairment.

processing in clinical patients. This type of study generally takes advantage of signal-averaging/evoked-response techniques, with data analysis strategies concentrating on clinically relevant changes in the latency and/or amplitude of particular response components.

For example, the pattern of activity evoked by electrical stimulation of the median nerve is found to be abnormal in several clinical conditions, the most notable of which is multiple sclerosis (MS). As shown by the work of Karhu et al., waveforms from patients with MS appear very different from waveforms from normal control subjects.[73] Of particular note is significant enhancement of the 60 msec evoked-response component, especially in patients with periventricular lesions (Fig. 9-64). In another interesting condition, progressive myoclonus epilepsy (PME), the magnitude of somatosensory evoked fields may be augmented up to sixfold what is observed in normal subjects. In the same patients, auditory evoked responses are of normal magnitude. These results imply that PME is associated with selective thalamocortical hyperreactivity of the somatosensory system.[74]

Other research in somatosensory processing has focused on issues of cortical reorganization associated with peripheral and/or central nervous system (CNS) pathology. For example, Yang and colleagues have provided evidence of cortical reorganization in patients with upper arm amputation.[75] Specifically, it is shown that the cortical representation for somatosensory processing of information of the face expands superiorly in these patients. Mogilnar and colleagues

have shown very-fine-grain changes in somatotopic organization in patients with syndactyly (webbing of adjacent fingers).[76] Evaluations of these subjects before and after restorative plastic surgery to separate fused digits show millimeter changes in cortical hand representation.

Cortical pathology can cause very significant reorganization, as shown in the work of Lewine et al.[77] These investigators examined an adult patient who had a neonatal infarct of the left middle cerebral artery. Despite complete loss of primary and secondary somatosensory areas of the left hemisphere, the subject had only a mild paresthesia of the right hand. Median nerve stimulation revealed unexpected somatosensory responses from intact portions of the left temporal lobe and from right mesial parietal cortex (Figs. 9-65 and 9-66).

Work on clinical aspects of auditory information processing is also prominent. Tinnitus (ringing in the ear) is a symptom often associated with a variety of middle and inner ear diseases, and it is a frequent, residual effect of head trauma. Its incidence is high in the general population (greater than 5%), and for some patients, its presence significantly compromises the quality of life.[78] Real internal sound sources can be specified in a few patients, but for most, tinnitus is a subjective experience that is difficult to evaluate objectively. Although traditional auditory evoked potential methods have failed to provide any evidence of auditory dysfunction in patients with tinnitus, work by Hoke and colleagues suggests that MEG monitoring can provide an objective measure.[79] Auditory

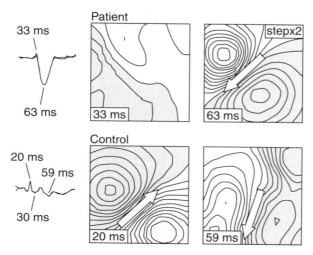

Fig. 9-64. Somatosensory evoked responses from a control subject and a patient with multiple sclerosis. Data show reduced early components (at 20 and 30 msec) and enhanced late component (at 60 msec) for the patient. (Modified from Karhu J, Hari R, Makela J et al: Somatosensory evoked magnetic fields in multiple sclerosis, Electroenceph Clin Neurophysiol 83:192-200, 1992.)

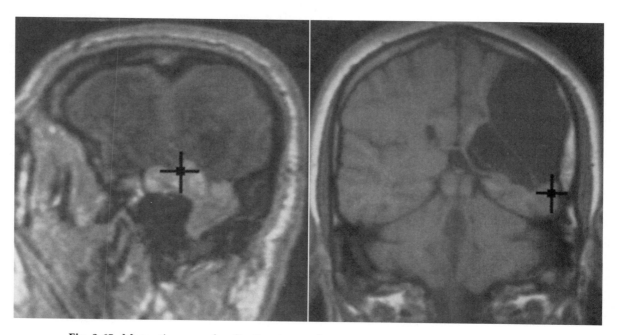

Fig. 9-65. Magnetic source localization image showing source location for early (30 msec) component of right median nerve response from an adult patient who had a neonatal infarct of the left middle cerebral artery. The source localizes to an intact region of left temporal cortex. (From Lewine JD, Astur RS, Davis LE et al: Cortical organization in adulthood is modified by neonatal infarct: a case study, Radiology 190:93-96, 1994.)

evoked fields are dominated by components at 100 and 200 msec, the M100 and M200, respectively. In normal subjects, these components have approximately the same amplitude, but Hoke et al. found reduced M200/M100 ratios in patients with unilateral tinnitus (Fig. 9-67).[79] Recently, these findings have been challenged in subsequent experiments by Jacob-

son et al.,[80] but methodologic differences may account for the discrepancies in findings.

Other work in the auditory system has focused on the effects of unilateral lesions of auditory cortex. If the lesion extends deep along the temporal plane, it can completely obliterate the M100 and M200 response from the damaged hemisphere.[81,82] Even more inter-

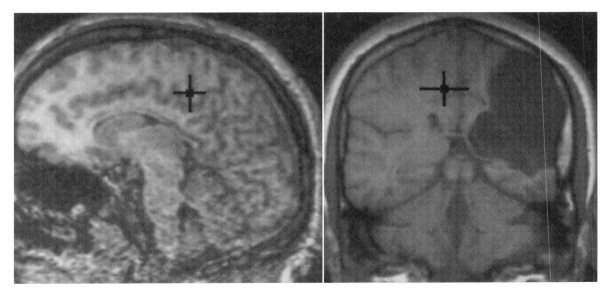

Fig. 9-66. Magnetic source localization image showing source of late (70 msec) component of right median nerve response from the same patient in Fig. 9-65. The source localizes to ipsilateral medial parietal cortex, inferior to the left leg region. (From Lewine JD, Astur RS, Davis LE et al: Cortical organization in adulthood is modified by neonatal infarct: a case study, Radiology 190:93-96, 1994.)

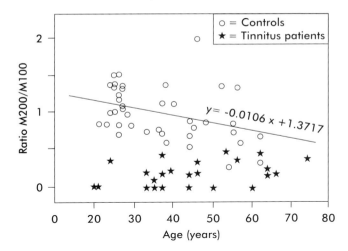

Fig. 9-67. M200/M100 ratios as a function of age and tinnitus. The data show reduced ratios in subjects with tinnitus. (From Hoke M, Feldman H, Pantev C et al: Objective evidence of tinnitus in auditory evoked magnetic fields, Hear Res 37:281-286, 1989.)

esting is that damage to one hemisphere alters the ipsilateral auditory response of the other, intact hemisphere. Specifically, the ipsilateral response displays reduced amplitude and increased latency with respect to that found for normal subjects. Although the exact mechanisms by which the ipsilateral auditory response is generated and modulated are unknown, these data suggest that transcallosal mechanisms (disrupted by the lesion) may normally facilitate ipsilateral reactivity.[83]

Another exciting area of clinical auditory research has focused on auditory evoked responses in psychiatric patients. Work by Reite and colleagues has demonstrated that normal subjects display significant left-right asymmetries in the positions of generators for the M50 and M100 components of auditory evoked responses.[84,85] This asymmetry appears to be lacking in schizophrenic males (but not females). Other lines of evidence also point to abnormal interhemispheric relationships in schizophrenic patients.[86-88] It remains to be determined if the lack of auditory asymmetry in male schizophrenic patients reflects anatomic factors (altered sulcal-gyral patterns) or a real physiologic difference. Regardless, simple and rapid MEG testing of asymmetries may become useful in classification of patient subpopulations.

Several investigators have recently suggested that the spatiotemporal dynamics and following characteristics of auditory evoked gamma activity (in the 35 to 45 Hz bandwidth) are altered in several pathologic conditions, including depression[89] and Alzheimer's dementia.[90,91] Gamma-band responses appear to reflect activity of multiple cortical and perhaps subcortical structures, an observation that has demanded the development of data analysis strategies that go beyond simple dipole modeling.[92,93] By examining coherence patterns across the sensors of large-array systems, it may become possible to detect early disruption of brain processing pathways before full-blown psychiatric and cognitive dysfunction occurs.

There has been relatively little clinical research on visual information processing, mostly because of technical complications (video screens cannot be

Fetal brain

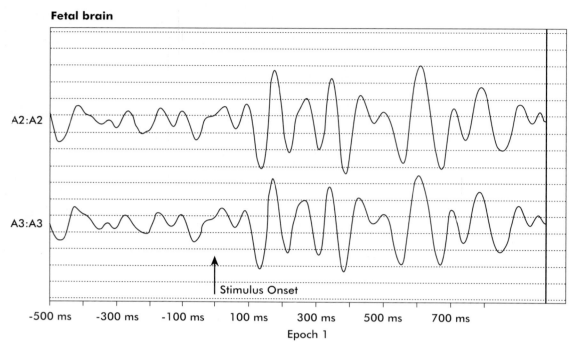

Fig. 9-68. Average neuromagnetic response ($n = 200$) of a 36-week-old fetus to presentation of an auditory stimulus. The data were recorded by placing the sensor unit over the mother's womb.

placed within the shielded room, and one is forced to resort to expensive fiberoptic projection systems) and the complexity of the visual evoked response. Nevertheless, Harding and colleagues have used visual flash and pattern evoked potentials to assess Alzheimer's disease.[94] These investigators have found normal pattern evoked magnetic fields but abnormal flash responses. This is believed to reflect selective dysfunction of visual association areas relative to primary calcarine cortex.

FUTURE DIRECTIONS

The clinical future for MEG appears bright. In the 3 years since large-array systems have become available for routine clinical use, tremendous progress has been made on a number of clinical fronts. Presurgical mapping of functional organization and epileptic activity are likely to remain the dominant clinical applications of MEG for some years to come, but new applications are developing rapidly. As the availability of large-array systems increases, it is anticipated that the number of investigations of abnormal information processing in clinical populations will grow rapidly.

Many data analysis strategies conceived during the days of single-channel systems are beginning to mature. For example, the availability of simultaneous MEG data from over the entire head has led to realization of data analysis strategies that focus on measures of coherence between channels. The inte-

gration of MRI and MEG data is beginning to move beyond the stage of mere mapping of MEG data onto MR images to a new stage in which neuroanatomic data are used specifically to constrain inverse modeling procedures.[95] This will undoubtedly lead to more accurate and realistic characterization of the generators of neuromagnetic signals. At the same time, multiple-dipole and distributed source analysis strategies are becoming more robust and will soon find their way into routine clinical use.

New technologic developments, including the development of superconducting shielding and the refinement of high-temperature SQUIDs, are also certain to play an important role in increasing the efficiency and efficacy of neuromagnetic procedures. The main challenge for MEG remains identification of a unique clinical position. MEG clearly has advantages over other imaging modalities, but the technology remains too expensive, especially in comparison with EEG. On the other hand, the ease and precision of MEG presurgical evaluations is beginning to secure its role in routine neurosurgical practice.[96]

One area of tremendous promise for MEG may be in the assessment of the developing brain. As first suggested by the work of Blum et al, MEG may be uniquely qualified for monitoring the fetal brain.[97] Work on this intriguing area is still at a very preliminary stage, but several other groups have now shown an ability to measure fetal responses to auditory stimuli (Dunajski, personal communication, 1993; Lewine and colleagues, unpublished observations; Fig. 9-68). If this ability can be refined and extended to an early period in gestation, MEG will play a critical role in the assessment of fetal well-being.

From the fetus to the patient with dementia, MEG affords a level of spatial and temporal resolution of brain activity that has previously been only dreamed of in science fiction novels. In both the clinic and the cognitive neuroscience laboratory, the spatial and temporal properties of MEG render it perhaps the single most promising technique for unraveling the mysteries of the human brain.

REFERENCES

1. Baule GM, McFee R: Detection of the magnetic field of the heart, Am Heart J 66:95-96, 1963.
2. Cohen D: Magnetoencephalography: evidence of magnetic fields produced by alpha rhythm currents, Science 161:784-786, 1968.
3. Zimmerman JE, Thiene P, Harding JT: Design and operation of stable rf-biased superconducting quantum interference devices and a note on the properties of perfectly clean metal contacts, J Appl Phys 41:1572-1580, 1970.
4. Cohen D, Edelsack EA, Zimmerman JE: Magnetocardiograms taken inside a shielded room with a superconducting point-contact magnetometer, Appl Phys Lett 16:278-280, 1970.
5. Cohen D: Magnetoencephalography: detection of the brain's electrical activity with a superconducting magnetometer, Science 175:664-666, 1972.
6. Brenner D, Williamson SJ, Kaufman L: Visually evoked magnetic fields of the human brain, Science 190:480-482, 1975.
7. Brenner D, Lipton J, Kaufman L, Williamson SJ: Somatically evoked magnetic fields of the human brain, Science 199:81-83, 1978.
8. Teyler TJ, Cuffin BN, Cohen D: The visual evoked magnetoencephalogram, Life Sci 17:683-691, 1975.
9. Hari R, Ilmoniemi, RJ: Cerebral magnetic fields, CRC Crit Rev. Biomed Eng 14:93-126, 1986.
10. Williamson SJ, Kaufman L: Analysis of neuromagnetic signals. In Gevins AS, Redmond A, editors: Handbook of electroencephalography and clinical neurophysiology, vol 1, Methods and analysis of brain electrical signals, Amsterdam, 1987, Elsevier.
11. Hari R: The neuromagnetic method in the study of the human auditory cortex. In Grandori F, Hoke M, Romani GL, editors: Auditory evoked magnetic fields and electric potentials, Basel, 1990, Karger.
12. Lewine JD: Neuromagnetic techniques for the noninvasive analysis of brain function. In Freeman SE, Fukushima E, Greene ER, editors: Noninvasive techniques in biology and medicine, San Francisco, 1991, San Francisco Press.
13. Weinberg H, Cheyne D, Crisp D: Electroencephalographic and magnetoencephalographic studies of motor function, Magnetoecephalogr Adv Neurol 54:193-206, 1990.
14. Swinney KR, Wikswo JP Jr: A calculation of the magnetic field of a nerve action potential, Biophys J 32:719-732, 1980.
15. Tripp JH: Biomagnetic fields and cellular current flow. In Erne SN, Hahlbohm HD, Lubbig H, editors: Biomagnetism, New York, 1981, Walter de Gruyter.
16. Wikswo JP Jr: Cellular action currents. In Williamson SJ, Romani GL, Kaufman L, Modena I, editors: Biomagnetism, an interdisciplinary approach, New York, 1983, Plenum.
17. Lorente de No R: Analysis of the distribution of action currents

of nerve in a volume conductor, Stud Rockefeller Inst Med Res 132:384-477, 1947.
18. Cuffin BN, Geselowitz DB: Computer model studies of the magnetocardiogram, Ann Biomed Eng 5:164-178, 1977.
19. Cohen D, Hosaka HJ: Magnetic field produced by a current dipole, J Electrocardiol 9:409-417, 1976.
20. Sarvas J: Basic mathematical and electromagnetic concepts of the biomagnetism inverse problem, Phys Med Biol 32:11-22, 1987.
21. Okada Y: Discrimination of localized and distributed current dipole sources and localized single and multiple sources. In Weinberg H, Stroink G, Katila T, editors: Biomagnetism, applications and theory, New York, 1985, Pergamon.
22. Supek S, Aine CJ: Simulation studies of multiple dipole neuromagnetic source localization: model-order and limits of resolution, IEEE Trans Biomed Eng 40:529-540, 1993.
23. Grynszpan F, Geselowitz DB: Model studies of the magnetocardiogram, Biophys J 13:911-925, 1973.
24. Hamalainen MS, Sarvas J: Feasibility of the homogeneous head model in the interpretation of magnetic fields, Phys Med Biol 32:91-97, 1987.
25. Meijs JWH, Bosch FGC, Peters MJ et al: On the magnetic field distribution generated by a dipolar current source situated in a realistically shaped compartment model of the head, Electroencephalogr Clin Neurophysiol 66:286-298, 1987.
26. Okada Y: Neurogenesis of evoked magnetic fields. In Williamson SJ, Romani GL, Kaufman L et al, editors: Biomagnetism, an interdisciplinary approach, New York, 1983, Plenum.
27. Spencer DD, Spencer SS, Mattson RH et al: Access to the posterior medial temporal lobe structures in the surgical treatment of temporal lobe epilepsy, Neurosurgery 15:667-671, 1984.
28. Shapiro WR: Intracranial neoplasms. In Rosenberg RN, Grossman RG, editors: The clinical neurosciences, New York, 1983, Churchill Livingstone.
29. Morris HH, Lueders H, Hahn JF et al: Neurophysiological techniques as an aid to surgical treatment of primary brain tumors, Ann Neurol 19:559-567, 1986.
30. Sobel DF, Gallen CC, Schwartz BJ et al: Central sulcus localization in humans: comparison of MRI-anatomic and magnetoencephalographic functional methods, AJNR 14:915-925, 1993.
31. Penfield W, Boldrey E: Somatic motor and sensory representation in the cerebral cortex of man as studied by electrical stimulation, Brain 60:389-443, 1937.
32. Black PM, Ronner S: Cortical mapping for defining the limits of tumor resection, Neurosurgery 20(6):914-919, 1986.
33. Berger MS, Kincaid J, Ojemann GA et al: Brain mapping techniques to maximize resection safety and seizure control in children with brain tumors, Neurosurgery 25(5):786-792, 1989.
34. Sutherling WW, Crandall PH, Darcey TM et al: The magnetic and electric fields agree with intracranial localizations of somatosensory cortex, Neurology 38:1705-1714, 1988.
35. Orrison WW Jr, Lewine JD: Magnetic source imaging in neurosurgical practice, Perspect Neurol Surg 4(2):141-148, 1993.
36. Galen CC, Sobel DF, Waltz T et al: Noninvasive pre-surgical neuromagnetic mapping of somatosensory cortex, Neurosurgery 33:260-268, 1993.
37. Lewine JD, Orrison WW, Maclin EL et al: Event-related magnetic fields and neurosurgical practice. In Advances in biomagnetism, 1993, Amsterdam, 1994, Elsevier.
38. Pantev C, Hoke M, Lehnertz K et al: Tonotopic organization of the human auditory cortex revealed by transient auditory evoked magnetic fields, Electroencephalogr Clin Neurophysiol 69:160-170, 1988.
39. Lewine JD, Edgar JC, Repa K et al: A physical phantom for simulating the impact of pathology on magnetic source imaging. In Advances in biomagnetism, 1993, Amsterdam, 1994, Elsevier.

40. Engel J, Ojemann GA: The next step. In Engel J, editor: Surgical treatment of the epilesies, ed 2, New York, 1993, Raven.

41. Rose DF, Smith PD, Sato S: Magnetoencephalography and epilepsy research, Science 238:329-335, 1987.

42. Sato S: Epilepsy research, NIH experience, Magnetoencephalogr Adv Neurol 54:223-230, 1990.

43. Sutherling WW, Barth DS: Magnetoencephalography in clinical epilepsy studies: the UCLA experience, Magnetoencephalogr Adv Neurol 54:231-246, 1990.

44. Ricci GB: Italian contributions to magnetoencephalographic studies on the epilepsies, Magnetoencephalogr Adv Neurol 54:247-260, 1990.

45. Stefan H, Schnieider S, Abraham-Fuchs K et al: Magnetic source localization in focal epilepsy; multichannel magnetoencephalography correlated with magnetic resonance brain imaging, Brain 113:1347-1359, 1990.

46. Stefan H, Schnieider S, Abraham-Fuchs K et al: The neocortico-to mesio-basal limbic propagation of focal epileptic activity during the spike-wave complex, Electroencephalogr Clin Neurophysiol 79:1-10, 1991.

47. Paetau R, Kajola M, Hari R: Magnetoencephalography in the study of epilepsy, Neurophysiol Clin 20:169-187, 1990.

48. Paetau R, Kajola M, Korkman M et al: Landau-Kleffner syndrome: epileptic activity in the auditory cortex, NeuroReport 2:201-204, 1991.

49. Paetau R, Kajola M, Karhu J et al: MEG localization of epileptic cortex—impact on surgical treatment, Ann Neurol 32:106-109, 1992.

50. Sutherling W, Crandall PH, Engel J et al: The magnetic field of complex partial seizures agrees with intracranial localizations, Ann Neurol 21:548-558, 1987.

51. Barth DS, Sutherling W, Engel J et al: Neuromagnetic localization of epileptiform spike activity in the human brain, Science 218:891-894, 1982.

52. Barth DS, Sutherling W, Engel J et al: Neuromagnetic evidence of spatially distributed sources underlying epileptiform spikes in the human brain, Science 223:293-296, 1984.

53. Scherg M, Vajsar J, Picton TW: A source analysis of the late human auditory evoked potentials, J Coqn Neurosci (4):336-355, 1989.

54. Ebersole JS, Squires K, Gamelin J et al: Simultaneous MEG and EEG provide complimentary dipole models of temporal lobe spikes, Epilepsia 34(6), 1993.

55. Ebersole JS, Squires K, Gamelin J et al: Dipole models of temporal lobe spikes from simultaneous MEG and EEG. In Abstracts, AEEGS, New Orleans, 1993.

56. Ebersole JS, Squires K, Gamelin J et al: Dipole models of temporal lobe spikes from simultaneous MEG and EEG, Abstracts, Biomagnetism '93, Vienna, 1993.

57. Vieth J: Magnetoencepalography in the study of stroke (cerebrovascular accident), Magnetoencephalogr Adv Neurol 54:261-269, 1990.

58. Gallen CC, Schwartz BJ, Pantev C et al: Detection and localization of delta frequency activity in human stroke. In Hoke M, Erne SN, Okada YC et al, editors: Biomagnetism: clinical applications, Amsterdam, 1992, Elsevier.

59. Lewine JD, Orrison WW, Astur RS et al: Explorations of pathophysiological spontaneous activity by magnetic source imaging. In Advances in Biomagnetism, 1993, Amsterdam, 1994, Elsevier.

60. Vieth J, Kober H, Sack G et al: The efficacy of the discrete and the quantified continuous dipole density plot (DDP) in multi-channel MEG. In Hoke M, Erne SN, Okada YC et al, editors: Biomagnetism: clinical applications, Amsterdam, 1992, Elsevier.

61. Vieth J, Grummich P, Kober H et al: Localization of slow and beta MEG waves associated with epileptogenic lesions, Epilepsia 34(6), 1993.

62. Reeve A, Knight J, Maclin E et al: Resting-state magnetoencephalography in schizophrenia. In Abstracts, International Congress for Schizophrenia Research, Colorado Springs, 1993.

63. Rieke K, Gallen CC, Sobel DF et al: Magnetic source imaging in cerebrovascular disease. In Abstracts, Biomagnetism '93, Vienna, 1993.

64. Gallen CC, Iragi V, Tecoma E et al: Identification of epileptic regions via MEG focal slow wave localizations: comparison with EEG monitoring, Abstracts, Biomagnetism '93, Vienna, 1993.

65. Lewine JD, Orrison WW, Halliday A et al: MEG functional mapping in epilepsy surgery. In Cascino GD, Jack CR, editors: Neuroimaging in epilepsy: principles and practice, Boston, 1994, Butterworth and Heinemann.

66. Oommen KJ, Galen C, Hirschkoff E et al: Inter-ictal magnetic source imaging and ictal subdural strip EEG: a comparison in source localization. In Abstracts, AEEGS, New Orleans, 1993.

67. Schwartz BJ, Gallen CC, Aung M et al: Magnetoencephalographic detection of focal slowing associated with head trauma. In Abstracts, Biomagnetism '93, Vienna, 1993.

68. Grummich P, Vieth J, Kober H et al: Localization of focal spontaneous beta wave activity associated with structural lesion in the brain. In Abstracts, Biomagnetism '93, Vienna, 1993.

69. Barkley GL, Tepley N, Nagel-Leiby S et al: Magnetoencephalographic studies of migraine, Headache 30:428-434, 1990.

70. Barkley GL, Tepley N, Moran JE et al: DC-MEG studies of migraine patients and controls. In Abstracts, Biomagnetism '93, Vienna, 1993.

71. Leao AAP, Morrison RS: The propagation of spreading cortical depression, J Neurophysiol 8:33-45, 1945.

72. Okada Y, Lauritzen M, Nicholson C: Magnetic field associated with spreading cortical depression: a model for detection of migraine, Brain Res 442:185-190, 1988.

73. Karhu J, Hari R, Makela J et al: Somatosensory evoked magnetic fields in multiple sclerosis, Electroencephalogr Clin Neurophysiol 83:192-200, 1992.

74. Karhu J, Hari R, Kajola M et al: Cortical reactivity in patients with progressive myoclonic epilepsy, Neurology 42(3):353, 1993.

75. Yang TT, Gallen CC, Ramachandran V et al: Noninvasive study of neural plasticity in adult human somatosensory system, Abstr Soc Neurosci 23, 1993.

76. Mogilnar A, Lopez L, Ribary U et al: Neuromagnetic assessment of somatosensory cortical organization following peripheral nerve injury and reconstruction, Abstr Soc Neurosci 17:1126, 1991.

77. Lewine JD, Astur RS, Davis LE et al: Cortical organization in adulthood is modified by neonatal infarct: a case study, Radiology 190:93-96, 1994.

78. Coles RRA: Epidemiology of tinnitus: prevalence, J Laryngol Otol Suppl 9:7-15, 1984.

79. Hoke M, Feldman H, Pantev C et al: Objective evidence of tinnitus in auditory evoked magnetic fields, Hear Res 37:281-286, 1989.

80. Jacobson GPB, Ahmad BK, Moran J et al: Auditory evoked cortical magnetic field (M100/M200) measurements of tinnitus and normal groups, Hear Res 56:44-52, 1980.

81. Leinonen L, Joutsiniemi S-L: Auditory evoked potentials and magnetic fields in patients with lesions of the auditory cortex, Acta Neurol Scand 79:316-325, 1989.

82. Makela JP, Hari R, Valanne L et al: Auditory evoked magnetic fields after ischemic brain lesions, Ann Neurol 30:76-82, 1991.

83. Makela JP, Hari R: Neuromagnetic auditory evoked responses after a stroke in the right temporal lobe, NeuroReport 3:94-96, 1992.

84. Reite M, Teale P, Goldstein L et al: Late auditory magnetic sources may differ in the left hemisphere of schizophrenic patients, a preliminary report, Arch Gen Psychiatry 46:565-572, 1989.

85. Reite M: Magnetoencephalography in the study of mental illness, Magnetoencephalogr Adv Neurol 54:207-222, 1990.

86. Dimond S, Scammell R, Pryce J et al: Some failures of intermodal and cross-lateral transfer in chronic schizophrenia, J Abnorm Psychol 89(3):505-509, 1980.

87. Coger R, Serafetinides E: EEG signs of lateralized cerebral dysfunction: relationship to cognitive impairment in alcoholics and to schizophrenic symptomatology. In Flor-Henry P, Gruzelier J, editors: Laterality and psychopathology, New York, 1983, Elsevier.

88. Nasrallah HA, McCalley-Whitters M, Bigelow L et al: A histological study of the corpus callosum in chronic schizophrenia, Psychiatry Res 8(4):251-260, 1983.

89. Ribary U, Weinberg H, Johnson B et al: EEG and MEG (magnetoencephalography) mapping of the auditory 40-Hz response: a study of depression, Soc Neurosci Abstr 14:339, 1988.

90. Ribary U, Llinas R, Kluger A et al: Neuropathological dynamics of magnetic, auditory, steady-state responses in Alzheimer's disease. In Williamson SJ, Hoke M, Stoink G et al, editors: Advances in biomagnetism, New York, 1989, Plenum.

91. Baumann SB, Papanicolaou AC, Levin HS et al: Auditory steady-state responses in subjects with early Alzheimer's disease. In Hoke M, Erne SN, Okada YC et al, editors: Biomagnetism: clinical applications, Amsterdam, 1992, Elsevier.

92. Ioannides AA, Bolton JPR, Clarke CJS: Continuous probabilistic solutions to the biomagnetic inverse problem, Inverse Probl 6:523-542, 1990.

93. Ribary U, Ioannides AA, Singh KD et al: Magnetic field tomography of coherent thalamo cortical 40-Hz oscillations in human subjects, Proc Natl Acad Sci USA 88:11,037-11,041, 1991.

94. Armstrong RA, Janday B, Slaven A et al: The use of flash and pattern evoked fields in the diagnosis of Alzheimer's disease. In Williamson SJ, Hoke M, Stoink G et al, editors: Advances in biomagnetism, New York, 1989, Plenum.

95. George S, Lewis P, Ranken DM et al: Anatomical constraints for neuromagnetic source models, SPIE Med Imaging V: Image Phys 1443:37-51, 1991.

96. Benzel EC, Lewine JD, Bucholz RC et al: Magnetic source imaging: a review of the Magnes system by Biomagnetic Technologies Incorporated, Neurosurgery 33:252-259, 1993.

97. Blum T, Bauer R, Arabin B et al: Prenatally recorded auditory evoked neuromagnetic fields of the human fetus. In Barber C, Blum T, editors: Evoked potentials III, Boston, 1987, Butterworth.

Magnetic Resonance Spectroscopy

John A. Sanders

M agnetic resonance spectroscopy (MRS) has been in use much longer than magnetic resonance imaging (MRI) and represents even more potential for impacting medical diagnosis, understanding, and treatment. MRS is a more general descriptor of the technology, with clinical proton MRI being only one narrow application of the rich physical phenomenon of nuclear magnetic resonance (NMR). This richness arises because many more interesting compounds exist in tissue than just the protons of water or fat. The characteristics of water and fat,

although very useful for diagnosis, have not been able to provide sufficient information for definitively discriminating between normal and pathologic tissue. Being able to noninvasively obtain information on specific metabolites and chemicals and on their uptake and changes at specific atomic locations within those compounds represents a vast amount of information useful for understanding and characterizing normal and pathologic processes. Rather than just being useful for diagnosis, the elucidation of the biochemical details of disease processes has the potential for significantly impacting the development of treatments.

The earlier chapters on MR in this book serve as a basic introduction to the tremendous diversity of the different types of information that can be obtained by MR techniques. We have seen that MR provides information regarding intrinsic T1 and T2 relaxation properties, spin density, blood and cerebrospinal fluid (CSF) flow, bulk motion, diffusion, diffusion anisotropy, perfusion, local oxygenation, local iron content, membrane permeability, and temporal dynamics of contrast agent interaction during imposed stresses or stimuli or with pathologic conditions. New developments and interpretations, such as localization of brain functional activation, continue to be developed. In principle, most of this information is available for each MRS-visible specific metabolite.

The additional information, which may be associated more often with MRS than MRI, results from the

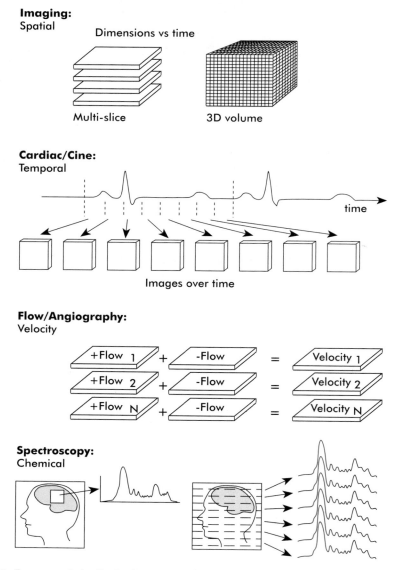

Fig. 10-1. Because of the limited amount of patient examination time, tradeoffs must be made among the different types of information available from nuclear magnetic resonance.

examination of nuclei other than protons, each of which has a spectrum of visible biomolecules and often represents different aspects of metabolism (e.g., energetics, compartmentalization, kinetics). Techniques are available to identify detailed molecular structures and conformations, local pH and temperature, biochemical pathways, and metabolite kinetics. These techniques can be applied toward assessing brain functional status and responses.

Obtaining MRS information generally involves giving up alternative types of information. This tradeoff is required because one cannot keep a patient comfortable in the magnet long enough to perform all the different measurements. In practice, one mostly trades spatial information (resolution) for chemical information (Fig. 10-1). As instrumentation and mea-

surement techniques are refined, the tradeoffs will be less severe. MRS procedures are evolving toward producing a detailed chemical spectra for each image voxel. Currently, the resolution of these voxels is limited by the desired signal-to-noise ratio (SNR), the tissue concentration of the metabolites of interest, and the amount of available scan time.

The concentration of water in tissue is on the order of 100 M, which is 10,000 times the millimolar concentrations of most metabolites of interest. This ratio explains why metabolite changes with physiologic events are not generally observed in images made from the net proton signals from tissue. It is also easy to see how images made of only the nonwater metabolites may be limited by signal strength. However, it is now feasible to obtain human

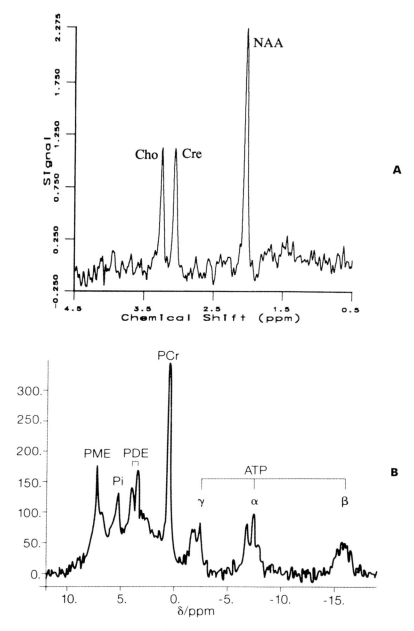

Fig. 10-2. Examples of **A**, ^{1}H, and **B**, ^{31}P MRS spectra of normal brain. (From Sauter R, Schneider M, Wicklow K et al: Current status of clinically relevant techniques in magnetic resonance spectroscopy, Electromedica 60:31-54, 1992.)

in vivo spectra from voxels as small as 8 ml with ^{31}P and smaller than 1 ml with [1]H. In addition, the feasibility of human in vivo ^{13}C, [23]Na, and ^{19}F images has been established.

The most common application of MRS is to the brain, somewhat reflecting the relative ease of implementation and its well-studied pathophysiology, neurobiology, and biochemistry (Fig. 10-2). The general findings from many studies indicate that spectra from pathologic tissue differ from those of healthy brain tissue and that these spectral changes are often greater

than the spectral variations observed throughout normal brain.

A particular focus has been MRS studies of brain tumors. These efforts are directed toward tumor differentiation according to the origin (cerebral or noncerebral) and the grade of malignancy. The results suggest that MRS is useful in clinical cancer management but that the diagnostic accuracy and prognostic value of MRS must be defined rigorously using well-designed multicenter trials examining large populations of patients.[1] With the establishment of routine examination procedures on available clinical scanners, these studies are underway.[2] A number of other pathologic processes have also been studied in vivo.

A natural extension of MRS brain studies is the development of techniques for examining chemical changes associated with neural activation. These techniques have been refined so that much information on cerebral blood flow (CBF), cerebral metabolic rate of oxygen extraction ($CMRO_2$), and glucose utilization, previously only available from radioisotope or positron emission tomography (PET) techniques, is now available from MRS studies. In addition, an increasing number of studies describe changes in metabolite concentrations resulting from activation. These functional MRS studies are often performed in conjunction with functional MRI to guide the placement of the MRS volumes of interest. The results from combined MRI and MRS functional examinations provide extraordinarily detailed information regarding the mechanisms of normal and pathologic neural activity.

MRS has a broad and extensive history of development and application, both in vitro and in vivo. The intention of this chapter is only to provide a brief introduction to the procedures and capabilities of this technology, particularly with respect to neurologic studies. Additional information on MRS is available in the references.[3-7]

HISTORY

The history of MRS is extensive and represents both the past and the future of MR as applied to medicine. The fundamentals of NMR spectroscopy were studied and developed for at least 30 years before being extended to clinical imaging. During this time, NMR spectroscopy was a principal tool of the physical and organic chemist for determining molecular structure. This extensive research and commercial history and the many years of development provide a firm basis of theory, technology, and methodology to support contemporary clinical applications.

As the sophistication of instrumentation and procedures evolved, application of spectroscopy to more and more complicated systems became possible. As MRS technology evolved to allow study of larger samples at higher field strengths, a logical step was to compare the spectral characteristics of normal and pathologic tissue specimens. In 1971, Damadian showed that differences existed between signals from normal and cancerous tissue samples and obtained a patent proposing a NMR scanning machine.[8] Shortly thereafter, in 1973, Lauterbur showed that images could be formed using NMR.[9] The excitement over x-ray computed tomography (CT) fueled this new development, and MRS applications to medicine were

eclipsed as MRI technology and clinical usefulness became firmly established. However, the goal of quick and easy cancer screening has not been fully realized using images formed from the relaxation characteristics of water and fat. The additional specificity offered by consideration of other tissue metabolites has led to a renewed interest in spectroscopic measurements. The ability to obtain these sensitive measurements routinely in vivo depends heavily on the availability of appropriate instrumentation. Some clinicians, used to the extraordinarily rapid deployment of MRI hardware and reimbursable procedures, may consider the progress toward clinical MRS to be slow.

MRS instrumentation development has followed a somewhat circular path to support current procedures. Initial imaging systems were converted spectrometers whose flexibility supported these new procedures but were perhaps difficult for people untrained in spectroscopy (i.e., radiologic technologists) to operate on a routine basis. Clinical imaging machines evolved toward specialized push-button instruments that made routine clinical operation efficient but offered less flexibility for new procedures. The instrumentation requirements for MRS are generally much more demanding than for MRI. Before MRI, the goal of magnet system design was to make the magnetic field homogeneity as pure as possible so that the slight frequency shifts of the signal would result from the specific nature of the chemical and not from the nonuniformity of the main magnetic field. As described more fully in Chapter 4, Lauterbur showed that by giving up the chemical information and applying a large field gradient, one could encode spatial position. Since the field homogeneity requirements for MRI are much less rigorous, the larger magnet systems needed for whole-body imaging systems could be constructed. However, the reduced homogeneity made MRS measurements difficult. Only recently have clinical whole-body magnet and instrumentation capabilities become sufficient to perform MRS studies effectively. Now that robust MRS localization and measurement techniques have been established, and the hardware and software demands of recent developments in high-speed MRI have become more exacting, instrument manufacturers have incorporated more flexibility and performance back into clinical systems, allowing further development of clinical spectroscopy.

In vitro MRS work is important for guiding and interpreting the in vivo results. However, continued development of in vivo techniques is essential in order to develop clinically relevant procedures, because notable differences often exist between in vivo metabolite ratios and those of in vitro extract work. For example, in vivo N-acetyl-L-aspartate (NAA)/Cr ratios are often greater than one, whereas they are less than

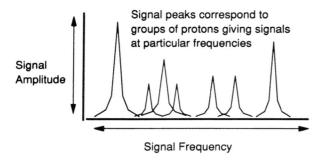

Fig. 10-3. A spectrum is a plot of signal intensity versus resonance frequency.

one in in vitro studies. In addition to the number of potential sources of metabolite level alterations during sample preparation and handling, it is known that metabolite levels change rapidly at death.[10]

BASIC PRINCIPLES

The basic principles for MRS are the same as those previously discussed for MRI (see Chapter 4). Imaging and spectral measurements are both aspects of the same physical phenomena of NMR. Specifically, all results in both spectroscopy and imaging follow directly from the fundamental relation that signal frequency is directly determined by magnetic field strength. The higher the field strength, the higher is the resonance frequency. The most significant procedural difference is that the MRS signal is collected in the absence of an applied magnetic field gradient (no frequency encoding of position), so the signal frequency distribution represents magnetic field differences other than those imposed by a gradient.

An MRS *spectrum* is a plot (intensity versus frequency) of the number of nuclei in different local magnetic field environments (Fig. 10-3). By convention, signal frequency increases to the left, reflecting the original measurement methods in which signal intensity was plotted relative to increasing applied magnetic field strength. The local magnetic environment results from an intrinsic *chemical shift* based on the electronic structure of the molecule in which the nuclei resides and the effects of any interactions with other nuclei. The signal recorded from the object volume of interest (VOI) is the sum of all the component signals at the different frequencies. As illustrated in Fig. 10-4, the now-familiar Fourier transform is used to convert the measured time-varying (time-domain) signal into a list of component frequency (frequency-domain) "peaks." This preoccupation with the measurement and interpretation of frequency spectra is where the term *spectroscopy* arises.

MRI is generally associated with the signals from hydrogen nuclei (i.e., protons) because of the relatively large amounts of these nuclei in biologic samples and the strong signals they provide. However, MRS

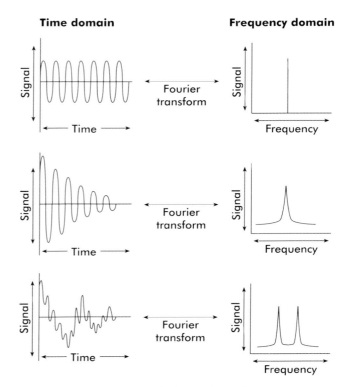

Fig. 10-4. The spectra result from taking the Fourier transform of the recorded time-domain data.

studies frequently make measurements of other nuclei, such as phosphorus (^{31}P), carbon (^{13}C), and fluorine (^{19}F). Table 10-1 shows the properties of the nuclei that are of most interest in biologic studies. As described in Chapter 4, three factors influence the ability to use nuclei for MRS studies: (1) the natural abundance of the atomic isotope having a MRS-visible nuclei (i.e., having net nuclear spin), (2) the amount of signal measureable from the particular nuclei, and (3) the natural occurrence or density of the nuclei in biologic systems.

As indicated in Table 10-1, nearly all hydrogen atoms (including both protons and deuterons) give an MRS signal, with the deuterium isotope (only 0.015% abundant) also being visible if the sample concentration is increased by administration of enriched compounds. Since the proton signals from water and fat are so large relative to other metabolites (Fig. 10-5), techniques must be employed to suppress these signals so that the other signals can be seen. Unfortunately, the MRS-visible isotope of carbon, ^{13}C, represents only 1.1% of all carbon atoms and requires either administered enriched compounds or sophisticated techniques to be effectively observed in vivo. All fluorine atoms are in the form of MRS-visible ^{19}F, but the naturally occurring amounts of fluorine are so low that administered compounds are also used in these measurements. The low natural background benefits

Table 10-1. NMR properties of biologic nuclei

Nucleus	Spin quantum number	Resonance frequency at 1.5 T (MHz)	Natural abundance (%)	Relative sensitivity at constant field
^{1}H	½	63.86	99.98	100
^{2}D	1	9.81	0.0156	1.5×10^{-4}
^{13}C	½	16.05	1.1	1.6×10^{-2}
^{14}N	1	4.62	99.6	1.0×10^{-2}
^{15}N	½	6.48	0.36	3.7×10^{-4}
^{19}F	½	66.0	100.0	83.0
^{23}Na	3/2	16.89	100.0	9.3
^{31}P	½	25.86	100.0	6.6
^{35}Cl	3/2	6.27	75.4	3.5×10^{-1}
^{39}K	3/2	2.97	9.1	4.6×10^{-2}

From Gadian DG: Nuclear magnetic resonance and its application to living systems, 1982, Oxford, UK, Clarendon Press.

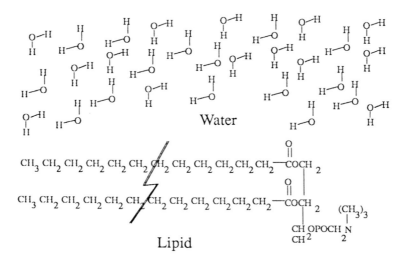

Fig. 10-5. Proton-rich water and fat give the dominant signals of in vivo ^{1}H MRS.

the use of fluorine in tracer studies. All sodium exists in the form of ^{23}Na, which provides large signals and is abundant in biologic systems. However, the biochemical information in a static sodium spectrum is limited. Phosphorus, ^{31}P, is the most frequently studied nuclei other than protons, and even though the sensitivity is low, the natural concentrations of phosphorus compounds are sufficient to allow a number of biologically important compounds to be studied (Fig. 10-6). When considering chemical species other than fat or water, the MRS measurement is always limited by SNR. The spatial resolution must be reduced or the acquisition time lengthened to obtain an adequate SNR.

Although protons are used here as an example, the basic principles of spectroscopy hold for all nuclei. Specific details are considered in the sections on each nuclear species.

Chemical Shifts

In 1946, the physicists Felix Bloch and Edward Purcell studied the environment of the nucleus and found that the resonance frequency of a particular nucleus ω_0, was directly proportional to the field strength experienced by the nuclei. In addition, the amount of signal (signal amplitude) was proportional to the number of nuclei being measured. As we have seen in Chapter 4, this simple relation can be expressed as

$$\omega_0 = \gamma B_0 \qquad (10\text{-}1)$$

where B_0 is the strength of the applied magnetic field and γ is a proportionality constant, the gyromagnetic ratio, that is characteristic for each different type of atomic nuclei. ^{1}H, ^{13}C, ^{31}P, and so on will have different resonance frequencies in the same magnetic field.

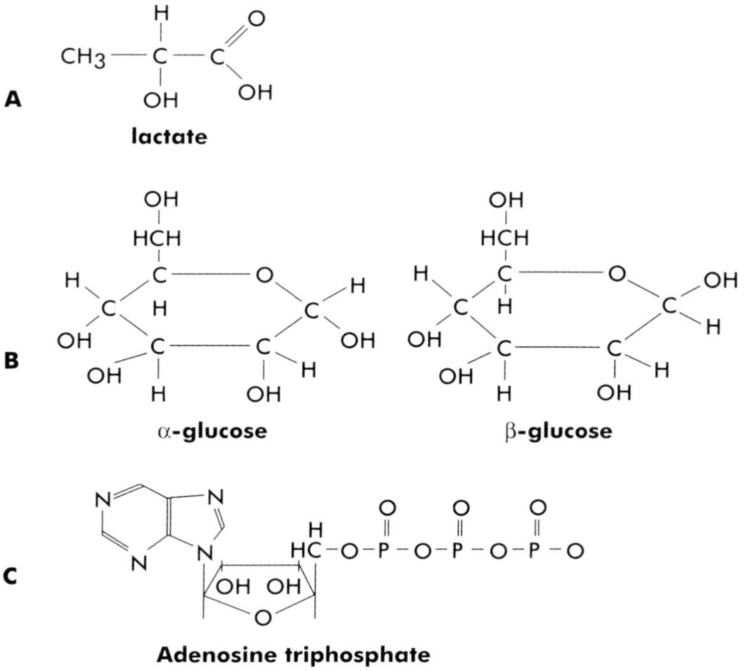

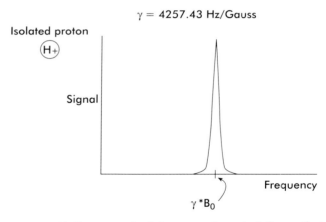

Fig. 10-6. The chemical structure of metabolites important in the MRS study of neural activation. **A**, Lactate; **B**, glucose; **C**, adenosine triphosphate (ATP).

This concept seems straightforward if we just consider bare protons in a magnetic field (Fig. 10-7). If all protons gave the same signal frequency, then little useful information would be available. However, an additional very important concept was soon recognized. If the same measurement is performed on protons that are part of a molecule, a difference exists in the resonance (and signal) frequency. This difference can be readily explained in terms of the basic principle of frequency being proportional to the magnetic field: a different measured frequency corresponds to the nuclei effectively experiencing a different magnetic field strength, B_{eff}:

$$B_{eff} = B_0 + B_{local} \qquad (10\text{-}2)$$

This local magnetic field contribution, B_{local}, can be either positive or negative and is primarily the result of two factors: (1) the magnetic fields of the circulating electrons around the nuclei and (2) the magnetic fields from nearby nuclei. Equation 10-1 also applies to this local field component. Therefore, the measured signal frequency, ω_{meas}, can be expressed as

$$\omega_{meas} = \gamma B_0 + \gamma B_{local} = \gamma B_0 (1 + \sigma) \qquad (10\text{-}3)$$

The second equality of the above expression reflects that the local field, B_{local}, produced is generally directly proportional to the strength of the applied magnetic field, B_0. The proportionality constant, σ, is called the *chemical shift* for the nucleus and is typically expressed

$\gamma = 4257.43$ Hz/Gauss

Fig. 10-7. If all protons had the same characteristics as that of a bare proton, little useful information available would be derived from proton MRS.

in terms of parts per million (ppm) of the frequency in the applied magnetic field. Expressed in this way, σ is independent of applied field strength and is fixed for the molecular environment (structure) of the nucleus. This also allows a somewhat instrument-independent measure for standardizing the reporting of results.

Electronic magnetic fields. In the absence of an applied magnetic field, the motions of the surrounding electrons produce no *net* magnetic field. However, in the presence of an applied magnetic field, a net

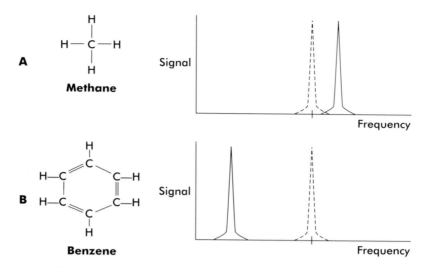

Fig. 10-8. A, Electrons surrounding the protons of methane shield the nucleus from the full applied magnetic field. **B,** The ring structure of benzene draws electrons from the protons, resulting in less shielding of the nuclei.

magnetic field is produced. Chemical shifts originate from the contribution by the electron magnetic fields.

The electron magnetic field produced by the application of an external magnetic field can be either *diamagnetic* (opposing the applied magnetic field) or *paramagnetic* (reinforcing the applied magnetic field). The type of field produced depends on the type and number of nearby electrons. Changes in field strength are also related to the electronic (chemical bond) interactions with other atoms. If the electron magnetic field induced by the applied field opposes the main magnetic field, the effective field at the nuclei is lessened and the nucleus is said to be "shielded" by the electronic fields (Fig. 10-8, **A**). Conversely, if the electron magnetic fields increases the field at the nucleus, the nucleus is said to be "deshielded" (Fig. 10-8, **B**).

A particular atomic species (e.g., hydrogen) is defined by the number of electrons that exist around it. If this electron density was always the same, all protons would still give signals at the same frequency, although slightly different from a bare proton, considering the local field generated by the associated electron(s). However, the actual electron density around the nuclei depends on the molecular environment (bonding structure) and the number of electronegative groups nearby. Protons of the body arise from two main sources: water (H_2O) and fat (primarily $-CH_2-$ groups). The electronegative oxygen atoms of H_2O tend to pull electrons away from the protons, so the applied field experienced by them is not shielded as much as the protons in fat. Thus, the proton signals from H_2O and the methylene protons of fat will be at frequencies that are separated by

approximately 3.5 ppm, regardless of the strength of the applied magnetic field.

The chemical shift of many compounds depends on the pH of the local environment. With the presence of a nearby titratable group, this property provides an important means of noninvasively ascertaining in vivo pH. This has been used particularly effectively in the case of ^{31}P spectroscopy, in which the location of the inorganic phosphate (P_i) peak is known to be very pH sensitive.[111] In proton spectra, the characteristic NAA peak is also pH sensitive, which can allow assessment of pH changes but also promote confusion with the nearby peak from acetate.[12]

Chemists immediately appreciated that such chemical shifts gave detailed information as to the chemical environment near the protons and the structure of the molecule in which the protons resided. As shown in Fig. 10-9, the relative peak amplitudes reflected the relative number of nuclei in the different environments. By examining the frequency spectra of the MRS signal of a sample of material, differences could be determined between molecules, giving information as to the chemical composition of the sample. The same process can also be applied to examining protons at different places within the same molecule. Protons in a molecule may be in different local field environments and so give rise to signals at different frequencies. Ratios of signals at the different frequencies indicate the relative numbers of protons at each location, providing basic information as to the molecular composition of a substance.

Imaging gradients. Typical proton chemical shifts represent a local magnetic field difference on the order

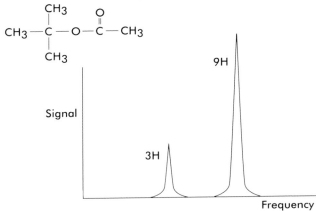

t-butyl acetate

Fig. 10-9. Relative peak amplitudes reflect the number of nuclei in the different magnetic environments.

of 10^{-7} tesla (T) for magnetic field strengths of 1 T. Magnetic field gradients used for imaging are on the order of 10^{-4} T/cm. Therefore, the frequency shifts caused by the gradient can be 1000 times greater than those from the chemical shifts. Furthermore, the homogeneity of the static magnetic field must be significantly less than this 10^{-7} T to observe frequency changes from the chemical shifts rather than from the magnet inhomogeneity.

Since chemical shifts are proportional to the applied magnetic field strength, they can be expressed in an instrument-independent fraction of the resonance frequency of some standard reference peak in the sample:

$$ppm = \frac{\left(\begin{array}{c}\text{Reference}\\\text{frequency}\end{array}\right) - \left(\begin{array}{c}\text{Metabolite}\\\text{frequency}\end{array}\right)}{(\text{Transmitter frequency})} \times 10^6 \quad (10\text{-}4)$$

The reference standard can be either added to the sample or, in the case of in vivo studies, can be a frequently appearing metabolite. For example, in proton MRS, water is an obvious standard and is often assigned a value of 4.7 ppm. Unlike external references, water is not an ideal shift reference because its precise resonant frequency can be influenced by the local environment. In phosphorus MRS, the phosphocreatine (PCr) peak is often used as a shift reference because its peak location does not appear to vary much with local conditions.

Fat and water "spectroscopy." It may be useful to point out how spectroscopic principles influence the appearance of fat and water in MRI. Basically, a simple spectroscopic measurement is being performed when the common occurrence of spatially misregistered fat

and water is observed in an image. Fig. 10-10 illustrates the mechanism for this process.

We have seen that the protons of fat and water are separated by 3.5 ppm because of differences in magnetic shielding by the electrons. In a 1.5 T magnet, this corresponds to an approximately 220 Hz difference in signal frequency. Given a typical frequency-encoding bandwidth of approximately 110 Hz/pixel, there will be a two-pixel offset of the fat from the water image in the frequency-encoding gradient direction. Since the signal from fat is strong relative to that of water, its appearance in the final summation image is noticeable. Every other proton metabolite behaves the same way and has a shifted appearance in the image. However, the small contribution of each shifted metabolite image to the final (blurred) image is usually not noticeable relative to those of fat and water. The gradient spatially distributes the signals along the gradient direction, superimposing with the shifted signals of other metabolites and allowing separation of metabolite contributions. This action of the frequency-encoding gradient is why imaging can be considered as typically trading spectral information for spatial information.

Peak splitting. Chemical information from MRS becomes even more detailed because of the process of peak splitting. If the spectral resolution of the measurement is adequate, the subdivision or splitting of many peaks into groups of individual peaks can be observed. Splitting of the signal peaks arises from the phenomenon of spin-spin coupling between nearby nuclei. Fig. 10-11 provides an example of these splitting cases.

In addition to the small electron magnetic fields influencing the net magnetic field at the nucleus, the small nuclear magnetic fields from nearby protons can also contribute to the net field strength. The precise field strength contribution to a nuclei depends on the neighboring nuclei and the chemical bonds between them. A resonance peak is often split into a number of equally spaced peaks, referred to collectively as a *multiplet*. The extent of the coupling depends on the proximity of the spins in space, with the most interaction occurring if the two spins are chemically bonded. However, spin-spin coupling can occur between spins that are two or more chemical bonds away.

The splitting occurs because protons tend to align themselves with or against the direction of the applied magnetic field. As seen in Chapter 4, the ambient thermal energy is sufficient to agitate rapidly the protons between the parallel and antiparallel orientations. Since this flipping process is so fast and frequent, the nuclei can be assumed to spend their time

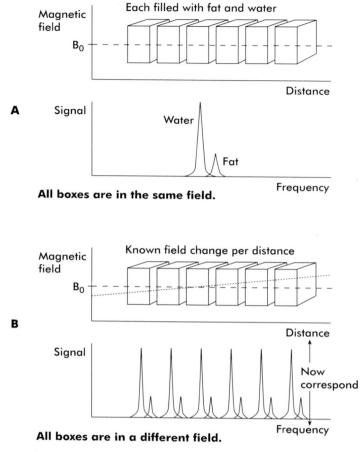

Fig. 10-10. A, Signals from the entire object reflect the relative proportions of fat and water protons. **B,** The application of an imaging gradient spreads the signals from each box along the gradient direction, leading to misregistration of the fat and water images.

approximately equally in both orientations. When a proton interacts with a nearby proton, they are influenced by each other's field. The net effect of this interaction depends on whether the respective fields are oriented with or against the applied magnetic field direction. Consider proton A being at one location within a molecule. If there is one neighboring proton, the neighbor's magnetic field can either add (+) or subtract (−) with proton A's field, and each case is equally likely. Therefore, the one neighboring proton will split proton A's signal into two equal and separate peaks.

If proton A now has two neighboring protons, the fields of the neighboring protons can add (+ +), be different (+ − or − +), or subtract (− −) from proton A's field. Being different is twice as likely as the other possibilities, so the peaks split in the same pattern as the likelihood, 1 : 2 : 1. From this splitting pattern, with the center of the triplet being twice as high, one can now tell the nature of the neighboring protons.

If there are N protons in the neighboring group, it splits the first group into $2NS + 1$ components, where

S is the atomic spin number of the particular nuclei (½ for proton; see Table 10-1). These splittings are small and are the same for both multiplets. The coupling constant, J, represents the distance expressed in hertz between the adjacent peaks of a multiplet and is characteristic of the type of chemical bond. Unlike chemical shifts, the coupling constants are independent of the applied field strength.

This splitting will not occur between identical protons having the same chemical shift, for example, with the three protons on a methyl group, since rapid spinning occurs around the carbon bond and therefore the average position of the three protons is the same. Signals from protons that exchange rapidly (i.e., they are rapidly replaced with a solvent proton), such as those of acid and some alcohol groups, are also not split. In addition, the centermost peak of a multiplet will slope upward in the direction of the set of peaks in the spectra with which it is coupled.

All these spectral clues allow organic chemists to determine what molecule/chemical is being measured. The pattern is unique, like a fingerprint, and the

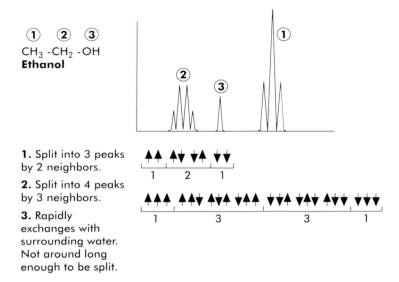

1. Split into 3 peaks by 2 neighbors.

2. Split into 4 peaks by 3 neighbors.

3. Rapidly exchanges with surrounding water. Not around long enough to be split.

Fig. 10-11. The splittings of ethanol protons reflect the number of neighboring protons.

pattern of an unknown compound can be compared with databases of spectral patterns. This technique has been used for more than 25 years to determine chemical structures. A huge number of theoretic and methodologic developments supported characterization of more and more complicated structures, including large macromolecules, biologic extracts, and isolated organ systems, and led to in vivo studies of animals and humans.

MEASUREMENT BASICS

The original and most basic measurement approach is to tune the radiofrequency (RF) transmitter and receiver to a specific frequency, measure the amplitude of the returned signal, make a slight change to the frequency, and remeasure. From this procedure, one can construct a plot of amplitude versus frequency, that is, the MR spectrum. Peaks in the spectrum occur at frequencies where a significant amount of the RF energy is absorbed and returned by nuclei, and these peaks correspond to the resonance frequency of that nuclei. A more current and efficient way is to transmit a wide range of RFs and measure the amplitudes throughout the returned range. The mixed returned signal can be separated into component frequencies using the Fourier transform.

Procedures

The primary difference between imaging and spectroscopy sequences is that the spectroscopy signals are collected in the absence of the readout gradient that is used for image frequency encoding. Although newer chemical shift imaging techniques use phase encoding, more typical MRS procedures do not use phase-encoding gradients for spatial localization. Since the signals from biochemicals other than fat or water are limited by SNR, most spectroscopy measurements employ a significant amount of repeated data-averaging measurements.

Echo time. Spin echo signal formation and collection are often employed. However, two major difficulties arise when using echo signals. The first concerns the loss of signal from compounds having short T2 relaxation times. Some of these are so short (e.g., ^{31}P of ATP) that free induction decay (FID) sequences are preferred to avoid loss of metabolite signals. The most frequently used proton localization sequences require the use of long echo times (TEs) of 135 to 270 msec to apply adequate water suppression measures and to avoid instrumental problems, such as residual eddy currents, after the application of magnetic field gradients for localization. Unfortunately, the long delay between excitation and acquisition allows T2 relaxation effects to reduce significantly the measured SNR. This can lead to almost complete signal loss for metabolites when TE is greater than two or three T2 intervals (e.g., mobile lipids). The use of shorter TEs reduces this source of signal loss (Fig. 10-12).

Second, long TEs may complicate the interpretation of signals from compounds having strongly spin-coupled groups, such as the methylene groups of glutamate and glutamine. Increasing TE may lead to irreversible spin dephasing from the complex modulation of the multiplet resonances. At short TEs, the metabolite peaks are seen as complex multiplet patterns because multiple components have less time to dephase in accordance with J-modulation.[13] The me-

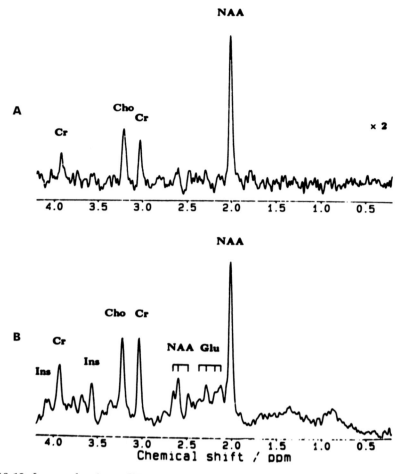

Fig. 10-12. Long echo times (TEs) lead to the loss of signals from metabolites having short T2s. White matter spectra at **A**, 270 msec, and **B**, 20 msec (From Frahm J, Bruhn H, Naenicke W et al: Localized proton NMR spectroscopy of brain tumors using short-echo time STEAM sequences, J Comput Assist Tomogr 15:915-922, 1991.)

thyl doublet resonance of lactate (and also alanine) is weakly coupled, and the TE is often lengthened (135 or 270 msec) to allow these signals to rephase.

Magnet. MRS magnets at MRS magnetic field strength are typically of superconducting designs. The magnet design should be such that the field is homogeneous to within 0.1 ppm and encompasses a region larger than the volume of interest in the object. The introduction of different study objects will affect the shim and require manual adjustment, but the adjustment is often limited by the static magnetic field inhomogeneity. The uniform field region must be stable over the course of the experiment.

Advantages of field strength. It is generally assumed that a 1.5 T or higher magnetic field strength is required to obtain adequate spectroscopy results, and MRS greatly benefits from measurement at higher applied magnetic field strengths (Fig. 10-13). In addi-

tion to SNR improvements with increasing fields, the spectrum is spread out so that overlapping signals from adjacent peaks do not obscure fine detail such as peak splittings. A 6 ppm chemical shift range of most proton metabolites is contained within a frequency range of approximately 380 Hz at 1.5 T. Those metabolite signals are spread out over approximately 1020 Hz at 4.0 T. These effects can also be observed in the imaging results at higher fields where fat and water chemical shift artifacts may become objectionable. The broadening of spectral features similarly improves the spectra from phosphorus (about 10 ppm range), fluorine (approximately 10 to 200 ppm range), and carbon (about 200 ppm range).

Also, it may be easier to study other nuclei at higher field strengths because the resonance frequency of other species increases and becomes closer to the resonance frequencies of protons in clinical imaging, allowing the use of somewhat more widely available instrumentation.

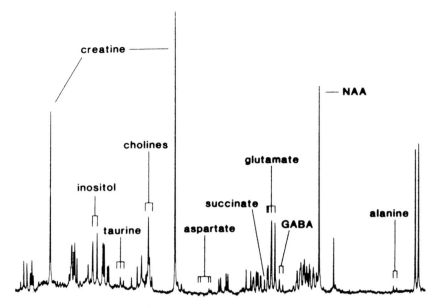

Fig. 10-13. High-field (7.0 T) ^{1}H spectra from an extract of gray matter. The spectral resolution and signal-to-noise ratio (SNR) increase with increasing field strength. (From Peeling J, Sutherland G: High-resolution ^{1}H NMR spectroscopy studies of extracts of human cerebral neoplasms, Magn Reson Med 24:123-126, 1992.)

Gradients. Eddy currents are small electrical currents and magnetic fields induced by changes in gradient strength and direction in nearby conducting structures within the magnet system. These currents persist during data collection and distort the recorded signals. MRS systems should incorporate gradient systems that allow fast rise and fall times without inducing eddy currents. Approaches to reduce eddy currents include: (1) tuned modifications to gradient waveform patterns that reduce eddy-current formation (precompensation), (2) actively shielded gradient coils that set up canceling magnetic fields outside the center of the magnet, and (3) improved magnet designs that do not have conductive materials near the gradient coils.

Since multiple repeated measurements are typically obtained for data averaging, the gradient system must be stable and reproducible so that it causes little variation from acquisition to acquisition.

Instrument requirements. A spectroscopy system generally requires broad-band RF transmitter and receiver systems to detect nuclei other than proton. Broad-band, rather than separate, systems are preferred because it is often of interest also to measure proton signals in order to form images to guide localization, to shim on the strong water signal, or to study simultaneously more than one nucleus.

A range of clinical imaging sequences is provided with the MR instrument, but only since the early 1990s

have spectroscopy sequences for clinical MRI scanners become available from instrument vendors. In general, a software facility is required to program and compile new sequences. The scanner programming language must have sufficient flexibility to accommodate the spectroscopy measurements. Even with provided sequences, spectroscopy measurements are often more sensitive to site-specific tuning (e.g., gradient balancing) than are imaging sequences, requiring some facility for adjustment.

Data-handling requirements. The data produced by MRS sequences and the required data processing are usually different from those of imaging studies, and the system must accommodate this type of data collection and processing. With the possible exception of sophisticated "four-dimensional" ("4D") MRS studies (three spatial, one spectral dimension), the size of MRS data sets is typically much smaller than that of imaging studies. The spectral information may contain approximately twice as much data as in one dimension of an imaging data set (twice the number of acquisition samples), but the spatial resolution of the measurements is often much reduced from that of imaging. Several differences exist in processing and display of MRS data, although the standard processing procedures do not require extraordinary computer facilities.

General MRS improvements to MRI instruments include increased stability, greater control over magnetic field gradients, finer frequency selectivity, reduced gradient-induced eddy currents, and optimized pulse modulation. Integration with imaging capabilities allows image-guided placement of spectroscopic regions of interest (ROIs). System improvements that are becoming more widely available include software-driven tools for rapid parameter optimization, optimized definition of (and data collection from) object ROIs, and faster postprocessing data analysis.

Coils. Measurement at different resonance frequencies typically means that different RF transmitter and receiver antenna coils must be designed and used. Because of the acute SNR limitations to MRS measurements, additional care needs to be taken with respect to coil efficiency and other areas of potential signal loss. The coil should be tuned to the object to maximize the efficiency of signal collection. The coil should also be uniformly sensitive throughout the VOI. Surface coils are often employed because the coil can be positioned closer to the signal-generating nuclei, and because the localized reception profile means that less noise will be collected from regions of the object (usually the dominant source of noise) remote from the coil.

Often, dual-tuned coils are used so that proton images can be obtained using the same coil. The much stronger proton signals allow the coil to be less optimized for these signals and still produce adequate images.

Homogeneity and shimming. In general, there is no way to distinguish between magnet inhomogeneity shifts and chemical shifts. The applied magnetic field inhomogeneity should be less than the desired spectral resolution to minimize the influence of the magnet system.

Although the area under a spectral peak is proportional to the number of contributing nuclei, the shape of the peak reflects the uniformity of the magnetic field. This directly follows from the basic proportionality of field and frequency. If all nuclei of a particular type are in exactly the same magnetic field (i.e., in a perfectly uniform field), they all will have exactly the same frequency and will show up in a spectra as a sharp spike at that frequency. In practice, the intrinsic exponential signal decay of their signal leads to the spike being slightly blurred into a lorentzian shape. More specifically, a lorentzian shape is the Fourier transform of an exponential decay, and this shape is convolved with each peak in the spectra, turning spikes into a more smooth shape.

If the magnetic field is not precisely uniform, the same type of nuclei at different locations in the measurement volume will be at a slightly different field and will have a slightly different frequency. The appearance of the spectral peak will therefore be

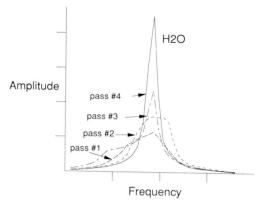

Fig. 10-14. Improvements in magnetic field homogeneity can be assessed by the shape of the water peak. The profile will become more narrow with improved shimming.

broader, even though the area under the peak is the same (Fig. 10-14). The amount of broadening reflects the distribution of magnetic fields throughout the measurement volume. When these applied magnetic field variations become greater than the field changes as a result of chemical shifting, the broad spectral peaks will overlap and make identification and analysis difficult.

The extent of inhomogeneity broadening is often measured using the shape of the large water peak. The amount of broadening is typically specified as the "FWHM line width," which is the full width of the peak (in ppm) at the half of the peak maximum. This parameter avoids some of the difficulties associated with measurement of the width of the broad "tails" characteristic of the bottom of lorentzian line shapes. Occasionally, a similar parameter for the full width at one-tenth maximum is specified to provide more detail about the shape of the peak and distribution of magnetic fields within the measurement region.

The magnetic field homogeneity strongly influences results obtained in MRS, and the FWHM values are useful for interpreting the results and in comparing results from other sites. Narrower spectral line shapes are more desirable to allow separation of closely spaced peaks. Most whole-body clinical magnet systems are designed with an approximately basketball-sized volume of high-field homogeneity in the center. In this volume, the lines of magnetic field intensity are uniformly spaced as they pass through.

The placement of an object into this region alters the uniformity of the region because of differences in magnetic field susceptibility within and between the object. MRS systems must have some provision for retuning the magnetic field strength for each object being studied. This process is called *shimming* because, as the name suggests, small mag-

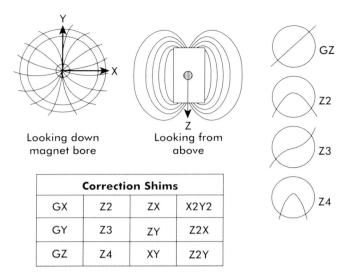

Correction Shims			
GX	Z2	ZX	X2Y2
GY	Z3	ZY	Z2X
GZ	Z4	XY	Z2Y

Fig. 10-15. Shimming uses a number of linear and higher-order field patterns to correct for nonuniform field distributions.

netic field offsets are added and subtracted to improve the homogeneity. During installation, the magnet system is "passively" shimmed using small pieces of metal to change the paths of the lines of magnetic field through the central volume. This proves adequate for imaging because the field homogeneity is only required to be significantly smaller than the relatively large field gradients applied for imaging. Spectroscopic measurements require shimming for each object being examined.

This important process is typically done interactively and may consume most of the total examination time. During this process, the currents through a number of different "active" shim coils within the magnet are adjusted to tailor the field within the measurement volume (Fig. 10-15). The availability and efficient adjustment of these coils are a primary hardware feature of MRS systems. These currents and the design of the shim coils set up small magnetic field patterns that are added or subtracted from the main magnetic field. Typically, both linear and higher-order gradient profiles are available. The linear shim profiles can be implemented as offsets to the currents in the normal linear gradients used for imaging. Specially shaped shim coils are used to generate the nonlinear patterns. Each profile may not need to be altered for each subject, and the lower-order patterns are somewhat more influential than the higher-order profiles.

Although shimming seems to be an appropriate procedure for automation, effective *autoshimming* methods have only recently been developed. Much of the complexity arises from the nonindependent nature of each shim profile. A change in one profile may affect the optimal setting of the other currents, and the

process becomes a difficult multidimensional (12, if there are 12 shim profiles) numerical optimization problem. An experienced operator can often obtain a good shim faster than an automated procedure. Mastering the "art" of shimming is the only significant operator-training issue for performing MRS studies routinely.

The basic procedure for shimming is to set up for repeated measurement of the water peak in the desired spatial regions. Since the peak line width is directly (through the Fourier transform) related to the decay time of the measured signal, either the time or the frequency domain of the measurement can be monitored as changes are made to the shim currents. Observing the decay envelope of the time signal is often easier if the transmitter is tuned 50 to 100 Hz off resonance. The adjustments to the shim currents are usually made to make the signal decay longer with a larger-amplitude integral, since a more uniform field will cause less signal dephasing because of $T2^*$-like cancellation. Adjustments are also made so that the shape of the signal decay appears more as an ideal exponential profile.

Water suppression. Since the concentration of water in tissue (100 M) is so much greater than the tissue concentration of most metabolites of interest (10 mM), the water signal would completely dominate the recorded signal unless measures were employed to reduce its signal (Fig. 10-16). The primary problem is the dynamic range of the receiver systems. The receiver gain needs to be set high enough so that the water signal does not saturate the system and severely distort the spectra. However, the sensitivity to changes in the much smaller metabolite signals is reduced by using the majority of the available measurement increments to accommodate the water signal. To use the available dynamic range more efficiently, several possible water signal reduction schemes are employed, each based on differences between the properties of water and those of the metabolites of interest.

Frequency-selective pulses. Several water suppression techniques take advantage of the chemical shift differences between water and other metabolites.[14-16] The most common approach is to use *che*mical *s*hift *se*lective (CHESS) RF pulses,[17] which are directly analogous to slice-selection pulses used in imaging sequences (Fig. 10-17). In this technique, a limited band of RF frequencies is transmitted to excite only those tissue compounds having a corresponding resonance frequency. The spins excited by imaging slice-selection pulses are determined by their position in an applied magnetic field gradient. The spins excited in the absence of an applied gradient are determined by their chemical shifts. For spectrally

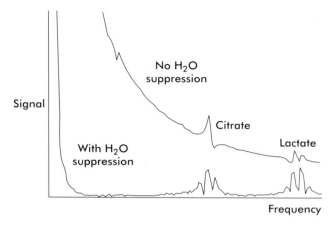

Fig. 10-16. The huge signal from water may obscure many metabolites of interest unless the water signal is suppressed.

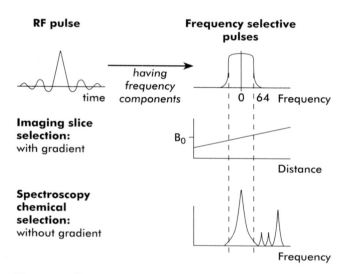

Fig. 10-17. Frequency-selective pulses use a radiofrequency (RF) pulse constructed to excite only a narrow band of frequencies corresponding to water in the sample. The principle is used for slice selection when combined with a field gradient.

(rather than spatially) selective pulses, the bandwidth of frequencies composing the RF pulse is typically chosen in order to select a limited number of chemical species. The most common application of this approach is to saturate and reduce the large water peak. In this procedure, a narrow bandwidth of frequencies centered on the water peak is transmitted, with the bandwidth determined by the line width of the water signal. One or more 90-degree excitations of water are followed by large dephasing gradients to eliminate the excited water signal. While the water magnetization is beginning to recover and is not available for excitation, the rest of the sample is excited and measured.

This approach can be used to reduce the signal from any unwanted peak in the sample (e.g., fat suppres-

sion). Alternatively, the selective RF pulse can be used to excite selectively any band of resonance frequencies. However, just as in slice selection, the nonideal frequency profiles available may not have sufficiently sharp frequency cutoffs to avoid having residual (tails of the frequency profile) excitation of the water signal or suppression of desired metabolite signals.

T1 methods. Other methods use the T1 relaxation differences between water and other metabolites. Inversion recovery sequences are often employed,[18-20] in which the water is selectively inverted by a frequency-selective 180-degree RF pulse. The magnetization of the metabolites of interest is excited after an appropriate delay until when the water magnetization passes through zero. A single inversion recovery procedure is sensitive to magnetic field inhomogeneity and variations in relaxation recovery rates. Shen and Saunders have demonstrated that better water suppression is obtained using repeated inversion recovery steps.[18]

Fat and tissue (water) T1s are different, so another method of reducing the appearance of fat in images is to perform an inversion recovery sequence with the inversion time, TI, adjusted to apply the 90-degree excitation pulse where fat is just crossing the zero line during its recovery from the 180-degree inversion pulse. At this point, fat has no longitudinal magnetization available for excitation, whereas the tissue magnetization is sufficiently recovered to give a water-only image.

Dixon method. A method developed by Dixon can also lead to the production of fat or water images.[21] His procedure of encoding chemical shift by signal phase is more general, but for fat suppression, typically two to four image acquisitions are used. This technique is based on the differences in precession frequency between fat and water and the phase difference that arises from the timing differences between echo signals formed by readout gradient area balance

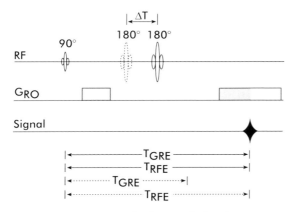

Fig. 10-18. The Dixon method uses slight changes in echo timing to cause differences between gradient and RF echoes, leading to fat and water acquiring a mutual phase shift.

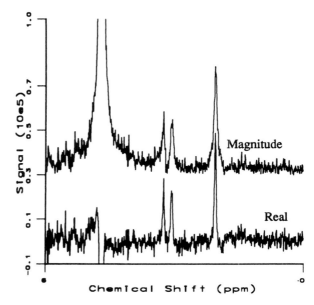

Fig. 10-19. The phase-corrected real part of the complex spectral values is typically used. Note that the peaks of the magnitude spectra are broader than those of the phase-corrected spectra.

(gradient echo) and the echo signal formed by the timing of the 180-degree pulse (RF echo). If the sequence is designed so that the gradient echo and RF echo occur simultaneously (as is usually done), all chemical shifts will have the same phase in the final image. If a short interval occurs between the two echoes, caused by moving the 180-degree pulse without changing the gradients (Fig. 10-18), the spins will be in phase at the RF echo and out of phase at the gradient echo and therefore in the image. The phase difference will be the difference in precession rates (about 3.5 ppm) times the echo mismatch interval. This can be adjusted so that the water and fat peaks are completely in phase or completely out of phase. Addition of these two (complex-valued) images leads to the cancellation of the fat, leaving a water image. Subtraction of the two images leads to the formation of a fat image.

Weisskoff and Kiihne[22] developed a similar technique for magnetic field and susceptibility mapping which is a more time efficient extension of Glover and Schneider's three-point technique.[23]

Zero/multiple quantum. Multiple-quantum filtering sequences[24-26] take advantage of water protons being noncoupled while some metabolites, such as lactate, contain coupled spin systems. These methods have been applied only relatively recently to human in vivo studies.

Data Processing

The production of spectral information from the collected data does not generally require extensive or complicated processing and follows basic signal-processing procedures. However, the postprocessing procedures associated with analyzing the results may be very sophisticated. MRS data processing consists of four basic steps: (1) initial preprocessing, (2) Fourier transform, (3) postprocessing and data corrections, and (4) data analysis.

Initial processing. During the preprocessing step, the raw time-domain data collected from the acquisition system analog-to-digital converters (ADCs) has any direct-current (DC) voltage offset and initial RF spikes removed. The data set is typically extended in length by addition of zero values (zero padding) to interpolate the spectrum after Fourier transform. Often, the data are multiplied by an exponential function (with a time constant of approximately $T2^*$) to reduce the noise contribution of later measurement samples obtained when little signal is available. This apodization or line-broadening operation improves the spectral SNR but at the cost of some broadening of the spectral line widths.

Fourier tranform. The second step consists of a Fourier transform that converts the collected complex time-domain data to the frequency domain and produces a complex-valued frequency spectrum.

Postprocessing. Postprocessing and data correction of the frequency spectra to remove artifacts are performed during the third processing step. Two frequently required operations are phase correction of the complex data and correction for the effects of eddy currents.

Phasing. Typically, phase corrections must be applied manually to the data to correct for both constant and linear phase shifts introduced during data collection (Fig. 10-19). The phase corrections are applied to obtain the corrected spectra in the real part of the Fourier-transformed complex data. This is done to

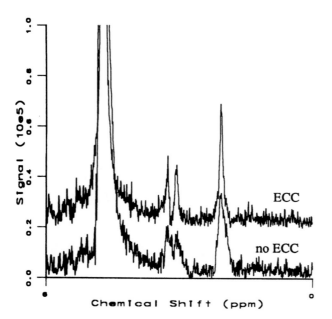

Fig. 10-20. Correction for eddy current–induced distortions leads to narrower peaks and improved peak profiles.

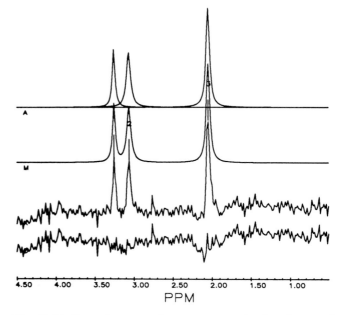

Fig. 10-21. To estimate peak areas accurately, the shapes of the spectra are fit with idealized peak functions. *Top to bottom*; model lorentzian peaks, resulting model spectra, actual acquired spectra, and difference between model and actual spectra.

avoid broadening the spectral peaks that result from computing a magnitude spectrum. The magnitude operation will always broaden the peaks unless the complete echo signal is obtained,[27] which rarely occurs in practice. The phasing may be difficult if both positive and negative peaks are in the spectra as a result of coupling. Spectroscopic imaging experiments are often accompanied by voxel-to-voxel phase shifts. Phased spectroscopic images are generally obtained by phasing the spectra from each voxel individually. However, manual phasing is not practical for large, multidimensional spectral images, and these cases must employ automatic phasing procedures.[28,29]

Eddy correction. Unless the magnet system incorporates active magnetic shielding, the eddy currents induced in the nearby metallic components (primarily the cryostat) cause phase distortion of the acquired spectra (Fig. 10-20). These problems may be even worse in spectrosopic imaging studies because these phase shifts may be combined with those from static field inhomogeneities. These effects limit the speed and amplitude of the gradient pulses employed in MRS sequences. The artifacts from these eddy currents are usually not as severe in magnitude images, even though imaging gradient activity may occur more rapidly. Pulse sequences with short TE are more sensitive to the effects of eddy currents.

Procedures for correcting the time-varying phase effects from eddy currents during acquisition have been proposed[30,31] and use a corresponding non-water-suppressed signal as a reference signal. This signal is obtained under otherwise identical conditions and allows estimation of the additional eddy-current

contribution to the suppressed signal. These methods have been further extended for application to chemical shift imaging (CSI) data.[32]

Several related techniques have been suggested for correcting the effects of static field inhomogeneity on acquired CSI data.[33-35]

Data analysis. The fourth processing step consists of quantitative spectral analysis of chemical shifts and computation of absolute or relative metabolite concentrations. The first activity is performed by identifying a known peak and assigning it a standard shift value. Using available information as to the measured spectral bandwidth and transmitter frequency, a chemical shift (in ppm) can be assigned to the remaining spectral peaks. Since the ppm shift value is largely instrument independent, the identity of the sample peaks may be determined by comparison with tabulated or in vitro experimental results.

The concentration of the metabolites generally are proportional to the area under the peak profile. In the case of isolated peaks, where the signal returns to baseline on both sides, the area can be obtained by simple numerical integration of the peak. For peaks that are close enough to overlap each other, the area under each peak can be estimated by numerically fitting an appropriately shaped curve (typically a lorentzian or gaussian profile) to the data points (Fig. 10-21). Absolute quantification requires a calibration measurement series or added internal standards of known concentration. This is often not available for in vivo measurements, so although the peaks within a spectrum reflect relative concentrations, determination of absolute concentrations may be problematic because the details of signal scaling during the measurement process are not known. Thus, direct comparison with spectra acquired from different experimental sessions is not feasible, and often only changes in metabolite ratios are used. Metabolite ratio changes can often be misleading if both metabolite levels are simultaneously changing. For example, even if both levels double, no change will occur in the ratio.

Furthermore, differences in T1 or T2 relaxation rates among the different metabolites will lead to errors in any analysis considering only peak ratios. In adults, metabolite peak signals do not decrease monoexponentially with increasing TE.[36] Longitudinal relaxation rates of the main peaks in the spectrum are not very different from each other,[36,37] so relative peak intensities are largely independent of the repetition rate (TR). The relaxation times reported (in seconds)[38] for common brain metabolites include water: T1 = 0.61, T2 = 0.11; choline: T1 = 1.20, T2 = 0.36; creatine: T1 = 1.60, T2 = 0.20; NAA: T1 = 1.50, T2 = 0.37; and lactate: T1 = 1.50, T2 = 0.37.

Quantitation. The spectral baseline may also be corrected to estimate accurately the relative areas of the spectral peaks. This baseline-leveling process must be done with care to avoid artificially introducing quantification errors. Poor water suppression leaves a large, broad signal, and the metabolite peaks of interest may occur on the shoulder of this signal. An alternative method for removing this water signal is to high-pass filter the data, with a spectral cutoff between water and desired peaks.

Even though quantitation is more difficult than observations of changing peak ratios, several procedures have been employed[36,39,40-42] to allow absolute quantitation of brain metabolite concentrations. Most of these procedures rely on the choice of some reference characteristic in the data, although in at least one report, the metabolite concentrations were calibrated by performing identical measurements on human autopsy samples.[43]

A semiquantitative analysis is available by calibration of the signal intensities to the noise level and assuming the measurement SNR does not change significantly. Although this technique is not expected to produce highly reliable quantitative values, the values may be sufficiently correct if the study intent is to show changes in patterns rather than fully evaluate the metabolite concentrations.

Procedures using the unsuppressed water signal as a reference are often employed.[36,44,45] Metabolite concentrations can be estimated by calculating the ratio of the metabolite and water signals and assuming a cerebral water content (e.g., 43.0 mmol/g wet weight[46]). Additional factors that may affect these and other procedures include (1) correction for any partial saturation from CHESS water suppression pulses, (2) diffusion losses in localization sequence, and (3) the coil sensitivity pattern.

Quantitative analysis must consider and/or correct the tissue composition of the voxel. For example, the measurement volume may contain mixtures of normal brain with tumor, CSF with normal brain, and so on. For methods that make comparisons with spectral data from additional, presumably normal tissue, the details of the patient treatment history must be considered.

A broad range of advanced signal-processing methods is available for analysis and comparison of spectral data. Fitting the individual peaks of the spectrum gives good results for estimating peak area but the Fourier transform may introduce distortions in the spectrum and in the subsequent quantification because of truncation of the measured signal. Sophisticated algorithms have been developed that combine data smoothing and estimation of signal parameters.[47] Multivariate statistical classification routines can be employed to use more fully all of the available peaks for discrimination between two sample classes.

Display methods. Effective presentation of the data from these methods is required for interpretation of the spectral results and for acceptance into clinical practice. This is a multidimensional data visualization problem, which has not even been adequately resolved for normal volumetric imaging.

Although only one-dimensional (1D) spectra are produced by localized volume methods, the relationship between the three-dimensional (3D) VOI and the surrounding tissue must be adequately represented. VOI results can be complicated by the presence of a mixture of tissue types within the measurement volume. Often, display of the VOI location in three orthogonal MR images is employed (Fig. 10-22), but adequate assessment of composition and potential signal contamination requires a more accurate representation of the actual VOI shape and spatial location of all parts of the VOI.

The limited spatial resolution of two-dimensional (2D) CSI data sets have allowed the frequently used display of an array of voxels, each with the spectra inside (Fig. 10-23). Data presented in this way can become difficult to interpret at higher matrix sizes. An alternative method is to restrict the information content to one (gray scale) or a few (color) measured chemical species and to form an image from the peak area under the compound (Fig. 10-24). In this way, an image can be made of any peak in the spectrum. Because of the limited CSI resolution, it can be difficult

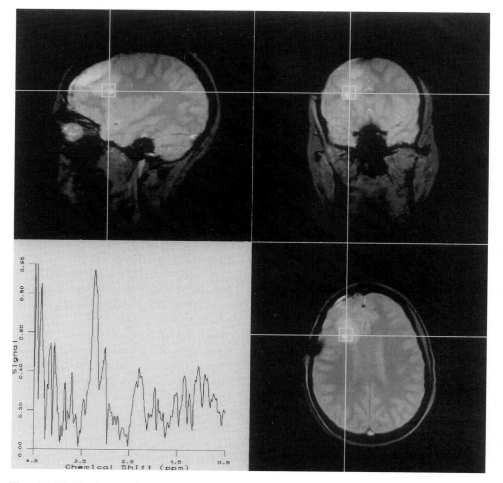

Fig. 10-22. Single-voxel spectroscopy region of interest (ROI) is displayed on the corresponding three image planes.

to identify anatomic structures, so these data are often superimposed on a corresponding high-resolution anatomic image. Interpolation of the metabolite image is often used liberally.

The use of contours to represent metabolite levels is also limited by the coarse CSI resolution and is seen less often. Effective presentation of full 3-D CSI information remains an unsolved problem.

Spectral Localization Methods

The long history of in vitro work with chemical solutions or prepared tissue samples has amply indicated how much useful information is available from MRS. The extension of this technology to in vivo work generally requires limiting the measurements to some specific and identifiable tissue region. This allows identification of the tissue of origin of the spectra and examination of regional differences in spectral characteristics. As spatial localization techniques have become more refined, spectroscopy measurements have moved closer to recovering some of the spatial resolution difference between MRI and MRS measure-

ments. Most current MRS localization methods use proton images to guide the placement of the regions or VOIs. Therefore, spectroscopy examinations typically include an MRI study.

Surface coils. To overcome the poor SNR of measurements of the low-concentration in vivo metabolites of interest, small surface coil antenna systems were initally employed.[48] The limited reception profile of the coils provides a measure of localization of the detected signal (Fig. 10-25). The shape of the sensitive region relative to the coil can be specified by alterations to the coil design. Selective RF excitations and other modifications to the RF characteristics can further improve the localization ability, but surface coils are effective primarily in relatively superficial regions of the body. Surface coils are still often used to utilize their SNR advantages, but their use in conjunction with other localization techniques has made the shape of the coil reception profile less critical.

Surface coils can be either transmit and receive or receive-only RF antennas. Often, another coil with a

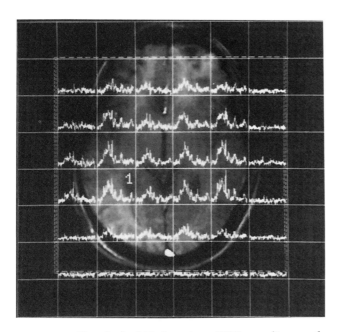

Fig. 10-23. Chemical shift imaging (CSI) results can be displayed to show the spectra recorded at each pixel location. (From Sauter R, Schneider M, Wicklow K et al: Current status of clinically relevant techniques in magnetic resonance spectroscopy, Electromedica 60:31-54, 1992.)

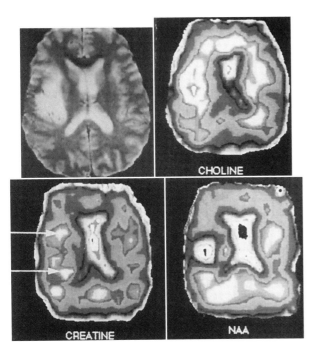

Fig. 10-24. Images can be made of any peak in the spectra recorded at each pixel location. (From Fulham MJ, Bizzi A, Dietz MJ et al: Mapping of brain tumor metabolites with proton MR spectroscopic imaging: clinical relevance, Radiology 185:675-686, 1992.)

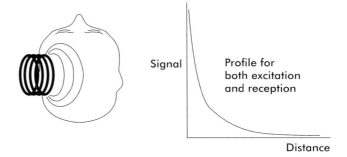

Fig. 10-25. The limited sensitivity profile of surface coils provides some localization of the recorded signals.

more uniform RF profile is used to transmit, and the surface coil is used for reception. The RF sensitivity pattern of the surface coil also applies to RF transmission, and this nonuniform distribution of excitation energy typically means that an RF pulse will result in a distribution of flip angles throughout the object. The effects from the application of nonuniform B_1 fields by these coils can be reduced through the use of adiabatic RF pulses showing flip angle insensitivity to field homogeneity and applied RF power.[49-53]

Chemical shift imaging. CSI[54,55] and spectroscopic imaging are the terms most often used to describe MRS acquisitions that employ phase encoding of spatial position. This use of phase encoding is very similar to the procedures used in regular 2D and 3D imaging applications. The acquisition of spectral information means that frequency encoding of position cannot be used. To obtain both spectral and spatial information, spatial information can be encoded in signal phase. However, as with most imaging sequences, phase encoding requires repeated acquisitions, which directly lengthens the required imaging times.

These procedures can be applied for 1D, 2D, or even 3D acquisition of brain spectra (Fig. 10-26). This occurs with only a slight reduction in SNR per unit volume and unit time.[56] The result of these studies is a complete chemical spectra for each voxel in the phase-encoded volume. The resolution and frequency width of these spectra are determined by the same data acquisition parameters as are nonimaging spectroscopic measurements. From this information, a complete image can be made using the area of any peak in the spectrum. Although the availability of this detailed information is attractive, the long imaging times required and limitations in metabolite signal strength usually result in the image spatial resolution being reduced from that of imaging-only studies.

Typically, a complete acquisition (of duration specified by TR) is obtained for each phase-encoding step. The set of entries in a phase-encode table is played out

1D CSI – spectra from each strip

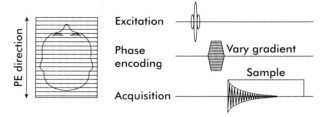

2D CSI – spectra from each pixel

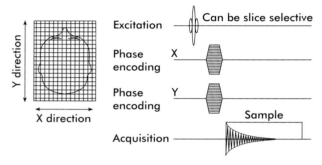

Fig. 10-26. Just as in imaging, phase encoding can be used in MRS to encode spatial position in either **A**, one dimension, or **B**, two dimensions.

for each encoded direction. However, it has been shown that this phase encoding can also be performed with appropriately modulated RF pulses.[57] A 1D CSI data set typically employs slice-selective excitation with orthogonal saturation bands to define a column through the structure of interest. The phase encoding is performed along the column. Just as in 3D volumetric imaging, a 2D CSI data set is obtained using two phase-encoding acquisition loops. Instead of using an applied readout gradient during data collection to frequency-encode the remaining spatial dimension, acquisition of the signal without a gradient allows the spectral dimension to be collected.

A primary and compelling advantage of CSI is the ability to define better the regions where the spectra are being measured. In addition, the localized spectra from many locations are acquired simultaneously, giving a larger detected signal and better SNR. Consequently, CSI can be significantly more efficient than single-voxel techniques. Instead of only averaging N different signals from a single voxel, the signal from an entire region is obtained N times, each with a different phase encoding. The Fourier transform is used to obtain the spectra from each phase-encoded region.

The CSI data allow easier evaluation of spatial differences in spectral features. Another important advantage for this type of data is that after examination, the position of the reconstruction voxels can be shifted in the phase-encoding direction[13] to match the desired measurement location.

A major disadvantage of CSI is that the signal from a voxel is prone to contamination by signal coming from the outside. This contamination is a consequence of the discrete and finite sampling, the artifacts from which are also seen in normal imaging using small matrix sizes. Since the number of phase-encoding steps is typically more limited than for normal imaging acquisitions, the point-spread function for each voxel will cause the signal from each voxel to contain a significant contribution from neighboring voxels (Fig. 10-27). This so-called voxel bleeding leads to less accurate spatial localization.

Another signficant difficulty for CSI studies is the large influence of static field inhomogeneity and gradient-induced eddy currents. These factors can distort the resonance frequency, the line width, and line shape (i.e., overall phase). Since spectral data are collected over a larger region than a single voxel, more demands are made on the homogeneity of the magnetic field and in the effectiveness of shimming with respect to the object. The variation in magnetic field and resonance frequency across the object makes effective application of frequency-selective pulses (e.g. CHESS pulses for water suppression) problematic and leads to individual spectra being offset in frequency.

The resolution of CSI images is determined by the magnetic field homogeneity and the pulse sequence details. If two spectral lines arising from a tissue region overlap because the field is inhomogeneous across the tissue, an empirically plausible approach may be to divide the tissue into smaller voxels, which have a more uniform field across each voxel. The spectra from each voxel can then be aligned (e.g., using water as a shift reference) and the voxel signals added back to improve the SNR of an overall spectra from the tissue. Unfortunately, even if the quality of the individual spectra is sufficient to allow mutual alignment, the addition of the voxel signals does not recover all the SNR that was lost by subdividing the tissue region. This is an important difference between MRS and nuclear medicine imaging techniques, in which pixel sizes can be increased after the measurement. Increasing the size of MRS pixels incurs a substantial noise penalty because all measurements have the same noise, whereas in particle-counting techniques, the noise increases with the number of measured counts.[58]

Since frequency encoding is not used, a 2D CS image requires phase encoding in two directions. A 2D CS image with $N \times M$ pixels requires $N \times M$ phase-encoding steps, with each measurement taking TR length of time. Therefore, a 2D CSI measurement can be obtained in approximately the same amount of time as a 3D imaging measurement. Furthermore, the limited signal strength of most metabolites requires delaying the next acquisition cycle long enough for T1 recovery to occur. For example, it would take approxi-

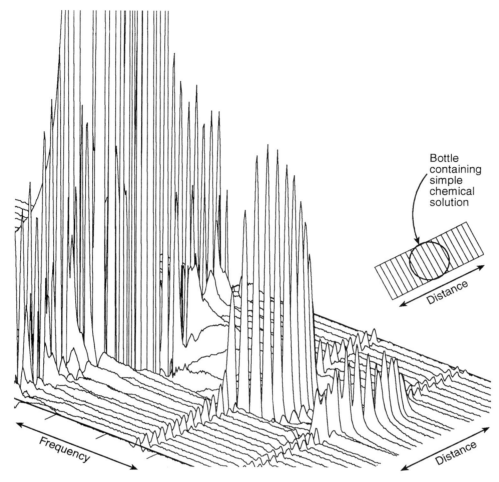

Bottle containing simple chemical solution

Distance

Frequency

Distance

Fig. 10-27. The small matrix sizes of some CSI experiments lead to contamination from signals from adjacent voxels. In the 1D CSI experiment shown, the amount of signal bleeding into adjacent voxels is greater for the large water peak (*left*) than the smaller peaks of citrate (*middle*) and lactate (*right*).

mately 4½ hours to produce 128 × 128 phase-encoding steps using a TR of 1 second. However, 32 × 32 phase-encoding steps can be obtained in only 17 minutes, which can be interpolated to give data on a 64 × 64 grid. These relatively long imaging times make these measurements susceptible to artifacts from patient motion during the examination.

Although one measurement is often sufficient for spatial encoding an imaging dimension, more than one measurement average often is required to obtain a sufficiently high SNR for the measurement of dilute compounds such as lactate or PCr. Therefore, the compromise is usually to increase the pixel sizes so that fewer phase-encoding steps are required. Since the time penalty for obtaining 3D CSI data sets is so severe, 2D CSI acquisition procedures have been extended to make measurements of multiple slices.[59] Duyn and Moonen further extended these techniques to use the signals from multiple spin echoes.[60] Since the T2* decay is typically much shorter than the

intrinsic T2 decay, the measurement efficiency can be increased by acquiring multiple spin echo signals. The optimal number of echoes, with respect to efficiency and spectral resolution, depends on the ratio of T2*/T2 and therefore on B_0 homogeneity.

Localized volume. Another very successful approach to spectral localization is to apply a series of slice-selective RF pulses so that only the spins in a localized VOI are properly excited to produce a signal. The position and size of the VOI is determined by the region defined by the intersection of the three orthogonal slices (Fig. 10-28). The shape of the intersection is considered as being a box, but the actual shape depends on the slice profiles of the selective pulses. Clinical imaging systems have long employed arbitrarily located saturation bands for reducing imaging artifacts and have developed efficient methods of placing these slices with respect to acquired scout images. The availability of these facilities and the

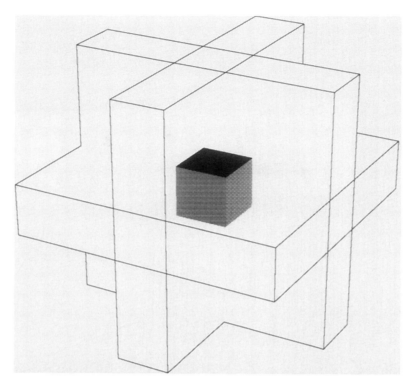

Fig. 10-28. In single-voxel spectroscopy, the measurement volume is defined by the intersection of three orthogonal slice planes.

relative ease of implementing these sequences have made these techniques widely available options on clinical instruments. This type of examination often obtains MRS data from more than one VOI placement to investigate spatial variations or to obtain reference data from uninvolved tissues. There are three principal variants of localized-volume procedures.

PRESS. *P*oint-*res*olved *s*pectroscopy (PRESS)[61,62] is a double spin echo technique in which three perpendicular slices are excited by one 90-degree and two 180-degree sinc-shaped pulses (Fig. 10-29). Only the spins in the volume defined by the intersection of the three excited slices experience all three pulses and create a second echo. Only the second echo generated is collected.

The initial 90-degree pulse produces the transverse magnetization, and throughout the entire sequence, the magnetization remains in the xy plane and contributes to the measured second-echo signal. The slice profiles of 180-degree pulses are often worse than those of a 90-degree pulse, so PRESS VOI definition and spectral localization may be worse than those of other techniques (e.g., STEAM) that use only 90-degree pulses. Furthermore, the repeated 180-degree pulses require more power than 90-degree pulses, which may be excessive for either large VOIs (i.e., thick slices) or large objects.

STEAM. *St*imulated *e*cho *a*cquisition *m*ode (STEAM) spectroscopy[63,64] is also frequently em-

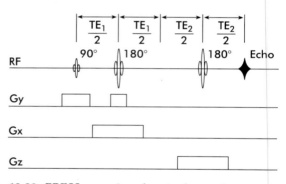

Fig. 10-29. PRESS, or spin-echo single-voxel spectroscopy, uses orthogonal 90-degree and 180-degree slice-selective pulses to define the volume of interest.

ployed for brain MRS studies. In this technique, three perpendicular slices are excited by three 90-degree sinc-shaped RF pulses (Fig. 10-30). Only the spins in the volume defined by the intersection of the three excited slices experience all three RF pulses and create a stimulated echo. All other echo signals generated are spoiled by gradient pulses, and only the stimulated echo from the VOI is collected.

The initial 90-degree pulse rotates all the magnetization into the xy (transverse) plane. The second 90-degree pulse rotates 50% of the magnetization back to the xz and yz planes. The remaining 50% of the magnetization remaining in the xy plane is dephased

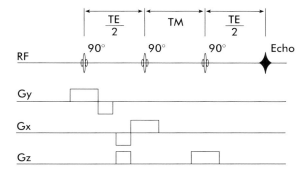

Fig. 10-30. STEAM localization uses three orthogonal 90-degree pulses to produce a signal from a volume of interest (VOI).

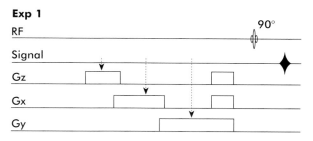

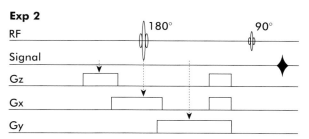

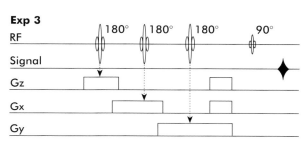

Fig. 10-31. ISIS uses combinations of multiple experiments to cancel signals from regions outside of the desired VOI.

during the middle TM interval between the second and third RF pulses and will not contribute to the stimulated-echo signal. Therefore, this method has a factor of 2 loss in SNR. The spoiler gradients must rephase the stimulated echo or second spin echo and dephase all FIDs and primary echoes. During the TM period, the magnetization in the xz or yz planes will decrease according to T1, but not T2, relaxation, and this period is kept short to avoid significant signal loss. The third 90-degree RF pulse rotates the magnetization back into the xy plane, where it refocuses after another TE/2 interval to give the stimulated-echo signal.

ISIS. *I*mage-selected *i*n vivo *s*pectroscopy (ISIS)[65] employs a series of repeated acquisitions, using up to three slice-selective 180-degree inversion pulses before a nonselective 90-degree excitation pulse, to define the VOI (Fig. 10-31). Eight different experiments must be performed, each preceded by a different preparation block, and the signals are subsequently combined in an addition/subtraction scheme that cancels the contributions of signals from outside the VOI. Depending on which planes are to be inverted, the preparation period consists of zero to three inversion pulses, applied at fixed timing points within the ISIS sequence. The eight on/off combinations of the three slice-selective inversion pulses define the eight possible different ISIS preparations. A 90-degree excitation pulse is applied after the preparation (Fig. 10-32). The particular order of the experiments is called a *phase cycle*, which can be optimized to avoid contamination from outside of the VOI.[66]

This technique usually uses a cubic VOI, defined from the intersection of the three slice planes. In contrast to other single-volume localizations, ISIS introduces essentially no T2 losses between signal preparation and detection, making ISIS an appropriate technique for localization with ^{31}P experiments. Unlike STEAM and PRESS, which combine acquisition and localization pulses, the ISIS sequence achieves

localization before the excitation sequence, allowing total echo evolution times (TE + TM) to be minimized. This reduction in echo evolution time maximizes SNR by minimizing T2 and *J*-modulation losses.

Hybrid techniques. Both single-voxel and CSI techniques have advantages. CSI methods are appropriate for observing regional variations of metabolites (e.g., tumor heterogeneity), whereas VOI techniques are useful for interrogating specific locations within the brain (e.g., neuronal metabolic alteration) and are easy to implement. It is natural that hybrid techniques would be developed to combine these advantages (Fig. 10-33).

Long examination times are required to obtain data from more than one VOI placement or to phase-encode a CSI slice adequately. Because the time penalties can be so severe, methods have been developed to obtain localized information from a specified region without having to phase-encode completely the spatial location of the signals. This allows more of the available examination time to be spent obtaining data for signal averaging and SNR

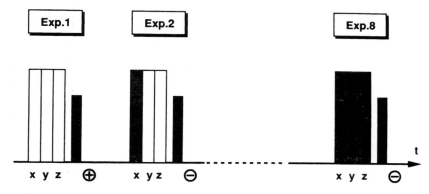

Fig. 10-32. Schematic representation of an ISIS measurement. The slice-selective inversion pulses are represented by empty rectangles if the pulse is omitted. The final pulse is the nonselective 90-degree excitation pulse. The required receiver phase is indicated by the + or − sign. (From Burger C, Buchli R, McKinnon G et al: The impact of the ISIS experiment order on spatial contamination, Magn Reson Med 26:218-230, 1992.)

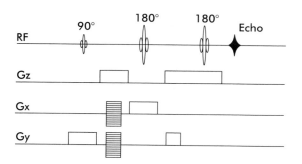

Fig. 10-33. Hybrid single-voxel/CSI sequence that uses spin echo excitation of a localized volume, which is then phase-encoded to give a CSI data set.

improvements. Often a volume-selective set of preparation pulses is applied to reduce the region where phase encoding is required.

Particularly with the VOI techniques that use 180-degree pulses, definition of a region for subsequent phase encoding generally involves increasing the slice thicknesses and RF power requirements. In general, spectra are desired from only a particular region in the slice field of view (FOV). Volume selection of a limited region allows fewer phase-encoding steps to be used to produce the desired CSI voxel resolution. This approach helps reduce the effects of voxel bleeding, particularly in order to avoid lipid contamination from scalp fat. VOI prepulses can also be employed in normal imaging to reduce the image FOV while avoiding aliasing.

CLINICAL APPLICATIONS

Spectroscopy is an important tool for investigating the concentrations and kinetics of tissue metabolites partly because of its completely noninvasive nature. Often, analytical biochemical extraction and analysis does not provide accurate values of metabolite levels (particularly for energy-related compounds such as P_i, ATP, and ADP) and does not allow repeated measurements on the same sample. MRS provides a wealth of information regarding biochemical processes underlying normal and diseased tissue. However, these measurements are technically demanding, and MRS is used mostly as a research tool at relatively few MR facilities.

With the development of robust procedures, MRS examination times of less than the typical 60 minutes for which a patient may remain comfortable can produce clinically relevant information. Within this time frame, patient motion does not appear to be a major limitation. However, the presence of superficial dural clips, large areas of hemorrhage, or metal fillings from previous surgery can cause significant artifact problems. Given the heterogeneous nature of most lesions, MRS is more likely to be most effective in conjunction with MRI studies.

Proton

Proton MRS benefits from having a strong signal, a variety of observable and biologically important metabolites, and ease of implementation on MRI systems. The main problem for proton MRS is dealing with the relatively huge signals from water and fat. Fortunately, little fat is present in the brain, but signal contamination by scalp fat requires careful spatial localization. Water suppression is required, and various techniques, ranging from readily implementable to quite esoteric, are available.

Much work in proton MRS has focused on the diagnosis and staging of brain tumors. Although not completely definitive, proton MRS may allow the distinction between low-grade and high-grade primary brain tumors by means of the degree of elevation of choline, reduction in creatine, or elevation of lactate.[1] This assessment may be easier to make in

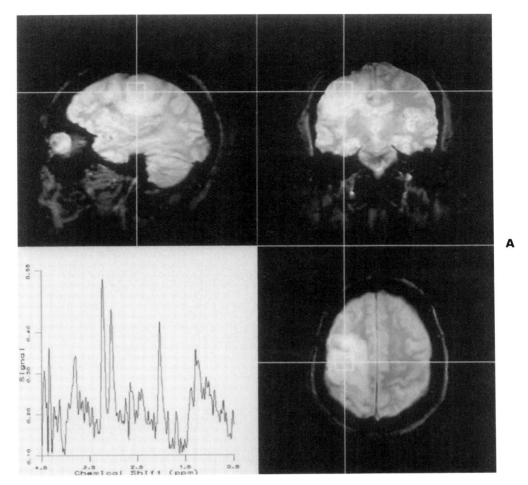

Fig. 10-34. Proton primary brain tumor spectra. **A,** Tumor.   *Continued.*

comparison with spectra from contralateral, uninvolved tissue (Fig. 10-34). However, this is complicated by systemic effects, and corresponding "normal" brain tissue is not available for metastatic lesions.

At 1.5 T, the proton chemical shift range normally of interest is approximately 6 ppm or 380 Hz. Three relatively prominent resonances are typically observed in proton spectra of the brain: choline, creatine, and N-acetyl-L-aspartate (NAA).

Choline. The $N(CH_3)_3$ group of choline (Cho) gives a strong peak at 3.2 ppm. In addition, there may also be contributions from glycerophosphocholine, phosphocholine, and possibly phosphatidylcholine, all of which are components of phospholipid metabolism and are constituents of cell membranes.[67] Thus, increased choline signal intensity may reflect increased membrane synthesis and cellularity.[68] Response to treatment may be followed by monitoring the decline in choline levels, which is most effective if a pretreatment baseline examination is performed.[67]

Based on their finding of a large choline concentration that decreases rapidly after birth, Kreis et al. suggest that levels of MRS-visible choline compounds may decrease in newborns because of incorporation of choline-containing compounds (e.g., phosphatidylcholine) into MRS-invisible macromolecules associated with myelin.[69] This would also be consistent with the high levels of choline observed with acute demyelinating diseases.[70,71]

Choline levels increase in most solid tumors, and solid high-grade gliomas generally have higher normalized choline values than solid low-grade tumors. However, a study by Fulham and colleagues found that the normalized choline levels were not a discriminator of tumor grade because necrotic high-grade lesions also had reduced choline values.[67]

Creatine. The $N(CH_3)$ group of creatine/phosphocreatine (Cr/PCr) provides a strong signal at 3.03 ppm. This peak may also contain some contribution from γ-aminobutyric acid (GABA), lysine, and glutathione. The separation achieved between Cr/PCr

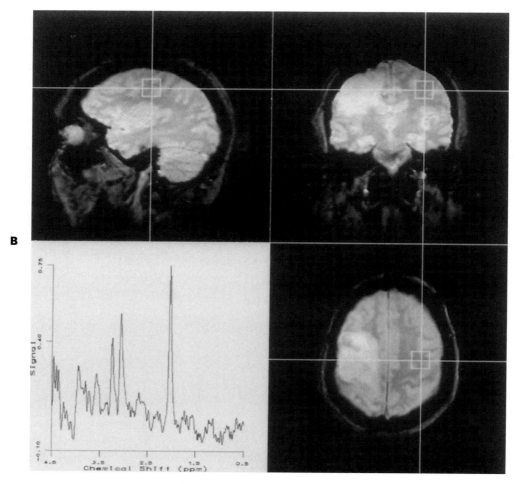

Fig. 10-34. cont'd. B, contralateral.

and the nearby choline peak provides an approximate assessment of the success of the shimming procedures. An additional creatine peak can be observed at 3.94 ppm.

Although creatine itself is of little direct biochemical interest, the equilibrium enzyme creatine kinase (converting Cr to PCr) appears to be crucial to the maintenance of energy-dependent systems in all brain cells.[69] Creatine may increase in hypometabolic tumors but decrease in hypermetabolic tumors.[67] This is somewhat different from studies using ^{31}P, which report that PCr remains the same or becomes decreased in tumors.

NAA. The *N*-acetyl methyl (CH_3) group of NAA gives a prominent peak at 2.0 ppm and is one of the most distinctive features in the spectrum from normal brain. This peak also contains contributions from *N*-acetylaspartylglutamate (NAAG) (in white matter) and other *N*-acetyl groups.[72] The aspartyl group of NAA gives resonances at 2.48, 2.60, and 2.64 ppm.

NAA is generally accepted to be a neuronal marker,[73-76] although some evidence suggests that other cell types contain NAA.[69,77] Noncerebral tumors show little or no NAA.[78] Therefore, destructive or infiltration diseases that selectively cause neuronal loss are likely to result in the decrease of NAA levels relative to other metabolites. NAA can be a marker of neuronal loss or damage in various disorders, including cerebrovascular accident (CVA, stroke), human immunodeficiency virus (HIV), or epilepsy, but this nonspecificity implies that NAA levels may be less effective in the evaluation of brain tumors. NAA has been generally observed to decrease in tumors and radiation necrosis.[67]

Lactate. Little lactate is observed in the spectra of normal brain. Therefore, the appearance of lactate can be an important indicator of tissue status, and this metabolite has been extensively studied by proton MRS. Its important role in energy metabolism has made lactate MRS particularly relevant for functional

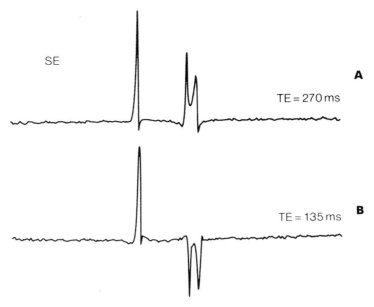

Fig. 10-35. A, The *J*-modulation of the lactate signal causes it to be inverted at an echo time of 135 msec. **B,** The signal rephases above the baseline at an echo time of 270 msec. (From Sauter R, Schneider M, Wicklow K et al: Current status of clinically relevant techniques in magnetic resonance spectroscopy, Electromedica 60:31-54, 1992.)

activation studies. Lactate apparently provides a use-responsive local energy store and also acts as a neuromodulator, altering the excitability of local neurons.[79]

Unfortunately, lactate identification and measurement can be technically difficult. One of lactate's two resonances, the CH resonance at 4.1 ppm, is very near to water and may be exposed to water suppression efforts. The other resonance, the characteristic doublet of the CH_3 resonance at 1.32 ppm, is near the strong peaks from fatty acid–$(CH_2)_n$–groups. Although little mobile lipid is present in the brain, lipid peaks may arise from contamination by scalp fat. Lipids are also known to occur in several different tumor types.[29,80,81] Longer TEs often lead to relatively reduced lipid signals.

Coupling. Because of *J*-coupling, the CH_3 signal of lactate appears as a doublet separated by 7 Hz, regardless of the magnetic field strength. Lactate assignment is facilitated by exploiting this phase modulation of the lactate echo signal in a spin echo experiment. Setting the spin echo delay TE equal to 1/*J* (*J* = 7.3 Hz), spectra can be obtained in which the 1.32 ppm CH_3 lactate resonance is inverted while uncoupled systems are not[82-85] (Fig. 10-35). This period approximately corresponds to the frequently used TE of 135 msec. A 270 msec TE produces a lactate doublet that is refocused but no longer inverted.

Editing. Fortunately, many spectral editing procedures are available for lactate to eliminate overlapping water and lipid resonances, although at the cost of additional sequence complexity. These homonuclear editing sequences typically employ three to six RF pulses and may inherently display some reduced sensitivity to lactate. (For a review, see references 86 or 87.) Difference editing methods include polarization transfer,[88,89] double-quantum coherence filtering,[90] and spin echo difference spectroscopy using selective decoupling,[91] selective inversion,[92,93] or zero quantum.[94] However, the selectivity of these methods may be influenced by patient motion, spectrometer instability, or dynamic range limitations.[95] Alternative single-acquisition techniques include homonuclear polarization transfer,[96-98] zero quantum,[99,100] or double quantum,[101] but these techniques only detect at most 50% of the available lactate signal. Newer techniques that edit lactate in a single scan with full sensitivity have been described[26,102-105] but may be more difficult to implement for in vivo studies.

Tumors. Lactate is more likely to be found in high-grade gliomas, but its presence is not a reliable indicator of malignancy.[67] This is particularly true in treated tumors, when one cannot distinguish lactate from the tumor itself and from treatment-induced ischemia in tumoral tissue. There seems to be no obvious relation to tumor grade,[38,67,78,106] and lactate levels depend on tumor vascularity, perfusion, and transport in addition to the rate of anaerobic glycolysis within the lesion.[38] Lactate accumulates in other abnormal regions as well, particularly in cysts, necrotic areas, or blood. It also has been reported in human studies that lactate accumulates in cystic

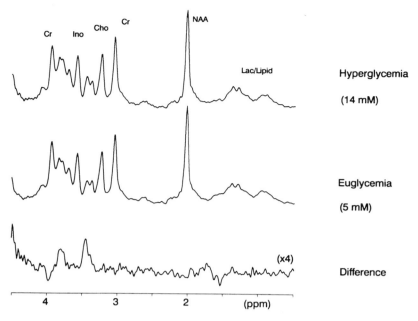

Fig. 10-36. A difference measurement method allows changes from glucose infusion to be observed, even though the glucose peak is not well resolved in the proton spectrum. (From Gruetter R, Rothman DL, Novotny EJ et al: Detection and assignment of the glucose signal in ¹H NMR difference spectra of the human brain, Magn Reson Med 27:183-188, 1992.)

compartments, even if is is produced in different regions.[107,108]

Metabolism. With loss of blood supply, local oxidative respiration quickly ends, and carbohydrate catabolism leads to the production of large amounts of lactate. Measurement of lactate turnover after relief from global ischemia can indicate levels of tissue metabolic activity and determine the viability of the tissue.[109] It is also possible that similar measurements can be made using glutamate.[110] Under these conditions, when oxidative production of adenosine triphosphate (ATP) is not sufficient to meet the energy demands of ATP utilization, the rate of anaerobic glycolysis may exceed oxidative metabolism, leading to the production of lactate. Therefore, the relatively low normal concentrations of brain lactate can be increased 10 to 20-fold by ischemia and epileptic seizure.[111-113]

Glucose. Gruetter et al. quantified brain glucose concentrations in humans using ¹³C MRS and intravenous infusions of D-[$1 - {}^{13}C$]glucose.[114] Although the use of ¹³C-enriched glucose has an advantage of allowing a direct peak observation in a region of the carbon spectrum that is free from overlap with other resonances, the method is limited by inherently low sensitivity and requires sophisticated and costly infusion protocols.[115]

Proton MRS offers an alternative method of measuring the brain glucose signal at a much higher sensitivity. However, direct observation of 3.43 and 3.80 ppm resonances is hampered by the proximity of the water signal and overlap with resonances from taurine, inositol, glutamate, and glutamine, all of which are more concentrated in the brain.[116] The α-glucose peak at 5.24 ppm is also visible, which should be free from overlap if water peak suppression is adequate.[117]

A difference method for measurement of glucose has been demonstrated in another study by Gruetter and colleagues.[115] This procedure obtains an isolated glucose proton spectra from the brain by taking the difference between spectra obtained from normal (5 mM) and glucose infusion (hyperglycemic 14-17 mM) conditions (Fig. 10-36). The difference spectrum contains only signals from glucose, allowing high-sensitivity proton measurements of changes in glucose levels with a 3-minute resolution. These authors estimated that resting glucose levels contribute at most a third to the amplitude of the peak at 3.44 ppm and suggest that this procedure may be useful for monitoring functional stimulation.

Previous PET studies have shown that the glucose utilization rate is correlated with glioma grade.[118-120] However, as described previously, it may be difficult to observe glucose peak changes directly by proton MRS. An alternate approach is to monitor glycolytic metabolism end products such as lactate. However, these results may be difficult to interpret because several tissue types may contribute to the observed lactate signal (e.g., active tumor cells versus necrotic pools). One approach to monitoring active lactate formation is by infusing a precursor with a ^{13}C label, which splits lactate proton resonances when the label is incorporated into the molecule.[121]

Lipid. Although most believe that little lipid exists in the brain, many cell types, including some tumor cells, do display significant lipid resonances.[122] Methyl and methylene resonances, perhaps from mobile lipids, have been reported in high-grade astrocytomas.[117,123-125] The origin of these signals is a subject of continuing research,[126,127] but they may be correlated with the presence of tumor necrosis and thus to tumor grade.

Protein. The spectral signals from relatively low-molecular-weight compounds are superimposed on top of low and broad signals from high-molecular-weight macromolecules. The macromolecular contribution must be considered in rigorously quantitative studies, particularly with sequences using short TEs (<20 msec).[128]

Disease states. An increasing number of studies on large patient populations have investigated proton MRS and pathologic conditions. Only a few results from these studies are mentioned here.

Tumors. In general, single-voxel methods may be difficult to interpret because CSI results often show a significant amount of heterogeneity within tumors.[67,108,129] In these cases, CSI may be appropriate for guiding biopsy. Unambiguous differentiation of intracranial tumors is not always possible on the basis of NAA/Cho and NAA/Cr ratios, but some characteristic patterns can be observed for different histologic tumor types. Meningiomas typically show a drastic decrease in NAA and Cr signals. In addition, there is a corresponding appearance of an alanine resonance at 1.47 ppm.[78] In vitro studies of astrocytomas show that choline concentration is higher in malignant (136 μmol/100 g tissue) than in benign (101 μmol/100 g tissue) tissue, whereas the NAA concentration is lower in malignant (21 μmol/100 g tissue) than in benign (58 μmol/100 g tissue) tissue.[130] Lactate is present in some gliomas, but the levels have not been directly correlated to grade. Characteristic findings for metastasis are signals at 1.3 and 1.0 ppm corresponding to lipids.[78]

Brain infarction. Elevated lactate and decreased Cho, Cr, and NAA levels are consistently observed after cerebral infarction.[131] These are probably the results of diminished cell activity in the infarcted region. The decrease in NAA can be larger than the decrease in Cr or Cho.[132] (Additional information can be found in references 131 to 135.)

Multiple sclerosis. In general, multiple sclerosis lesions show a decrease in NAA, presumably reflecting secondary axonal loss or damage.[136-139] MRS studies may be useful for staging disease progression.

Epilepsy. Proton MRS studies of epilepsy have reported decreases of NAA and increases in the Cho/NAA ratio in regions that appear normal in MR images.[140,141] The decrease in NAA correlates to the neuronal loss characteristic of this disease. In most patients, increased lactate levels are also reported, indicating that lactate accumulates as a result of seizure activity even in the absence of ischemia.

AIDS. Applications of MRS to the study of acquired immunodeficiency syndrome (AIDS) have recently been reported. Menon and colleagues observed a reduction in NAA/Cho and NAA/Cr ratios in AIDS patients.[142] These abnormal findings were obtained from brain regions having approximately normal MRI appearance, suggesting that MRS may offer a sensitive method for detecting early pathologic changes. Jarvik et al. studied a population of HIV-positive subjects and found that 87% had significantly abnormal features compared with measurements made on control subjects.[143] These authors suggest that a combination of MRI and MRS may be useful in characterizing disease progression.

Phosphorus

The spectra of phosphorus-containing compounds provide valuable information regarding the energy metabolism in tissue that is largely complementary to the information from ^1H. ^{31}P MRS represents an accurate method for noninvasively monitoring changes in energy metabolite levels under normal and pathologic conditions. Unfortunately, ^{31}P MRS may have limited use in the clinical environment because of its poor spatial resolution,[144] which restricts measurements in brain to tissue volumes not smaller than approximately 20 ml using current methods. Heterogeneity within larger tumors cannot be easily resolved, and spectra from smaller tumors cannot be obtained without significant contamination from surrounding edema or nontumor tissue. Measurements that use lengthy multiple data-averaging acquisitions to improve resolution are more susceptible to motion artifacts.

Several metabolites can be measured with ^{31}P MRS (Fig. 10-37). PCr, at 0 ppm, is a storage site for high-energy phosphate groups used in metabolism and is often taken as the reference for chemical shift because its position does not change with local conditions. P_i provides a sharp peak at 4.8 ppm. The shift of the P_i peak relative to PCr is often used as an indicator of tissue pH[6] and has been used for the study of pH gradients across tumor cell membranes.[145] Adenosine diphosphate (ADP) and ATP represent the primary energetic currency of metabolism. All three phosphorus atoms of ATP are visible, with the alpha resonance peak at -7.6 ppm, the beta peak at -16.3 ppm, and the gamma resonance at -2.6 ppm. Additional visible peaks are from phosphomonoesters (PMEs) at 6.8 ppm, phosphodiesters (PDEs) at 2.9 ppm, diphosphodiesters (DPDEs) at -8.1 ppm, and uridine diphosphoglucose (UDPG) at -9.6 ppm.

Energy metabolism. The components of oxidative metabolism are well represented in ^{31}P MRS spectra of the brain. This process can be described as[146]

$$3ADP + 3P_i + NADH + H^+ + \frac{1}{2}O_2 =$$
$$3ATP + NAD^+ + H_2O \qquad (10\text{-}5)$$

where NADH and NAD$^+$ are the reduced and oxidized forms of nicotinamide-adenine dinucleotide, respectively, all these components have the potential to regulate the rate of this reaction. As shown in Table 10-2, several aspects of energy metabolism can be

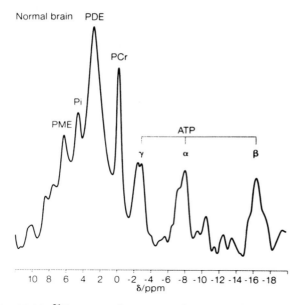

Fig. 10-37. ^{31}P spectra from normal region of brain. (From Sauter R, Schneider M, Wicklow K et al: Current status of clinically relevant techniques in magnetic resonance spectroscopy, Electromedica 60:31-54, 1992.)

monitored with ^{31}P MRS. Neuronal activity after stimulation results from transmembrane sodium and potassium movements that require ion pumping to reestablish the ion gradients and membrane potentials. The energy is provided by the breakdown of ATP into ADP and P$_i$. A transient energy transfer from PCr restores ATP and is indicated by a reduction in PCr peak area and an increase in the P$_i$ peak. Steady-state ATP levels during sustained activation are maintained by the 36-fold less efficient glycolytic phosphorylation. When glycolysis rates of pyruvate production are greater than that which mitochondrial respiration is consuming, an undesirable production of lactate and intracellular acidosis ensues.[146] Lactate levels can be monitored by proton MRS while the position of the P$_i$ peak indicates local pH levels. If intracellular and extracellular compartments are at different shift locations, membrane kinetics can be monitored. Enzyme kinetics can be assessed through the selective excitation of individual peaks and measurement of intensity and relaxation changes in neighboring metabolite levels. These saturation transfer experiments can be used to study steady-state, unidirectional fluxes through enzyme-catalyzed reactions in cells and tissues.

A classic application of ^{31}P MRS is to study muscle physiology. Changes in absolute metabolite levels, pH levels, and recovery rates have been observed in response to exercise or pathology.[147,148]

Tumors. Human cancer cells typically have a higher pH than normal cells and also have low PCr, high PME, and high PDE levels[1] (Fig. 10-38). Reports from in vivo patient studies have shown differences in spectra originating from meningiomas, pituitary adenomas, and gliomas.[149,150] Phosphoethanolamine appears in high levels (about 10 mM) in malignant neuroblastoma tumors in human infants[151] and may represent a marker for invasiveness.

Tumor pH values reflect the local environment and may not provide sufficiently specific information regarding tumor grade. Local pH depends on the rate of delivery of acid-producing metabolic substrate, the rate of removal of acid products of metabolism, the perfusion of the tissue, and the level of oxygen available for the metabolic functions of the cell.

Table 10-2. Aspects of cell metabolism that are particularly suited for ^{31}P MRS investigation

Metabolism	Pathway
Energy cost paid	$ATP \rightarrow ADP + P_i$
Energy recharge from PCr	$3ADP + PCr \leftrightarrow ATP + Cr$
Oxidative phosphorylation	$3ADP + 3P_i + NADH + \frac{1}{2}O_2 + H^+ \rightarrow NAD^+ + H_2O + 3ATP$
Glycolytic phosphorylation	$Glucose + 2ADP + 2P_i + 2NAD^+ \rightarrow 2Pyruvate + 2ATP + 2NADH + 2H^+$

From Chance B, Leigh JS, McLaughlin AC et al: Phosphorus-31 spectroscopy and imaging. In Partain CL, Price RR, Patton JA et al, editors: Magnetic resonance imaging, ed 2, Philadelphia, 1988, Saunders.

Sodium

The in vivo ^{23}Na signal is surprisingly strong, reflecting the 100% natural abundance of the MRS-visible isotope and the high sodium concentration in biologic systems. The sodium concentration in the human body is 44 mM, compared with 387 mM of phosphorus and approximately 99.9 M of protons. The overall sensitivity of ^{23}Na in the body is 4.1×10^{-5}, whereas it is 25.7×10^{-5} for ^{31}P, assuming a unit sensitivity for ^{1}H.[152,153] However, in practice, the overall NMR sensitivity of ^{23}Na may be better than of ^{31}P because the signal of ^{31}P is spread out among several metabolite peaks, whereas the ^{23}Na spectrum is much simpler (Fig. 10-39). In addition, sodium generally has a shorter T1 relaxation time, which

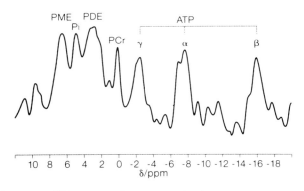

Fig. 10-38. ^{31}P spectra from a meningioma. (From Sauter R, Schneider M, Wicklow K et al: Current status of clinically relevant techniques in magnetic resonance spectroscopy, Electromedica 60:31-54, 1992.)

allows shorter TRs and more data averages per amount of measurement time.[152]

The ^{23}Na intracellular concentration is small relative to the extracellular compartment, but under normal circumstances, all ions resonate at the same frequency. This concentration of signal into a single peak allows images to be formed of regional sodium levels, although the images are of low resolution and generally have poor contrast. One can see differences between intracellular and extracellular sodium ions through the use of paramagnetic shift reagents that alter the chemical shift of the ions in the different compartments. This allows study of membrane transport because shift reagents change the chemical shift of the ions that enter or leave the compartments. In this case, the ^{23}Na spectrum consists of only two major features: peaks corresponding to extracellular and intracellular cation levels. Even though the spectral diversity is limited, ^{23}Na studies are often used to investigate membrane transport dynamics and the compartmentalization of sodium concentrations.[152] The cellular concentrations of sodium and sodium concentration gradients across cellular membranes are very important in many physiologic processes. ^{23}Na MRS offers a way of noninvasively measuring and monitoring these processes.

Carbon

The low (1.1%) natural abundance of ^{13}C often requires administration of supplementary labeled compounds to obtain adequate signal strength. Only certain storage compounds that are rich in carbon, such as triacylglycerols or glycogen, can be directly detected by ^{13}C MRS unless small-bore and high-field magnet systems are employed.

However, ^{13}C offers very rich spectra, as would be expected from so fundamental a constituent of organic compounds (Fig. 10-40). In addition, the low natural abundance allows the metabolic fate of administered labeled compounds to be followed. Furthermore, the

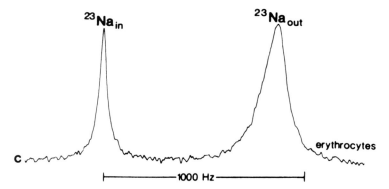

Fig. 10-39. The use of paramagnetic shift reagents allows ^{23}Na spectra to identify separate peaks corresponding to intracellular and extracellular ions. (From Partain CL, Price RR, Patton JA et al, editors: Magnetic resonance imaging, ed 2, Philadelphia, 1988, Saunders, p 1543.)

many visible peaks are distributed throughout a chemical shift range that is much wider than that of proton or phosphorus. The in vitro ^{13}C MRS spectra of biologic systems generally show many sharp metabolite peaks with distinct chemical shifts.[154] However, in vivo surface coils used to examine rat brains generally show only lipid resonances.[154-156] ^{13}C MRS provides a very powerful method of investigating metabolic pathways and kinetics but, as described later, these studies are often performed in conjunction with ^{1}H techniques to increase measurement sensitivity.

Deuterium

Deuterium (^{2}H) is a stable isotope of hydrogen commercially available as D_2O. Similar to ^{13}C, the low natural abundance of deuterium requires enrichment through the administration of labeled compounds for effective MRS detection. The potentially high concentration of labeled water and the short T1 relaxation time help compensate for the low natural abundance (0.0156%), providing substantial sensivity for MRS.[157] D_2O is toxic at high levels, but the toxicity in mammals does not appear to be consequential at lower levels.[157,158] Several MRI/MRS studies have demonstrated the use of deuterium labeling in animal models.[157-161]

Fluorine

Although 100% of fluorine atoms are MRS visible, fluorine has very little biologic natural abundance. Most of the body's fluorine is not in soft tissues but rather is a constituent of bone minerals such as fluoroapatite.[162] Under normal imaging conditions (i.e., non-solid-state MRI), these atoms are held relatively immobile, have a very short relaxation time, and produce spectral peaks that are too broadened to be observed readily on clinical instrumentation.

^{19}F has a relatively high gyromagnetic ratio (40.05 MHz/T), a spin of ½, and a high relative (to proton) sensitivity of 0.83. The resonance frequency of ^{19}F is near enough to that of protons that normal electronics can be used. The low natural background and high signal strength make this nucleus very appropriate for studies of administered fluorine-labeled compounds such as the antidepressant drug fluoxetine.[163] The retention of fluorinated anesthetics (e.g., halothane, isoflurane) has been studied spectroscopically in rabbit brains by Wyrwicz et al. using surface coil ^{19}F MRS methods.[164,165]

Although PET studies with radioactive ^{18}F-fluorodeoxyglucose (FDG) have been used widely for metabolic studies, the concentration required for ^{19}F-FDG is prohibitively high and requires single-spectrum acquisition times on the order of hours.[162] In animal studies of glucose metabolism, 2-FDG has a relatively high toxicity (median lethal dose [LD_{50}] = 600 mg/kg) compared with 3-FDG (nontoxic at 5 g/kg levels).[162,166]

Fluorinated blood substitutes. A natural application of ^{19}F MRS is in the measurement of signal from highly fluorinated organic compounds known as perfluorocarbons (PFCs) (Fig. 10-41). These compounds have shown potential for use as blood substitutes because of their ability to dissolve up to 60 vol % of oxygen and 120 vol % of carbon dioxide.[162,167,168] It has been demonstrated that it is possible to image administered PFCs in vivo.[169-171] Further applications of this technique are based on the

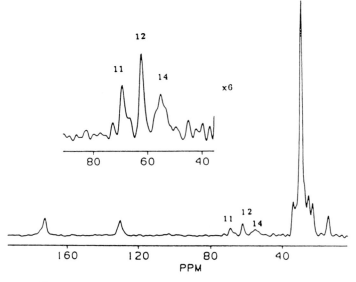

Fig. 10-40. In vivo ^{13}C spectra from normal brain. (From Seelig J, Burlina AP: Clin Chim Acta 206:125, 1992.)

sensitivity of the PFC chemical shifts to local environmental factors such as pH and temperature. Several of these factors can be expected to change with brain functional activation, making these methods very suitable for following these processes.

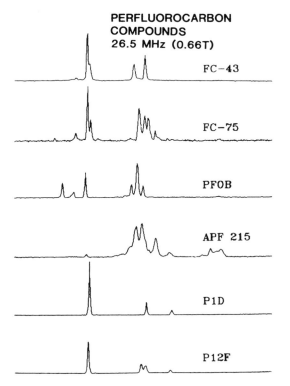

PERFLUOROCARBON COMPOUNDS
26.5 MHz (0.66T)

FC−43

FC−75

PFOB

APF 215

P1D

P12F

Fig. 10-41. Spectra (at 0.66 T) for several different perfluorocarbon compounds. (From Partain CL, , Price RR, Patton JA et al, editors: Magnetic resonance imaging, ed 2, Philadelphia, 1988, Saunders, p 1543.)

Oxygenation state. Measurement of PFC chemical shifts with MRS has the potential for the in vivo monitoring of the oxygen tension (P_{O_2}) in tissue.[172-176] This potential is based on the intrinsic paramagnetism of O_2, which significantly affects the spin lattice T1 of the PFC. It is well known that the relaxation of individual resonances of PFCs depends on the local (P_{O_2})[162,176-178] (Fig. 10-42). The relaxation rate, $T1^{-1}$, has been found to increase linearly with P_{O_2}, leading to image contrast enhancement in regions of increased P_{O_2}.

Temperature. Another useful application of ^{19}F and PFCs is based on the temperature dependence of PFC compounds.[162,179-182] The relative position, magnitude, and shape of various chemical shift spectral lines for a given PFC as a function of temperature may be used to monitor temperature gradients in vivo. Temperature measurement may be important for monitoring hyperthermia tumor treatment.

Local blood volume. For proton MRI blood volume measurements based on T1 changes of the tissue with an applied diffusible contrast material,[183] assumptions are required regarding the exchange and equilibrium of the agent between intravascular and extravascular spaces. Alternatively, the extravascular $T2^*$ or T2-mediated effects from intravascular concentrations of Gd-DTPA are difficult to quantify.[184] [19]F methods have an advantage over proton techniques because the signal amplitude is directly proportional to the quantity of fluorine (e.g., using administered PFCs) in the vascular system. This method allows small voxels, on the order of 21 mm³,[185] allowing high-resolution blood volume maps to be formed (Fig. 10-43). The PFC

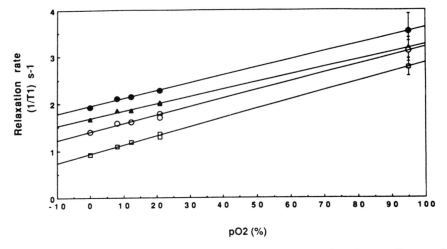

Fig. 10-42. T1 relaxation rate with respect to oxygenation for the perfluorocarbon compound FC-43. Separate curves are shown for each resonance of the compound. (From Mason RP, Nunnally RL, Antich PP: Tissue oxygenation: a novel determination using 19-F surface coil NMR spectroscopy of sequestered perfluorocarbon emulsion, Magn Reson Med 18:71-79, 1991.)

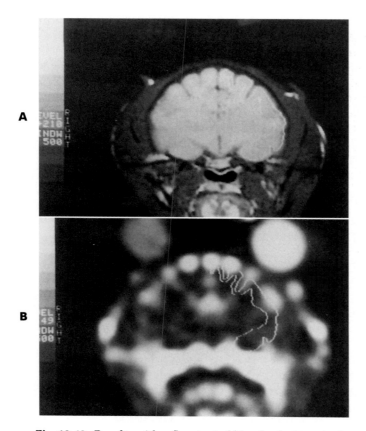

Fig. 10-43. Results with a fluorinated blood substitute in the cat showing **A**, the ^{1}H image, and **B**, the ^{19}F local cerebral blood volume map. (From Lu D, Joseph PM, Greenberg JH et al: Use of ^{19}F magnetic resonance imaging to measure local cerebral blood volume, Magn Reson Med 29:179-187, 1993.)

suspensions are considered to remain completely intravascular.

Multinuclear

Several methods are available for simultaneously acquiring data from multiple nuclei.[146,186,187] These methods are particularly useful for observing both energy metabolites and lactate production.

Carbon. Methods are available to overcome the sensitivity limitations of ^{13}C spectroscopy by using *proton-detected carbon editing* (PDCE).[188-191] Rather than detecting the carbon signal directly, these methods detect the much larger signals from protons interacting with the carbon. These proton MRS techniques exploit the magnetic coupling between ^{13}C and the protons bonded to it to detect ^{13}C in certain chemical structures. This method can be used to monitor the time course of ^{13}C enrichment of a particular C–H group after administration of ^{13}C-labeled compounds. This powerful method has many potential applications, including the estimation of specific cerebral metabolic rates.[192]

In demonstrating high-quality in vivo imaging of glucose (Fig. 10-44), van Zijl et al. suggest that this type of MRS has sufficient sensitivity to monitor glucose metabolism.[193] Furthermore, these methods are not as sensitive as PET FDG studies for nonmetabolic uptake or metabolite trapping. These MRS methods may also have a better-defined spatial localization than PET methods.

Phosphorus. ^{1}H/^{31}P double resonance techniques have demonstrated improved sensitivity to phosphorus metabolites.[194] In these studies, the capability of simultaneously exciting at both resonance frequencies is used to decouple ^{31}P nuclei from the influence of protons in order to resolve components of the PME and PDE peaks, including phosphocholine, phosphoethanolamine, glycerophosphocholine, and glycerophosphoethanolamine.

FUNCTIONAL APPLICATIONS
Indicator Dilution

Tissue exchange. The basic principles describing the mechanism for exchange between capillaries and tissue were first proposed by Starling almost 100 years ago.[195] He postulated that the net exchange between tissue compartments is determined primarily by the difference between the hydraulic (blood) pressure and the oncotic pressure generated by water diffusing to dilute the protein confined in the plasma by the semipermeable membrane. Under normal conditions, the sum of the outward forces exceeds that of the inward forces at the arterial end of the capillary, and the opposite is true at the venous end of the capillary. On the average, the outward forces and the inward forces almost balance, and a lymphatic system serves to drain any excess filtrate out of the tissue. In brain, the ventricular system and CSF serve a part of the function provided by lymphatics in other organs.

Thus, several components determine the exchange of compounds between intravascular and extravascular tissue compartments. Blood flow for maintenance of concentration gradients and the diffusion rate of the compound within and between compartments are particularly important for indicator dilution measurements.

Diffusible indicators. The use of diffusible indicator substances for measurement of tissue blood flow dates back to 1945 and the studies by Kety and Schmidt using nitrous oxide (N_2O).[196] Since that time, much work has established experimental and quantitative analysis procedures that underlie current methods. (These procedures are reviewed in references 197 to 201.) Similar to the intravascular tracer studies introduced in Chapter 7, these techniques depend on the central volume principle:[202]

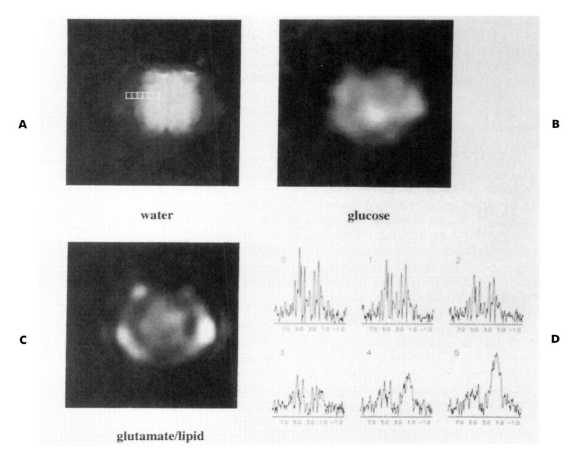

water   glucose

glutamate/lipid

Fig. 10-44. A to **C**, Results in the cat showing how proton-detected ^{13}C studies can provide chemical shift images of water, glucose, and other metabolites. **D**, Spectra from inside to outside at locations indicated in **A**. (From van Zijl PCM, Chesnick AS, DesPres D et al: In vivo proton spectroscopy and spectroscopic imaging of {1 − ^{13}C} − glucose and its metabolic products, Magn Reson Med 30:544-557, 1993.)

$$F = \frac{V_d}{\text{MTT}} \qquad (10\text{-}6)$$

where F is the tissue perfusion (ml/min), V_d is the accessible volume in the tissue (ml), and MTT is the mean transit time for the tracer. This expression can be rewritten as

$$F_t = \frac{\lambda}{\text{MTT}} \qquad (10\text{-}7)$$

where F_t is the flow rate per amount of tissue (typically in units of ml/[min 100 g]) and λ is the tissue-to-blood partition coefficient; λ is defined as the ratio of tracer concentration in tissue and in blood. This value is determined independently of the blood flow measurement and is assumed to be a constant parameter for the flow measurements. The availability of this parameter allows blood flow to be directly related to the tissue volume and distinguishes diffusible methods from previously discussed intravascular tracer studies. With purely intravascular tracers, a significant difference

exists between accessible (vascular) tissue volume and the entire tissue volume being measured using residue detection. This difference is largely responsible for the additional analysis and assumptions required to obtain tissue flow measurements with intravascular tracers.

The fundamental assumption for diffusible tracer studies is that the tracer is freely diffusible between the intravascular and extravascular spaces. This is required so that the clearance of the tracer from the tissue depends on the blood flow removing the tracer rather than diffusive processes. If the tracer is diffusion limited, the washout kinetics become independent of flow rate, and the analysis models will not apply. There is evidence of diffusion-limited washout patterns at flows greater than 60 ml/(min 100 g) from H$_2$^{15}O studies of baboon brain.[201,203] Given adequate measurement of temporal resolution, some correction of diffusion limiting is possible using the concept of extraction fraction.[203] With (correctable) freely diffusible tracers and a value for λ, measurement of tissue blood flow becomes a matter of measuring the tracer MTT.[201]

The tracer material can be administered either as an bolus injection or, if there is no tracer recirculation, by constant infusion. In the simplest bolus-injection, first-order kinetic model (corresponding to a single-compartment tissue model), the tracer washout will follow a monoexponential decay of this form:[201,204]

$$I(t) = I(0) \exp(-kt) \qquad (10\text{-}8)$$

where $I(t)$ is the time course of the tracer signal intensity detected in the tissue of interest (i.e., residue detection), $I(0)$ is the initial intensity at time 0, and k is the first-order exponential time constant describing the washout. If a nonideal bolus administration is implemented, as seen in Chapter 7, the measured time course will be the convolution of the washout exponential and the (measured) arterial input function.

It can be shown that the exponential washout time constant, k, is the inverse of the tracer MTT. The value of k can be obtained by fitting an exponential curve to the experimental time course data, and the inverse of k (= MTT) can then used in Equation 10-7 to obtain the tissue blood flow. More sophisticated models can be used to consider the effects of recirculation or multiple tissue compartments. Information regarding compartmental structure and exchange is available through a detailed analysis of the multiexponential washout time course. (The fundamentals of these methods, including constant infusion protocols, are fully described in reference 199.)

Tracer compounds. To use tracer methods, the relationship between measured signal and sample concentration must be available. At least four MRS tracers are in use for measurement of CBF[205]: trifluoromethane, D_2O, $H_2^{17}O$, and protons of water in arterial blood. Unfortunately, the MRS sensitivity to the tracer compounds can be low, and cost can be a factor.

In considering a tracer compound for CBF measurements, as in every other type of MRS measurement, the SNR is of primary concern. Interacting with SNR considerations, and with each other, are considerations regarding the total imaging time, the maximal tolerable concentration of tracer, and the spatial resolution of the results.[205] Measurement sensitivity may be enhanced with the use of nuclear species (e.g., ^2H or ^{19}F) that have little biologic natural abundance and background signal. As mentioned earlier, it is important that the tracer material is not diffusion limited at the flow rates expected in the tissue of interest. This is why several tracers are labeled water, which has relatively free movement in tissue. The movement of tritiated water (^3H_2O) across the red blood cell (RBC) membranes has been measured to be

very rapid, with a half-time of approximately 4 msec.[206] As mentioned in Chapter 7, the structure of the blood-brain barrier (BBB) also may restrict the movement of water. In general, the entire brain water space (cellular plus extracellular) functions as one well-mixed compartment.[206] When the diffusion gradient favors tissue loss to blood, labeled water is rapidly cleared from cells and the interstitium across the BBB with a half-life (70 to 90 seconds[207,208]), indicating that blood flow in the vessel is the primary rate-limiting step in the process.

The MTT of blood flow from small arterioles through the capillary bed and small venules (less than 50 μm diameter) has been estimated under normal conditions to be 0.3 to 0.6 second for gray matter and 0.6 to 0.9 second for white matter.[209,210] Therefore, the time that water resides in the capillary bed is long compared with the membrane exchange time.[206] The major mechanism of blood flow change appears to be altered flow velocity and not capillary recruitment.[209-211] When blood flow increases, the average flow velocity increases and this may lead to diffusion limiting.

Deuterium. Deuterium-labeled water (D_2O) is likely to satisfy the freedom of movement requirements for a diffusible tracer substance, and its use for measurement of perfusion has been demonstrated in animals.[158,212,213] The absence of background signals helps make this an effective method. In general, rapid pulse repetition (since the quadrupole relaxation is relatively fast) and surface coil detection are used to increase the measurement SNR. Recent articles by Kim and Ackerman detail the theory and use of D_2O in compartmental analysis and quantification of blood flow.[200,204]

Measurement of perfusion with radiolabeled microspheres represents the "gold standard" for tissue flow techniques. Neil obtained good agreement between deuterium and microsphere techniques in rat muscle, but, particularly for flows greater than 250 ml/(min 100 g), the D_2O method underestimated flow in the rat brain.[201] These results suggest that additional diffusion limitation is imposed by the BBB membranes on the free movement of D_2O. Corbett et al. also obtained good agreement at lower flow rates between these two techniques in piglet brain and suggested that the method is still useful with the understanding that it underestimates flow at higher rates.[214]

Fluorine. Fluorine is often a constituent of volatile compounds (e.g., Freon, halothane) that can be administered as gases. One frequently employed substance is gaseous trifluoromethane. The use of these materials as tracer compounds is closely related to the routinely used xenon-133 inhalation radiotracer techniques.[215,216] Although noninvasive, administration by inhalation typically requires arterial sampling to obtain arterial input function. However, it may also be possible to obtain this information through analysis of expired air.[217]

In cat brain, the in situ ^{19}F method using Freon gas as a tracer compared well with simultaneous measurements using invasive inlet/outlet detection.[217] Note, however, that these studies depend heavily on the accuracy of the value of λ used. These techniques have been extensively developed in animal models by Branch et al.,[218,219] most recently in primates.[220]

Methods. After proton imaging, the MRI coil is retuned to the ^{19}F frequency and the indicator administered. Gradient-refocused techniques are used to localize CBF estimates to a 2 cm^3 voxel.[205] Other approaches have employed STEAM volume localization and phase encoding to image flow in a volume as small as 0.4 cm^3.[221] The uptake and clearance of trifluoromethane can be followed by rapidly imaging its cerebral concentration during the entire administration period. Since there is no background signal, the signal strength is directly proportional to the concentration in the brain. The end-tidal record of indicator concentration in expired air provides an estimate of arterial input function, and multicompartmental models are iteratively fitted to the data to find the maximal likelihood estimates of those parameters.[205]

Toxicology. A number of side effects of Freon administration are known, including hypotension and bradycardia after administration of 40% Freon-22 to anesthetized cats and tachycardia after the washout.[201,217] In addition, perfusion increased by approximately 50% after administration. Use of other Freon compounds may result in less susceptibility to these effects.[222,223]

While trifluoromethane is generally considered to have low toxicity, these properties are under study in cats,[224] primates,[220] and humans.[205] The relatively high concentrations required and the current understanding of the toxicology of trifluoromethane may limit application of ^{19}F techniques in humans. Based on cat studies with breathing mixtures of 70% v/v, Ewing and colleagues estimated the saturation concentration of ^{19}F in the brain to be approximately 30 mM.[205] Even given the good sensitivity of ^{19}F, this concentration yields an SNR of 4 : 1 in a 16-second interval in a 2 cm^3 volume. The authors concluded that concentrations of less than 30% v/v may not allow useful imaging resolutions. The availability of high-field (i.e., greater than 1.5 T field strengths) systems should improve SNR and allow reduced in vivo concentrations to be used.

17-Oxygen. ^{17}O MRI can be used to follow the time course of H$_2$^{17}O in the brain after a arterial bolus injection and the results can be analyzed to obtain an image of CBF.[225,226] Furthermore, measurements made in combination with $^{17}O_2$ inhalation allow the calculation of the oxygen consumption within the voxel. This approach is based on the incorporation of $^{17}O_2$ gas into H$_2$^{17}O by oxidative metabolism.[227] Since labeled water produced elsewhere in the body may circulate to the brain, corrections are required to measure CBF and tracer recirculation. Pekar et al., in studies of cat brain, showed that the results from this technique agreed reasonably well with those from simultaneous autoradiographic techniques.[225]

Additional methods for measuring CBF use ^{17}O-labeled water as a proton-imaging contrast agent.[228,229] These methods enjoy the SNR advantages and convenience of proton imaging. ^{17}O is a stable isotope of oxygen with a nuclear spin of 5/2, which enhances water proton T2 relaxation rates through its scalar-coupled interactions.[229] The presence of H$_2$^{17}O can be monitored by observation of local T2 relaxation changes. Kwong et al. demonstrated this technique in dogs but obtained an underestimate of the actual CBF because of identifiable experimental issues.[229] They further noted that clinical application of this potentially useful technique is limited by the high cost of the labeled water.

Simultaneous ^{17}O and ^{19}F. PET studies often employ the radioactive tracers H$_2$^{15}O[230] and CH$_3$^{18}F[231] for measurements of regional CBF. ^{15}O can also be used[230] to measure the CMRO$_2$ by following the rate of H$_2$^{15}O production through the following reaction[232]:

$$C_6H_{12}O_6 + 6O_2 \rightarrow 6CO_2 + 6H_2O \quad (10\text{-}9)$$

The availability of MRS-visible analogs of these reactants allows many of the PET procedures to be performed using MRS techniques.

The ^{17}O methods for measurement of CBF described earlier have several important limitations.[232] Simultaneous CBF and CMRO$_2$ measurements are not feasible because both processes result in a change in the measured H$_2$^{17}O concentrations. In addition, arterial bolus injections of tracers is not appropriate for human studies. An independent measurement of CBF is available through the use of ^{19}F trifluoromethane techniques, as discussed previously. Arterial injections are avoided through the use of these inhalation gas techniques.

The time course of the ^{19}F NMR signal is directly measured in the brain, and the arterial input concentration time course is obtained from analysis of expired air (Fig. 10-45). Pekar et al. measured the time course of the ^{19}F signal from 0.4 cm^3 voxels in a cat brain before, during, and after inhalation of a gas mixture containing 57% trifluoromethane, CHF$_3$.[221] The con-

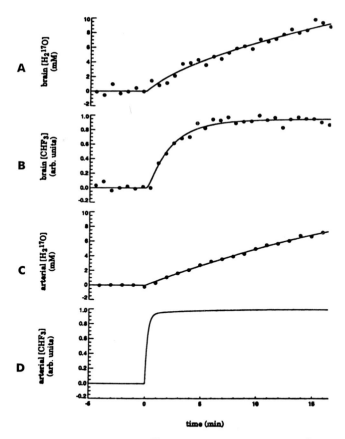

Fig. 10-45. A, Excess $H_2^{17}O$ concentration in a 0.8 cm³ voxel in the cat brain. **B,** CHF_3 concentration in the same voxel. **C,** Excess $H_2^{17}O$ concentration in arterial blood. **D,** arterial CHF_3 concentration obtained from mass spectrometer gas analysis of expired air. Analysis of these measured curves leads to an estimation of $CMRO_2$. (From McLaughlin AC, Pekar J, Sinwell T et al: ^{17}O and ^{19}F magnetic resonance imaging of cerebral blood flow and oxygen consumption, Syllabus, SMRM FMRI Workshop, Arlington, Va, 1993.)

centration of CHF_3 in arterial blood, $C_a(t)$, was measured simultaneously using mass spectrometer gas detection of expired air. The CBF, F_t, can be obtained by fitting the data with the following PET relation[230]:

$$C_b(T) = F_t \int_0^T C_a(t) \exp \left[\frac{Ft}{\lambda(t - T)} \right] dt \quad (10\text{-}10)$$

where $C_b(T)$ is the concentration of CHF_3 in the brain voxel, and λ is the brain/blood partition coefficient for CHF_3 ($\lambda = 0.9$ ml/g).[222,223]

Oxygen consumption. The production of $H_2^{17}O$ from $^{17}O_2$ can be used to estimate the rate of oxygen consumption,[225,226,233-235] but the interpretation of measured $H_2^{17}O$ changes is complicated by venous circulation washout of $H_2^{17}O$ formed locally and by washin of $H_2^{17}O$ formed in other organs. These effects can be corrected for if the CBF and the arterial

concentration of $H_2^{17}O$ are measured during the inhalation protocol.[225,232] Simultaneous inhalation of $^{17}O_2$ and CHF_3 and simultaneous measurement of ^{19}F and ^{17}O signals allow simultaneous determination of $H_2^{17}O$ and CHF_3 in brain voxels. Combined with concurrent arterial sampling for $H_2^{17}O$ and gas analysis of CHF_3, this approach allows simultaneous imaging of CBF and $CMRO_2$.[232,236]

Limitations. Compared with PET radiotracer studies, a relatively high concentration of tracer material is required to obtain adequate SNR and imaging resolution. The potential for clinical $^{17}O/^{19}F$ measurements of $CMRO_2$ and CBF depends on the toxicity of the tracers for human use. $^{17}O_2$ and $H_2^{17}O$ are generally considered to be nontoxic and safe for human studies,[232] whereas preliminary results indicate that CHF_3 is safe at low levels.[205] However, an additional consideration is the cost of the ^{17}O isotopes, which can be very high.

Spectral Changes

Direct observations of spectral changes with brain activity using proton MRS has focused primarily on detection of lactate and glucose because these compounds are so central to energy metabolism.

Lactate. ^{13}C infusion studies have indicated that blood and brain lactate compartments are not exchanging rapidly. Prichard suggests that the function of sequestered lactate may be to shorten the response time for local energy generation.[79] Local lactate elevation by previous activity would prime a region to deliver its maximal response to sudden demand in the period while the glycolytic rate is increasing. Simultaneous ^1H and ^{31}P MRS measurements during bicuculline-induced seizures in rabbit[112] or anoxic stress in rats[237] demonstrated that increased lactate levels are not necessarily accompanied by increased tissue pH. However, a significant pH shift with seizure activity was observed by Schnall et al. using simultaneous ^1H, ^{31}P, and ^{23}Na measurements.[238]

In many cases, the poststimulation lactate elevation persists longer than would be expected. In MRS experiments using direct cortical electroshock, 1 to 10 seconds of stimulation leads to elevated lactate levels for the following 1 to 2 hours.[239] Further proton-detected ^{13}C studies showed that 90% of this elevated pool of lactate turned over,[240] indicating that it is not trapped in dead cells or in some other nonmetabolizing compartment.[79]

Functional stimulation. The MRS results of functional stimulation experiments are consistent with previous PET interpretations that some types of stimulation within the range of normal brain function preferentially activate nonoxidative glycolysis.[241]

Prichard et al., using an ISIS technique, showed that

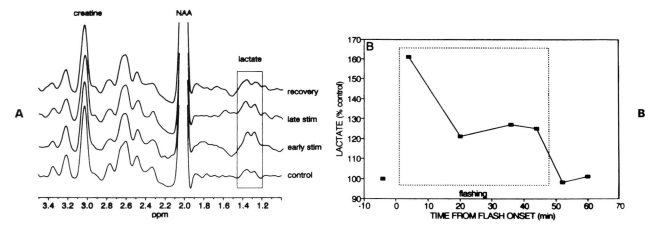

Fig. 10-46. Changes in lactate concentration with visual stimulation. **A,** Example spectra. **B,** Time course of lactate recovery. (From Prichard J, Rothman D, Novotny E et al: Lactate rise detected by ^{1}H NMR in human visual cortex during physiological stimulation, Proc Natl Acad Sci USA 88:5829-5831, 1991.)

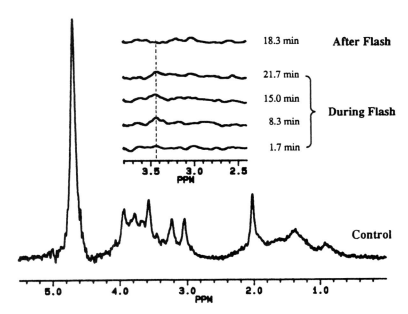

Fig. 10-47. Difference measurements of glucose levels obtained during photic stimulation. (From Chen W, Novotny EJ, Zhu XH et al: Localized ^{1}H NMR measurement of glucose consumption in the human brain during visual stimulation, Proceedings, 12th SMRM Annual Meeting, New York, 1993, p 1528.)

photic stimulation does cause a transient elevation in lactate levels in the human visual cortex (Fig. 10-46).[242] This is consistent with PET reports showing that photic stimulation results in a 50% increase in blood flow and glucose uptake, but only a 5% increase in oxygen extraction.[241] In these experiments, the maximal lactate rise occurred shortly after the onset of stimulation and gradually declined as stimulation continued. These results suggest that initially glycolysis provides the necessary energy, but the mismatch between glycolysis and respiration does not continue

with sustained activation. Sappey-Marinier and colleagues also measured visually evoked potentials and showed that a decrease in the P_{100} peak correlates to lactate changes during photic stimulation.[243] They suggested that adaptation or fatigue leads to diminished neural activity and decreased lactate production.

A subsequent study by Merboldt et al. did not observe significant lactate changes with photic stimulation but noted great measurement variability.[244] Further studies have detected changes in lactate levels with visual stimulation but noted that the slight

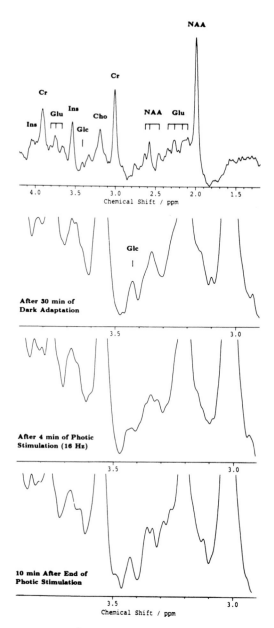

Fig. 10-48. Direct ^{1}H MRS observation of glucose changes during visual stimulation. (From Merboldt KD, Bruhn H, Hanicke W et al: Decrease of glucose in the human visual cortex during photic stimulation, Magn Reson Med 25:187-194, 1992.)

changes may be masked by partial volume averaging, low SNR, and the limited temporal resolution of the MRS measurements.[243,245,246]

Preliminary results from Xue et al. indicate that a surprisingly large decrease in NAA and increase in lactate accompany motor stimulation.[247]

Singh and colleagues have shown that lactate changes with auditory stimulation can be observed on 1.5 T instruments.[248,249] These measurements used a 40 Hz presentation of a 1 kHz tone. Given the noise from the gradients, no true nonstimulus control measurements were available. The results were consistent with

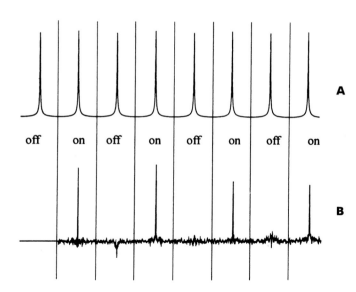

Fig. 10-49. A, Water peak observed with and without visual stimulation. **B,** Note the sensitivity to activation-induced changes in the difference spectra. (From Hennig J, Ernst TH, Speck O et al: Detection of brain activation using oxygenation sensitive functional spectroscopy, Magn Reson Med 31:85-90, 1994.)

those from other stimuli, in that the lactate levels increased initially and then gradually decreased.

Glucose. Oxygen can freely diffuse from blood into brain, whereas glucose must be transported across the endothelial cell membranes of the BBB. If energy demands by the tissue increase, the rate of metabolism may be limited by transport such that energy production is insufficient to maintain normal brain function. Thus, intracerebral glucose metabolism is a function of metabolism and bidirectional transport rates across the BBB.[115,250]

Chen et al. demonstrated a difference method for measuring changes in glucose consumption during activation.[251] Building on their experience with ^{13}C glucose measurements, they measured an average increase in glucose consumption of 22% during 8 Hz photic stimulation (Fig. 10-47). The difference from PET reports of 51%[241] was attributed to partial volume effects (a 13 cm^3 VOI was used), and the time course of the changes was noted to be similar to that observed for lactate. These results are consistent with a decoupling of glucose metabolism from oxygen uptake during photic stimulation. This study demonstrated the feasibility of using ^{1}H MRS to measure directly the change in glucose consumption during brain functional activity in individual subjects.

An assessment of changes in glucose levels with photic stimulation has been demonstrated using short-TE (20 msec) STEAM MRS.[252] At this TE, the 3.43 ppm resonance of glucose can be adequately observed (Fig. 10-48). Changes in lactate during stimulation were not consistent (as in reference 244,

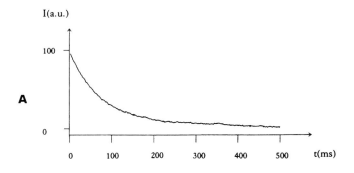

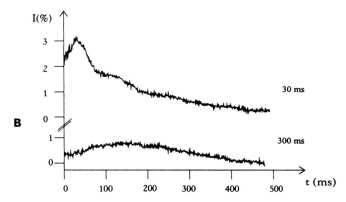

Fig. 10-50. A, Measured functional spectroscopic free induction decay (FID) signal. **B**, Difference between signals with and without stimulation for two different echo times. (From Hennig J, Ernst TH, Speck O et al: Detection of brain activation using oxygenation sensitive functional spectroscopy, Magn Reson Med 31:85-90, 1994.)

but contrary to other reports), but 50% glucose decreases were reported.

Functional Spectroscopy

A novel spectroscopic approach to measurement of functional activation has been demonstrated by Hennig et al. with visual, motor, and medial nerve stimulation.[253] This method uses PRESS single-voxel localization of the high SNR water signal and forms difference spectra between activated and nonactivated acquisitions. Unlike most proton spectroscopic techniques, only the characteristics of the water peak are monitored (Fig. 10-49). The advantages of this technique include fast observation times (25 to 100 msec acquisitions) and a high sensitivity to changes occurring with activation. Similar to echo planar image acquisition, the short imaging times reduce the influences of motion or flow.

The primary disadvantage of this technique is the requirement of a priori knowledge for the voxel placement. The demonstration of this technique for both visual and motor stimulation used gradient-recalled echo functional MRI procedures to identify functionally active regions and to guide the voxel positioning. The size of the voxel (20 mm^3) may also

lead to partial volume effects if the positioning is not optimal. However, the authors suggest that with the very high measurement SNR and effect-to-noise ratio, the size of the voxel may be reduced and/or multivoxel or CSI methods may be used.

Fig. 10-50 shows examples of the FID and difference FID signals, which show a distinctive change in T2* with activation. The effect-to-noise ratio of a nonaveraged difference FID was estimated to be in the range of 10 to 50 : 1. Gated 100 msec acquisition intervals were used throughout the cardiac cycle.

These studies only observe the unsuppressed water signal, ignoring the rest of the proton spectrum. Given the slow changes in other metabolites such as lactate, this may not be a significant compromise. This technique should provide temporal and spatial resolution adequate to characterize the time course of activation responses.

• • •

People unfamiliar with MRS often consider it to be a rare and exotic technology, extremely remote from clinical application. The intention of this chapter has been to introduce MRS and show that this is not necessarily the case. MRS and MRI both are aspects of the same fundamental principles, and both have contributions to make to clinical practice, especially to the study of brain functional activation. The unfortunate distinction between MRS and MRI, resulting in part from the patchwork implementation of MRS on clinical scanners, will become less apparent with the increasing availability of integrated MRI/MRS systems. Although MRS has long had the potential for clinical impact, realization of the potential has been slow. The new systems should allow faster progress toward the important goal of clinically reimbursable MRS examination procedures.

MRS can characterize metabolite changes with pathologic conditions or brain functional stimulation, but the detailed significance of the findings may not be completely known. Currently, the use of MRS is limited in identifying and staging tumors or guiding clinical treatment. However, these limitations also are caused by limitations in the detailed understanding of tumor biochemistry.

MRS measurements of a variety of nuclear and chemical species have been demonstrated to provide information regarding the biochemical mechanisms of brain function. Rate and uptake information, previously only available by radiotracer methods, can now be obtained with NMR methods, and the MRS biochemical information produced is tightly integrated with anatomic MRI results. The potential for routine clinical application of these methods, extending the usefulness of the large, installed base of MRI instruments, will drive continued investigation into these techniques.

MRS/MRI technology is perhaps similar to that of biotechnology and genetic engineering in that powerful tools have been developed, but full realization of a vast potential depends on improvements in the detailed understanding of the complex mechanisms involved in normal and disease processes. The continuing development and application of these tools will expand this required understanding and help advance physiology and medicine from an empirical to a quantitative basis.

REFERENCES

1. Negendank WG, Brown TR, Evelhoch JL et al: Proceedings of a National Cancer Institute workshop: MR spectroscopy and tumor cell biology, Radiology 185:875-883, 1992.
2. Negendank W, Zimmerman R, Gotsis E et al: A cooperative group study of 1H MRS of primary brain tumors, Proceedings, 12th SMRM Annual Meeting, New York, 1993, p 1521.
3. Farrar TC, Becker ED: Pulse and Fourier transform NMR, San Diego, 1971, Academic Press.
4. Fukishima E, Roeder SB: Experimental pulse NMR, Reading, Mass, 1981, Addison-Wesley.
5. Mansfield P, Morris PG: NMR imaging in biomedicine, San Diego, 1982, Academic Press.
6. Gadian DG: Nuclear magnetic resonance and its application to living systems, Oxford, UK, 1982, Clarendon Press.
7. Partain CL, Price RR, Patton JA, editors: Magnetic resonance imaging, Philadelphia, 1988, Saunders.
8. Damadian RV: Tumor detection by nuclear magnetic resonance, Science 171:1151-1153, 1971.
9. Lauterbur PC: Image formation by induced local interactions: examples employing nuclear magnetic resonance, Nature 242:190-191, 1973.
10. van Zijl PCM, Moonen CTW: *In situ* changes in purine nucleotide and *N*-acetyl concentrations upon inducing global ischemia in cat brain, Magn Reson Med 29:381-385, 1993.
11. Moon RB, Richards JH: Determination of intracellular pH by ^{31}p MR, J Biol Chem 248:7276-7278, 1973.
12. Martin M, Labouesse J, Canioni P, Merle M: *N*-acetyl-L-aspartate and acetate ^{1}H NMR signal overlapping under mild acidic pH conditions, Magn Reson Med 29:692-694, 1993.
13. Sauter R, Schneider M, Wicklow K, Kolem H: Current status of clinically relevant techniques in magnetic resonance spectroscopy, Electromedica 60:31-54, 1992.
14. Hore PJ: Solvent suppression in Fourier transform nuclear magnetic resonance, J Magn Reson 55:283-300, 1983.
15. Bottomley PA, Edelstein WA, Foster TH, Adams WA: *In vivo* solvent-suppressed localized hydrogen nuclear magnetic resonance spectroscopy: a window to metabolism? Proc Natl Acad Sci USA 82:2148-2152, 1985.
16. Dumoulin CL: A method of chemical-shift-selective imaging, Magn Reson Med 2:583-585, 1985.
17. Haase A, Frahm J, Hanicke W, Matthei D: ^{1}H NMR chemical shift selective (CHESS) imaging, Phys Med Biol 30:341-344, 1985.
18. Shen JF, Saunders JK: Double inversion recovery improves water suppression, Magn Reson Med 29:540-542, 1993.
19. Patt SL, Sykes BD: Water eliminated Fourier transport NMR spectroscopy, J Chem Phys 11:3182-3184, 1972.
20. Haasnoot CAG: Selective solvent suppression in ^{1}H FT NMR using a DANTE pulse: its application in normal and NOE measurements, J Magn Reson 52:153-158, 1983.
21. Dixon WT: Simple proton spectroscopic imaging, Radiology 153:189-194, 1984.
22. Weisskoff RM, Kiihne S: MRI susceptometry: image-based measurements of absolute susceptibility of MR contrast agents and human blood, Magn Reson Med 24:375-383, 1992.
23. Glover GH, Schneider E: Three-point Dixon technique for true water/fat decomposition with B_0 inhomogeneity correction, Magn Reson Med 18:371-383, 1991.
24. Dumoulin CL: The application of multiple quantum techniques for the suppression of water signals in ^{1}H NMR spectra, J Magn Reson 64:38-46, 1985.
25. Sotak CH, Freeman DM: A method for volume localized lactate editing using zero quantum coherence created in a stimulated echo pulse sequence, J Magn Reson 77:382-388, 1988.
26. Trimble LA, Shen JF, Wilman AH, Allen PS: Lactate editing by means of selective-pulse filtering of both zero and double quantum coherence signals, J Magn Reson 86:191-198, 1990.
27. Bax A, Mehlkopf AF, Smidt J: Absorption spectra from phase-modulated spin echoes, J Magn Reson 35:373-377, 1979.
28. van Waals JJ, van Gerven PHJ: Novel methods for automatic phase correction of NMR spectra, J Magn Reson 86:127-147, 1990.
29. Lefur Y, Ziegler D, Bourgeois D et al: Phased spectroscopic images: application to the characterization of the ^{1}H 1.3-ppm resonance in intracerebral tumors in the rat, Magn Reson Med 29:431-435, 1993.
30. Klose U: *In vivo* proton spectroscopy in the presence of eddy currents, Magn Reson Med 14:26-30, 1990.
31. Riddle WR, Gibbs SJ, Willcott MR: Removing effects of eddy currents in proton MR spectroscopy, Med Phys 19:501-509, 1992.
32. Roebuck JR, Hearshen DO, O'Donnell M, Raidy T: Correction of the phase effects produced by eddy currents in solvent suppressed ^{1}H-CSI, Magn Reson Med 30:277-282, 1993.
33. Webb P, Spielman D, Macovski A: Inhomogeneity correction for in vivo spectroscopy by high-resolution water referencing, Magn Reson Med 23:1-11, 1992.
34. Spielman D, Webb P, Macovski A: Water referencing for spectroscopic imaging, Magn Reson Med 12:38-49, 1989.
35. Maudsley AA, Hilal SK: Field inhomogeneity correction and data processing for spectroscopic imaging, Magn Reson Med 2:218-233, 1985.
36. Kreis R, Ernst T, Ross BD: Absolute quantitation of water and metabolites in the human brain. II. Metabolite concentrations, J Magn Reson B 102:9-19, 1993.
37. Frahm J, Bruhn H, Gyngell ML et al: Localized proton NMR spectroscopy in different regions of the human brain *in vivo*: relaxation times and concentrations of cerebral metabolites, Magn Reson Med 11:47-63, 1989.
38. Barker PB, Blackband SJ, Chatham JC et al: Quantitative proton spectroscopy and histology of a canine brain tumor model, Magn Reson Med 30:458-464, 1993.
39. Hennig J, Pfister H, Ernst T, Ott D: Direct absolute quantification of metabolites in the human brain with *in vivo* localized proton spectroscopy, NMR Biomed 5:193-199, 1992.
40. Christiansen P, Henriksen O, Stubgaard M et al: In vivo quantification of brain metabolites by ^{1}H-MRS using H_2O as an internal standard, Magn Reson Imaging 11:107-124, 1993.
41. Provencher SW, Michaelis T, Hanicke W, Frahm J: Automated detection of metabolite concentrations from localized *in vivo* proton NMR spectra, Proceedings, 11th SMRM Annual Meeting, Berlin, 1992, p 670.
42. Barker PB, Blackband SJ, Chatham JC et al: Quantitation of ^{1}H NMR spectra of the human brain, Proceedings, 10th SMRM Annual Meeting, San Francisco, 1991, p 388.
43. Juppi PS, Posse S, Lazeyras F et al: Magnetic resonance in

preterm and term newborns: [1]H-spectroscopy in developing human brain, Pediatr Res 30:574-578, 1991.

44. Tofts PB, Christiansen P, Pryds O et al: Absolute concentrations of brain metabolites in childhood measured by [1]H-magnetic resonance spectroscopy, Proceedings, 11th SMRM Annual Meeting, Berlin, 1991, p 2001.

45. Ernst T, Kreis R, Ross BD: Absolute quantitation of water and metabolites in the human brain. I. Compartments and water, J Magn Reson B 102:1-8, 1993.

46. Diem K, Lentner C: Documenta Geigy: scientific tables, Basel, 1970, Ciba-Geigy.

47. Nelson SJ, Brown TR: The accuracy of quantification from 1D NMR spectra using the PIQABLE algorithm, J Magn Reson 84:95-109, 1989.

48. Ackerman JJH, Grove TH, Wong GG et al: Mapping of metabolites in whole animals by ^{31}P NMR using surface coils, Nature 283:167-170, 1980.

49. Silver MS, Joseph RI, Hoult DI: Highly selective pi/2 and pi-pulse generation, J Magn Reson 59:347-351, 1984.

50. Hardy DJ, Edelstein WA, Vatis D: Efficient adiabatic fast passage for NMR population inversion in the presence of radiofrequency field inhomogeneity and frequency offsets, J Magn Reson 66:470-482, 1986.

51. Ugurbil K, Garwood M, Bendall MR: Amplitude modulated and frequency modulated pulses to achieve 90 degrees plane rotation with inhomogeneous B1 fields, J Magn Reson 72:177-185, 1987.

52. Bendall MR, Garwood M, Ugurbil K, Pegg DT: Adiabatic refocussing pulse which compensates for variable rf power and off-resonance effects, Magn Reson Med 4:493-499, 1987.

53. Garwood M, Merkle H: Heteronuclear spectral editing with adiabatic pulses, J Magn Reson 94:180-185, 1991.

54. Brown TR, Kincaid BM, Ugurbil K: NMR chemical shift imaging in three dimensions, Proc Natl Sci USA 79:3523-3626, 1982.

55. Maudsley AA, Hilal SK, Perman WH, Simon HE: Spatially resolved high resolution spectroscopy by "four dimensional" NMR, J Magn Reson 51:147-152, 1983.

56. Maudsley AA: Sensitivity in Fourier imaging, J Magn Reson 68:363-366, 1986.

57. Hennig J: Chemical shift imaging with phase-encoding RF pulses, Magn Reson Med 25:289-298, 1992.

58. Dixon WT: Chemical shift imaging. In Budinger TF, Margulis AR, editors: Medical magnetic resonance imaging and spectroscopy: a primer, Berkeley, Calif, 1986, Society of Magnetic Resonance in Medicine.

59. Spielman D, Pauley JM, Macovski A et al: Lipid-suppressed single- and multisection proton spectroscopic imaging of the human brain, J Magn Reson Imaging 2:253-262, 1992.

60. Duyn JH, Moonen CTW: Fast proton spectroscopic imaging of human brain using multiple spin echoes, Magn Reson Med 30:409-414, 1993.

61. Bottomley P: Selective volume method for performing localized NMR spectroscopy, US Patent 4,480,228, Assigned to General Electric, Schnectady, NY 1984.

62. Bottomley PA: Spatial localization in NMR spectroscopy *in vivo*, Ann NY Acad Sci 508:333-348, 1987.

63. Frahm J, Bruhn H, Gyngell ML et al: Localized high-resolution proton NMR spectroscopy using stimulated echoes: initial application to human brain *in vivo*, Magn Reson Med 9:79-93, 1989.

64. Frahm J, Michaelis T, Merboldt KD et al: Improvements in localized proton NMR spectroscopy of human brain: water suppression, short echo times, and 1 ml resolution, J Magn Reson 90:464-463, 1990.

65. Ordidge RJ, Connelly A, Lohman JAB: Image-selected *in vivo* spectroscopy (ISIS)—a new technique for spatially selective NMR spectroscopy, J Magn Reson 66:283-294, 1986.

66. Burger C, Buchli R, McKinnon G et al: The impact of the ISIS experiment order on spatial contamination, Magn Reson Med 26:218-230, 1992.

67. Fulham MJ, Bizzi A, Dietz MJ et al: Mapping of brain tumor metabolites with proton MR spectroscopic imaging: clinical relevance, Radiology 185:675-686, 1992.

68. Agris PF, Campbell ID: Proton nuclear magnetic resonance of intact Freund leukemia cells: phosphorylcholine increase during differentiation, Science 216:1325-1327, 1982.

69. Kreis R, Ernst T, Ross BD: Development of the human brain: *in vivo* quantitification of metabolite and water content with proton magnetic resonance spectroscopy, Magn Reson Med 30:424-437, 1993.

70. van der Knaap MS, van der Grond J, Luyten PR et al: [1]H and ^{31}P magnetic resonance spectroscopy of the brain in degenerative cerebral disorders, Ann Neurol 31:202-211, 1992.

71. Arnold DL, Matthews PM, Francis GS et al: Proton magnetic resonance spectroscopic imaging for metabolite characterization of demyelinating plaques, Ann Neurol 31:235-241, 1992.

72. Frahm J, Michaelis T, Merboldt KD et al: On the *N*-acetyl methyl resonance in localized ^{1}H-NMR spectra of the human brain *in vivo*, NMR Biomed 4:201-204, 1991.

73. Fleming MC, Lowry OH: The measurement of free and *N*-acetylated aspartic acid in the nervous system, J Neurochem 13:779-783, 1966.

74. Nadler JV, Cooper JR: *N*-acetyl-L-aspartic acid content of human neural tumors and bovine peripheral nervous tissues, J Neurochem 19:313-319, 1972.

75. Miller BL: A review of chemical issues in ^{1}H NMR spectroscopy: *N*-acetyl-L-aspartate, creatine and choline, NMR Biomed 4:47-52, 1991.

76. Birken DL, Oldendorf WH: *N*-acetyl-L-asparatic acid: a literature review of a compound prominent in ^{1}H-NMR spectroscopic studies of the brain, Neurosci Biobehav Rev 13:23-31, 1989.

77. Urenjak J, Williams SR, Gadian DG: Specific expression of *N*-acetylaspartate in neurons, oligodendrocyte-type-2 astrocyte progenitors, and immature oligodendrocytes *in vitro*, J Neurochem 59:55-61, 1992.

78. Kugel H, Heindel W, Ernestus RI et al: Human brain tumors: spectral patterns detected with localized H-1 MR spectroscopy, Radiology 183:701-709, 1992.

79. Prichard JW: Brain function and lactate MRS, Syllabus, SMRM FMRI Workshop, Arlington, Va, 1993, pp 95-101.

80. Remy C, Von Kienlin M, Lotito A et al: *In vivo* ^{1}H NMR spectroscopy of an intracerebral glioma in the rat, Magn Reson Med 9:395-401, 1986.

81. Bourgeois D, Remy C, Lefur Y et al: Proton spectroscopic imaging: a tool for studying intracerebral tumor models in rat, Magn Reson Med 21:10-20, 1991.

82. Le Fur Y, Ziegler A, Bourgeois D et al: Phased spectroscopic images: application to the characterization of the [1]H 1.3-ppm resonance in intracerebral tumors in the rat, Magn Reson Med 29:431-435, 1993.

83. Luyten PR, Marien JH, den Hollandar JA: Acquisition and quantitation in proton spectroscopy, NMR Biomed 4:64-69, 1991.

84. Williams SR, Gadian DG, Proctor EA: A method for lactate detection *in vivo* by spectral editing without the need for double irradiation, J Magn Reson 66:562-567, 1986.

85. Chang LH, Cohen Y, Weinstein PR et al: Interleaved ^{1}H and ^{31}P spectroscopic imaging for studying regional brain imaging, Magn Reson Imaging 9:223-227, 1991.

86. Hetherington HP: Homo- and heteronuclear editing in proton spectroscopy, NMR Basic Principles Prog 27:179-198, 1992.

87. Freeman D, Hurd R: Metabolite specific methods using

double quantum coherence transfer spectroscopy, NMR Basic Principles Prog 27:199-222, 1992.

88. Wokaun A, Ernst RR: Selective detection of multiple quantum transitions in NMR by two-dimensional spectroscopy, Chem Phys Lett 52:407-412, 1977.

89. Dumoulin CL, Williams EA: Suppression of uncoupled spins by single quantum homonuclear polarization transfer, J Magn Reson 66:86-92, 1986.

90. Knuttel A, Kimmich R: Double-quantum filtered volume-selective NMR spectroscopy, Magn Reson Med 10:404-410, 1989.

91. Rothman DL, Behar KL, Hetherington HP, Shulman RG: Homonuclear ¹H double-resonance difference spectroscopy of the rat brain *in vivo,* Proc Natl Acad Sci USA 81:6330-6334, 1984.

92. Hetherington HP, Avison MJ, Shulman RG: ¹H homonuclear editing of rat brain using semiselective pulses, Proc Natl Acad Sci USA 82:3115-3118, 1985.

93. Williams SR, Gadian DG, Proctor E: A method for lactate detection *in vivo* by spectral editing without the need for double irradiation, J Magn Reson 66:562-567, 1986.

94. Sotak CH, Freeman D: A method for volume-localized lactate editing using zero-quantum coherence created in a stimulated-echo pulse sequence, J Magn Reson 77:382-388, 1988.

95. Bourgeois D, Kozlowski P: A highly sensitive lactate editing technique for surface coil spectroscopic imaging *in vivo,* Magn Reson Med 29:402-406, 1993.

96. von Kienlin M, Albrand JP, Authier B et al: Spectral editing *in vivo* by homonuclear polarization transfer, J Magn Reson 75:371-377, 1987.

97. Knuttel A, Kimmich R: Single scan volume-selective spectral editing by homonuclear polarization transfer, Magn Reson Med 9:254-260, 1989.

98. Stryjewski D, Oschkinat H, Liebfritz D: Detection of metabolites in body fluids and biological tissue by a 1D soft COSY technique, Magn Reson Med 13:158-161, 1990.

99. Doddrell DM, Brereton IM: A selective excitation/B0 gradient technique for high-resolution ¹H NMR studies of metabolites via zero quantum coherence and polarization transfer, NMR Biomed 2:39-43, 1989.

100. Doddrell DM, Brereton IM, Moxon LN, Galloway GJ: The unequivocal determination of lactic acid using a one-dimensional zero-quantum coherence-transfer technique, Magn Reson Med 9:132-138, 1989.

101. McKinnon GC, Boesiger P: A robust method for localized lactate detection in the presence of strong fat signals, Proceedings, 8th SMRM Annual Meeting, Amsterdam, 1989, p 222.

102. Sotak CH, Freeman DM, Hurd RE: The unequivocal determination of *in vivo* lactic acid using two-dimensional double quantum coherence-transfer spectroscopy, J Magn Reson 78:355-361, 1988.

103. McKinnon GC, Boesiger P: A one-shot lactate-editing sequence for localized whole-body spectroscopy, Magn Reson Med 78:355-361, 1988.

104. Brereton JM, Galloway GJ, Rose SE, Doddrell DM: Metabolite editing via correlated *z* order with total inherent coherence: ECZOTIC, J Magn Reson 83:190-196, 1989.

105. Reddy R, Subramanian VH, Clark BJ, Leigh JS: Longitudinal spin-order-based pulse sequence for lactate editing, Magn Reson Med 19:477-482, 1991.

106. Alger JR, Frank A, Bizzi A et al: Metabolism of human gliomas: assessment with H-1 MR spectroscopy and F-18 flurodeoxyglucose PET, Radiology 177:633-641, 1990.

107. Frahm J, Bruhn H, Hanicke W et al: Localized ¹H NMR spectroscopy in fifty cases of newly diagnosed intracranial tumors, J Comput Assist Tomogr 15:67-76, 1991.

108. Herholz K, Heindel W, Luyten P et al: *In vivo* imaging of glucose consumption and lactate concentration in human gliomas, Ann Neurol 31:319-327, 1992.

109. Rothman DL, Howseman AM, Graham GD et al: Localized proton NMR observation of 3-¹³C-lactate in stroke after 1-¹³C-glucose infusion, Magn Reson Med 21:302-307, 1991.

110. Rothman DL, Novotny EJ, Shulman GI et al: ¹H-[¹³C] NMR measurements of [4-¹³C]glutamate turnover in human brain, Proc Natl Acad Sci USA 89:9603-9606, 1992.

111. Prichard JW, Shulman RG: NMR spectroscopy of brain metabolism *in vivo,* Ann Rev Neurosci 9:61-85, 1986.

112. Petroff OAC, Prichard JW, Ogino T et al: Combined ¹H and ³¹P nuclear magnetic resonance studies of bicuculline-induced seizures in vivo, Ann Neurol 20:185-193, 1986.

113. Myers RE: Lactate measurements in cerebral ischemia, In Fahn S, Davis JN, Rowland LP, editors: Advances in neurology, New York, 1979, Raven Press.

114. Gruetter R, Novotny EJ, Boulware SD et al: Direct measurement of brain glucose concentration in humans by ¹³C NMR spectroscopy, Proc Natl Acad Sci USA 89:1109-1112, 1992.

115. Gruetter R, Rothman DL, Novotny EJ et al: Detection and assignment of the glucose signal in ¹H NMR difference spectra of the human brain, Magn Reson Med 27:183-188, 1992.

116. Petroff OAC, Spencer DD, Alger JR, Prichard JW: High-field proton magnetic resonance spectroscopy of human cerebrum obtained during surgery for epilepsy, Neurology 39:1197-1202, 1989.

117. Frahm J, Bruhn H, Haenicke W et al: Localized proton NMR spectroscopy of brain tumors using short-echo time STEAM sequences, J Comput Assist Tomogr 15:915-922, 1991.

118. DiChiro G, DeLaPaz RL, Brooks RA et al: Glucose utilization of cerebral gliomas measured by [¹⁸F] fluorodeoxyglucose and positron emission tomography, Neurology 32:1323-1329, 1982.

119. DiChiro G: Positron emission tomography using [¹⁸F] fluoro-deoxyglucose in brain tumors: a powerful diagnostic and prognostic tool, Invest Radiol 22:360-371, 1987.

120. Alavi JB, Alavi A, Chawluk J et al: Positron emission tomography in patient with glioma, Cancer 62:1074-1078, 1988.

121. Schupp DG, Merkle H, Ellerman JM et al: Localized detection of glioma glycolysis using editied ¹H MRS, Magn Reson Med 30:18-27, 1993.

122. May GL, Wright LC, Holmes KT et al: Assignment of methylene proton resonances in NMR spectra of embryonic and transformed cells to plasma membrane triglyceride, J Biol Chem 261:3048-3055, 1986.

123. Ott D, Hennig J, Ernst T: Human brain tumors: assessment with *in vivo* proton MR spectroscopy, Radiology 186:745-752, 1993.

124. Posse S, Schuknecht B, Smith ME et al: Short echo time proton MR spectroscopic imaging, J Comput Assist Tomogr 17:1-14, 1993.

125. Kuesel AC, Sutherland GR, Halliday W, Smith ICP: ¹H MRS of high grade astrocytomas: mobile lipid accumulation in necrotic tissue, NMR Biomed 7(3):149-155, 1994.

126. May GL, Sztelma K, Sorrell TC: The presence of cytoplasmic lipid droplets is not sufficient to account for neutral lipid signals in the MR spectra of neutrophils, Magn Reson Med 31:212-217, 1994.

127. Callies R, Sri-Pathmanathan RM, Ferguson DYP, Brindle KM: The appearance of neutral lipid signals in the ¹H NMR spectra of a myeloma cell line correlates with the induced formation of cytoplasmic lipid droplets, Magn Reson Med 29:546-550, 1993.

128. Fitzpatrick SM, Hetherington HP, Behar KL, Shulman RG: Effects of acute hyperammonemia on cerebral amino acid metabolism and pH *in vivo* measured by H-1 and P-31 nuclear MR, J Neurochem 20:741-749, 1989.

129. Luyten PR, Marien AJH, Leindel W et al: Metabolic imaging of patients with intracranial tumors: H-1 MR spectroscopic imaging and PET, Radiology 176:791-799, 1990.

130. Peeling J, Sutherland G: High-resolution ¹H NMR spectroscopy studies of extracts of human cerebral neoplasms, Magn Reson Med 24:123-136, 1992.

131. Bruhn H, Frahm J, Gyngell ML et al: Cerebral metabolism in man after acute stroke: new observations using localized proton NMR spectroscopy, Magn Reson Med 9:126-131, 1989.

132. Duijn JH, Matson GB, Maudsley AA et al: Human brain infarction: proton MR spectroscopy, Radiology 183:711-718, 1992.

133. Luyten PR, van Ryen PC, Tulleken CAF, den Hollander JA: Metabolite mapping using ¹H NMR spectroscopic imaging in patients with cerebrovascular disease, Proceedings, 8th SMRM Annual Meeting, Amsterdam, 1989, p 452.

134. Berkelbach, van der Sprenkel JW, Luyten PR et al: Cerebral lactate detected by regional proton magnetic resonance spectroscopy in a patient with cerebral infarction, Stroke 19:1556-1560, 1988.

135. Hubesch B, Sappey-Marinier D, Hetherington HP et al: Clinical MRS studies of the brain, Invest Radiol 24:1039-1042, 1989.

136. Wolinsky JS, Ponnada A, Narayana PA, Fenstermacher MU: Proton magnetic resonance spectroscopy in multiple sclerosis, Neurology 40:1764-1769, 1990.

137. Arnold DL, Matthews PM, Francis G, Antel J: Temporal profile of regional chemical-pathological changes in demyelinating lesions defined by MRSI, Proceedings, 10th SMRM Annual Meeting, San Francisco, 1991, p 80.

138. Husted CA, Hugg JW, Duyn JH et al: ¹H and ³¹P MR spectroscopic imaging (MRSI) of multiple sclerosis, Proceedings, 10th SMRM Annual Meeting, San Francisco, 1991, p 83.

139. van Hecke PK, Marchal G, Johannik K et al: Human brain proton localized NMR spectroscopy in multiple sclerosis, Magn Reson Med 18:199-206, 1991.

140. Matthews PM, Andermann F, Arnold DL: A proton magnetic resonance spectroscopy study of focal epilepsy in humans, Neurology 40:985-989, 1990.

141. Luyten PR, van Rijen PC, Meiners LC et al: Identifying epileptic foci by ¹H NMR spectroscopic imaging in patients with therapy resistant epilepsy, Proceedings, 9th SMRM Annual Meeting, New York, 1990, p 1009.

142. Menon DK, Baudouin CJ, Tomlinson D, Hoyle C: Proton MR spectroscopy and imaging of the brain in AIDS: evidence of neuronal loss in regions that appear normal with imaging, J Comput Assist Tomogr 14:882-885, 1990.

143. Jarvik JG, Lenkinski RE, Grossman RI et al: Proton MR spectroscopy of HIV-infected patients: characterization of abnormalities with imaging and clinical correlation, Radiology 186:739-744, 1993.

144. Barker PB, Glickson JD, Bryan RN: In vivo magnetic resonance spectroscopy of human brain tumors, Top Magn Reson Imaging 5:32-45, 1993.

145. Navon G, Ogawa S, Shulman RG, Yamane T: ³¹P nuclear magnetic resonance studies of Ehrilich ascites tumor cells, Proc Natl Acad Sci USA 74:87-91, 1977.

146. Chance B, Leigh JS, McLaughlin AC et al: Phosphorus-31 spectroscopy and imaging. In Partain CL, Price RR, Patton JA et al, editors: Magnetic resonance imaging, Philadelphia, 1988, Saunders.

147. Ross BD, Radda GK, Gadian DG et al: Examination of a case of suspected McArdles's syndrome by ³¹P nuclear magnetic resonance, N Engl J Med 304:1338-1342, 1981.

148. Edwards RHT, Dawson MJ, Wilkie DR et al: Clinical use of nuclear magnetic resonance in the investigation of myopathy, Lancet 2:725-731, 1982.

149. Arnold DL, Shoubridge EA, Villemure JG, Feindel W: Proton and phosphorus magnetic resonance spectroscopy of human astrocytomas in vivo: preliminary observations on tumor grading, NMR Biomed 3:184-189, 1990.

150. Heindel W, Bunke J, Glathe S et al: Combined ¹H-MR imaging and localized ³¹P-spectroscopy of intracranial tumors in 43 patients, J Comput Assist Tomogr 12:907-916, 1988.

151. Maris JM, Evans AE, McLaughlin AC et al: ³¹P Nuclear magnetic resonance spectroscopic investigation of human neuroblastoma in situ, N Engl J Med 312:1500-1505, 1985.

152. Narayana PA, Kulkarni MV, Mehta SD: NMR of ²³Na in biological systems. In Partain CL, Price RR, Patton JA et al, editors: Magnetic resonance imaging, Philadelphia, 1988, Saunders.

153. Springer C: Measurement of metal cation compartmentalization in tissue by high-resolution metal cation NMR, Ann Rev Biophys Chem 15:375-399, 1987.

154. Cohen SM: Carbon-13: NMR spectroscopy. In Partain CL, Price RR, Patton JA et al, editors: Magnetic resonance imaging, Philadelphia, 1988, Saunders.

155. Reo NV, Ewy CS, Siegfried BA, Ackerman JJH: High-field ¹³C NMR spectroscopy of tissue in vivo: a double-resonance surface-coil probe, J Magn Reson 58:76-84, 1984.

156. Alger JR, Sillerud LO, Behan KL et al: In vivo carbon-13 nuclear magnetic resonance studies of mammals, Science 214:660-662, 1981.

157. Ewy CS, Ackerman JJH, Balaban RS: Deuterium NMR cerebral imaging in situ, Magn Reson Med 8:35-44, 1988.

158. Ackerman JJH, Ewy CS, Becker NN, Shalwitz RA: Deuterium nuclear magnetic resonance measurements of blood flow and tissue perfusion employing ²H₂O as a freely diffusible tracer, Proc Natl Acad Sci USA 84:4099-4102, 1987.

159. Brereton IM, Irving MG, Field J, Doddrell DM: Preliminary studies on the potential of in vivo deuterium NMR spectroscopy, Biochem Biophys Res Commun 137:579-584, 1986.

160. Irving MG, Brereton IM, Field J, Doddrell DM: In vivo determination of body iron stores by natural abundance deuterium magnetic resonance spectroscopy, Magn Reson Med 4:88-92, 1987.

161. Muller S, Seelig J: In vivo NMR imaging of deuterium, J Magn Reson 72:456-466, 1987.

162. Thomas S: The biomedical applications of fluorine-19 NMR. In Partain CL, Price RR, Patton JA et al, editors: Magnetic resonance imaging, Philadelphia, 1988, Saunders.

163. Komoroski RA, Newton JEO, Cardwell D et al: In vivo ¹⁹F spin relaxation and localized spectroscopy of fluoxetine in human brain, Magn Reson Med 31:204-211, 1994.

164. Wyrwicz AM, Pszenny MH, Schofield JC et al: Noninvasive observation of fluorinated anesthetics in rabbit brain by fluorine-19 nuclear magnetic resonance, Science 222:428-430, 1983.

165. Wyrwicz AM, Ryback K, Pszenny MH: In vivo ¹⁹F NMR study of fluorinated anesthetics elimination from a rabbit brain, Proceedings, Third SMRM Annual Meeting, New York, 1984, p 763.

166. Bessel EM, Courtenay VD, Foster AB et al: Some in vivo and in vitro antitumor effects of the deoxyfluoro-ᴅ-glucopyranoses, Eur J Cancer 9:463-470, 1973.

167. Clark LC, Gollan F: Survival of mammals breathing organic liquids equilibrated with oxygen at atmospheric pressure, Science 152:1755-1756, 1966.

168. Wessler EP, Iltis R, Clark LC: The solubility of oxygen in highly fluoridated liquids, J Fluor Chem 9:137-146, 1977.

169. McFarland E, Koutcher JA, Rosen BR et al: In vivo ¹⁹F NMR imaging, J Comput Assist Tomogr 9:8-15, 1985.

170. Joseph PM, Fishman JE, Mukherji B, Sloviter HA: In vivo ¹⁹F NMR imaging of the cardiovascular system, J Comput Assist Tomogr 9:1012-1019, 1985.

171. Thomas SR, Clark LC, Ackerman JL et al: MR Imaging of the lung using liquid perfluorocarbons, J Comput Assist Tomogr 10:1-9, 1986.

172. Clark LC, Ackerman JL, Thomas SR et al: High contrast tissue and blood oxygen imaging based on fluorocarbon ^{19}F NMR relaxation times, Magn Reson Med 1:135-136, 1984 (abstract).

173. Clark LC, Ackerman JL, Thomas SR et al: Perfluorinated organic liquids and emulsions as biocompatible NMR imaging agents for ^{19}F and dissolved oxygen. In Bruley D, Bicher HI, Reneau D, editors: Advances in experimental medicine and biology, New York, 1985, Plenum.

174. Parhami P, Fung BM: Fluroine-19 relaxation study of perfluoro chemicals as oxygen carriers, J Phys Chem 87:1928-1931, 1983.

175. Lai CS, Stair SJ, Miziorko H et al: Effect of oxygen and the lipid spin label TEMPO-laruate on fluorine-19 and proton relaxation rates of the perfluorochemical blood substitute, FC-43 emulsion, J Magn Reson 57:447-452, 1984.

176. Reid RS, Koch CJ, Castro ME et al: The influence of oxygenation in the ^{19}F-spin-lattice relaxation rates of fluosol-DA, Phys Med Biol 30:677-686, 1985.

177. Mason RP, Nunnally RL, Antich PP: Tissue oxygenation: a novel determination using 19-F surface coil NMR spectroscopy of sequestered perfluorocarbon emulsion, Magn Reson Med 18:71-79, 1991.

178. Parhami P, Fung BN: Fluorine-19 relaxation study of perfluorochemicals as oxygen carriers, J Phys Chem 87:1928-1931, 1983.

179. Ackerman JL, Clark LC, Thomas SR et al: NMR thermal imaging, Proceedings, Third SMRM Annual Meeting, New York, 1984, p 1.

180. Dieckman SL, Kreishman GP, Pratt RG et al: 19-F NMR thermal imaging utilizing perfluorocarbons, Proceedings, 6th SMRM Annual Meeting, New York, 1987, p 815.

181. Fishman JE, Joseph PM, Carvlin MJ et al: *In vivo* measurement of vascular oxygen tension in tumors using MRI of a fluorinated blood substitute, Invest Radiol 24:65-71, 1989.

182. Taylor J, Deutsch CJ: 19F-Nuclear magnetic resonance: measurements of [O_2] and pH in biological systems, Biophys J 53:227-233, 1988.

183. Kent TA, Quast MJ, Kaplan BJ et al: Cerebral blood volume in a rat model of ischemia by MR imaging at 4.7 T, AJR 10:335-338, 1989.

184. Villringer A, Rosen BR, Belliveau JW et al: Dynamic imaging with lanthanide chelates in normal brain: contrast due to magnetic susceptibility effects, Magn Reson Med 6:164-174, 1988.

185. Lu D, Joseph PM, Greenberg JH et al: Use of ^{19}F magnetic resonance imaging to measure local cerebral blood volume, Magn Reson Med 29:179-187, 1993.

186. Schnall MD, Subramanian HV, Leigh JS et al: A technique for simultaneous ^{1}H and ^{31}P NMR at 2.2 T *in vivo,* J Magn Res 63:401-405, 1985.

187. Styles P, Grathuchl C, Brown F: Simultaneous multinuclear NMR by alernate scan recording of ^{31}P and ^{13}C spectra, J Magn Res 35:329-336, 1979.

188. Rothman DL, Behar KL, Hetherington HP et al: [1]H observed ^{13}C decoupled spectroscopic measurements of lactate and glutamate in the rat brain *in vivo,* Proc Natl Acad Sci USA 82:1633-1637, 1985.

189. Fitzpatrick SM, Hetherington HP, Behar KL et al: The flux from glucose to glutamate in the rat brain *in vivo* as determined by ^{1}H-observed, ^{13}C-edited NMR spectroscopy, J Cereb Blood Flow Metab 10:170-179, 1990.

190. Rothman DL, Howseman AM, Graham GD et al: Localized proton NMR observation of [3-^{13}C] lactate in stroke after [1-^{13}C] glucose infusion, Magn Reson Med 21:302-307, 1991.

191. Rothman DL, Novotny EJ, Shulman GI et al: ^{1}H-[^{13}C] NMR measurement of [4-^{13}C] glutamate turnover in human brain, Proc Natl Acad Sci USA 89:9603-9606, 1992.

192. Mason GF, Rothman DL, Behar KL et al: NMR determination of the TCA cycle rate and alpha-ketoglutarate exchange rate in rat brain, J Cereb Blood Flow Metab 12:434-447, 1992.

193. van Zijl PCM, Chesnick AS, DesPres D et al: *In vivo* proton spectroscopy and spectroscopic imaging of [1-^{13}C]-glucose and its metabolic products, Magn Reson Med 30:544-551, 1993.

194. Bachert-Baumann P, Ermark F, Zabel HJ et al: *In vivo* nuclear Overhauser effect in [31]P-^{1}H double resonance experiments in a 1.5 T whole-body MR system, Magn Reson Med 15:165-172, 1990.

195. Starling EH: On the absorption of fluids from the connective tissue spaces, J Physiol (Lond) 19:312-326, 1896.

196. Kety SS, Schmidt CF: The determination of cerebral blood flow in man by the use of nitrous oxide in low concentrations, Am J Physiol 143:53-66, 1945.

197. Lassen NA, Perl W: Tracer kinetic methods in medical physiology, New York, 1978, Raven Press.

198. Zierler KL: Equations for measuring blood flow by external monitoring of radioisotopes, Circ Res 16:309-321, 1965.

199. Lassen NA, Henriksen O, Sejrsen P: Indicator methods for measurement of organ and tissue blood flow. In Shepherd JT, Abboud FM, editors: Handbook of physiology, Bethesda, Md, 1983, American Physiological Society.

200. Kim SG, Ackerman JJH: Quantification of regional blood flow by monitoring of exogenous tracer via nuclear magnetic resonance spectroscopy, Magn Reson Med 14:266-282, 1990.

201. Neil JJ: The validation of freely diffusible tracer methods with NMR detection for measurement of blood flow, Magn Reson Med 19:299-304, 1991.

202. Robertson GW, Larson KB, Speath EE: The interpretation of mean transit time measurements for multiphase tissue systems, J Theor Biol 39:447-475, 1973.

203. Raichle ME, Martin WRW, Hershovitch P et al: Brain blood flow measured with intravenous H_2[15]O. II. Implementation and validation, J Nucl Med 24:790-798, 1983.

204. Kim S, Ackerman J: Multicompartmental analysis of blood flow and tissue perfusion employing D_2O as a freely diffusible tracer: a novel deuterium NMR technique demonstrated via application with murine RIF-1 tumors, Magn Reson Med 8:410-426, 1988.

205. Ewing JR, Branch CA, Helpern JA et al: Tracer approaches: problems and limitations, Syllabus, SMRM FRMI Workshop, Arlington, Va, 1993, p 53.

206. Fenstermacher JD: The flow of water in the blood-brain-cerebrospinal fluid system, Syllabus, SMRM FMRI Workshop, Arlington, Va, 1993, p 9.

207. Bradbury M, Patlak C, Oldendorf W: Analysis of brain uptake and loss of radiotracers after intracarotid injection, Am J Physiol 229:1110-1115, 1975.

208. Patlak C, Fenstermacher J: Measurements of dog blood-brain transfer constants by ventriculocisternal perfusion, Am J Physiol 229:877-884, 1975.

209. Bereczki D, Wei L, Otsuka T et al: Hypoxia increases velocity of blood flow through parenchymal microvascular systems in rat brain, J Cereb Blood Flow Metab 13:475-486, 1993.

210. Wei L, Otsuka T, Acuff V et al: The velocities of red cell and plasma flows through parenchymal microvessels of rat brain are decreased by pentobarbital, J Cereb Blood Flow Metab 13:487-497, 1993.

211. Gobel U, Klein B, Schrock H, Kuschinsky W: Lack of capillary recruitment in the brains of awake rats during hypercapnia, J Cereb Blood Flow Metab 9:491-499, 1989.

212. Ackerman J, Ewy C, Kim S, Shalwitz RA: Deuterium magnetic resonance *in vivo:* the measurement of blood flow and tissue perfusion, Ann NY Acad Sci 508:89-98, 1987.

213. Detre J, Subramanian V, Mitchell M et al: Measurement of regional cerebral blood flow in cat brain using intracarotid [2]H_2O and ^{2}H NMR imaging, Magn Reson Med 14:389-395, 1990.

214. Corbett RT, Laptook AR, Olivares E: Simultaneous measurement of cerebral blood flow and energy metabolites in piglets

using deuterium and phosphorus nuclear magnetic resonance, J Cereb Blood Flow Metab 11:55-65, 1991.

215. Obrist W: Determination of regional cerebral blood flow by inhalation of 133-xenon, Circ Res 20:124-135, 1967.

216. Obrist W, Thompson H, Wang H, Wilkinson W: Regional cerebral blood flow estimated by 133-xenon inhalation, Stroke 6:245-256, 1975.

217. Ewing JR, Branch CA, Helpern JA et al: Cerebral blood flow measured by NMR indicator dilution in cats, Stroke 20:259-267, 1989.

218. Branch C, Helpern J, Ewing J, Welch K: ^{19}F NMR imaging of cerebral blood flow, Magn Reson Med 20:151-157, 1991.

219. Branch C, Ewing J, Helpern J et al: Atraumatic quantitation of cerebral perfusion in cats by ^{19}F magnetic resonance imaging, Magn Reson Med 28:39-53, 1992.

220. Branch CA, Ewing JR, Butt SM et al: Signal-to-noise and acute toxicity of a quantitative NMR imaging measurement of cerebral perfusion in baboons, J Cereb Blood Flow Metab 11:s778, 1991.

221. Pekar J, Ligeti L, Sinnwell T et al: ^{19}F NMR imaging of cerebral blood flow with 0.4 cc resolution, Proceedings, 11th SMRM Annual Meeting, Berlin, 1992, p 1814.

222. Baranco D, Sutton L, Florin S et al: Use of ^{19}F NMR spectroscopy for measurement of cerebral blood flow: comparative study using microspheres, J Cereb Blood Flow Metab 9:886-891, 1989.

223. Ewing J, Branch C, Fagan S et al: Fluorocarbon-23 measure of cat cerebral blood flow by nuclear magnetic resonance, Stroke 21:100-106, 1990.

224. Branch C, Ewing J, Fagan S et al: Acute toxicity of a nuclear magnetic resonance cerebral blood flow indicator in cats, Stroke 21:1172-1177, 1990.

225. Pekar J, Ligeti L, Ruttner Z et al: *In vivo* measurement of cerebral oxygen consumption and blood flow using 17-O magnetic resonance imaging, Magn Reson Med 21:313-319, 1991.

226. Fiat D, Ligeti L, Lyon RC et al: *In vivo* 17-O NMR study of rat brain during 17-O_2 inhalation, Magn Reson Med 24:370-374, 1992.

227. Arai T, Nakao S, Mori K et al: Cerebral oxygen utilization analyzed by the use of oxygen-17 and its nuclear magnetic resonance, Biochem Biophys Res Commun 169:153-158, 1990.

228. Hopkins AL, Haacke EM, Tkach J et al: Improved sensitivity of proton MR to oxygen-17 as a contrast agent using fast imaging: detection in brain, Magn Reson Med 7:222-229, 1988.

229. Kwong KK, Hopkins AL, Belliveau JW et al: Proton NMR imaging of cerebral blood flow using $H_2{}^{17}O$, Magn Reson Med 22:154-158, 1991.

230. Frackowiak RSJ, Lenzi G, Jones T, Heather JD: Quantitative measurement of regional cerebral blood flow and oxygen metabolism in man using ^{15}O and positron emission tomography: theory, procedure, and normal values, J Comput Assist Tomogr 4:727-736, 1980.

231. Herholz K, Pietrzyk U, Wienhard K et al: Regional cerebral blood flow measurement with intravenous [^{15}O] water bolus and [^{18}F] fluoromethane inhalation, Stroke 20:1174-1181, 1989.

232. McLaughlin AC, Pekar J, Sinnwell T et al: ^{17}O and ^{19}F magnetic resonance imaging of cerebral blood flow and oxygen consumption, Syllabus, SMRM FMRI Workshop, Arlington, Va, 1993, p 69.

233. Mateescu GD, LaManna JC, Lust WD et al: Oxygen-17 magnetic resonance: *in vivo* detection of nascent mitochondrial water in animals breathing $^{17}O_2$ enriched air, Proceedings, 10th SMRM Annual Meeting, San Francisco, 1991, p 1031.

234. Hopkins AL, Barr RG: Oxygen-17 compounds as potential NMR T2 contrast agents: enrichment effects of $H_2{}^{17}O$ on

protein solutions and living tissues, Magn Reson Med 4:399-403, 1987.

235. Lasker SE, Bupte P, Arai T: Proton NMR imaging of myocardial reperfusion injury by visualization of metabolites of oxygen-17, Proceedings, 9th SMRM Annual Meeting, New York, 1990, p 1202.

236. Pekar J, Sinnwell TM, Ligeti L et al: Double-label tracer experiments using multinuclear MRI: mapping cerebral oxygen consumption and blood flow using ^{17}O and ^{19}F MRI, Proceedings, 12th SMRM Annual Meeting, New York, 1993, p 1388.

237. Hida K, Suzuki N, Kwee IL, Nakada T: pH-lactate dissociation in neonatal anoxia: proton and ^{31}P NMR spectroscopic studies in rat pups, Magn Reson Med 22:128-132, 1991.

238. Schnall MD, Yoshizaki K, Chance B, Leigh JS: Triple nuclear NMR studies of cerebral metabolism during generalized seizure, Magn Reson Med 6:15-23, 1988.

239. Prichard JW, Petroff OA, Ogino T, Shulman RG: Cerebral lactate elevation by electroshock: a ^{1}H magnetic resonance study, Ann NY Acad Sci 508:54-63, 1987.

240. Petroff OAC, Novotny EJ, Avison MJ et al: Cerebral lactate turnover after electroshock: *In vivo* measurements by ^{1}H/^{13}C magnetic resonance spectroscopy, J Cereb Blood Flow Metab 12:1022-1029, 1992.

241. Fox PT, Raichle ME, Mintun MA, Dence C: Nonoxidative glucose consumption during focal physiologic neural activity, Science 241:462-464, 1988.

242. Prichard J, Rothman D, Novotny E et al: Lactate rise detected by ^{1}H NMR in human visual cortex during physiological stimulation, Proc Natl Acad Sci USA 88:5829-5831, 1991.

243. Sappey-Marinier D, Calabrese G, Fein G et al: Effect of photic stimulation on human visual cortex lactate and phosphates using ^{1}H and ^{31}P magnetic resonance spectroscopy, J Cereb Blood Flow Metab 12:584-592, 1992.

244. Merboldt KD, Bruhn H, Gyngell ML et al: Variability of lactate in normal human brain *in vivo*: localized proton MRS during rest and photic stimulation, Proceedings, 10th SMRM Annual Meeting, San Francisco, 1991, p 392.

245. Jenkins BG, Belliveau JW, Rosen BR: Confirmation of lactate production during photic stimulation, Proceedings, 11th SMRM Annual Meeting, Berlin, 1992, p 2145.

246. Watanabe H, Kuwabara T, Tsuji S et al: Prolonged lactate elevation after photic stimulation in the visual cortex of patients of mitochondrial encephalomyopathy, Proceedings, 12th SMRM Annual Meeting, New York, 1993, p 1527.

247. Xue M, Ng TC, Comair YG, Modic M: Decreased NAA and increased lactate in the activated motor cortex detected with localized spectroscopy guided with functional MRI, Proceedings, 12th SMRM Annual Meeting, New York, 1993, p 59.

248. Singh M: Toward proton MR spectroscopic imaging of stimulated brain function, IEEE Trans Nucl Sci 39:1161-1164, 1992.

249. Singh M, Kim H, Huang KT: Effect of stimulus rate on lactate in the human auditory cortex, Proceedings, 11th SMRM Annual Meeting, Berlin, 1992, p 2146.

250. Lund-Andersen H: Transport of glucose from blood to brain, Physiol Rev 59:305-352, 1979.

251. Chen W, Novotny EJ, Zhu XH et al: Localized ^{1}H NMR measurement of glucose consumption in the human brain during visual stimulation, Proceedings, 12th SMRM Annual Meeting, New York, 1993, p 1528.

252. Merboldt KD, Bruhn H, Hanicke W et al: Decrease of glucose in the human visual cortex during photic stimulation, Magn Reson Med 25:187-194, 1992.

253. Hennig J, Ernst TH, Speck O et al: Detection of brain activation using oxygenation sensitive functional spectroscopy, Magn Reson Med 31:85-90, 1994.

Index